Recent Results in Cancer Research

Volume 225

This book series presents comprehensive, high-quality updates on areas of current interest in basic, clinical, and translational cancer research. The scope of the series is broad, encompassing epidemiology, etiology, pathophysiology, prevention, diagnosis, and treatment. Each volume is devoted to a specific topic with the aim of providing readers with a thorough overview by acclaimed experts. While advances in understanding of the cellular, genetic, and molecular mechanisms of cancer and progress toward personalized cancer care are a particular focus, subjects such as the lifestyle, psychological, and social aspects of cancer and public policy are also covered. *Recent Results in Cancer Research* is accordingly of interest to a wide spectrum of researchers, clinicians, other health care professionals, and stakeholders. The series is listed in PubMed/Index Medicus.

Otmar Schober • Fabian Kiessling
Jürgen Debus
Editors

Molecular Imaging in Oncology - Volume 2

Advanced Solutions to Acquire Disease-Specific Biomarkers - Clinical Applications

Third Edition

Springer

Editors
Otmar Schober
Department of Nuclear Medicine
University of Münster
Münster, Northrhein-Westphalia, Germany

Jürgen Debus
Department of Radiation Oncology
Heidelberg University
Heidelberg, Baden-Württemberg, Germany

Fabian Kiessling
Institute for Experimental
Molecular Imaging
University Hospital
RWTH Aachen University
Nordrhein-Westfalen, Germany

ISSN 0080-0015 ISSN 2197-6767 (electronic)
Recent Results in Cancer Research
ISBN 978-3-032-21414-0 ISBN 978-3-032-21415-7 (eBook)
https://doi.org/10.1007/978-3-032-21415-7

This Springer imprint is published by the registered company Springer Nature Switzerland AG
The registered company address is: Gewerbestrasse 11, 6330 Cham, Switzerland

Preface

What does “molecular imaging” mean? There are several definitions, but the authors of this handbook define it as the visualization, characterization, and quantification of biological processes at the molecular and cellular level. “Oncology” is the leading specialty for the prevention, diagnosis, and treatment of cancer. One of the most important prerequisites for fighting cancer is understanding the underlying molecular processes and combating them at the earliest possible stage.

This has been described by experts from various disciplines in the well-received previous second edition of this handbook. One of the lessons learned and feedback on the topics covered are that the associations and challenges of molecular imaging in oncology are very similar to those in diseases of the cardiovascular, neurological and immune systems. This inter- and transdisciplinary approach is reflected at best and not solely in the Technology and Probe Design section.

The established sections are still: Technology and Probe Design, Preclinical Studies, Clinical Applications, and Future Challenges.

All chapters of this third edition have been updated, and the book has been supplemented by five chapters about “Total Body PET,” “Artificial Intelligence and Radiomics,” “Potential Clinical Applications of Hyperpolarized ^{13}C and ^{2}H MRI,” “Imaging of Immunotherapy,” and “Theranostics.”

One rational challenge and motive should be mentioned, that is to bring or keep together the disciplines radiology, nuclear medicine, and radiotherapy/radiooncology.

Münster, Germany	Otmar Schober
Aachen (Aix-la-Chapelle), Germany	Fabian Kiessling
Heidelberg, Germany	Jürgen Debus

Contents

Part III

Clinical Applications

Quantitative SPECT/CT: Technique and Clinical Applications

19

Stijn De Schepper, Tim Van den Wyngaert, Philipp Ritt, and Torsten Kuwert

19.1 Introduction

Single photon emission computed tomography (SPECT) is widely used in the field of Nuclear Medicine for various purposes. The most important diagnostic applications are skeletal imaging using Tc-99m-labeled polyphosphonates, assessment of cardiac perfusion using Tc-99m-MIBI, and thyroid imaging using Tc-99m-pertechnetate. Additionally, SPECT is frequently applied for the confirmation of desired tracer distribution under I-131 therapy or the diagnosis of diseases of the neuronal system like Tc-99m-HMPAO for epilepsy or Alzheimer's disease or I-123-FP-CIT for dopamine transporter function.

Another established field of application is the individualized dosimetry, for example, I-131 or Lu-177 labeled radioligands. For this purpose, an exact

S. De Schepper (✉) · T. Van den Wyngaert
Department of Nuclear Medicine, Antwerp University Hospital, Edegem, Belgium

Faculty of Medicine and Health Sciences (MICA – IPPON), University of Antwerpen, Wilrijk, Belgium
e-mail: stijn.deschepper@uza.be; Tim.vandenwyngaert@uza.be

P. Ritt
Chair for Clinical Nuclear Medicine, Friedrich-Alexander-Universität Erlangen-Nürnberg, Erlangen, Germany
e-mail: Philipp.ritt@fau.de

T. Kuwert
Nuclear Medicine, Friedrich-Alexander-Universität Erlangen-Nürnberg, Erlangen, Germany
e-mail: Torsten.kuwert@uk-erlangen.de

O. Schober et al. (eds.), *Molecular Imaging in Oncology - Volume 2*, Recent Results in Cancer Research 225, https://doi.org/10.1007/978-3-032-21415-7_1

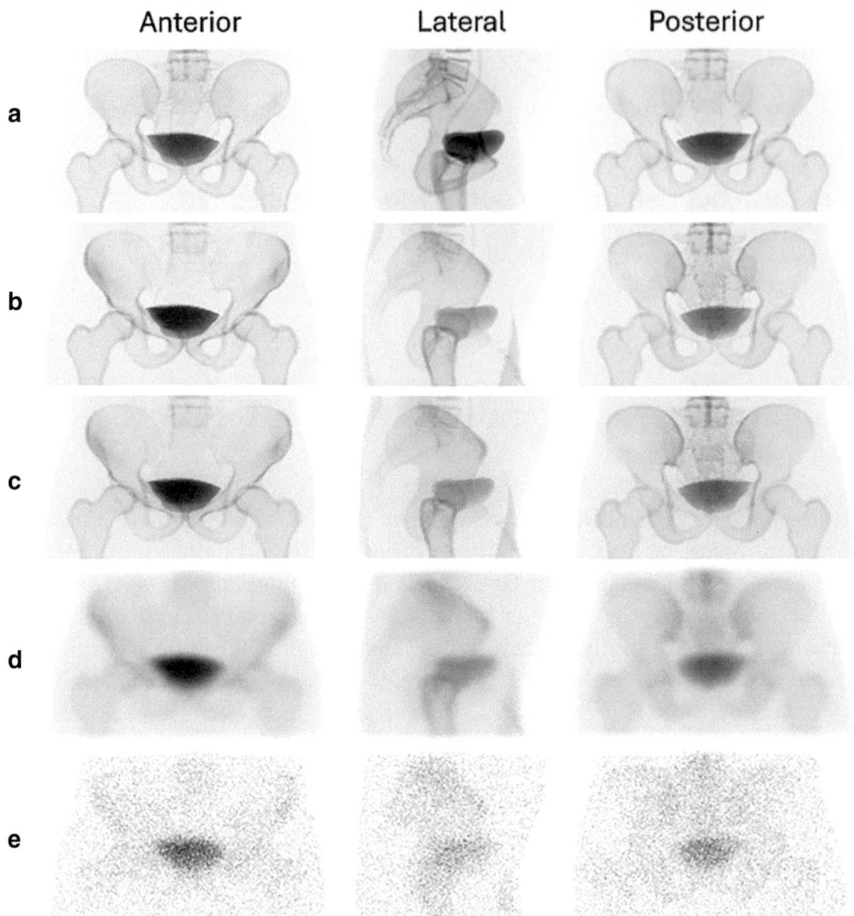

Fig. 19.1 Illustration of several image degrading effects based on simulated SPECT projection data. (**a**) perfect image, no degrading factors, (**b**) added photon attenuation, especially deep organs such as bladder appear at lower intensities, (**c**) added photon scatter, effect is noticeable as slight blurring, for example, at the edge of bony structures. (**d**) realistic spatial resolution, depending on the activity distribution, counts are distributed outside (spill-out) or integrated into (spill-in) a region-of-interest and (**e**) realistic photon count level and noise

representation of the radiopharmaceutical distribution is especially desirable, which leads to the need for absolute quantification with SPECT. This process is compromised by photon scatter, photon attenuation and partial volume artefacts (see Fig. 19.1 for an overview of image degrading effects). Thus, the following paragraphs are focused on SPECT/CT instrumentation, correction techniques of the aforementioned effects and additional steps that are necessary for quantitatively accurate absolute quantification in clinical applications.

19.2 Quantitative SPECT/CT

SPECT allows the visualization of the distribution of radioactivity within the human body. The modality is widely used for clinical purposes [1]. SPECT also holds the promise to exactly quantify the concentration of radioactivity within a given volume in absolute units, for example, as kBq/cm^3. This process is heavily compromised by photon scatter, photon attenuation and partial volume artefacts. In SPECT, technical progress in overcoming these hurdles has been considerably slower than in PET.

In this paragraph, we outline the current state-of-the-art for SPECT/CT. A simplified diagram of the image generation chain for quantitative SPECT is given in Fig. 19.2 for the purpose of orientation. We will begin with the reconstruction methods that nowadays incorporate many corrections mentioned in the latter paragraphs. We will then focus on scatter and partial volume artefacts: in each of these paragraphs, a short explanation of the underlying physical effect and an overview of the appropriate correction techniques are given. In addition, we will briefly introduce an intuitive calibration technique.

Please note that it has to be assumed that the kinetics of the radioactive tracer of interest are slow with respect to the imaging time. If this is not true, significant quantification errors are very likely to occur, and other approaches (e.g. dynamic SPECT) should be considered.

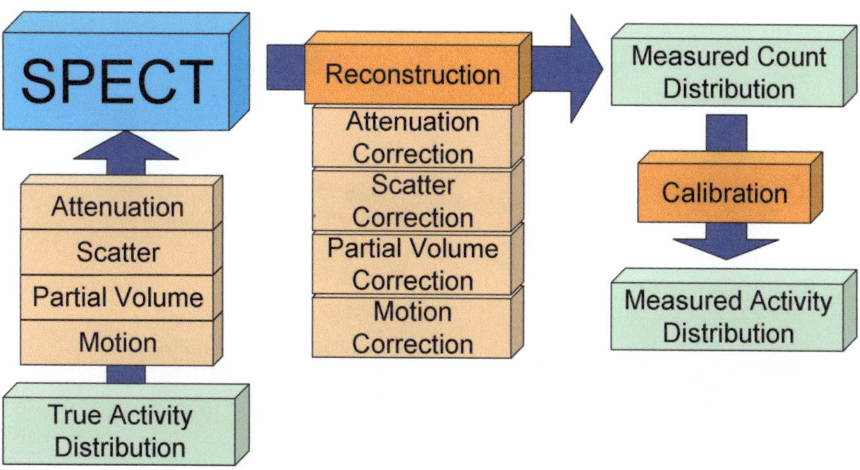

Fig. 19.2 Illustration of a simplified image formation chain. The image of the true activity distribution is influenced by several effects, namely attenuation, scatter, partial volume and motion. The SPECT reconstruction, along with possible corrections for those effects, results in a measured, three-dimensional count distribution. By calibration, the count distribution can be translated into a measured activity distribution

19.2.1 SPECT/CT Instrumentation

Modern SPECT devices are mostly based on the gamma camera principle by Hal Anger. Its main components are a collimator, a scintillation crystal (mainly NaI), which is read out by photomultipliers, and subsequent electronics. The unit of these components is commonly referred to as a detector. The detector itself is mounted onto a gantry, which allows movements of the detector head. For SPECT, nowadays the application of dual detector head cameras is the standard (Fig. 19.3a, b), with triple detector head cameras being more uncommon.

An important property of any imaging system is spatial resolution which is defined as the full-width half maximum (FWHM) of a point source. In SPECT, this is mainly limited by collimator performance. SPECT utilizes absorptive collimation to identify the direction of the photon line-of-response (LOR). Only a small fraction of the gamma photons that reach the collimator surface pass through it. As a consequence, the detection efficiency of SPECT is limited. It is important to notice that there is always a trade-off between spatial resolution and detection efficiency in SPECT. The collimators are typically designed with the maximum allowable resolution in order to partially compensate for the limited detection efficiency.

The achievable spatial resolution is also influenced by the detectors´ intrinsic resolution, defined as the spatial resolution of the detector without a collimator. The

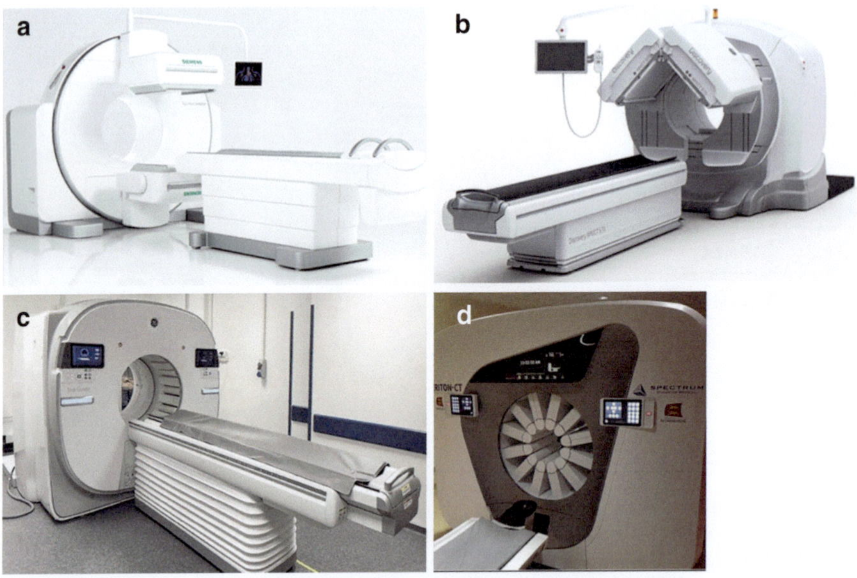

Fig. 19.3 Examples of SPECT/CT systems. (**a**) Siemens Symbia Intevo, (**b**) GE Healthcare NM/CT 670 DR, (**c**) GE Healthcare Starguide and (**d**) Spectrum Dynamics Medical Veriton-CT. Image (**c**) reproduced from Zorz et al. [2] under the terms of the Creative Commons Attribution 4.0 International License. Image (**d**) reproduced from Desmonts et al. [3] under the terms of the Creative Commons Attribution 4.0 International License

detectors of most clinical SPECT systems are made of a single crystal plate of NaI, which acts as a scintillator and illuminates an array of photomultipliers. The intrinsic resolution of the detector depends on the photopeak energy of the radionuclide used and the crystal thickness of the NaI. Higher gamma photon energy allows a better intrinsic resolution due to the higher light output of the scintillation. In contrast, larger crystal thickness decreases intrinsic resolution. This is a consequence of the broader spread of the scintillation light before it exits the crystal and is detected with the photomultipliers.

In recent years, alternatives to the Anger camera, where the detectors are mounted in a ring geometry (Fig. 19.3c, d), have been introduced into clinical practice [4]. Solid-state detectors, relying on materials like cadmium telluride (CdTe) and cadmium zinc telluride (CZT), convert the gamma photons directly into electrical signals; this leads to an increased energy resolution (~5% vs ~10% at 140 keV) as compared to the Anger technique. Additionally, the linear attenuation coefficient of CZT is slightly higher than that of NaI (~3 cm^{-1} vs ~2 cm^{-1} at 140 keV), which could potentially lead to an increased sensitivity, although this benefit is often foregone when it is decided, for economic reasons, to limit the thickness of the semiconductors. In fact, the considerable advantages in terms of the photon sensitivity (regularly reported to be four to eight times higher) and resolution of these cameras are achieved through changes to features other than just the detector material, for example, through special geometries, adapted collimation and pixelated detectors.

Typical SPECT detectors have an intrinsic spatial resolution in the range of 3–5 mm for Tc-99 m. However, the image resolution for the whole SPECT system depends mainly on the collimator design and the source-to-collimator distance. For parallel-hole collimation of Tc-99 m and typical source-to-collimator distances, the FWHM ranges from 7 to 15 mm. This is considerably larger than that seen in PET (2–5 mm FWHM). However, by using other collimator geometries, for example, (multi-) pinhole, spatial resolution better than in PET can be achieved [5]. However, these collimator geometries are exclusively used in systems dedicated to a single application that requires only a narrow field of view, such as small animal or cardiac imaging.

Novel 360° CZT systems employ a collimator which forms an integral unit with the detector similar to the ones used in the dedicated cardiac systems. While the collimator designs are mostly optimized for Tc-99m imaging, as performed in cardiac imaging, this results in considerable septal penetration for higher-energy imaging, already at 208 keV photons from Lu-177 [6]. As the collimator forms an integral unit with the detector, it cannot be changed for higher-energy applications. An in-depth description on collimator geometries can be found in [7]. Collimators are a major, but not the sole, cause for degradation of the system's spatial resolution; a more general review on improvement techniques was written by Cheng et al. [8].

The advantage of combining a SPECT camera with an X-ray computed tomography (CT) allows for diagnostic use, anatomical correlation and provides data for image correction techniques. The SPECT and CT are installed in a sequential manner, sharing a common bed. The following paragraph will discuss how hybrid imaging can be achieved using SPECT/CT systems.

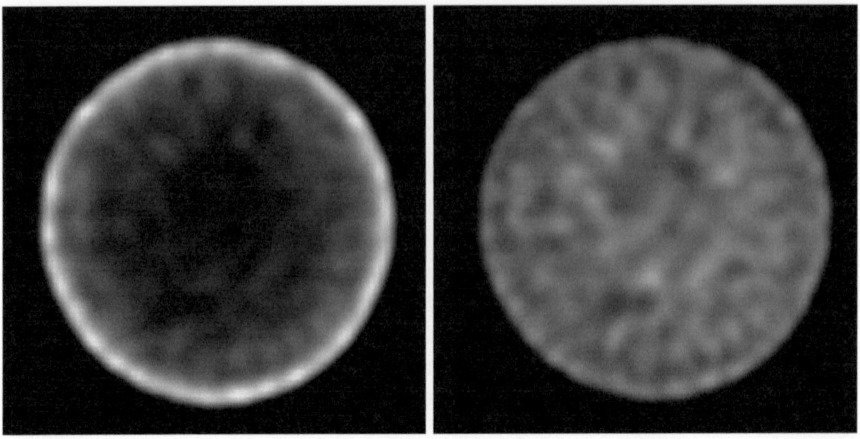

Fig. 19.4 A reconstructed SPECT image of a homogenously filled phantom (Tc-99 m). The uncorrected image (left side) shows a relative overestimation of the activity at the rim of the phantom and an underestimation at the centre. The attenuation-corrected image (right side) restores the homogenous distribution

19.2.2 Attenuation Correction of SPECT

SPECT images are heavily affected by the effect of photon attenuation (see Fig. 19.4).

The probability P_{Det} for gamma photon emitted at position d for reaching a detector at position D (under the assumption that it is emitted in the proper direction) is calculated according to Eq. 19.1:

$$P_{\text{det}} = \exp\left\{ \int_{\vec{d}}^{\vec{D}} -\mu(\vec{r})\,d\vec{r} \right\} \tag{19.1}$$

The line integral covers the path of the radiation from its origin through the object, to the location of its detection (see Fig. 19.5 for a simplified illustration).

For SPECT imaging, the probability depends on the (unknown) location of the decay d and on the linear attenuation coefficients $\mu(r)$ of the object.

For the correction of attenuation, the spatial distribution of the attenuation coefficients of the examined object for the photon energy of the used radionuclide needs to be known. The distribution of attenuation coefficients (called attenuation map) can be generated through a simple transformation of a transmission scan. First, the transmission images need to be converted to the attenuation factors valid at the effective energy of the emission scan (140 keV for Tc-99m); then, they need to be corrected for the spatial registration between the emission and transmission images. The resulting attenuation map can, for example, be integrated into the reconstruction step in order to correct for photon attenuation.

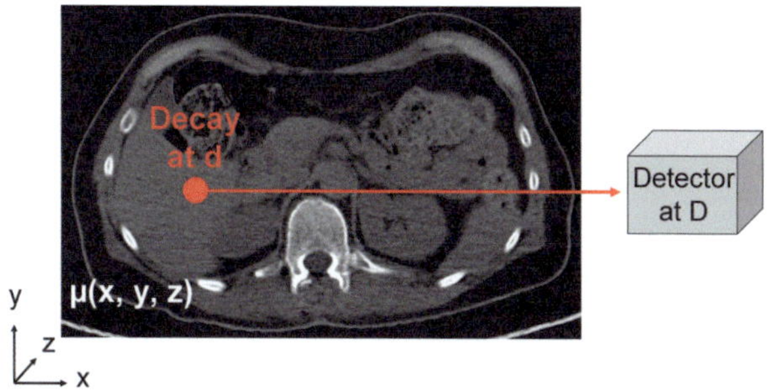

Fig. 19.5 A simplified illustration of the detection of a decay event: The signal from the decay at position *d* is lowered by photon attenuation. The amount of attenuation depends on the spatially non-constant linear attenuation coefficients $\mu(x,y,z)$ and on the distance between the detector and the decay, |*D-d*|

With the availability of SPECT/CT hybrid devices, and with their ability to perform highly correlated high-quality X-ray CT transmission scans, it is the clinical standard to use these scans for attenuation correction. The CT scans are obtained in Hounsfield units. These units have to be converted to the linear attenuation coefficients valid at the respective photon energy of the radionuclide, which is, for example, Tc-99m 140 keV.

In some cases, patient motion could occur between the emission and transmission acquisitions in a hybrid system. This can lead to artefacts in reconstructed attenuation-corrected images, which in turn could lead to false readings of the corrected SPECT images. A manual post-registration could help to prevent such artefacts. Similar risk of artefacts exists near high-density objects, for example, prosthetics.

Still, the methods that rely on the segmentation of contours in SPECT can be sufficient for SPECT quantification in predictable and/or relatively uniform anatomies like the brain. Nevertheless, the attenuation correction by SPECT/CT has become the clinical standard and is, in general, highly recommended. Attenuation and other corrections are obligatory for accurate quantification with SPECT/CT, which will be discussed in the following paragraph.

19.2.3 Image Reconstruction

Image reconstruction is the technique used to transform the measured 2-D projection data into a 3-D activity distribution. Iterative reconstruction techniques are the current standard in both SPECT and CT. For a review of the different algorithms in SPECT, see [9].

Most iterative techniques rely on mathematical models which assume a linear dependency of the image $\boldsymbol{f}$ (vector with elements f_j representing the voxels of the activity distribution) and the projection data $\boldsymbol{p}$ (vector with elements p_i representing detector pixels) via the system matrix $\boldsymbol{A}$. Each element A_{ij} describes the probability that a photon originating from voxel j is detected at pixel i. The projection data thus can be expressed as a multiplication of the system matrix $\boldsymbol{A}$ by $\boldsymbol{f}$ (Eq. 19.2):

$$\boldsymbol{Af} = \boldsymbol{p} \tag{19.2}$$

The most common iterative techniques are the Maximum Likelihood Expectation Maximization (MLEM) algorithm and its accelerated version, Ordered-Subsets Expectation Maximization (OSEM). It is based on the fact that the image $\boldsymbol{f}$ consists of Poisson-distributed random variables, and it seeks to maximize the likelihood of the observed data given the source $\boldsymbol{f}$. The well-known update rule of the iterative MLEM algorithm is given in Eq. 19.3:

$$f_j^{\text{new}} = \frac{f_j^{\text{old}}}{\sum_l a_{lj}} \sum_i a_{ij} \frac{p_i}{\sum_k a_{ik} f_k^{\text{old}}} \tag{19.3}$$

Besides explicit Poisson-noise modelling, an important additional advantage of MLEM is its capacity to implement the crucial attenuation and scatter corrections and to model the collimator-detector response (CDR) directly into the reconstruction. While the attenuation and scatter corrections model the interaction of the photons with the imaged object, the latter represents their interaction with the detection

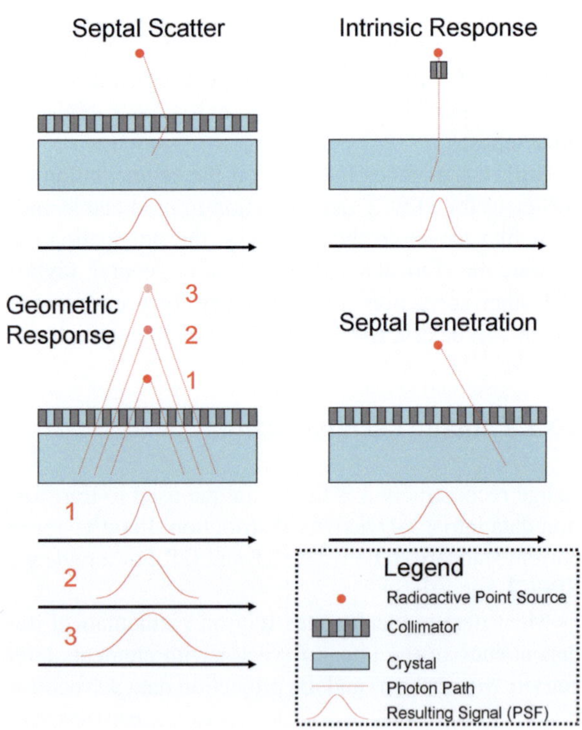

Fig. 19.6 Illustration of the different components that form the collimator-detector response function. *Lower left:* The geometric response function models source-to-collimator distance effects: The measured response in the crystal varies with source-to-collimator distance. *Upper right:* The intrinsic response function describes the effects of interactions in the detector crystal (please note: the point source is collimated to form a pencil beam). *Upper left and lower right:* The septal scatter and septal penetration functions model the interactions between the photons and the collimator

system (collimator, crystal and electronics). As illustrated in Fig. 19.6, the most important components of the CDR are: (a) the intrinsic response that is caused by scatter occurring in the crystal itself and the uncertainty of the position estimation of the detected photon, (b) the geometric response which represents a distance-dependent spatial resolution caused by the finite bore length and width of the collimator, (c) scatter in the collimator itself and (d) septal penetration when photons are detected after passing through the walls of the collimator holes.

The CDR is commonly assumed to be Gaussian and modelled as such in the reconstruction. In general, it has been demonstrated that this leads to significantly improved image quality [10]. Several studies found that with iterative reconstruction techniques, the acquisition time or patient dose could be reduced by a factor of up to two compared to FBP, for example, in skeletal examinations [11].

Still, it is clear that the Gaussian modelling approach has only limited precision since significant differences between the model and the real CDR can be found, especially in regions on the edge of the geometric response. There, the Gaussian model systematically underestimates the number of detected counts. Moreover, methods using deconvolution with a Gaussian introduce ring artefacts more commonly known as Gibbs artefacts, which artificially increase activity concentration for objects with sharp edges. Additionally, a rotationally invariant function like the Gaussian cannot express the contours found in real CDRs which mimic the shape of the collimator bore. Multiple solutions have been proposed for further improving the modelling: Monte Carlo (MC) simulations can be used to calculate the CDR during reconstruction [12] or prior to reconstruction [13]. In later approaches, a set of distance-dependent CDRs is calculated, stored and then used in the iterative reconstruction. Other approaches rely on more sophisticated mathematical models and fit their free parameters to a set of point source measurements [14]. Nevertheless, Gaussian modelling is the method that is applied in most clinically available tools.

19.2.4 Scatter Correction

Scatter is another factor which degrades the quality of SPECT images, although its correction is somewhat less important than the corrections for the collimator-detector response or for photon attenuation. However, since very accurate technical solutions for these latter problems are already available in clinical practice, scatter remains a major limiting factor of the image quality and quantitative accuracy of current SPECT systems, particularly when using isotopes with complex emission spectra. There exist numerous techniques for scatter correction; describing them all is beyond the scope of this chapter, but an extensive review can be found in [15].

The Compton Effect is the dominant process for scattering of photons in the patient and in the collimators at clinically relevant energies in Nuclear Medicine. Coherent scattering, an interaction between the photons and atoms or molecules, which is another phenomenon capable of deflecting photons from their original direction, is important only for energies below 50 keV. With Compton scattering, the photon transfers part of its energy to an electron and should be detected at lower energies in an ideal detector with perfect energy resolution. In a real detector, the uncertainty of energy determination limits the detectable energy loss. In general, the amount of energy loss depends on the scatter angle. The result of this relationship is that scattered photons are often detected at locations unrelated to their initial trajectories, leading to a loss of information about the activity distribution being imaged. The proportion of scattered photons in a particular acquisition is object dependent but can be rather high. The amount of Compton scatter originating in the collimators is most likely negligible for 140 keV Tc-99m imaging but increases with increasing energy and thus is considerably higher for I-131 at 364 keV [16]. In order to minimize the amount of scatter and to exclude photons that do not originate from the decay of the respective radionuclide, energy windows around the photopeak of interest are applied. Nevertheless, due to the limited energy resolution of SPECT detectors and the typical width of the photopeak windows, a considerable amount of scattered photons is still recorded.

A very common approach in clinical routine is based on utilizing dual-, triple- or even multi-energy windows. The additional scatter energy windows are placed below and/or above the photopeak energy window. Additional projections are acquired at those windows simultaneously to the image at the photopeak window. Subsequently, for each pixel of the projections at the photopeak window, the amount of scattered radiation can be estimated from the scatter window images. This amount is subtracted from the projections or incorporated in the iterative reconstruction.

This underlines the fact that additional techniques are necessary to account and correct for scatter. First, the amount of scattered photons in the photopeak window needs to be estimated. Here, two paradigms are possible: estimates based on directly measured data or estimates based on modelling. The most common approach, that is, that of measuring the counts in multiple additional energy windows adjacent to the photopeak window, belongs to the former paradigm. For the triple energy window (TEW) technique, the scattered photons in the photopeak can be calculated according to Eq. 19.4 for every pixel. Here, n_s are the counts of the pixel that were scattered and n_l, n_u are the measured counts in the lower and upper scatter windows. The widths of the photopeak, the lower scatter, and the upper scatter window are denoted by w_p, w_l and w_u:

$$n_s = \left(\frac{n_l}{w_l} + \frac{n_u}{w_u} \right) * \frac{1}{2} w_p \tag{19.4}$$

The calculated amount of scattered photons is then incorporated into the image reconstruction. This can be achieved in multiple ways. The simplest approach is to subtract the counts from the photopeak window. However, it was found [17] that incorporating the amount of scatter directly into the forward projector in the MLEM algorithm is a superior approach in terms of image quality and quantitative accuracy. This is to a large extent explained by the high amount of noise in the scatter window data which is due to the generally low count number in these windows.

As an extension of the TEW method, so-called spectral models can be applied. Such methods try to improve the accuracy and the noise properties of the scatter estimates via a finer sampling of the energy distribution of the photons that reach each detector pixel. Ideally, one would record the energy of each photon individually (list-mode acquisition). With this information, models that predict the amount of scatter in the photopeak window could be estimated with good confidence and low noise [18]. With the introduction of CZT-based systems, list-mode acquisitions have become more routine in clinical practice, opening opportunities for future research.

Scatter estimation and correction with the help of full Monte Carlo (MC) simulations has been a popular topic in research. These simulations are supported by the availability of faster computational hardware and the development of accelerated versions of the MC algorithms [19]. Two important prerequisites for these simulations are the estimates of the spatial distributions of the radioactive source and of the probability that scatter occurs. For this reason, MC simulations are usually carried out in each step of the iterative SPECT reconstruction, since the source distribution is not known a priori and is therefore updated at each iteration. The probability that scatter occurs can be estimated using transmission scans of the object, which are readily available with SPECT/CT systems. Drawbacks of these methods are the still comparatively long calculation times and the inability to account for photons that originate from outside the camera's field of view. A faster method that relies on partial MC simulations and approximated scatter patterns is called effective source scatter estimation [20].

However, despite the availability of very sophisticated scatter correction methods, the estimation of scatter by either TEW or DEW (the dual energy window approach that neglects upper scatter) and its correction in the MLEM or in the OSEM algorithm is still the standard approach in clinical SPECT.

19.2.5 Partial Volume Correction

Partial volume effects are caused by the limited spatial resolution of the SPECT device. Radioactivity concentration in regions of interest (ROI) in structures smaller than approximately 2–3 times of the FWHM is misquantified: the activity in ROIs of that size is either under- or over-estimated, depending on the combination of 'spill-in' and 'spill-out' effects. Spill-in means that activity from outside the ROI or structure, due to the limited spatial resolution, is integrated (added) to the activity inside the ROI; the activity inside the ROI is erroneously increased. Spill-out implies that the activity of the ROI or structure is distributed over its borders (again due to limited spatial resolution) and therefore 'lost': the activity measured inside the ROI is then underestimated. Patient motion can be another cause for increased partial volume effects, especially in clinical settings.

The approaches for a correction of the partial volume effect are divided into two groups: approaches that are based on additional information from images (e.g. CT and MR) of the structures in question and methods that work solely on the emission images.

If only the average activity concentration in a sufficiently large object is of interest, like, for example, in organ-based dosimetry, one simple way of compensating the partial volume effect is by careful definition of the region/volume of interest (ROI/VOI) for the evaluation of the activity. As mentioned above, the counts registered by the detector are distributed over an area which is larger than the physical extent of the object of interest. Thus, for 'hot' objects in a comparably 'cold' background, one could dilate the VOI over the actual physical extent as given by CT and partially recover the counts otherwise lost due to spill-out. The extent of dilation should be carefully chosen based on the target-to-background ratio and the spatial resolution of the SPECT acquisition. The accuracy of this method is varying strongly, depending on the activity distribution that surrounds the VOI. Alternatively, for large objects that can be assumed having homogenous tracer uptake, one could draw a smaller spherical VOI, in a sub-region unaffected by partial volume effect and extrapolate to the whole VOI [21].

Another common and still simple post-reconstruction approach in the latter group is founded on measurements with physical phantoms, simulation studies or theoretical derivations: as outlined by Kessler et al. [22] recovery coefficients (the ratio of apparent activity concentration to true activity concentration) for simple geometries (e.g. spheres, discs and cylinders) can be measured or estimated and consequently be used to calculate corrected values for the amount of radioactivity in those structures. However, a major limitation is the geometry dependence of the activity recovery. Even simple geometries like the NEMA phantom spheres will have a different recovery depending on their position compared to the detector [23]. This approach is therefore very limited in its applicability; in general, the radioactivity distribution in a patient will render this approach not very useful. Another method is the deconvolution-based partial volume correction. When attempting this approach for Lu-177, Liu et al. [24] found an increased accuracy, however, limited to 17.8%.

Every technique that results in an improved spatial resolution of the imaging system helps to lower the influence of the partial volume effect. For example, some methods that are described in the *Image Reconstruction* paragraph which incorporate information about the collimator-detector response function will improve the systems spatial resolution to some extent and therefore can be interpreted as a partial volume correction technique. For example, Hutton et al. [25] report improved accuracy for the simulated Mathematical Cardiac Torso (MCAT) phantom for their implementation of the detector response modelling into the MLEM and OSEM reconstruction.

The other group of methods utilizes structural and anatomical information in the form of segmented images from another imaging modality (CT, MR and US) for partial volume correction. The segmentation itself can be done in a fully automatic fashion or by manually outlining ROIs. The simple methods rely on multiple two-class segmentation (regions with activity and regions without activity). For example, Pretorius et al. [26] apply this approach to co-registered myocardial CT images on the MCAT phantom and are able to obtain improved visual characteristics as well as a higher quantitative accuracy of the corrected SPECT data.

19.2.6 Noise Reduction

OSEM is notorious for increasing the noise in the image with every iteration, while quantitative accuracy increases with each iteration. This intricate balance can be improved upon by applying noise reduction techniques after or during image reconstruction. Traditionally, noise has been reduced through the application of a low-pass filter similar to those used in FBP such as Butterworth or Hamming filters to reduce the high-frequency noise. Noise can also be reduced in the reconstruction process by penalizing solutions that include more noise. For this purpose a prior is introduced that promotes local smoothness [27]. One of the proposed priors takes the simplified form of Eq. 19.6 where λ_j is the activity in pixel j, N_j is the set of neighbours of pixel j and β is the weight given to the prior.

$$M(\lambda) = -\sum_{j}\sum_{k \in N_j} \beta \phi(\lambda_j - \lambda_k), \tag{19.6}$$

These algorithms can run to full convergence without noise amplification in each step. This increases quantitative accuracy. This algorithm was shown to yield no significant difference in activity concentration when compared to OSEM by the same vendor; however, noise amplification was significantly reduced [6].

More recently, new approaches leveraging artificial intelligence have become of interest. Currently, two solutions are commercially available for bone SPECT/CT in combination with 360° CZT cameras [28, 29]. Both use a 3D residual UNet convolutional neural network architecture with the mean square error as a loss function. The noise reduction step can be either applied post-reconstruction or in the iterative reconstruction algorithm. DLNR showed an increasing contrast-to-noise ratio while preserving the SUVmax in clinical datasets. Clarify DL showed an improved rating in clinical image quality as evaluated by multiple readers, while also improving quantitative accuracy in phantom measurements compared to factory preset reconstruction.

Similarly to the above-mentioned application for bone SPECT/CT, the interest in noise reduction in other fields of (quantitative) SPECT/CT such as myocardial perfusion imaging has increased [30], although to the best of our knowledge, these applications are not yet commercially available.

19.2.7 Calibration

An important requirement for quantitative accurate SPECT is the determination of the system volume sensitivity S_{Vol} (Eq. 19.7):

$$S_{\mathrm{Vol}} = \frac{R}{V_{\mathrm{VOI}} \cdot c_{\mathrm{Vol}}} \times \exp\left(\frac{T_0 - T_{\mathrm{cal}}}{T_{1/2}} \cdot \ln 2\right) \times \left(\frac{T_{\mathrm{acq}}}{T_{1/2}} \cdot \ln 2\right) \times \left(1 - \exp\left(-\frac{T_{\mathrm{acq}}}{T_{1/2}} \cdot \ln 2\right)\right)^{-1} \tag{19.7}$$

This is needed for the calibration of the scanner to absolute values and is typically obtained by a correlation of measured results to a calibrated well counter and/or radionuclide calibrator. This process is intuitive, standardized and its description can be found in detail, for example, in the NEMA protocols [31]. Its principle is briefly outlined in the following: in order to avoid partial volume effects, a large cylindrical phantom (larger than 20 cm in diameter and length) with known activity concentration c_{Vol} is scanned with the SPECT system. Subsequently, corrections for attenuated and scattered photons are applied and a large VOI with volume V_{VOI} is defined in the reconstructed image. T_0 is the start time, T_{acq} the duration of the acquisition. $T_{1/2}$ is the half time of the used radionuclide, T_{cal} the time of the activity calibration, and R represents the counting rate measured in the VOI. Finally, based on Eq. 19.7, a calibration factor, which allows conversion from detected counts per second to becquerel, is calculated. This calibration factor is specific to every radionuclide as well as for different intrinsic detector sensitivities and collimators. It is possible and in some cases beneficial to have count rate-dependent calibration factors. Reasons for this are thought to be non-linearities of the detector at the different count rates and dead time effects at high activities. Those effects will be stronger for higher-energy radionuclides (e.g. I-131). Dewaraja et al. [32] report on dead time and pulse pile-up effects for the SPECT quantification of therapeutic activities of 2–6 GBq I-131.

Currently, all new SPECT/CT systems and reconstruction workstations which are commercially available can provide images in quantitative units (often Bq/mL) as output. For most of these systems, one first needs to determine a proper calibration factor which is then applied in the image reconstruction. One notable exception relies on NIST-traceable quantitative sources and currently offers quantitative capabilities for the radionuclides (Tc-99m, I-123, In-111 and Lu-177) [33]. This promises to minimize the variability of quantitative data obtained at different centres/hospitals and helps to standardize quantitative SPECT, which could be advantageous for multi-centre studies.

19.3 Standardization and Harmonization

Once quantitative values have been derived, the true power of these values lies in the clinical meaning that can be assigned to them. However, the discussions in previous paragraphs have demonstrated that there can be a large variability in the quantitative capabilities of different systems depending on system properties, corrections and reconstruction settings. This variability can be countered by standardization and harmonization efforts. These efforts rely on two phantom measurements: a uniform cylinder to test the calibration of the systems towards a primary standard and a NEMA IEC Body Phantom (or equivalent) to assess the quantitative performance over different-sized spheres, capturing the effective resolution of the system. Multiple groups have investigated the possibility of standardization and harmonization in SPECT/CT for different isotopes, most importantly Tc-99m and Lu-177. The effective resolution is geometry-dependent which complicates the use of recovery coefficients for standardization and harmonization. Nonetheless, an accreditation programme for Lu-177 SPECT/CT will be introduced by EARL, a European Association for Nuclear Medicine subsidiary, which uses the spherical recovery coefficients [1].

19.4 Validation

To validate applications of quantitative imaging, we would need access to ground truth. This is difficult to achieve in vivo, as this would require sampling human tissue. However, this can also be achieved through measurements of phantoms representing a geometry relevant for imaging.

19.4.1 Phantoms

We have already mentioned the more generic phantoms such as the uniform cylinder and NEMA IEC Body Phantom with different-sized spherical inserts which are important in quality control. While these phantoms provide a valuable tool for standardization and harmonization through their widespread availability, they are not suitable for validation of clinical applications. Validation requires phantoms representative of human structures. Several phantoms representing simplified structures are commercially available including phantoms representing the myocardium, brain and torso.

The increased availability of 3D printing technology has created the ability to develop more realistic phantoms representing patient geometries rather than simplified or generic shapes [34]. For example, kidneys are organs at risk in radioligand therapies, and the accuracy of activity concentration is important for dosimetry calculations. As a result, we have seen an increase in complexity for kidney phantoms over the past decade. The first phantoms were simplified single-compartment mode [35, 36]. This approach was extended to include a second compartment, separating the cortex and medulla as they both show a different uptake of tracer in PRRT [37]. The models can be further refined by including a grid inside the compartment to locally decrease tracer concentration [38].

19.4.2 Ex Vivo

While the phantom studies are interesting and have improved our understanding of quantitative imaging in general, we must sometimes be reminded that phantoms are still not human. In the ideal circumstances, we would be able to verify our in vivo imaging by ex vivo measurement in, for example, a gamma counter. Such an ex vivo validation was performed by Zeintl et al. by measuring the urinary bladder activity concentration on SPECT/CT and verifying the concentration after urinary sampling for Tc-99m [39]. Later, Kennedy et al. repeated this experiment on a flat panel CZT

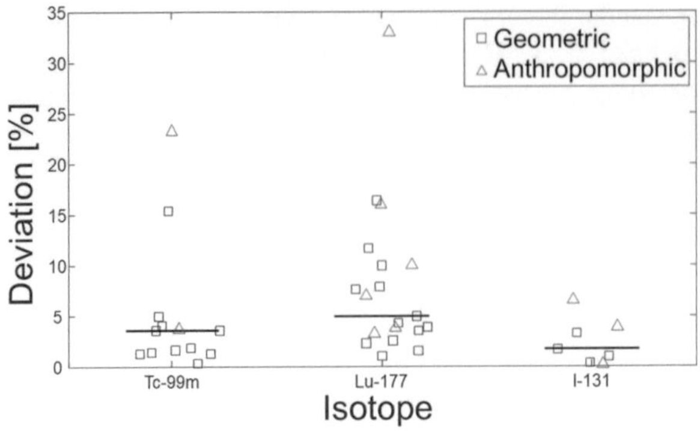

Fig. 19.7 Overview of the results of 24 studies reporting on the quantitative accuracy of SPECT, by radionuclide. Markers indicate the average deviation between ground truth and imaging-derived quantitative values, as reported by the respective study. Additionally, mean values are provided for each group

camera [40] and afterwards extended the approach to Lu-177 [41], demonstrating quantitative accuracy within 20% for both isotopes.

Overall quantitative accuracy of SPECT/CT was evaluated for Tc-99m, Lu-177 and I-131 based on 24 studies [36–39, 42–61]. The results are summarized in Fig. 19.7. In general, reasonable accuracy can be achieved for the selected isotopes with a deviation from the true value of 5.1 ± 6.7%, 7.6 ± 7.7% and 2.3 ± 2.5% for Tc-99m, Lu-177 and I-131, respectively. Notable outliers are measurements in anthropomorphic phantoms of the mandibular condyles [61] or the renal cortex [37], which have challenging geometries due to their small size or complex geometry. The increased interest in Lu-177 quantitative accuracy for dosimetry is clear from the number of studies evaluating its accuracy. Three SPECT-only studies were omitted which results in a relatively low number of studies evaluating I-131 accuracy. The accuracy achieved for Lu-177 has a larger variation, which can be explained at least in part by the higher scatter fraction and the septal penetration for the higher-energy photons. Generally, quantitative accuracy in PET is in the same range, at least for sufficiently large structures. Nevertheless, for smaller structures, PET will most likely achieve better quantitative accuracy due to its higher spatial resolution. Generally, a quantitative accuracy of within 10% error could be achieved with SPECT/CT.

19.5 Clinical Applications of Quantitative SPECT

19.5.1 Dosimetry

Radionuclide therapy with ^{131}I has been a major success in the treatment of benign and malignant thyroid diseases even since before quantitative SPECT/CT was available. Results from the SEL-I-METRY suggest quantitative I-123 pre-therapy imaging and dosimetry can be useful to determine whether I-131-refractory patients could be successfully retreated [62].

From the mid-2010s, there has been an increase in Lu-177 radioligand therapies driven by the results of the NETTER-1 and NETTER-2 trials which showed increased progression-free survival for patients with advanced midgut neuroendocrine tumours after treatment with Lu-177-DOTATATE [63, 64] and by the VISION and PSMAfore trials for patients with metastatic castration-resistant prostate cancer after administration of Lu-177-PSMA-617 [65, 66]. These landmark trials have ushered in a new era in radioligand therapies, quantitative imaging to accurately assess tracer distribution, dosimetry to optimize treatment and toxicity evaluation [67]. The MRTDosimetry project proposed a calibration procedure which resulted in deviation of 10% and 6% for the kidneys and spleen respectively [60]. Several groups have since investigated the accuracy for Lu-177 imaging on ring-geometry systems reporting accuracies of within 10% [6, 48]. Diagnostic imaging for PRRT theranostics is performed at a single timepoint within 1–2 h after injection which cannot capture long term uptake important for dose delivery. Nevertheless, by combining diagnostic Ga-68-DOTATATE PET/CT with machine learning, Akhavanallaf et al. showed an improved correlation with posttherapy dosimetry compared to diagnostic PET/CT by itself [68]. Once accurate quantification and dose predictive models are established, the final piece of the puzzle to establish truly personalized medicine is the dose-effect relationship. Currently, such a relationship is still lacking.

With the recent success of Lu-177-based radioligand therapies, the quest for improvement has also sparked interest in different isotopes which are currently not available on a scale required for clinical translation but can be used for SPECT imaging. Examples are Ac-225, At-211, Tb-161, Cu-64/67 and Sc-47 [69].

19.5.2 Cardiology

In cardiology, quantitative SPECT/CT has not yet been adopted in standard imaging protocols. However, there are currently three major applications where it is suggested that quantitative SPECT/CT could provide benefit compared to the current relative scoring systems: myocardial perfusion, coronary flow reserve and transthyretin cardiac amyloidosis.

Myocardial perfusion SPECT/CT is performed to evaluate coronary artery disease (CAD) using Tc-99m-sestamibi or Tc-99m-tetrofosmin. Through relative quantification, the perfusion of the different regions of the left ventricle receives a score. However, global hypoperfusion can lead to underestimation of the CAD. It has been suggested that absolute quantification is a promising technique in myocardial perfusion imaging [70]. The fast acquisition times of dedicated cardiac and 360° CZT cameras allow dynamic SPECT imaging, which can be used to calculate the coronary flow reserve. A dynamic acquisition is performed starting at the moment of tracer injection for both the stress and rest perfusion imaging. Through segmentation of the right pulmonary artery, the arterial input function is calculated for estimation of the coronary flow reserve. This measurement was shown to agree with an invasive measurement through intracoronary Doppler [71].

Transthyretin cardiac amyloidosis is a subtype of cardiac amyloidosis which is a progressive disease where continued accumulation of misfolding transthyretin leads to a loss of contractility and conductivity, and ultimately to heart failure. Scintigraphy using bone-seeking tracers like Tc-99m-HMDP, Tc-99m-DPD or Tc-99m-PYP has a high sensitivity and specificity for the diagnosis of TTR cardiac amyloidosis [72]. Nevertheless, semiquantitative or qualitative scoring on planar scintigraphy can result in misdiagnosis when blood pool activity is high. Adding SPECT/CT increases specificity and allows for quantitative analysis. It was shown that absolute quantification can distinguish normal hearts from hearts with amyloid deposition [73]. Quantitative metrics are promising for the assessment of amyloid burden. With several therapies available for treatment of ATTR-CM, it is important to assess treatment response and quantitative SPECT/CT has been studied as part of this, where a decrease in tracer uptake has been shown to correlate with an increase in cardiac function [74].

19.5.3 Neurology

Presynaptic dopamine transporter imaging using I-123-FP-CIT is an essential part of distinguishing several diagnoses with clinical presentations similar to Parkinson's disease, such as essential tremor or Lewy Body dementia. Current clinical practice is visual interpretation which can be combined with a semiquantitative analysis of tracer uptake in ROIs of the striatum and putamen [75]. These semiquantitative metrics are then compared to age-matched normal values. There is a natural reduction of tracer uptake with ageing, which is taken into account by calculating semiquantitative ratios of uptake in the striata and the occipital or cerebellar cortex. Besides demonstrating the applicability of the striatal-to-background ratio, Tokiihara et al. demonstrated the potential of SUV as a parameter to distinguish between disease with or without presynaptic dopamine transporter deficit [76].

19.5.4 Bone Imaging

Bone imaging spans a large variation in bone-seeking tracers and pathologies. 99mTc labelled bisphosphonates bind where there is active bone remodelling through osteoblast activity. Many bone pathologies are associated with a change in bone remodelling [77].

19.5.4.1 Bone Metastases

Measuring bone metastases on CT or MRI is difficult, given the lack of a sharp boundary between tumour and healthy bone, while the presence of bone remodelling can be assessed using bone-seeking tracers. In a recent review, it was suggested that imaging of bone disease is one of the main applications of quantitative SPECT/CT [78]. While SUV cutoffs have been proposed, bone remodelling of bone metastases has been shown to be variable in time [79] and previous experiences with PET/CT have demonstrated that absolute values are only transferable after harmonization and standardization of acquisition and reconstruction settings.

19.5.4.2 Mandibula

In rare cases, a difference in growth rate between both mandibular condyles results in facial asymmetry and malocclusion which can require surgical correction. It is essential this correction is only performed after growth has ended. The asymmetry in growth is assessed by comparing the tracer uptake in both condyles, while bilateral growth is assessed by comparing uptake in both condyles. However, variability in reported diagnostic performance for SPECT suggests not all aspects are understood. It has been shown that quantitative SPECT/CT improves accuracy in anthropomorphic phantoms and sensitivity in patient scans, while suggesting improvement in specificity [61].

19.5.4.3 Osteoarthritis and Arthroplasty

In an advanced stage, osteoarthritis can be effectively treated by arthroplasty. There is no single specific biomarker for the evaluation of the severity of osteoarthritis, but it has been suggested that quantitative bone SPECT/CT can be a valuable tool for patient selection in severe osteoarthritis of the knee [80]. After arthroplasty, quantitative SPECT/CT was shown to outperform visual reading for loosening of symptomatic hip and knee joint prostheses [81]. In both studies the bone uptake was normalized to patient body weight, which could potentially overestimate uptake in obese patients. Adding a correction term to take into account age and bone density improved robustness of normal tracer uptake in a retrospective study [82].

19.6 Summary and Outlook

The continuous development of SPECT and SPECT/CT over the past 50 years has led to remarkable improvements in image quality and diagnostic confidence. The most influential developments include, to name but a few, the realization of hybrid SPECT/CT devices, the implementation of attenuation correction, and iterative reconstruction techniques.

In recent years, some interesting approaches in detector technology have found their way into commercial products. For example, some SPECT cameras dedicated to specific organs use semi-conductive materials like CZT as detector material. It has been shown that this could help to further increase the obtainable image quality.

New trends in the ongoing development of SPECT/CT are quite diverse. For example, whole-body SPECT/CT images consisting of acquisitions from multiple consecutive bed positions, similar to PET/CT, have begun to increase. The limitation of the relatively long SPECT acquisition times (typically 15 min per bed position and 30–45 min for the trunk) can be overcome with the 360° CZT SPECT/CT systems. Even though new reconstruction techniques already allow for a reduction in acquisition times, in the future, new collimator and detector designs with higher photon sensitivity could further support this development. Additionally, this trend could be facilitated by the incorporation of low-dose concepts applicable to CT, like, for example, the use of iterative CT reconstruction in SPECT/CT.

With the availability of SPECT list-mode data on newer systems, there is potential to gain information. This information could be used to improve estimation and correction of confounding factors like patient motion and scattered radiation.

Information can also be gained from other modalities. When more information than only attenuation is incorporated from the CT images into the SPECT reconstruction, the partial volume effect can also be decreased. This development could lead to improved spatial resolution. While the focus of manufacturers has shifted towards theranostic applications; this technique has been commercially introduced for Tc-99m bone scans only. However, it could be extremely useful with other tracers as well.

Similarly, noise reduction through deep learning has been commercialized for bone SPECT/CT first. Another important aspect of SPECT/CT is the fact that the technique, like PET, allows quantification of the amount of tracer in terms of Bq/mL or as an SUV. Numerous publications have shown that absolute quantification is feasible. This can be expected to further boost diagnostic confidence.

The ever-increasing number of publications on SPECT/CT shows that this modality is of great clinical interest. New technical developments will strengthen this trend and ensure that SPECT/CT remains the workhorse of nuclear medicine, even when compared to other strong contenders like PET/CT.

References

1. Dickson JC, Armstrong IS, Gabina PM, Denis-Bacelar AM, Krizsan AK, Gear JM et al (2023) EANM practice guideline for quantitative SPECT-CT. Eur J Nucl Med Mol Imaging 50(4):980–995
2. Zorz A, Rossato MA, Turco P, Colombo Gomez LM, Bettinelli A, De Monte F et al (2024) Performance evaluation of the 3D-ring cadmium-zinc-telluride (CZT) StarGuide system according to the NEMA NU 1-2018 standard. EJNMMI Phys 11(1):69
3. Desmonts C, Bouthiba MA, Enilorac B, Nganoa C, Agostini D, Aide N (2020) Evaluation of a new multipurpose whole-body CzT-based camera: comparison with a dual-head Anger camera and first clinical images. EJNMMI Phys 7(1):18
4. Van den Wyngaert T, Elvas F, De Schepper S, Kennedy JA, Israel O (2020) SPECT/CT: standing on the shoulders of giants, it is time to reach for the sky! J Nucl Med 61(9):1284–1291
5. Schramm NU, Ebel G, Engeland U, Schurrat T, Behe M, Behr TM (2003) High-resolution SPECT using multipinhole collimation. Nucl Sci IEEE Trans 50(3):315–320
6. Danieli R, Stella M, Leube J, Tran-Gia J, Marin C, Uribe CF et al (2023) Quantitative (177) Lu SPECT/CT imaging for personalized dosimetry using a ring-shaped CZT-based camera. EJNMMI Phys 10(1):64
7. Cherry SR, Sorenson JA, Phelps ME (2003) Physics in nuclear medicine, 3rd edn. Elsevier, Philadelphia

8. Cheng Z, Chen P, Yan J (2025) A review of state-of-the-art resolution improvement techniques in SPECT imaging. EJNMMI Phys 12(1):9
9. Bruyant PP (2002) Analytic and iterative reconstruction algorithms in SPECT. J Nucl Med 43(10):1343–1358
10. Aldridge MD, Waddington WW, Dickson JC, Prakash V, Ell PJ, Bomanji JB (2013) Clinical evaluation of reducing acquisition time on single-photon emission computed tomography image quality using proprietary resolution recovery software. Nucl Med Commun 34(11):1116–1123
11. Stansfield EC, Sheehy N, Zurakowski D, Vija AH, Fahey FH, Treves ST (2010) Pediatric 99mTc-MDP Bone SPECT with ordered subset expectation maximization iterative reconstruction with isotropic 3D resolution recovery. Radiology 257(3):793–801
12. Liu S, Farncombe TH eds (2007) Collimator-detector response compensation in quantitative SPECT reconstruction. In: Nuclear science symposium conference record, 2007 NSS '07 IEEE; 2007 Oct. 26 2007–Nov. 3 2007
13. Du Y, Tsui BM, Frey EC (2006) Model-based compensation for quantitative 123I brain SPECT imaging. Phys Med Biol 51(5):1269–1282
14. Se Young C, Fessler JA, Dewaraja YK (2013) Correction for collimator-detector response in SPECT using point spread function template. IEEE Trans Med Imaging 32(2):295–305
15. Hutton BF, Buvat I, Beekman FJ (2011) Review and current status of SPECT scatter correction. Phys Med Biol 56(14):R85–R112
16. Zaidi H, Koral KF (2004) Scatter modelling and compensation in emission tomography. Eur J Nucl Med Mol Imaging 31(5):761–782
17. King MA, DeVries DJ, Pan TS, Pretorius PH, Case JA (1997) An investigation of the filtering of TEW scatter estimates used to compensate for scatter with ordered subset reconstructions. Nucl Sci IEEE Trans 44(3):1140–1145
18. Buvat I, Rodriguez-Villafuerte M, Todd-Pokropek A, Benali H, Di Paola R (1995) Comparative assessment of nine scatter correction methods based on spectral analysis using Monte Carlo simulations. J Nucl Med 36(8):1476–1488
19. Sohlberg A, Watabe H, Iida H (2008) Acceleration of Monte Carlo-based scatter compensation for cardiac SPECT. Phys Med Biol 53(14):N277–N285
20. Frey EC, Tsui BMW, eds (1996) A new method for modeling the spatially-variant, object-dependent scatter response function in SPECT. In: Nuclear science symposium, 1996 conference record, 1996 IEEE; 1996 2–9 Nov 1996
21. Vicente EM, Lodge MA, Rowe SP, Wahl RL, Frey EC (2017) Simplifying volumes-of-interest (VOIs) definition in quantitative SPECT: beyond manual definition of 3D whole-organ VOIs. Med Phys 44(5):1707–1717
22. Kessler RM, Ellis JRJ, Eden M (1984) Analysis of emission tomographic scan data: limitations imposed by resolution and background. J Comput Assist Tomogr 8(3):514–522
23. Leube J, Claeys W, Gustafsson J, Salas-Ramirez M, Lassmann M, Koole M et al (2024) Position dependence of recovery coefficients in (177)Lu-SPECT/CT reconstructions – phantom simulations and measurements. EJNMMI Phys 11(1):52
24. Liu Y, Lu Z, Chen G, Shi K, Mok GSP (2024) Partial volume correction for Lu-177-PSMA SPECT. EJNMMI Phys 11(1):93
25. Hutton BF, Lau YH (1998) Application of distance-dependent resolution compensation and post-reconstruction filtering for myocardial SPECT. Phys Med Biol 43(6):1679
26. Pretorius PH, King MA (2009) Diminishing the impact of the partial volume effect in cardiac SPECT perfusion imaging. Med Phys 36(1):105–115
27. Nuyts J, Beque D, Dupont P, Mortelmans L (2002) A concave prior penalizing relative differences for maximum-a-posteriori reconstruction in emission tomography. Nucl Sci IEEE Trans 49(1):56–60
28. Ziv O, Yuzefovich B, Sachs J, Kovalski G (2024) White paper: clarify DL – deep learning image reconstruction for bone SPECT scans
29. Bahloul A, Verger A, Lamash Y, Roth N, Dari D, Marie PY et al (2024) Ultra-fast whole-body bone tomoscintigraphies achieved with a high-sensitivity 360 degrees CZT camera and a dedicated deep-learning noise reduction algorithm. Eur J Nucl Med Mol Imaging 51(5):1215–1220

30. Aghakhan Olia N, Kamali-Asl A, Hariri Tabrizi S, Geramifar P, Sheikhzadeh P, Farzanefar S et al (2022) Deep learning-based denoising of low-dose SPECT myocardial perfusion images: quantitative assessment and clinical performance. Eur J Nucl Med Mol Imaging 49(5):1508–1522
31. Performance Measurements of Gamma Cameras (2007) NEMA NU 1-2007. National Electrical Manufacturers Association, Rosslyn
32. Dewaraja Y, Ljungberg M, Koral K (2008) Effects of dead time and pile up on quantitative SPECT for I-131 dosimetric studies. J Nucl Med Meeting Abstracts 49(MeetingAbstracts_1):47P-c
33. Vija AH (2013) White paper: introduction to xSPECT technology: evolving multi-modal SPECT to become context-based and quantitative. Siemens Medical Solutions USA, Inc
34. De Schepper S, Gnanasegaran G, Dickson JC, Van den Wyngaert T (2021) Absolute quantification in diagnostic SPECT/CT: the phantom premise. Diagnostics (Basel) 11(12):2333
35. Gear JI, Long C, Rushforth D, Chittenden SJ, Cummings C, Flux GD (2014) Development of patient-specific molecular imaging phantoms using a 3D printer. Med Phys 41(8):082502
36. Tran-Gia J, Schlogl S, Lassmann M (2016) Design and fabrication of kidney phantoms for internal radiation dosimetry using 3D printing technology. J Nucl Med 57(12):1998–2005
37. Tran-Gia J, Lassmann M (2018) Optimizing image quantification for (177)Lu SPECT/CT based on a 3D printed 2-compartment kidney phantom. J Nucl Med 59(4):616–624
38. Jessen L, Gustafsson J, Ljungberg M, Curkic-Kapidzic S, Imsirovic M, Sjogreen-Gleisner K (2024) 3D printed non-uniform anthropomorphic phantoms for quantitative SPECT. EJNMMI Phys 11(1):8
39. Zeintl J, Vija AH, Yahil A, Hornegger J, Kuwert T (2010) Quantitative accuracy of clinical 99mTc SPECT/CT using ordered-subset expectation maximization with 3-dimensional resolution recovery, attenuation, and scatter correction. J Nucl Med 51(6):921–928
40. Kennedy JA, Reizberg I, Lugassi R, Himmelman S, Keidar Z (2019) Absolute radiotracer concentration measurement using whole-body solid-state SPECT/CT technology: in vivo/in vitro validation. Med Biol Eng Comput 57(7):1581–1590
41. Kennedy JA, Lugassi R, Gill R, Keidar Z (2020) Digital solid-state SPECT/CT quantitation of absolute (177)lu-radiotracer concentration: in vivo/in vitro validation. J Nucl Med. https://doi.org/10.2967/jnumed.119.239277
42. Zimmerman BE, Grosev D, Buvat I, Coca Perez MA, Frey EC, Green A et al (2017) Multicentre evaluation of accuracy and reproducibility of planar and SPECT image quantification: an IAEA phantom study. Z Med Phys 27(2):98–112
43. Wilson LJ, Belko S, Gingold E, Wan S, Monane R, Pugliese R et al (2025) 3D-printed organ-realistic phantoms to verify quantitative SPECT/CT accuracy for 177Lu-PSMA-617 treatment planning. Pharmaceuticals (Basel) 18(4):550
44. Willowson K, Bailey DL, Bailey EA, Baldock C, Roach PJ (2010) In vivo validation of quantitative SPECT in the heart. Clin Physiol Funct Imaging 30(3):214–219
45. Willowson K, Bailey DL, Baldock C (2008) Quantitative SPECT reconstruction using CT-derived corrections. Phys Med Biol 53(12):3099–3112
46. van Gils CA, Beijst C, van Rooij R, de Jong HW (2016) Impact of reconstruction parameters on quantitative I-131 SPECT. Phys Med Biol 61(14):5166–5182
47. Uribe CF, Esquinas PL, Tanguay J, Gonzalez M, Gaudin E, Beauregard JM et al (2017) Accuracy of (177)Lu activity quantification in SPECT imaging: a phantom study. EJNMMI Phys 4(1):2
48. Stenvall A, Ceric Andelius I, Nilsson E, Lindvall A, Larsson E, Gustafsson J (2024) Bias and precision of SPECT-based (177)Lu activity-concentration estimation using a ring-configured solid-state versus a dual-headed anger system. EJNMMI Phys 11(1):91
49. Shcherbinin S, Piwowarska-Bilska H, Celler A, Birkenfeld B (2012) Quantitative SPECT/CT reconstruction for (1)(7)(7)Lu and (1)(7)(7)Lu/(9)(0)Y targeted radionuclide therapies. Phys Med Biol 57(18):5733–5747
50. Shcherbinin S, Celler A, Belhocine T, Vanderwerf R, Driedger A (2008) Accuracy of quantitative reconstructions in SPECT/CT imaging. Phys Med Biol 53(17):4595–4604

51. Sanders JC, Kuwert T, Hornegger J, Ritt P (2015) Quantitative SPECT/CT imaging of (177) Lu with in vivo validation in patients undergoing peptide receptor radionuclide therapy. Mol Imaging Biol 17(4):585–593
52. Mezzenga E, D'Errico V, D'Arienzo M, Strigari L, Panagiota K, Matteucci F et al (2017) Quantitative accuracy of 177Lu SPECT imaging for molecular radiotherapy. PLoS One 12(8):e0182888
53. Marin G, Vanderlinden B, Karfis I, Guiot T, Wimana Z, Flamen P et al (2017) Accuracy and precision assessment for activity quantification in individualized dosimetry of (177) Lu-DOTATATE therapy. EJNMMI Phys 4(1):7
54. Koral KF, Yendiki A, Dewaraja YK (2007) Recovery of total I-131 activity within focal volumes using SPECT and 3D OSEM. Phys Med Biol 52(3):777–790
55. Desy A, Bouvet GF, Croteau E, Lafreniere N, Turcotte EE, Despres P et al (2021) Quantitative SPECT (QSPECT) at high count rates with contemporary SPECT/CT systems. EJNMMI Phys 8(1):73
56. de Nijs R, Lagerburg V, Klausen TL, Holm S (2014) Improving quantitative dosimetry in (177) Lu-DOTATATE SPECT by energy window-based scatter corrections. Nucl Med Commun 35(5):522–533
57. D'Arienzo M, Cazzato M, Cozzella ML, Cox M, D'Andrea M, Fazio A et al (2016) Gamma camera calibration and validation for quantitative SPECT imaging with (177)Lu. Appl Radiat Isot 112:156–164
58. Beauregard JM, Hofman MS, Pereira JM, Eu P, Hicks RJ (2011) Quantitative (177)Lu SPECT (QSPECT) imaging using a commercially available SPECT/CT system. Cancer Imaging 11(1):56–66
59. Adam DP, Grudzinski JJ, Bormett I, Cox BL, Marsh IR, Bradshaw TJ et al (2022) Validation of Monte Carlo (131) I radiopharmaceutical dosimetry workflow using a 3D-printed anthropomorphic head and neck phantom. Med Phys 49(8):5491–5503
60. Tran-Gia J, Denis-Bacelar AM, Ferreira KM, Robinson AP, Calvert N, Fenwick AJ et al (2021) A multicentre and multi-national evaluation of the accuracy of quantitative Lu-177 SPECT/CT imaging performed within the MRTDosimetry project. EJNMMI Phys 8(1):55
61. De Schepper S, Gnanasegaran G, De Vos W, Van de Casteele E, Dickson JC, Van den Wyngaert T (2024) From SPECT/CT towards absolute quantification? – the case of unilateral condylar hyperplasia of the mandible. EJNMMI Phys 11(1):74
62. Taprogge J, Abreu C, Yusuf S, Ainsworth G, Phillip RH, Gear JI et al (2023) The role of pretherapy quantitative imaging and dosimetry in radioiodine therapy for advanced thyroid cancer. J Nucl Med 64(7):1125–1130
63. Strosberg J, El-Haddad G, Wolin E, Hendifar A, Yao J, Chasen B et al (2017) Phase 3 trial of (177)Lu-Dotatate for midgut neuroendocrine tumors. N Engl J Med 376(2):125–135
64. Singh S, Halperin D, Myrehaug S, Herrmann K, Pavel M, Kunz PL et al (2024) [(177) Lu]Lu-DOTA-TATE plus long-acting octreotide versus high-dose long-acting octreotide for the treatment of newly diagnosed, advanced grade 2-3, well-differentiated, gastroenteropancreatic neuroendocrine tumours (NETTER-2): an open-label, randomised, phase 3 study. Lancet 403(10446):2807–2817
65. Sartor O, de Bono J, Chi KN, Fizazi K, Herrmann K, Rahbar K et al (2021) Lutetium-177-PSMA-617 for metastatic castration-resistant prostate cancer. N Engl J Med 385(12):1091–1103
66. Morris MJ, Castellano D, Herrmann K, de Bono JS, Shore ND, Chi KN et al (2024) (177) Lu-PSMA-617 versus a change of androgen receptor pathway inhibitor therapy for taxane-naive patients with progressive metastatic castration-resistant prostate cancer (PSMAfore): a phase 3, randomised, controlled trial. Lancet 404(10459):1227–1239
67. Sjogreen Gleisner K, Chouin N, Gabina PM, Cicone F, Gnesin S, Stokke C et al (2022) EANM dosimetry committee recommendations for dosimetry of 177Lu-labelled somatostatin-receptor – and PSMA-targeting ligands. Eur J Nucl Med Mol Imaging 49(6):1778–1809
68. Akhavanallaf A, Peterson AB, Fitzpatrick K, Roseland M, Wong KK, El-Naqa I et al (2023) The predictive value of pretherapy [(68)Ga]Ga-DOTA-TATE PET and biomarkers in [(177) Lu]Lu-PRRT tumor dosimetry. Eur J Nucl Med Mol Imaging 50(10):2984–2996

69. Radzina M, Saule L, Mamis E, Koester U, Cocolios TE, Pajuste E et al (2023) Novel radionuclides for use in nuclear medicine in Europe: where do we stand and where do we go? EJNMMI Radiopharm Chem 8(1):27
70. van de Burgt A, Dibbets-Schneider P, Slump CH, Scholte A, Atsma DE, de Geus-Oei LF et al (2021) Experimental validation of absolute SPECT/CT quantification for response monitoring in patients with coronary artery disease. EJNMMI Phys 8(1):48
71. Petretta M, Soricelli A, Storto G, Cuocolo A (2008) Assessment of coronary flow reserve using single photon emission computed tomography with technetium 99m-labeled tracers. J Nucl Cardiol 15(3):456–465
72. Ahluwalia N, Roshankar G, Draycott L, Jimenez-Zepeda V, Fine N, Chan D et al (2023) Diagnostic accuracy of bone scintigraphy imaging for transthyretin cardiac amyloidosis: systematic review and meta-analysis. J Nucl Cardiol 30(6):2464–2476
73. Ramsay SC, Lindsay K, Fong W, Patford S, Younger J, Atherton J (2018) Tc-HDP quantitative SPECT/CT in transthyretin cardiac amyloid and the development of a reference interval for myocardial uptake in the non-affected population. Eur J Hybrid Imaging 2(1):17
74. Rettl R, Wollenweber T, Duca F, Binder C, Cherouny B, Dachs TM et al (2023) Monitoring tafamidis treatment with quantitative SPECT/CT in transthyretin amyloid cardiomyopathy. Eur Heart J Cardiovasc Imaging 24(8):1019–1030
75. Morbelli S, Esposito G, Arbizu J, Barthel H, Boellaard R, Bohnen NI et al (2020) EANM practice guideline/SNMMI procedure standard for dopaminergic imaging in parkinsonian syndromes 1.0. Eur J Nucl Med Mol Imaging 47(8):1885–1912
76. Toriihara A, Daisaki H, Yamaguchi A, Kobayashi M, Furukawa S, Yoshida K et al (2018) Semiquantitative analysis using standardized uptake value in (123)I-FP-CIT SPECT/CT. Clin Imaging 52:57–61
77. Van den Wyngaert T, Strobel K, Kampen WU, Kuwert T, van der Bruggen W, Mohan HK et al (2016) The EANM practice guidelines for bone scintigraphy. Eur J Nucl Med Mol Imaging 43(9):1723–1738
78. De Schepper S, Ritt P, Van den Wyngaert T, Kuwert T (2019) Quantitative radionuclide imaging of bone metastases. Q J Nucl Med Mol Imaging 63(2):129–135
79. Yamane T, Fukushima K, Shirotake S, Nishimoto K, Okabe T, Oyama M et al (2021) Test-retest repeatability of quantitative bone SPECT/CT. Ann Nucl Med 35(3):338–346
80. Kim J, Lee HH, Kang Y, Kim TK, Lee SW, So Y et al (2017) Maximum standardised uptake value of quantitative bone SPECT/CT in patients with medial compartment osteoarthritis of the knee. Clin Radiol 72(7):580–589
81. Braun M, Cachovan M, Kaul F, Caobelli F, Baumer M, Hans Vija A et al (2021) Accuracy comparison of various quantitative [(99m)Tc]Tc-DPD SPECT/CT reconstruction techniques in patients with symptomatic hip and knee joint prostheses. EJNMMI Res 11(1):60
82. Damian T, Spielhofer N, Heimer J, Sauter AW, Popescu C, Hausmann D et al (2024) Quantification of [(99m)Tc]Tc-HDP bone SPECT/CT: can we improve the body weight based standardized uptake value with a more robust normalization? EJNMMI Res 14(1):111

Fluorescence Imaging of Cancer

20

Dirk Grosenick

20.1 Introduction

Optical imaging of head, breast, and skin, as well as of inner cavities of the human body, for example, bladder or colon, is a powerful diagnostic tool with high potential for early detection of tumors. Besides the measurement of intrinsic tissue optical parameters like absorption, scattering, hemoglobin (Hb) concentration, and blood oxygen saturation, fluorescence imaging has attracted increasing interest in medical diagnostics and therapy over many years. First developments of cancer-specific molecular probes equipped with fluorescent molecules for visualization seemed to open an excellent way for early detection of cancer [41]. These probes were expected to strongly increase the image contrast because of a high cancer-to-background fluorescence ratio. Over the years, fluorescence imaging on small animal models became an important tool for the evaluation of such probes, and many preclinical studies with targeted conjugates were conducted. On the other hand, there are only a few clinical studies so far [29].

The translation of molecular probes to the clinics is also limited by the difficulties in imaging fluorescent objects through overlaying tissue structures. Compared to visible light, near-infrared radiation can penetrate several centimeters of tissue. However, light intensity is strongly decreasing with each millimeter of tissue thickness. Accordingly, fluorescence imaging works best for superficial tissue structures.

This chapter is based on chapter Fluorescence Imaging of Breast Tumors and Gastrointestinal Cancer from the previous edition, written by Dirk Grosenick and Christoph Bremer.

D. Grosenick (✉)
Physikalisch-Technische Bundesanstalt (PTB), Berlin, Germany
e-mail: dirk.grosenick@ptb.de

O. Schober et al. (eds.), *Molecular Imaging in Oncology - Volume 2*, Recent Results in Cancer Research 225, https://doi.org/10.1007/978-3-032-21415-7_2

In this case, scattering of light in the tissue is of low importance, and wavelengths across the whole spectrum of light can be applied to excite fluorescence of appropriate exogenous contrast agents or endogenous markers. Typically, the tissue region of interest is homogeneously illuminated with a laser or LED to excite the fluorophores, and a sufficiently sensitive camera equipped with a long pass or bandpass filter for blocking the excitation light is employed to record the fluorescence images in reflection. Often, this flat-field fluorescence imaging approach is combined with white-light imaging, and the fluorescent tissue structures are overlaid on the conventional color image. Besides endoscopes with a fluorescence detection channel, several new research and commercial devices have been developed for flat-field fluorescence imaging, with the main focus on application for fluorescence-guided open surgery of cancer and fluorescence-assisted sentinel lymph node detection [28].

When deeper tissue layers have to be investigated, the strong scattering of light in biological tissue plays an important role. Both the excitation light and the emitted fluorescence light are scattered multiple times, and the corresponding optical path lengths are significantly increased. To obtain a sufficient penetration depth of the excitation light and a measurable fluorescence signal, excitation and emission wavelengths have to fall into the so-called diagnostic window between approximately 650 and 1000 nm, where light absorption of the tissue is moderate. Recent developments in experimental methods have allowed the extension of the application of fluorescence imaging to diseases of highly scattering tissue such as breast cancer [3, 10, 38], stroke, or rheumatoid arthritis. These techniques offer ways to translate corresponding probes for molecular imaging from preclinical research to clinical application.

In the following, we discuss two applications for fluorescence-assisted clinical diagnosis and therapy of tumors. As an example for imaging in highly scattering tissue we review results on the detection of carcinomas in the female breast. We focus on the nonspecific contrast agents indocyanine green (ICG) and omocianine and report on a recently explored method to characterize differences in the extravasation of ICG between malignant and benign breast lesions utilizing vessel permeability. Then, we discuss first results with targeted and activatable probes aiming at the reliable detection of tumor margins in breast surgery. As an example of superficial lesions, tumor detection in the gastrointestinal tract by fluorescence endoscopy will be explained. We report on results with protoporphyrin IX which acts as an endogenous specific target for malignancy. Finally, we briefly discuss exogenous targeted and activatable probes for esophageal and colorectal tumors.

20.2 Fluorescence Imaging of Breast Cancer

Due to the high prevalence of breast cancer, many efforts are undertaken to develop targeted contrast agents for the early detection of this disease. Hereby, optical imaging plays an important role in understanding the properties of the agent and its action on the cellular level. By adding a fluorescent moiety to the carrier molecule of the probe fluorescence imaging can be applied as a sensitive method to detect the probe in the tissue. Basic investigations on new probes are often performed on small animal models. Due to the small dimensions of such animal models, tumors are easily accessible by optical methods, since they are situated directly on or close to the tissue surface. Accordingly, simple wide-field fluorescence imaging is sufficient for their detection. In contrast, optical imaging of a molecular contrast agent in the human breast is much more challenging due to the drastically enlarged tissue dimensions compared to a small animal breast tumor model.

Numerous investigations have shown that the human breast can be transilluminated by near-infrared light due to the low absorption of breast tissue in this spectral range [9]. The challenge in generating optical images of the breast is the separation of tissue absorption and fluorescence on one side and tissue scattering properties on the other side. Compared to X-ray mammography and magnetic resonance (MR) imaging of the breast, optical imaging is not able to visualize morphological characteristics in the breast with adequate spatial resolution. Instead, important physiological properties of the tissue can be derived.

20.2.1 Basics of Breast Optical Imaging and Endogenous Tumor Contrast

The original idea of optical mammography comprised the diagnosis of breast cancer by exploiting endogenous contrast arising from differences in the total Hb concentration and the blood oxygen saturation (StO_2) between carcinomas and the surrounding healthy tissue. Near-infrared light is an almost perfect tool to determine the tissue concentrations of oxygenated (HbO_2) and deoxygenated hemoglobin (HbR) since these two substances dominate the absorption of light in breast tissue for wavelengths between about 650 and 900 nm. The expected higher concentration of Hb is a direct implication of neoangiogenesis in the carcinoma. Accordingly, all relevant in vivo studies confirmed the increased Hb concentration in breast carcinomas. On average, the increase was estimated to be about two to threefold with respect to the surrounding healthy tissue [9].

For blood oxygen saturation, a decrease was originally expected for carcinomas due to their high metabolic activity and the related demand on energy. This expectation was supported by measurements of the O_2 tension in breast carcinomas showing hypoxic behavior. However, several clinical studies revealed that blood oxygen saturation is not a characteristic biomarker for breast cancer. There are carcinomas with decreased blood oxygen saturation as well as carcinomas with no characteristic deviation of this parameter from the surrounding healthy tissue [9].

Besides oxygenated and deoxygenated Hb, other tissue constituents with absorption in the near-infrared range were considered as possible biomarkers for the detection of carcinomas. In particular, an increased content of water and collagen was reported for breast carcinomas. Furthermore, several groups could show an increased scattering coefficient of breast carcinomas compared to healthy tissue [9]. To assess the diagnostic potential of the endogenous contrast in breast optical imaging, it is necessary to evaluate the differentiation between carcinomas and benign alterations. Corresponding investigations on arbitrary patient populations revealed a limited specificity only [30], in particular, since many benign tissue alterations show increased Hb concentration, similar to carcinomas. Whereas the endogenous optical contrast seems to be insufficient for cancer diagnosis and differentiation, it has high potential for monitoring the progress of neoadjuvant chemotherapy. In this application, the shrinking of a known lesion prior to surgery is studied by frequent observation of the Hb concentration. Another possible application of intrinsic near-infrared breast imaging is the assessment of tumor risk by considering the tissue collagen content. Also, several groups pursue optical breast imaging as an adjunct modality to X-ray mammography, MR breast imaging or ultrasound [9].

20.2.2 Contrast Agents for Breast Cancer

To improve the diagnostic and differentiation of breast cancer, and, more recently, to improve the detection of tumor margins during breast cancer surgery, several contrast agents have been investigated. Most of the diagnostic studies were performed with ICG. This dye is clinically approved and well accepted as a safe contrast agent in various clinical applications for many years. It is routinely used for ocular fundus fluorescence angiography, for examination of the hepatic function, for cardiac output measurements and, to a lower extent, for the diagnosis of rheumatic diseases. Besides these applications with intravenous injection, ICG has been used in many studies on sentinel lymph node detection for various types of tumors, where it is directly injected into the tumor or the adjacent tissue.

The spectral properties of ICG are almost perfect for the application in near-infrared diffuse optical imaging, since it shows absorption around 760 nm and fluorescence around 830 nm (in tissue). After intravenous injection, ICG binds immediately to plasma proteins and is distributed in the vascular compartment. Since carcinomas are characterized by a locally increased vessel density, a higher tissue concentration of ICG in the carcinoma compared to healthy breast tissue should be detectable. After about 10 min of circulation, ICG has been cleared from the blood by the liver. Clinical studies that looked at the increased ICG concentration during the circulation (vascular phase) are discussed in Sect. 20.2.3. A more promising method is the detection of extravasated ICG that settled in the carcinoma during the vascular phase. Corresponding investigations are discussed in Sect. 20.2.4.

The research on new contrast agents for the diagnosis of breast cancer by optical imaging has already been started at a time when basic experimental concepts and theoretical models for diffuse optical imaging of the human breast were still under development. In particular, fluorescence imaging systems for the breast were not yet available. The agents were derived from ICG with the aims to overcome the short plasma lifetime of ICG, its low fluorescence quantum yield, and its instability in aqueous solution which all were considered as disadvantages for fluorescence-assisted breast cancer detection. Finally, the new dye omocianine found the way to clinical trials [26, 38]. Compared to ICG, omocianine (also known as TSC) has a weaker binding to plasma proteins and a higher fluorescence quantum yield. Furthermore, the absorption and emission bands are slightly shifted to shorter wavelengths. Whereas ICG is washed out from the blood by the liver within typically 10 min, omocianine remains in the blood vessels for more than 24 h. Clinical results on this dye are presented in Sect. 20.2.5.

ICG and omocianine do not exhibit specific binding to tumor cells. In contrast, molecular probes exploit specific properties of cancer cells. Up to date, such probes did not yet find application for breast cancer diagnostics by optical imaging. A promising field of their application is the detection of tumor margins during breast cancer (as well as other cancers) surgery [13]. The probe bevacizumab-IRDye800CW targets the vascular endothelial growth factor A (VEGF-A). It is a conjugation of the therapeutic agent bevacizumab (Roche AG) and the near-infrared dye IRDye800CW (LI-COR Biosciences Inc.). The target protein VEGF-A is involved in tumor angiogenesis and frequently overexpressed in breast cancer. The molecular probe EC17 (On Target Laboratories LLC, West Lafayette, USA) targets the tumor-specific overexpression of the folate receptor alpha. It consists of a folate analogue conjugated to 5-fluorescein isothiocyanate (FITC), which fluoresces at 520–530 nm. Because of this short wavelength, EC17 seems to be preferably suited for imaging of superficial structures. It was already investigated on several types of cancer [13].

LUM015 (pegulicianine) is a protease-activatable probe that consists of a polyethylene glycol, the near-infrared dye Cy5 (emission wavelength about 665 nm), and a fluorescence quencher. Cathepsins, being overexpressed by tumors, cleave the probe, thus enabling tumor-specific fluorescence of Cy5 [13]. AVB-620 is another protease-activatable fluorescent probe. It utilizes the increased proteolytic activity from matrix metalloproteinases (MMPs) in tumors and the surrounding stromal microenvironment. AVB-620 contains Cy5 and Cy7 fluorescent molecules. The intact agent shows fluorescence by Cy7. Its hydrolysis by MMPs results in a shift of fluorescence emission to Cy5 [12].

Besides molecular probes, also the classical perfusion type contrast agents ICG [34] and methylene blue [35] have been investigated in clinical trials for tumor margin detection in breast surgery.

20.2.3 Breast Tumor Detection by ICG Using Vascular Contrast

The first application of ICG in optical mammography was demonstrated by Ntziachristos et al. [22] who compared ICG absorption contrast with Gadolinium (Gd) enhancement in concurrently recorded MR images. Hereby, a time-domain NIR imager with a fixed grid of source and detector optical fibers was implemented into a 1.5 T MR breast imager with slight compression of the breast between two parallel plates. The investigations comprised Gadolinium enhanced MR imaging of the breast followed by optical imaging prior to, during, and after a bolus injection of ICG. The optical measurements were restricted to the tumor region known from the MR images. The increase in absorption at 830 nm observable about 3 min after ICG bolus injection was reconstructed for a slice selected at the known tumor position using a perturbation model of diffusion theory.

These absorption images showed good correlation to the structures with Gd enhancement in the MR images for all three cases investigated. A 1 cm invasive ductal carcinoma was optically visible by a local absorption increase of about 0.05 cm^{-1}, and a 1.5 cm fibroadenoma by an absorption increase of about 0.03 cm^{-1}. ICG induced absorption enhancement in other regions as well as for the third case without a lesion did not exceed 0.025 cm^{-1}. The authors discussed that the ICG molecules (due to their binding to the large plasma proteins) behave like macromolecules, and that extravasation of these macromolecules through leaky tumor capillaries should be a slow process not yet being visible at the early time of measurement. Accordingly, the absorption images are vascularization maps. As discussed in Sect. 20.2.2, such maps have been recorded by several groups exploiting the intrinsic Hb contrast. Ntziachristos et al. suggested measurements of ICG absorption over a longer time period to study ICG kinetics and to possibly quantify vessel permeability as an additional feature for cancer differentiation [22].

Intes et al. used a single-wavelength continuous-wave optical imager to measure the kinetics of an ICG bolus on three patients [11]. The 2D circular tomographic arrangement of light sources and detectors was positioned around the freely hanging breast such that it covered the lesion position known from palpation. A perturbation model was used to reconstruct 2D maps of the absorption change due to the ICG bolus. Figure 20.1 displays the ICG kinetics for the three cases investigated.

The adenocarcinoma and the invasive ductal carcinoma are characterized by a significantly slower inflow, and the invasive ductal carcinoma, in addition, by a strongly delayed washout compared to the healthy tissue reference data. The benign fibroadenoma behaves similarly to the healthy tissue. Obviously, the vessels in the two carcinomas have an increased resistance to blood flow, possibly arising from a

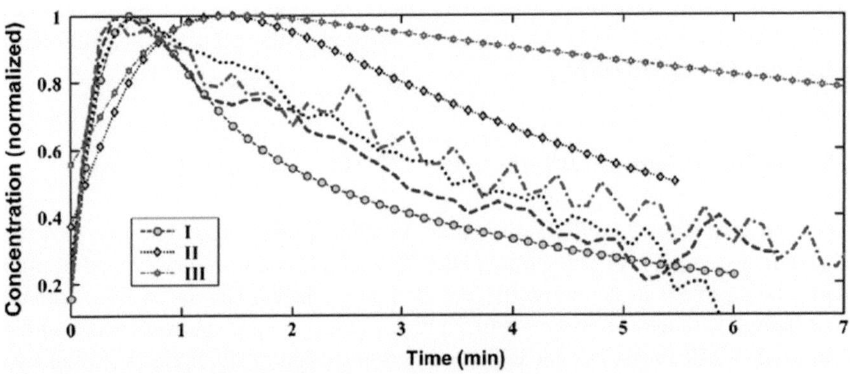

Fig. 20.1 ICG concentration kinetics for three patients with breast tumors; case I: fibroadenoma (diameter 1–2 cm), case II: adenocarcinoma (diameter 2–3 cm), case III: invasive ductal carcinoma (size 4 cm × 3 cm); curves with markers: tumors, curves without markers: healthy tissue of the suspicious breast. (Reprinted with permission from Intes et al. [11])

chaotic vessel structure in the carcinomas. The delay in the washout could be an indicator of extravasation of the ICG-plasma protein macromolecules.

Rinneberg et al. performed a study on ICG bolus kinetics on 11 patients with breast cancer using a time-domain optical mammograph [30]. Before bolus injection, the positions of the carcinomas were determined by recording transmission optical mammograms at 675 and 785 nm. Then, transmission at 785 nm was sampled continuously at the tumor position and at two reference positions to observe ICG inflow and washout. These measurements showed a strong patient-to-patient variation in the washout time. However, the temporal characteristics of the carcinoma and the reference positions of the same breast were almost identical in each case.

Figure 20.2a shows an example of the absorption change induced by the ICG bolus illustrating the higher ICG concentration in the carcinoma compared to the two healthy tissue reference positions. To compare the temporal characteristic, the three curves were normalized to the total Hb concentration at each position derived from the intrinsic absorption maps at 675 and 785 nm. Figure 20.2b shows that the normalized ICG absorption is essentially the same for the carcinoma and the healthy references during the about 10 min long measurement time. This result corresponds

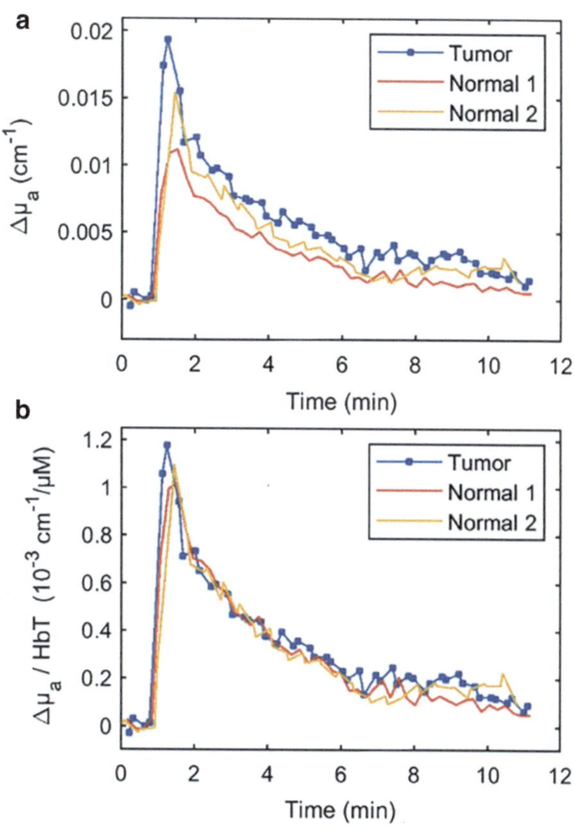

Fig. 20.2 Washout kinetics of ICG for an invasive carcinoma (size 2 cm) and two (healthy) reference positions with different vascularizations in the same breast; (**a**) absorption change $\Delta\mu_a$ by ICG bolus and (**b**) absorption change $\Delta\mu_a$ normalized to local total Hb concentration HbT

to the expectation that almost all ICG is contained in the vessels due to the strong plasma binding. Similar ICG kinetics were obtained for the other 10 cases. Hence, the carcinomas in this study did not show increased resistance to blood flow, in contrast to the two carcinomas discussed in Fig. 20.1.

The signal-to-noise ratio in the measurement of ICG absorption is limited due to the high intrinsic tissue absorption. Fluorescence imaging of ICG offers the advantage of an almost background-free measurement. On the other hand, the fluorescence signal is expected to be small due to the low fluorescence quantum yield of ICG in tissue, making its detection challenging. The first successful detection of ICG fluorescence in patients with breast cancer was reported by Corlu et al. [3]. Using a frequency-domain parallel plate optical mammograph and 3D reconstruction, the ICG concentrations were determined 10.2 min after bolus injection. For the three patients with invasive ductal carcinomas investigated in this study a 4:1 to 6:1 contrast of the ICG concentration between carcinoma and healthy tissue was obtained whereas the contrast in the total Hb concentration was about 1.3:1 only. This result has been interpreted as an indicator for remarkable extravasation of ICG around 10 min after bolus injection due to high permeability of the tumor vessels for macromolecules.

The different studies with ICG discussed so far give a nonuniform picture about the advantages of the contrast agent. Corlu et al. reported ICG extravasation about 10 min after bolus injection, whereas Rinneberg et al. obtained ICG contrast comparable to Hb contrast at this time. And Intes et al. observed a remarkably delayed inflow of ICG into the malignant lesion. One case with a delayed ICG inflow was reported also in a later study conducted by Poellinger et al. [25]. This delay was explained by histologically confirmed necrotic tissue in the tumor, whereas the other lesions in this study did not show such an abnormality. Since the study by Poellinger et al. differs in several aspects from the investigations discussed above, it is presented in detail in the next section.

20.2.4 Breast Tumor Imaging and Differentiation by ICG Using Vessel Permeability

The clinical results discussed in the preceding section could not yet fully elucidate the role of ICG extravasation. In general, due to its high binding to plasma proteins, ICG should act as a macromolecule. According to the enhanced permeability and retention (EPR) effect, this macromolecule is expected to extravasate in a malignant tumor, and to stay in the extracellular space for a longer time. In contrast, vessels in the healthy tissue, and most likely in benign lesions, too, should not allow extravasation of the macromolecules.

The absorption or fluorescence signal detected in the above investigations is dominated by the large number of ICG molecules circulating in the vessels. In this way, a strong signal is obtained which can easily be measured. However, the small contribution from extravasated ICG molecules is hidden. The way to get a signal from extravasated ICG exclusively is a measurement with high fluorescence detection sensitivity at a sufficiently late time when ICG has been totally washed out from the vascular system. This way was pursued in the study by Poellinger et al. [25], already briefly mentioned above. The device used in this study was designed to detect the fluorescence of ICG as well as the absorption and scattering properties of the tissue at selected near-infrared wavelengths [10]. Figure 20.3 illustrates the block diagram.

Images of the breast being gently compressed between two parallel glass plates were generated within about 3–10 min by continuously moving source and detector fibers in tandem across the tissue. Fluorescence of the contrast agent was excited by a module with four synchronized picosecond diode lasers (wavelength 780 nm, 15 mW average power at the breast surface). The central detection fiber bundle was bifurcated to guide the transmitted light to the fluorescence and the excitation wavelength detection channels. Time-correlated single-photon counting ensured a high light detection sensitivity. Fluorescence and excitation light information were combined in a fluorescence ratio mammogram. Without this normalization (or an appropriate reconstruction) fluorescent lesions appear with reduced contrast, or contrast could even be cancelled out due to the absorption of fluorescence photons by the locally enhanced Hb in the lesion. The optical mammograph was equipped with six more detection fiber bundles and photomultipliers (not shown in Fig. 20.3) to derive 3D information about the breast tissue and with four additional picosecond diode lasers (660, 797, 934, and 1066 nm) for spectroscopic measurements.

The device was used in a feasibility study on 20 patients with malignant and benign lesions [25]. This study differed from the previous trials with ICG discussed in Sect. 20.2.3 by two main points: (i) imaging of ICG extravasated from the blood vessels was done at a late time when ICG had been completely washed out from the vascular system, and (ii) ICG was injected by a combination of a bolus and a 20 min

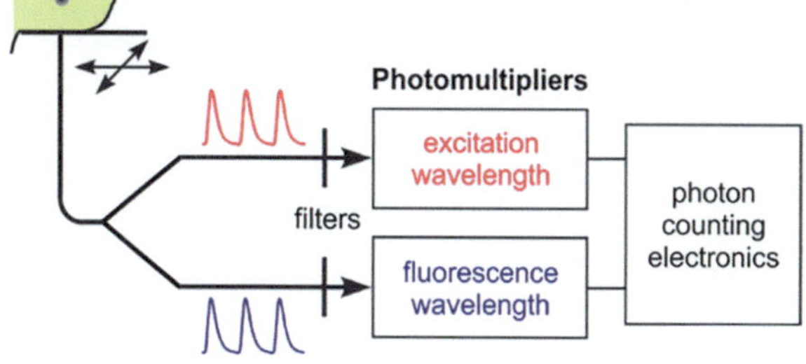

Fig. 20.3 Block diagram of the PTB fluorescence mammograph developed by Hagen et al. [10]

long infusion to elongate the interaction time with the vessels. Figure 20.4 summarizes the examination protocol of the study.

Mammograms of the suspicious breast were recorded at three different times: (i) prior to application of ICG (native phase), (ii) two times during the infusion period (when the dye was distributed in the blood vessels—vascular phase), and (iii) two times starting about 20 min after the end of the infusion (when the dye had been washed out from the blood by the liver—extravascular phase). During the examination, the plasma level of ICG was monitored by conventional transcutaneous pulse densitometry using a finger clip.

To demonstrate typical results of the approach, we consider two cases with invasive ductal carcinomas, an older and a younger woman, and a third example with a fibroadenoma as a benign tumor. The first case is a 72-year-old patient with a histologically proven moderately differentiated invasive ductal carcinoma with a maximum extension of 1.6 cm in the right breast. Since the breast of this older woman consisted mainly of adipose tissue, it was radiologically transparent, and the carcinoma was clearly visible in the X-ray mammogram. Similarly, the breast is highly transparent for optical radiation. Figure 20.5a, b shows the intrinsic absorption maps at 660 and 797 nm recorded prior to the application of ICG. Data refer to normalized photon counts in the so-called "late time window" of the time-domain technique [10].

At 660 nm, the carcinoma is clearly visible at high contrast, and at 797 nm, it has a contrast compared to the superficial blood vessels, which appear as elongated structures. Since 797 nm is close to the isosbestic point of oxy- and deoxyhemoglobin absorption, Fig. 20.5b is a qualitative map of the total Hb concentration, that is, the lesion has an increased Hb concentration as expected. The stronger tumor absorption at 660 nm reflects a high concentration of deoxyhemoglobin, that is, the carcinoma is characterized by a decrease in blood oxygen saturation compared to the surrounding tissue which is a sign of high metabolic activity. Figure 20.5c shows the breast absorption at the excitation wavelength (780 nm) for the first scan during

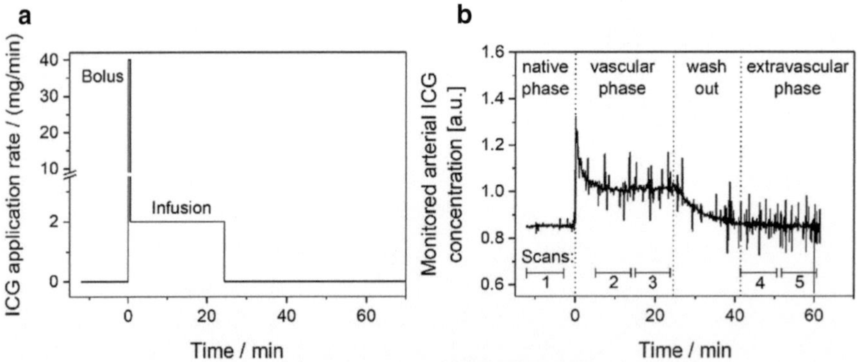

Fig. 20.4 Examination protocol: (**a**) temporal profile of ICG application and (**b**) monitored arterial ICG concentration (finger clip) with labeling of the various phases of the examination and of the time intervals of the five breast scans performed. (Data refer to the case in Fig. 20.5)

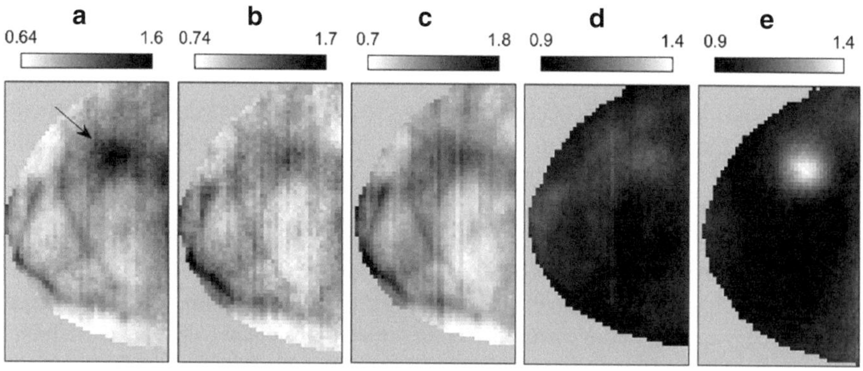

Fig. 20.5 Optical mammograms (case 1, craniocaudal view) of a 72-years-old patient with an invasive ductal carcinoma in the right breast, indicated by the arrow; (**a**) intrinsic absorption at 660 nm (native phase), (**b**) intrinsic absorption at 797 nm, (**c**) contrast-enhanced absorption during vascular phase, (**d**) fluorescence ratio mammogram of the vascular phase, and (**e**) fluorescence ratio mammogram of the extravascular phase. The absorption mammograms (**a**–**c**) display normalized reciprocal photon counts in a late time window

the vascular phase. Now, absorption is enhanced by ICG which is distributed in the vessels at this measurement time. According to the discussion in Sect. 20.2.3, the mammogram gives the same information as the intrinsic absorption image at the nearby wavelength of 797 nm (cf. Fig. 20.5b) due to the strong binding of ICG to plasma proteins.

Figure 20.5d shows the corresponding fluorescence ratio mammogram for the vascular phase, and Fig. 20.5e displays the fluorescence ratio mammogram for the second scan of the extravascular phase. For comparison, these two images are given with the same grayscale. Bright structures in the mammograms indicate a locally enhanced concentration of ICG. In Fig. 20.5d, fluorescence can be seen at the site of the (vascularized) carcinoma, as well as for the superficial blood vessels. The visibility of the carcinoma is comparable to Fig. 20.5b, c. The fluorescence ratio mammogram for the extravascular phase (Fig. 20.5e) displays the carcinoma with the highest contrast due to extravasation of ICG and its retention in the carcinoma. All other structures that appear in the native phase absorption mammograms and during the vascular phase are suppressed now. It should be noted, however, that a fluorescence background signal was obtained at all scan positions, which indicates a low extravasation in all parts of the breast.

The second patient is a 51-year-old woman with a well-differentiated invasive ductal carcinoma. The size given by histology was $1.1 \times 1.0 \times 0.8$ cm^3. The suspicious lesion was found by ultrasound. The X-ray mammogram revealed dense glandular tissue and showed only a poorly visible architectural distortion. The expected position of the lesion in the optical mammograms was derived from dynamic contrast-enhanced MRI measurements which showed the lesion at the lateral side of the breast close to the chest wall. MRI offered a second lesion nearby, which was histologically classified as low-grade ductal carcinoma in situ.

Figure 20.6a, b displays the absorption at 660 and 797 nm without a contrast agent (native phase). Both images show a lesion of strongly increased absorption in the upper left part in accordance with the location expected from MR imaging. However, the location differs between the two wavelengths, which makes it difficult to decide on the lesion visibility for the native phase. As for the first case, the contrast-enhanced absorption mammogram for the vascular phase (Fig. 20.6c) is very similar to the intrinsic absorption mammogram at 797 nm. Figure 20.6d, e displays the fluorescence ratio mammograms for this patient. Similarly to case 1, the image for the vascular phase is of flat contrast only when compared to the extravascular phase. The latter mammogram clearly displays the strong enrichment of the contrast agent at the expected tumor position. Besides the carcinoma, we observe a moderate fluorescence signal from the tissue close to the chest wall in the lower left part of the mammograms in Fig. 20.6d, e, and some contrast behind the nipple position. Compared to the carcinoma, these regions did not essentially change contrast from the vascular to the extravascular phase. The deviation of the shape of the breast in Fig. 20.6e from the other mammograms is caused by slightly different positioning of the breast during recompression for the extravascular phase measurements. Therefore, the location of the lesion in Fig. 20.6e cannot be directly transferred to the other mammograms.

The third case is an example of a benign lesion. The 52-year-old patient had a fibroadenoma in her left breast, which was finally validated by histology. From the ultrasound examination, the size of the lesion was estimated as 1.8 cm × 1.0 cm. The X-ray image did not show any abnormality. For this patient, data were recorded in

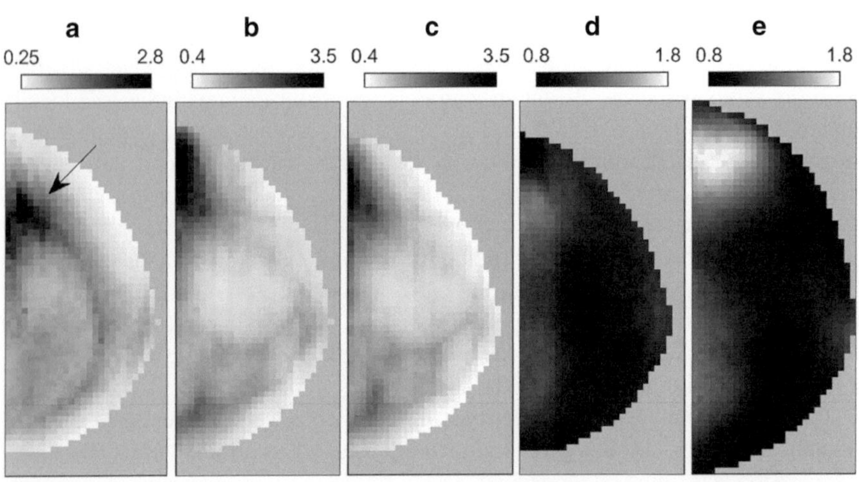

Fig. 20.6 Optical mammograms (case 2, craniocaudal view) of a 51-years-old patient with an invasive ductal carcinoma in the left breast, indicated by the arrow; (**a**) intrinsic absorption at 660 nm (native phase), (**b**) intrinsic absorption at 797 nm, (**c**) contrast-enhanced absorption at 780 nm during vascular phase, (**d**) fluorescence ratio mammogram for the vascular phase, and (**e**) fluorescence ratio mammogram for the extravascular phase. The absorption mammograms (**a–c**) display normalized reciprocal photon counts in a late time window

the native phase at the excitation wavelength (780 nm, see Fig. 20.7a). It was known from ultrasound that the fibroadenoma lies in the left part of the breast. Having in mind that fibroadenomas often exhibit increased absorption due to an increased hemoglobin concentration, their position most probably corresponds to the absorbing region in the left part of the breast, indicated by the arrow in Fig. 20.7a. However, there remains some uncertainty in this decision. Similar to the other two cases, the contrast-enhanced absorption mammogram for the vascular phase in Fig. 20.7b shows the same structures as the intrinsic absorption mammogram in Fig. 20.7a.

In Fig. 20.7c, d, the fluorescence ratio mammograms for the vascular and the extravascular phase are displayed. Apart from the blood vessels, which are only visible in Fig. 20.7c, both images are very similar. Hence, the fibroadenoma does not show any particular enrichment of ICG due to extravasation. This result corroborates the expectation that the capillary walls in benign lesions are not sufficiently leaky to allow enhanced extravasation of macromolecules.

Confirmed by the results on the other cases of the trial, the study has shown that fluorescence images recorded in the extravascular phase enable the detection of extravasated ICG, which offers a way to improve the specificity in breast cancer detection by exploiting vessel permeability for macromolecules to differentiate malignant from benign lesions [25]. Furthermore, this study enabled a comparison of the permeability-specific images with endogenous contrast optical mammograms of the same patients representing total Hb or deoxyhemoglobin distributions, and with ICG-enhanced vascular contrast mammograms. In this way, the advantages of the permeability-specific measurements could be convincingly demonstrated. Larger clinical studies are required to confirm the potential of the method.

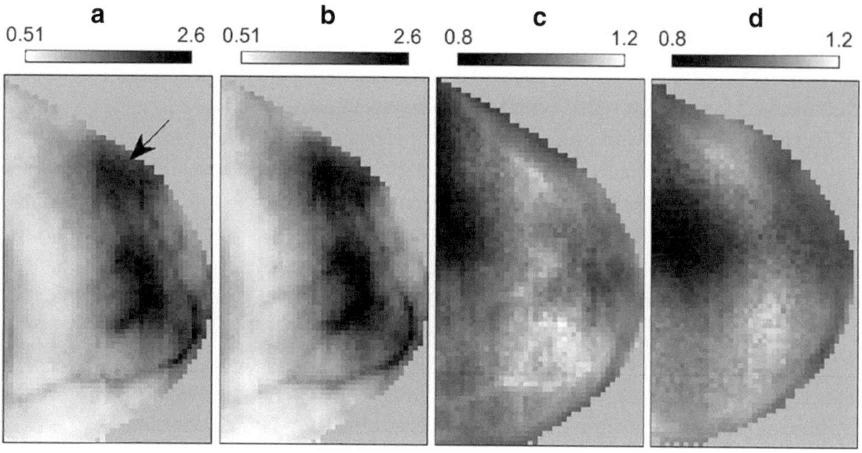

Fig. 20.7 Optical mammograms (case 3, craniocaudal view) of a 52-year-old patient with a fibroadenoma in the left breast. The presumed position of the lesion is indicated by the arrow; (**a**) intrinsic absorption at 780 nm (native phase), (**b**) contrast-enhanced absorption during vascular phase, (**c**) fluorescence ratio mammogram for the vascular phase, and (**d**) fluorescence ratio mammogram for the extravascular phase. Absorption mammograms display normalized reciprocal photon counts in a late time window

The EPR effect is also considered for improving the specificity in MR imaging of breast tumors. Gd-based contrast agents used in clinical routine act as small molecules that non-selectively extravasate in tumors as well as in healthy tissue. To obtain a more specific enhancement, several macromolecular contrast agents for MRI are under development. Up to now, no such agent has become available for clinical applications. A main problem is safety concerns related to the slow excretion and high tissue accumulation of toxic Gd ions [42]. In contrast, the approved contrast agent ICG offers a safe way to exploit the EPR effect. However, visualization of ICG in the breast by fluorescence imaging is hampered by the low spatial resolution of diffuse optical imaging.

20.2.5 Imaging of Breast Cancer with Omocianine

The small molecular contrast agent omocianine was used in two pilot studies. One study comprised the examination of 11 patients with a continuous-wave (CW) fluorescence and absorption tomography system developed by Philips Healthcare (Best, The Netherlands) [38]. This device uses a high-density source-detector fiber system arranged around a cup unit for the investigation of the freely pending breast. Optical contact is supported by a matching fluid.

Omocianine was administered intravenously as a bolus. Four different doses were used with three cases in each group (two cases for the highest dose). At the two lowest doses, five out of six malignant lesions were detected in the reconstructed fluorescence images, whereby the missed lesion was out of the field of view. No lesions could be seen in the two highest dose groups, for which reconstruction was problematic due to the non-negligible absorption of the contrast agent. The best lesion-to-background contrast was obtained 8 h after injection, ranging between 1.8 and 2.8. Figure 20.8 shows the reconstructed fluorescence image for a case with a 2.5 cm diameter invasive lobular carcinoma. The result for the contralateral breast is given as well.

Besides the lesion (green arrow) other fluorescent structures are visible such as the nipples of both breasts (red circles) and glandular tissue. The study showed that glandular tissue generally exhibited an enhancement pattern similar to the carcinomas making a reliable detection of carcinomas with omocianine probably problematic. The authors concluded that target-specific contrast agents will be crucial to translate fluorescence molecular breast imaging to clinical application.

The second study was a multicenter clinical trial with 52 patients who received omocianine and 9 patients who got placebos instead [26]. Fluorescence and absorption images of the freely pending suspicious breast were acquired with a tomographic device from Imaging Diagnostics Systems, Inc. (Ft. Lauderdale, FL, USA) using a vertically movable ring arrangement of light sources and detectors. Omocianine was administered at five different doses. The best performance was obtained at a dose of 0.1 mg omocianine per kg body weight which was the highest dose in the first study discussed above. All 7 malignant lesions were detected, whereas the two benign lesions in this group did not show enhanced fluorescence. However, the neighboring dose groups of 0.2 and 0.05 mg/kg yielded carcinoma

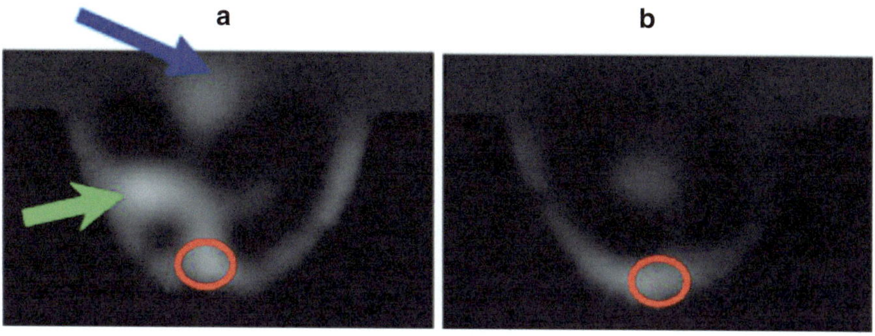

Fig. 20.8 Reconstructed fluorescence images of a patient with an invasive lobular carcinoma obtained 8 h after administration of omocianine; (**a**) left breast with carcinoma (green arrow) and a reconstruction artifact at the chest wall (blue arrow) and (**b**) right breast. The red circles indicate the nipple positions. (Reprinted with permission from van de Ven et al. [38])

detection rates of about 50% only, and 1 false positive result each. Furthermore, the time point of the best lesion contrast in this study showed a strong spread. On average, the optimal detection time lay between 3 and 4 h compared to the stable result of 8 h observed by van de Ven et al. There was a tendency for earlier imaging time points for malignant lesions in contrast to the visible benign lesions. Eventually, the authors concluded the need for improvements in the technique and the development of cancer-specific, targeted contrast agents [26].

The studies with omocianine revealed some preliminary technical problems that limited the value of the results. These problems may be overcome by improving data acquisition and reconstruction. However, both studies ended up with significant limitations due to the nonspecific nature of this contrast agent. In comparison, the contrast agent ICG has the advantage that the vessel permeability can be exploited as a characteristic feature of malignant tumors.

20.2.6 Fluorescence-Guided Breast Cancer Surgery

During breast-conserving cancer surgery, it is required to reliably recognize the borders between tumor and healthy tissue. Commonly, surgeons have to rely on visual inspection. Along with this technique, incomplete resections were reported for 20–40% of the patients [24]. Near-infrared fluorescence imaging is a promising technique to improve intraoperative tumor margin detection. Hereby, the fluorescent contrast agent should either actively or passively accumulate in the tumor, but not in the surrounding healthy tissue.

The extravasation of ICG in carcinomas according to the EPR effect offers potential to delineate tumor margins during surgery. As reviewed by Tipirneni et al., several clinical trials have been conducted to study the visualization of tumor margins with ICG [34]. For one study, results were recently published [27]. Fluorescence from the tumor bed after excision of the cancer was observed in 15 out of the 35 cases investigated. Five of these cases were confirmed by pathohistology to have positive tumor margins; the other 10 cases had negative margin status. The 20 patients without fluorescence from the tumor bed were all negative in the pathological investigation of the excised tissue. Consequently, a negative predictive value and a sensitivity of 100% were achieved, while the specificity was only 67%.

Tummers et al. investigated the application of methylene blue for tumor margin detection [35]. Intraoperative fluorescence imaging was conducted with a combined white-light and fluorescence detection system. Fluorescence was searched in the wound bed and on the surface of the resected specimens. Two out of the 24 cases in this study showed fluorescence at these locations after conventional cancer resection. For both cases, histopathology finally confirmed positive resection margins. As an example, Fig. 20.9 displays intraoperatively taken images for one of these cases.

Overall, 20 out of the 24 resected carcinomas in this study contained methylene blue as confirmed by fluorescence measurements after pathological bisection of the specimens. In one of the remaining four cases without methylene blue enrichment, histology revealed positive resection margins, too.

The four molecular probes listed in Sect. 20.2.2 were investigated in exploratory studies on tumor margin detection. The probe bevacizumab-IRDye800CW targeting the vascular epithelial growth factor VEGF-A was applied in a study on 20 patients [16]. Fluorescence and white-light images were recorded with a custom-made device with an excitation laser at 750 nm and a high-end cooled EMCCD camera for sensitive fluorescence detection. The contrast agent was administered intravenously at a microdose level. During surgery, fluorescence images were recorded at several predefined time points. After tumor removal, the surgical field was inspected again for fluorescence, and the excised specimens were imaged, too. Histopathology identified two patients with incomplete tumor removal. For both these cases, positive resection margins were visible in the fluorescence images recorded from the tissue lumps directly after removal. However, no residual fluorescence was seen in the wound bed. Final investigations on excised and sliced specimens showed IRDye800CW fluorescence in 19 of the 20 carcinomas. Microscopy

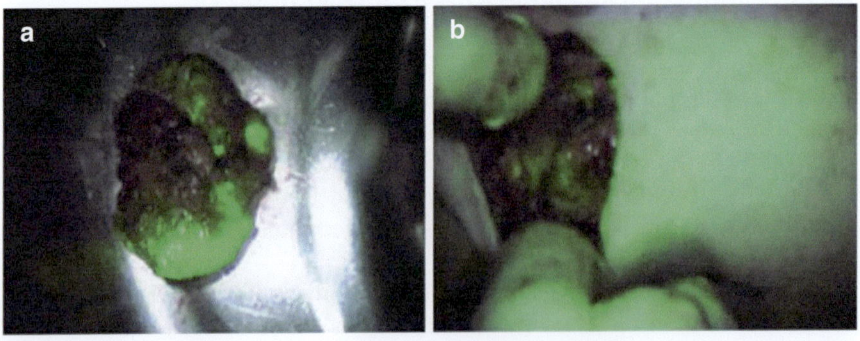

Fig. 20.9 (**a**) Resected breast cancer specimen and (**b**) wound bed after resection. Both images show fluorescence from methylene blue (overlaid as green color), indicating incomplete cancer removal. (Reprinted with permission from Tummers [35])

revealed complete overlap of the molecular probe and VEGF-A regions in 6 cases and adjacent location in 12 cases. In the remaining two cases, IRDye800CW and VEGF-A positions did not overlap.

The folate receptor alpha targeting agent EC17 was applied for intraoperative imaging on 3 patients with breast cancer [36]. Images of the surgical field, the excised specimens and of the wound bed were recorded with the Artemis fluorescence imaging system (Quest Medical Imaging, The Netherlands), specially configured to generate excitation light for EC17 at 490 nm. Tumor-specific fluorescence could be observed during surgery for all three cases. However, the autofluorescence of normal breast tissue strongly hampered tumor identification. Autofluorescence was also visible in fluorescence microscopy of the sliced tissue specimens. Nevertheless, a clear accumulation of EC17 in tumor cells could be seen here.

The activatable probe LUM015 (pegulicianine) was investigated in several consecutive studies. The final prospective multicenter clinical trial with 357 patients undergoing fluorescence imaging showed that about 10% of the patients had a favorable impact from the molecular probe by removal of residual cancer tissue not visible by standard margin detection, or by avoiding a second surgery. Ten patients with negative findings from LUM015 showed cancer in reexcisions. The specificity was about 85%. The sensitivity of about 49% was finally not fulfilling the expectations [32].

The activatable probe AVB-620 was applied in a study on 27 patients who underwent surgical excision of breast cancer [37]. The probe was administered by an infusion 2–20 h before surgery. Fluorescence images were taken from the surgical field as well as from the excised specimens. The study demonstrated measurable changes between tumor-positive and tumor-negative tissue classified by pathology.

In summary, the first results with specific molecular probes for breast cancer applied on humans show tumor-specific fluorescence signals. Contrast seems not yet sufficiently stable for a reliable detection of tumor margins during surgery, and further research is required. Furthermore, it remains an open question whether molecular probes could help to develop fluorescence imaging toward a diagnostic tool with high sensitivity and specificity for breast cancer. In fact, a highly specific molecular probe will be suitable for only a small fraction of cancer entities, since the pathology of tumor tissue differs widely among breast cancer patients.

20.3 Cancer and Early Malignancies of the Gastrointestinal Tract

The characterization of breast tumors discussed in the preceding section requires the use of near-infrared light in combination with advanced light detection techniques. In contrast, tumors of the gastrointestinal (GI) tract are superficial lesions that can easily be accessed in reflection geometry by light from the whole visible spectral range. The conventional technique for the detection of premalignant changes and early-stage carcinomas in the esophagus, colon, and rectum is white-light endoscopy. Since patients with inflammations of the GI tract have a high risk of developing malignancies, they are advised to regularly undergo surveillance examinations. However, the detection of lesions developing from inflamed tissue is difficult since the mucosa appears flat in the endoscopic images. Thus, for patients with ulcerative colitis, about 30% of flat intraepithelial neoplasias are not visible by conventional white-light endoscopy [31]. Similarly, the detection rate of neoplasia for patients with Barrett's esophagus is insufficient so far [39].

Over the years, enhanced optical imaging techniques have been developed for GI endoscopy. Narrowband imaging and autofluorescence imaging use endogenous tissue contrast. Recent studies suggested that narrowband imaging does not really improve neither the detection of esophageal neoplasia [7] nor the detection of colorectal dysplasia [17]. Likewise, autofluorescence imaging of the esophagus was found to be of limited value only for early detection of lesions [7]. Chromoendoscopy uses a dye spray to improve lesion detection. In 2015, this method became part of a consensus statement on surveillance and management of dysplasia in inflammatory bowel disease. In a recent study, Mooiweer et al. assessed more critically that chromoendoscopy of the colon does not yield enhanced performance compared to white-light endoscopy [20].

Another advanced technique is confocal laser endomicroscopy which provides microscopic details of the gastrointestinal mucosa in vivo. Studies on patients with Barrett's esophagus and with ulcerative colitis, performed in combination with chromoendoscopy using intravenous injection of fluorescein, demonstrated high diagnostic accuracy [8], whereas a later study on patients with Crohn's disease showed a lower diagnostic yield [40]. A main limitation of confocal laser endoscopy is that this technique is not suited for the investigation of the full hollow organ. It requires preselection of suspicious regions by, for example, white-light or chromoendoscopy, where it is then applied as a point technique to improve diagnosis.

Similar to other organs, further improvements of performance and diagnostic accuracy in endoscopy of the GI tract are expected by the application of tumor-specific molecular probes. In the following, we start with a discussion of 5-aminolevulinic acid, which is transformed into protoporphyrin IX preferentially in tumor tissue. Then we review recent results obtained with targeting peptides and antibodies, as well as activatable probes.

20.3.1 Protoporphyrin IX as Tumor Marker

Protoporphyrin IX (PpIX) is a natural precursor in the synthesis of heme. Its conversion to heme by insertion of a ferrous ion is catalyzed by the enzyme ferrochelatase. Tumor cells show an accumulation of PpIX which is assumed to be caused by a reduced activity of ferrochelatase and a relative enhancement of porphobilinogen deaminase activity. The endogenous small molecule 5-aminolevulinic acid (5-ALA) acts as a precursor in the biosynthesis of PpIX. When 5-ALA is additionally administered as an exogenous agent, the synthesis of PpIX is enforced and its accumulation in tumor cells is increased. PpIX can be made visible by fluorescence imaging using blue or green light for excitation. 5-ALA-supported PpIX accumulation has been applied for investigations on oral cancer, bladder cancer, lung cancer, skin cancer and brain tumors. Also, several studies were conducted on tumors of the GI tract.

Mayinger et al. investigated 22 patients with known or treated malignant and precancerous lesions of the esophagus [18]. 5-ALA was orally administered at a dose of 15 mg/kg body weight. Fluorescence and white-light endoscopy were conducted about 6 h later. The fiberoptic endoscope was connected to a light source capable of emitting violet-blue light and a CCD camera for the detection of the red fluorescence light. In this study, 85% of the biopsy sites with histologically confirmed premalignant or malignant tissue exhibited PpIX fluorescence. In contrast, only 25% of them were detected with white light.

The study by Brand et al. aimed at differentiating between Barrett's mucosa with and without dysplasia [1]. Twenty patients obtained 10 mg/kg of 5-ALA orally 3 h before endoscopy of the esophagus. Fluorescence was excited with a wavelength of 400 nm from a dye laser, and fluorescence intensities were measured quantitatively at 635 and 480 nm to account for PpIX and autofluorescence, respectively. By using the PpIX fluorescence intensity alone, high-grade dysplasia could be distinguished from nondysplastic tissue with a sensitivity of 77% and a specificity of 71%. Since the study showed a decreased autofluorescence intensity for nodular high-grade dysplasia, too, Brand et al. calculated the fluorescence intensity ratio of 635 and 480 nm signals. In this way, high-grade dysplasia could be differentiated from nondysplastic tissue with 100% sensitivity and 100% specificity. This result demonstrates the necessity to consider the fluorescence of PpIX with respect to the autofluorescence background.

20.3.2 Time-Gated Fluorescence Imaging of Protoporphyrin IX

Another approach to obtain a high sensitivity and specificity in dysplasia detection of the esophagus and the colon is time-gated fluorescence imaging and spectroscopy. This method utilizes the fluorescence lifetime as an additional parameter to improve the detection of PpIX fluorescence versus the tissue autofluorescence background. Figure 20.10 illustrates the main components of the research setup for time-gated fluorescence endoscopy developed at the PTB [23].

The endoscope in this setup has two working channels. The first one contains an optical fiber to guide the excitation light to the tissue. This fiber was also used to collect fluorescence light from the tissue for spectral analysis. The second working channel was equipped with an auxiliary image guide for the acquisition of fluorescence images by an intensified CCD camera. A bandpass filter in front of the camera suppressed the excitation light. The image guide was fixed in such a way that nearly the same field of view was covered by fluorescence and white-light images. The excitation light pulses were generated by an optical parametric oscillator (OPO), pumped by the third harmonic of a Q-switched Nd:YAG laser. Generally, the OPO could be tuned between 410 nm and 2.2 μm. For the investigations on PpIX fluorescence, a wavelength of 505 nm was chosen. The pulse duration was about 3 ns.

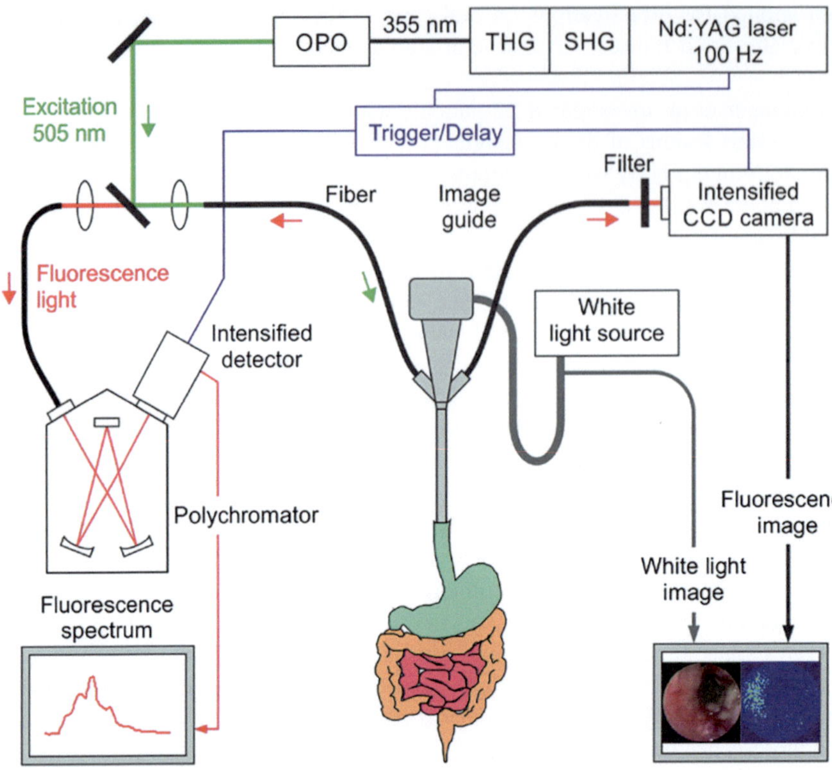

Fig. 20.10 Typical scheme of a setup for endoscopic investigation of time-delayed fluorescence of the gastrointestinal tract after topical application of 5-aminolevulinic acid

After attenuation to the appropriate power, the light pulses were guided through a dichroic beam splitter into the illumination fiber of the endoscope.

To record fluorescence spectra, the fluorescence light collected by the illumination fiber was guided through the dichroic beam splitter to a polychromator. Similar to the intensified CCD camera for imaging, the cooled detector array of the polychromator was equipped with an intensifier. This intensifier was opened for 20 ns after each laser pulse. Furthermore, an electrical delay enabled the start of the recording of fluorescence spectra either immediately or with a delay time of 20 ns with respect to the excitation pulse. Figure 20.11 illustrates the differences in the fluorescence spectra of normal mucosa and of a carcinoma of the colon obtained in this way. Data were acquired about 2 h after topical administration of 5-ALA.

Normal mucosa shows a broad and flat emission spectrum. When the delay of 20 ns is applied, then the fluorescence emission is almost down due to the short autofluorescence lifetime of about 3 ns [19]. The immediate spectrum of the carcinoma has the well-defined fluorescence peak of PpIX around 633 nm and a second minor band at about 700 nm. Both are overlaid on the flat autofluorescence background, similar to that of normal mucosa. The delayed spectrum is almost

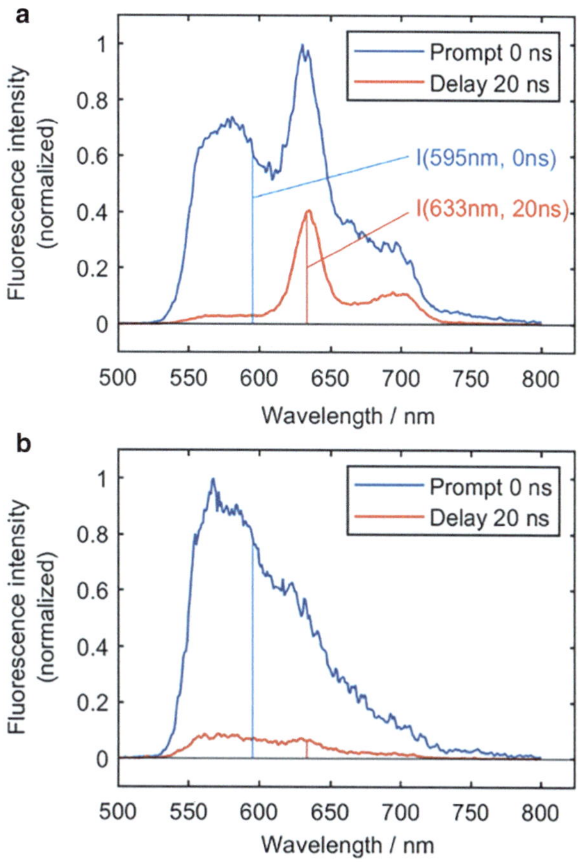

Fig. 20.11 Normalized fluorescence intensity of PpIX and autofluorescence background in dependence on wavelength. (**a**) Immediate and time-delayed fluorescence spectrum of a carcinoma in vivo and (**b**) immediate and time-delayed fluorescence spectrum of normal mucosa in vivo

free of the autofluorescence background, and the tumor-specific fluorescence bands at 633 and 700 nm are clearly visible due to the longer fluorescence lifetime of PpIX (about 16 ns). In order to quantify the tumor-specific fluorescence, the ratio R of the delayed fluorescence intensity at 633 nm and of the immediate fluorescence intensity at 595 nm, according to $R = I(633\text{ nm}, 20\text{ ns})/I(595\text{ nm}, 0\text{ ns})$ can be utilized [19].

The time-gated laser-induced fluorescence endoscopy technique was applied in clinical trials on the esophagus [23] and the colon [5]. In both studies, 5-ALA was topically administered to the patient about 2 h before the measurement. The investigations on a total of 141 esophageal lesions showed that the above-defined ratio R enables reliable differentiation of low-grade dysplasia from nondysplastic mucosa in Barrett's esophagus. Furthermore, the higher performance of the time-gated technique could clearly be demonstrated. Compared to screening white-light endoscopy, dysplasia was detected at a 2.8-fold higher rate. In addition, three early carcinomas were visible from the time-gated technique only [23]. Besides spectroscopic investigations, the time-gated technique can also be used to take prompt and delayed fluorescence images of lesions together with white-light images. Due to the short gate time, there is no significant background to the fluorescence signal from the white-light source.

As an example, Fig. 20.12 shows the delayed fluorescence image of a carcinoma in the esophagus together with the white-light image. The fluorescence image displays the carcinoma with its strong PpIX signal almost free of autofluorescence background. The slight discrepancy between the two images in Fig. 20.12 is caused by the slow refresh rate of the fluorescence image (2 images/s). The images were processed in real time in order to identify malignant spots in the white-light image for biopsy. Using this technique, the number of biopsies could be decreased.

The study on time-gated fluorescence colonoscopy was conducted on 42 patients with long-standing ulcerative colitis. Conventional white-light endoscopy with four-quadrant biopsies detected invisible flat intraepithelial neoplasia in three patients, and time-gated fluorescence endoscopy in 10 patients. With the time-gated fluorescence ratio technique, dysplastic and nondysplastic mucosa could be discriminated with a sensitivity and specificity of 73% and 81%, respectively [5]. Overall, the results on time-gated fluorescence endoscopy with PpIX as a tumor marker underline that this technique is superior to conventional white-light endoscopy. In particular, the detection limit is clearly improved after suppression of the short-lifetime tissue autofluorescence. As demonstrated on colorectal cancers and their metastases, PpIX fluorescence can even be detected without amplification by 5-ALA administration [19]. However, time-gated fluorescence endoscopy requires advanced detection systems together with pulsed lasers which are expensive and, thus, hamper its translation to clinical routine.

5-ALA and PpIX have also been considered for the detection of other tumors, including bladder cancer, glioma, and squamous cell carcinoma. Some studies on the brain have shown that PpIX can accumulate in nonmalignant tissue too, making its specificity for malignant tissue questionable [13]. Besides their application in diagnostics, 5-ALA and PpIX play an important role in photodynamic therapy.

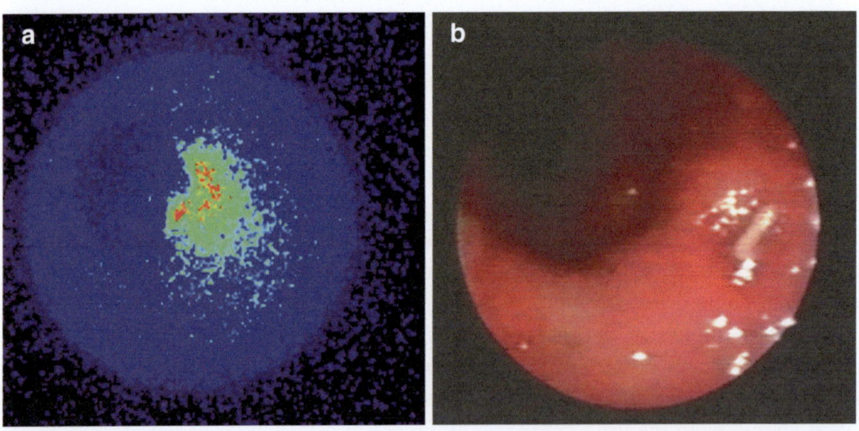

Fig. 20.12 (**a**) Fluorescence image taken with 20 ns delay and (**b**) corresponding white-light image of an esophageal carcinoma

20.3.3 Targeted Molecular Imaging in Gastrointestinal Endoscopy

As for cancer in general, targeted molecular probes are also considered as a promising approach for the early detection of tumors in the GI tract by fluorescence measurements. The targeted antibody bevacizumab-IR800CW and the activatable peptide LUM015 which have both been applied for fluorescence-guided surgery of breast cancer (cf. Sects. 20.2.2 and 20.2.6), are also investigated for the detection of cancer in the GI tract. Bevacizumab-IR800CW, which targets the vascular epithelial growth factor A, was applied in a study on 14 patients with Barrett's esophagus having known lesions [21]. For this study, the working channel of a high-definition white-light endoscope was equipped with a fiber bundle connected to a custom-built fluorescence imaging setup with a 750 nm laser for fluorescence excitation and a short-pass filtered white-light LED for the generation of overlay images. Two cameras positioned behind a dichroic beam splitter were used to acquire fluorescence and (short-pass restricted) white-light images simultaneously in real time. Five patients received the agent through an intravenous bolus 2 days before endoscopy, and the other nine patients topically by spraying immediately before fluorescence endoscopy.

Fluorescence imaging visualized 16 out of the 17 dysplastic and neoplastic lesions detected by conventional white-light endoscopy. Hereby, the missed lesion was not accessible, since its position at the gastric cardia could not be reached by the separate fiber bundle due to bending restrictions. In addition, fluorescence imaging found four more dysplastic and neoplastic lesions. As an example, Fig. 20.13 displays images of an early adenocarcinoma that was seen exclusively by fluorescence imaging. The smaller field of view in the overlay and the fluorescence image compared to the conventional endoscopic image is caused by the smaller aperture of the inserted fiber bundle. Compared to systemic administration, the topical administration was found to give a slightly higher tumor-to-background ratio of 4.30 ± 0.41. The high number of lesions found only after administration of

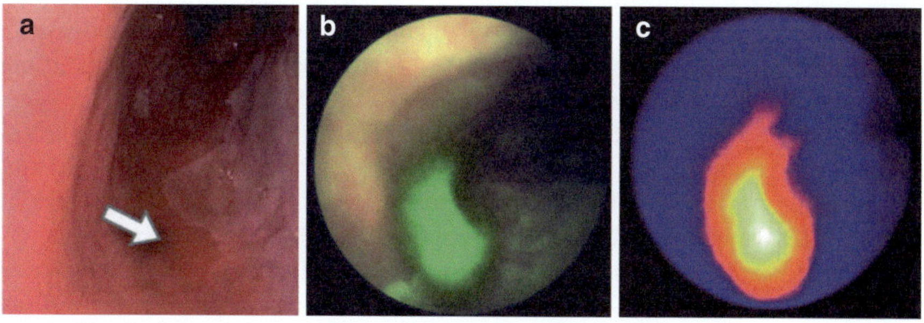

Fig. 20.13 In vivo detection of an early esophageal adenocarcinoma by targeted imaging with bevacizumab-IR800CW; (**a**) conventional white-light image without abnormality at the carcinoma position (arrow), (**b**) overlay image with fluorescence indicated in green, and (**c**) fluorescence image. (Reprinted with permission from Nagengast et al. [21])

bevacizumab emphasizes the high potential of targeted imaging for early detection of esophageal cancer.

Bevazizumab-IR800CW was also applied in a study on 8 patients with colorectal cancer [6]. SGM-101 and cRGD-ZW800-1 are further tumor-targeted fluorescent agents, which were investigated in early-phase clinical studies for colorectal cancer. SGM-101 targets the carcinoembryonic antigen. In a phase 2 study on 37 patients fluorescence led to resection of malignant lesions in 7 patients, which were not identified by conventional white-light endoscopy. In two other cases, fluorescence classified lesions correctly as benign, which were considered as cancer positive by conventional surgery [6]. cRGD-ZW800-1 targets various integrins that are overexpressed in colorectal cancer. So far, a study on 12 patients has been conducted, demonstrating feasibility [6].

The probe LUM015 which is activated by cathepsins, currently undergoes a phase 1/phase 2 clinical trial for assessing its safety and efficacy on patients with colorectal, pancreatic, and esophageal cancers [13]. As part of this study, fluorescence signals from specimens of resected tumors will be compared to histological findings (clinical trial number NCT02584244, clinicaltrials.gov). Likewise, the lectin wisteria floribunda which has been labeled with fluorescein is currently being evaluated in a phase 1 clinical trial for early detection of colorectal cancer. Lectins are expected to specifically detect cell-surface glycans that are altered in cancer [13]. Another activatable probe, ONM-100, exploits the acidic tumor environment. It becomes activated when the pH falls below 6.9. This probe undergoes a phase 2 clinical trial on colorectal cancer [6].

There are also several peptides under consideration for tumor detection in the GI tract. Compared to antibodies, peptides have the advantages of lower costs and limited immunogenicity. The peptide GE-137 (EMI-137) shows specific binding to c-Met, a protooncogene that encodes a transmembrane receptor tyrosine kinase to stimulate tumor progression and metastases. Fluorescence is emitted by the conjugated dye Cy5. Intravenously injected GE-137 is well-tolerated in humans. A pilot study using white-light and fluorescence colonoscopy has shown that GE-137 enabled visualization of all 38 neoplastic colon polyps that were visible with white light. Moreover, the detection of nine additional polyps demonstrated that GE-137 may enable the detection of polyps missed by other techniques [2]. In a study on 15 patients with Barrett's neoplasia, EMI-137 did not appear as an ideal marker; the fluorescence contrast was only moderate [4].

The specific peptides QRHKPRE and KSPNPRF are in the phase of first clinical trials for safety and efficacy evaluation [13]. QRHKPRE is considered for colorectal and esophageal cancers. It binds to the epidermal growth factor receptor (EGFR) overexpressed in epithelial cancers. The peptide KSPNPRF has undergone a clinical trial on esophageal cancer. It targets the epidermal growth factor receptor 2 (Her2) which is known to be overexpressed in colon and esophageal as well as several other cancers.

Several peptides have been identified empirically using phage display by screening against cancer [13]. The peptide VRPMPLQ was found to bind to premalignant rather than normal colonic crypts. Using confocal endomicroscopy on 20 patients, a high tumor-to-background ratio of 17.9 ± 4.2 between adenomas and normal colonocytes was found after topical administration. However, this peptide has not yet been successfully applied in wide-field fluorescence endoscopy. The suspicious sites for performing endomicroscopy were selected by white-light endoscopy.

Sturm et al. selected the peptide ASYNDA and labeled it with FITC for fluorescence imaging [33]. The peptide was investigated in a study on 25 patients with Barrett's esophagus having a history of biopsy-proven high-grade dysplasia of esophageal adenocarcinoma. Suspicious regions were selected by white-light endoscopy. The peptide was sprayed to the corresponding site by a catheter. After a waiting time of 5 min an endomicroscope was placed in contact to take confocal fluorescence images of the lesion and normal-appearing squamous mucosa. By using a tumor-to-background fluorescence intensity ratio of 4.2 as a threshold, high-grade dysplasia and adenocarcinoma could be differentiated from normal tissue with a sensitivity and specificity of 75% and 97%, respectively.

ASYNDA was used later by the same research group in a study with a multimodal wide-field endoscope [14]. Besides white-light images, this endoscope collected fluorescence images and reflectance images in an alternating manner at 20 frames per second. The reflectance measured with illumination at 540–560 nm was used to normalize the fluorescence images in order to correct the shadowing of the raw data due to the large acceptance angle in image acquisition. Figure 20.14 shows a representative example of the three images for a region with a histologically confirmed high-grade dysplasia. The dysplasia can already be seen in the raw fluorescence image whereas Barrett's esophagus and squamous epithelium are almost free of fluorescence. In the lower part, some fluorescence from the gastroesophageal junction is visible. Using the normalized fluorescence images, sensitivity and specificity for the detection of high-grade dysplasia and early adenocarcinoma amounted to 76% and 94%, respectively.

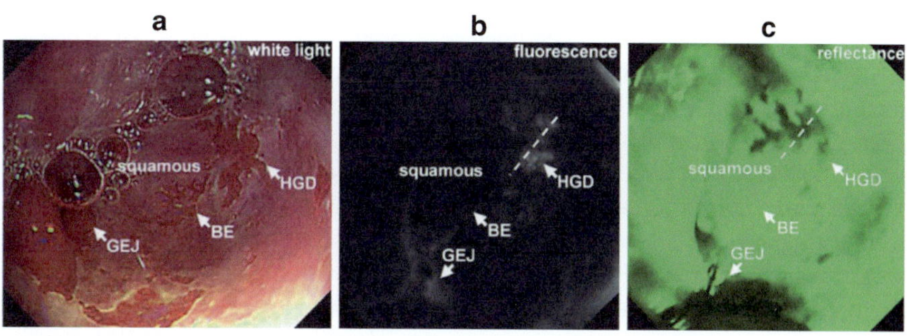

Fig. 20.14 In vivo detection of a high-grade dysplasia in the esophagus by targeted imaging with ASYNDA: (**a**) white-light image with several areas of Barrett's esophagus (BE), a high-grade dysplasia (HGD), squamous epithelium, and the gastroesophageal junction (GEJ); (**b**) fluorescence image; and (**c**) reflectance image co-registered with the fluorescence image. The dashed line indicates a cut through the lesion used for further analysis. (Reprinted with permission from Joshi et al. [14])

The peptide KCCFPAQ was found to bind specifically to sessile serrated adenomas of the colon [15]. It did not show any toxic effects in animals and patients. KCCFPAQ was topically administered in a pilot study on 38 patients, having a high risk for colorectal cancer, or having a suspected unresected proximal colonic polyp. Using wide-field fluorescence endoscopy, regions of sessile serrated adenomas were found to have a 2.4-fold higher mean fluorescence intensity than normal colonic mucosa. They could be distinguished with 89% sensitivity and 92% specificity. As described above for wide-field endoscopy with ASYNDA, this study used the same concept of fluorescence-to-reflectance ratio images to improve lesion detection.

In summary, there is a growing number of molecular probes that have entered clinical trials for the detection of carcinomas in the GI tract. In particular, the antibodies bevacizumab-IR800CW and SGM-101 or the specifically binding peptide EMI-137, could already reveal their high potential by visualizing lesions that would have been missed by conventional white-light microscopy. Furthermore, the application of molecular probes in confocal endomicroscopy could become a way for the evaluation of suspicious regions without the necessity of taking biopsy samples.

20.4 Outlook

The discussed results on molecular imaging of carcinomas in the breast and GI tract underline the huge efforts undertaken to improve the early detection of cancer. Promising results on optical detection and differentiation of breast cancer have been obtained by exploiting the enhanced permeability and retention effect of solid carcinomas using the nontargeted contrast agent ICG. Specific binding markers as well as activatable probes have not yet been applied for breast cancer diagnosis, although proposed more than 20 years ago. In part, this slow development could be caused by the general limitations in optical imaging of the breast arising from the diffusive nature of light propagation in tissue. The detection of small concentrations of a tumor marker through several centimeters of tissue is a challenging task requiring advanced and expensive fluorescence imaging techniques. Furthermore, the spatial resolution of diffuse optical imaging will never be competitive with other imaging modalities. However, structural features (requiring high spatial resolution) are highly important for early clinical diagnosis of breast cancer.

The situation is different when the cancerous tissue in the breast has to be visualized during surgery. In this scenario, the cancer tissue is directly exposed to the surgical site and optical imaging is the best-suited method for the surgeon. Accordingly, there is significant progress in the development of molecular probes for fluorescence-guided breast cancer surgery. Here we should expect the translation of molecular probes to clinical routine in the near future. This expectation is supported by the increasing number of fluorescence imaging systems approved for intraoperative use. However, the clinical development of highly specific molecular probes is limited by the selectivity of these contrast agents, making them (commercially) relevant only for a defined subgroup of patients.

High-grade dysplasia and early carcinomas of the GI tract are superficial lesions as well. Whereas the intrinsic tumor marker PpIX was of high interest for years, molecular probes are now more and more entering the field of GI tract imaging. Having the number of probes in mind, currently undergoing safety investigations, we can expect that several probes will find their way into clinical routine over the next few years. These probes may considerably improve the early detection of carcinomas in the GI tract. However, the same basic considerations concerning clinical probe development as pointed out for breast cancer apply to GI tumors as well.

Present results indicate that a tumor-to-background fluorescence ratio between 2:1 and 4:1 will be realistic. Since this contrast is not big, we can expect that quantitative imaging methods will become of high importance here. Similarly, the decision on tumor margins will depend on threshold values. Overall, quantification in fluorescence imaging might be an important step for the characterization of tumor grades as well as for the reliable resection of tumors.

References

1. Brand S, Wang TD, Schomacker KT, Poneros JM, Lauwers GY, Compton CC, Pedrosa MC, Nishioka NS (2002) Detection of high-grade dysplasia in Barrett's esophagus by spectroscopy measurement of 5-aminolevulinic acid-induced protoporphyrin IX fluorescence. Gastrointest Endosc 56(4):479–487. https://doi.org/10.1067/mge.2002.128172
2. Burggraaf J, Kamerling IMC, Gordon PB, Schrier L, de Kam ML, Kales AJ, Bendiksen R, Indrevoll B, Bjerke RM, Moestue SA, Yazdanfar S, Langers AMJ, Swaerd-Nordmo M, Torheim G, Warren MV, Morreau H, Voorneveld PW, Buckle T, van Leeuwen FWB et al (2015) Detection of colorectal polyps in humans using an intravenously administered fluorescent peptide targeted against c-Met. Nat Med 21(8):955–961. https://doi.org/10.1038/nm.3641
3. Corlu A, Choe R, Durduran T, Rosen M a, Schweiger M, Arridge SR, Schnall MD, Yodh AG (2007) Three-dimensional in vivo fluorescence diffuse optical tomography of breast cancer in humans. Opt Express 15(11):6696–6716. https://doi.org/10.1364/oe.15.006696
4. de Jongh SJ, Voskuil FJ, Schmidt I, Karrenbeld A, Kats-Ugurlu G, Meersma GJ, Westerhof J, Witjes MJH, van Dam GM, Robinson DJ, Nagengast WB (2020) C-Met targeted fluorescence molecular endoscopy in Barrett's esophagus patients and identification of outcome parameters for phase-I studies. Theranostics 10(12):5357–5367. https://doi.org/10.7150/THNO.42224
5. Fusco V, Ebert B, Weber-Eibel J, Jost C, Fleige B, Stolte M, Oberhuber G, Rinneberg H, Lochs H, Ortner M-A (2012) Cancer prevention in ulcerative colitis: long-term outcome following fluorescence-guided colonoscopy. Inflamm Bowel Dis 18(3):489–495. https://doi.org/10.1002/ibd.21703
6. Galema HA, Meijer RPJ, Lauwerends LJ, Verhoef C, Burggraaf J, Vahrmeijer AL, Hutteman M, Keereweer S, Hilling DE (2022) Fluorescence-guided surgery in colorectal cancer; a review on clinical results and future perspectives. Eur J Surg Oncol 48(4):810–821. https://doi.org/10.1016/J.EJSO.2021.10.005
7. Giacchino M, Bansal A, Kim RE, Singh V, Hall SB, Singh M, Rastogi A, Moloney B, Wani SB, Gaddam S, Mathur SC, Wallace MB, Kanakadandi V, Balasubramanian G, Gupta N, Sharma P (2013) Clinical utility and interobserver agreement of autofluorescence imaging and magnification narrow-band imaging for the evaluation of Barrett's esophagus: a prospective tandem study. Gastrointest Endosc 77(5):711–718. https://doi.org/10.1016/j.gie.2013.01.029
8. Goetz M, Kiesslich R (2008) Confocal endomicroscopy: in vivo diagnosis of neoplastic lesions of the gastrointestinal tract. Anticancer Res 28:353–360. http://www.ncbi.nlm.nih.gov/pubmed/18383869

9. Grosenick D, Rinneberg H, Cubeddu R, Taroni P (2016) Review of optical breast imaging and spectroscopy. J Biomed Opt 21(9):091311. https://doi.org/10.1117/1.JBO.21.9.091311
10. Hagen A, Grosenick D, Macdonald R, Rinneberg H, Burock S, Warnick P, Poellinger A, Schlag PM (2009) Late-fluorescence mammography assesses tumor capillary permeability and differentiates malignant from benign lesions. Opt Express 17(19):17016. https://doi.org/10.1364/OE.17.017016
11. Intes X, Ripoll J, Chen Y, Nioka S, Yodh AG (2003) In vivo continuous-wave optical breast imaging enhanced with indocyanine green. Med Phys 30(6):1039. https://doi.org/10.1118/1.1573791
12. Ito R, Kamiya M, Urano Y (2022) Molecular probes for fluorescence image-guided cancer surgery. Curr Opin Chem Biol 67. https://doi.org/10.1016/J.CBPA.2021.102112
13. Joshi BP, Wang TD (2018) Targeted optical imaging agents in cancer: focus on clinical applications. Contrast Media Mol Imaging 2018:2015237. https://doi.org/10.1155/2018/2015237
14. Joshi BP, Duan X, Kwon RS, Piraka C, Elmunzer BJ, Lu S, Rabinsky EF, Beer DG, Appelman HD, Owens SR, Kuick R, Doguchi N, Turgeon DK, Wang TD (2016) Multimodal endoscope can quantify wide-field fluorescence detection of Barrett's neoplasia. Endoscopy 48(2):A1–A13. https://doi.org/10.1055/s-0034-1392803
15. Joshi BP, Dai Z, Gao Z, Lee JH, Ghimire N, Chen J, Prabhu A, Wamsteker EJ, Kwon RS, Elta GH, Stoffel EM, Pant A, Kaltenbach T, Soetikno RM, Appelman HD, Kuick R, Turgeon DK, Wang TD (2017) Detection of sessile serrated adenomas in the proximal colon using wide-field fluorescence endoscopy. Gastroenterology 152(5):1002–1013.e9. https://doi.org/10.1053/j.gastro.2016.12.009
16. Lamberts LE, Koch M, de Jong JS, Adams ALL, Glatz J, Kranendonk MEG, Terwisscha van Scheltinga AGT, Jansen L, de Vries J, Lub-de Hooge MN, Schröder CP, Jorritsma-Smit A, Linssen MD, de Boer E, van der Vegt B, Nagengast WB, Elias SG, Oliveira S, Witkamp AJ et al (2017) Tumor-specific uptake of fluorescent bevacizumab-IRDye800CW microdosing in patients with primary breast cancer: a phase I feasibility study. Clin Cancer Res 23(11):2730–2741. https://doi.org/10.1158/1078-0432.CCR-16-0437
17. Leifeld L, Rogler G, Stallmach A, Schmidt C, Zuber-Jerger I, Hartmann F, Plauth M, Drabik A, Hofstädter F, Dienes HP, Kruis W, Büttner R, Löser H, Drebber U, Dignass A, Terjung B, Sauerbruch T, Schreiber S, Lanyi B et al (2015) White-light or narrow-band imaging colonoscopy in surveillance of ulcerative colitis: a prospective multicenter study. Clin Gastroenterol Hepatol 13(10):1776–1781.e1. https://doi.org/10.1016/j.cgh.2015.04.172
18. Mayinger B, Neidhardt S, Reh H, Martus P, Hahn EG (2001) Fluorescence induced with 5-aminolevulinic acid for the endoscopic detection and follow-up of esophageal lesions. Gastrointest Endosc 54(5):572–578. https://doi.org/10.1067/mge.2001.118642
19. Moesta KT, Ebert B, Handke T, Nolte D, Nowak C, Haensch WE, Pandey RK, Dougherty TJ, Rinneberg H, Schlag PM (2001) Protoporphyrin IX occurs naturally in colorectal cancers and their metastases. Cancer Res 61(3):991–999. http://www.ncbi.nlm.nih.gov/pubmed/11221895
20. Mooiweer E, van der Meulen-de Jong AE, Ponsioen CY, Fidder HH, Siersema PD, Dekker E, Oldenburg B (2015) Chromoendoscopy for surveillance in inflammatory bowel disease does not increase neoplasia detection compared with conventional colonoscopy with random biopsies: results from a large retrospective study. Am J Gastroenterol 110(7):1014–1021. https://doi.org/10.1038/ajg.2015.63
21. Nagengast WB, Hartmans E, Garcia-Allende PB, Peters FTM, Linssen MD, Koch M, Koller M, Tjalma JJ, Karrenbeld A, Jorritsma-Smit A, Kleibeuker JH, van Dam GM, Ntziachristos V (2019) Near-infrared fluorescence molecular endoscopy detects dysplastic oesophageal lesions using topical and systemic tracer of vascular endothelial growth factor A. Gut 68(1):7–10. https://doi.org/10.1136/gutjnl-2017-314953
22. Ntziachristos V, Yodh AG, Schnall MD, Chance B (2000) Concurrent MRI and diffuse optical tomography of breast after indocyanine green enhancement. Proc Natl Acad Sci USA 97(6):2767–2772. https://doi.org/10.1073/pnas.040570597
23. Ortner M-A, Ebert B, Hein E, Zumbusch K, Nolte D, Sukowski U, Weber-Eibel J, Fleige B, Dietel M, Stolte M, Oberhuber G, Porschen R, Klump B, Hörtnagl H, Lochs H, Rinneberg

H (2003) Time gated fluorescence spectroscopy in Barrett's oesophagus. Gut 52(1):28–33. https://doi.org/10.1136/gut.52.1.28
24. Pleijhuis RG, Graafland M, de Vries J, Bart J, de Jong JS, van Dam GM (2009) Obtaining adequate surgical margins in breast-conserving therapy for patients with early-stage breast cancer: current modalities and future directions. Ann Surg Oncol 16(10):2717–2730. https://doi.org/10.1245/s10434-009-0609-z
25. Poellinger A, Burock S, Grosenick D, Hagen A, Lüdemann L, Diekmann F, Engelken F, Macdonald R, Rinneberg H, Schlag PM (2011a) Breast cancer: early-and late-fluorescence near-infrared imaging with indocyanine green—a preliminary study. Radiology 258(2):409–416. https://doi.org/10.1148/radiol.10100258
26. Poellinger A, Persigehl T, Mahler M, Bahner M, Ponder SL, Diekmann F, Bremer C, Moesta KT, Dye F (2011b) Near-infrared imaging of the breast using omocianine as a fluorescent dye: results of a placebo-controlled, clinical, multicenter trial. Investig Radiol 46(11):697–704. https://doi.org/10.1097/RLI.0b013e318229ff25
27. Pop FC, Veys I, Vankerckhove S, Barbieux R, Chintinne M, Moreau M, Donckier V, Larsimont D, Bourgeois P, Liberale G (2021) Absence of residual fluorescence in the surgical bed at near-infrared fluorescence imaging predicts negative margins at final pathology in patients treated with breast-conserving surgery for breast cancer. Eur J Surg Oncol 47(2):269–275. https://doi.org/10.1016/j.ejso.2020.09.036
28. Preziosi A, Cirelli C, Waterhouse D, Privitera L, De Coppi P, Giuliani S (2024) State of the art medical devices for fluorescence-guided surgery (FGS): technical review and future developments. Surg Endosc 38(11):6227–6236. https://doi.org/10.1007/S00464-024-11236-5/TABLES/1
29. Refaat A, Yap ML, Pietersz G, Walsh APG, Zeller J, del Rosal B, Wang X, Peter K (2022) In vivo fluorescence imaging: success in preclinical imaging paves the way for clinical applications. J Nanobiotechnol 20(1):1–22. https://doi.org/10.1186/S12951-022-01648-7
30. Rinneberg H, Grosenick D, Moesta KT, Wabnitz H, Mucke J, Wübbeler G, Macdonald R, Schlag PM (2008) Detection and characterization of breast tumours by time-domain scanning optical mammography. Opto-Electron Rev 16(2):147–162. https://doi.org/10.2478/s11772-008-0004-5
31. Rubin DT, Rothe JA, Hetzel JT, Cohen RD, Hanauer SB (2007) Are dysplasia and colorectal cancer endoscopically visible in patients with ulcerative colitis? Gastrointest Endosc 65(7):998–1004. https://doi.org/10.1016/j.gie.2006.09.025
32. Smith BL, Hunt KK, Carr D, Blumencranz PW, Hwang ES, Gadd MA, Stone K, Dyess DL, Dodge D, Valente S, Dekhne N, Clark P, Lee MC, Samiian L, Lesnikoski B-A, Clark L, Smith KP, Chang M, Harris DK et al (2023) Intraoperative fluorescence guidance for breast cancer lumpectomy surgery. NEJM Evidence 2(7). https://doi.org/10.1056/EVIDOA2200333
33. Sturm MB, Joshi BP, Lu S, Piraka C, Khondee S, Elmunzer BJ, Kwon RS, Beer DG, Appelman HD, Turgeon DK, Wang TD (2013) Targeted imaging of esophageal neoplasia with a fluorescently labeled peptide: first-in-human results. Sci Transl Med 5(184):184ra61. https://doi.org/10.1126/scitranslmed.3004733
34. Tipirneni KE, Warram JM, Moore LS, Prince AC, de Boer E, Jani AH, Wapnir IL, Liao JC, Bouvet M, Behnke NK, Hawn MT, Poultsides GA, Vahrmeijer AL, Carroll WR, Zinn KR, Rosenthal E (2017) Oncologic procedures amenable to fluorescence-guided surgery. Ann Surg 266(1):36–47. https://doi.org/10.1097/SLA.0000000000002127
35. Tummers QRJG, Verbeek FPR, Schaafsma BE, Boonstra MC, van der Vorst JR, Liefers G-J, van de Velde CJH, Frangioni JV, Vahrmeijer AL (2014) Real-time intraoperative detection of breast cancer using near-infrared fluorescence imaging and methylene blue. Eur J Surg Oncol 40(7):850–858. https://doi.org/10.1016/j.ejso.2014.02.225
36. Tummers QRJG, Hoogstins CES, Gaarenstroom KN, de Kroon CD, van Poelgeest MIE, Vuyk J, Bosse T, Smit VTHBM, van de Velde CJH, Cohen AF, Low PS, Burggraaf J, Vahrmeijer AL (2016) Intraoperative imaging of folate receptor alpha positive ovarian and breast cancer using the tumor specific agent EC17. Oncotarget 7(22):32144–32155. https://doi.org/10.18632/oncotarget.8282

37. Unkart JT, Chen SL, Wapnir IL, González JE, Harootunian A, Wallace AM (2017) Intraoperative tumor detection using a ratiometric activatable fluorescent peptide: a first-in-human phase 1 study. Ann Surg Oncol 24(S3):3167–3173. https://doi.org/10.1245/s10434-017-6028-7
38. van de Ven SMWY, Wiethoff A, Nielsen T, Brendel B, van der Voort M, Nachabé R, van der Mark MB, Van Beek M, Bakker L, Fels L, Elias S, Luijten P, Mali W (2010) A novel fluorescent imaging agent for diffuse optical tomography of the breast: first clinical experience in patients. Mol Imaging Biol 12(3):343–348. https://doi.org/10.1007/s11307-009-0269-1
39. Vieth M, Ell C, Gossner L, May A, Stolte M (2004) Histological analysis of endoscopic resection specimens from 326 patients with Barrett's esophagus and early neoplasia. Endoscopy 36(9):776–781. https://doi.org/10.1055/s-2004-825802
40. Wanders LK, Kuiper T, Kiesslich R, Karstensen JG, Leong RW, Dekker E, Bisschops R (2016) Limited applicability of chromoendoscopy-guided confocal laser endomicroscopy as daily-practice surveillance strategy in Crohn's disease. Gastrointest Endosc 83(5):966–971. https://doi.org/10.1016/j.gie.2015.09.001
41. Weissleder R, Tung CH, Mahmood U, Bogdanov A (1999) In vivo imaging of tumors with protease-activated near-infrared fluorescent probes. Nat Biotechnol 17(4):375–378. https://doi.org/10.1038/7933
42. Yan Y, Sun X, Shen B (2017) Contrast agents in dynamic contrast-enhanced magnetic resonance imaging. Oncotarget 8(26):43491–43505. https://doi.org/10.18632/oncotarget.16482

FDG PET Hybrid Imaging

21

Caner Civan, Wolfgang P. Fendler, Bernd J. Krause, and Ken Herrmann

21.1 Introduction

Molecular imaging with positron emission tomography (PET) using tumour-seeking radiopharmaceuticals has gained wide acceptance in oncology with many clinical applications. Since its first in vivo application in the 1970s [4, 52], the glucose analogue 18-F-fluorodeoxyglucose (FDG) is the most common PET radiopharmaceutical in clinical routine, especially in oncology. In vivo FDG acts similar to glucose, but is trapped within the cells ('metabolic trapping') and is not metabolised any

This chapter is based on chapter FDG PET Hybrid Imaging from the previous edition, written by Juliane Becker and Sarah M. Schwarzenböck.

C. Civan (✉) · W. P. Fendler · K. Herrmann
Department of Nuclear Medicine, DKTK and NCT University Hospital Essen, Essen, Germany
e-mail: caner.civan@ext.uk-essen.de; Wolfgang.Fendler@uk-essen.de; Ken.Herrmann@uk-essen.de

B. J. Krause
Department of Nuclear Medicine, University Medicine Rostock, Rostock, Germany
e-mail: bernd.krause@med.uni-rostock.de

O. Schober et al. (eds.), *Molecular Imaging in Oncology - Volume 2*, Recent Results in Cancer Research 225, https://doi.org/10.1007/978-3-032-21415-7_3

further. Increased consumption of glucose is a characteristic of most tumour cells and is mainly related to overexpression of the GLUT-1 glucose transporters and increased hexokinase activity [93, 146]. FDG enables to visualise regional glucose metabolism with high sensitivity but somewhat lower specificity. Despite the high sensitivity of FDG PET/computed tomography (CT), false-positive findings may occur due to physiologic processes such as brown fat, colonic and gynaecologic activity, infectious and inflammatory processes and rebound thymus hyperplasia. False-negative findings can occur, for example, in the assessment of brain lesions as a consequence of physiologically high glucose uptake by surrounding normal brain. FDG accumulation can be assessed visually, semi-quantitatively and quantitatively. The most commonly used technique is the standardised uptake value (SUV): a semi-quantitative index of tumour uptake normalised to injected dose and a measure of the total volume distribution, such as the patient's body weight.

The hybrid imaging modality PET/CT was clinically introduced in the late 1990s. PET/CT imaging allows assessing molecular as well as morphologic information at the same time. Nowadays, PET/CT represents a state-of-the-art tool for whole-body staging and restaging in oncology within one imaging modality. PET/CT outperforms PET or CT alone by improving lesion localisation and lesion characterisation in oncology imaging.

21.2 Clinical Applications of FDG PET/CT in Oncology

This chapter provides an overview of the main clinical applications of FDG PET/CT in oncology.

FDG PET/CT plays an integral role in diagnosis, staging and restaging of disease in oncology. In addition, growing evidence suggests that FDG PET/CT can significantly contribute to the evaluation of therapy response and tumour control and to the prediction of prognosis in oncologic patients [59]. Conventional imaging modalities have limited utility in assessing therapy response. FDG has been proposed as an imaging surrogate for therapy effectiveness, providing highly reproducible quantitative measures of tumour glucose metabolism. Changes in tumour glucose uptake can therefore serve as indicators of metabolic response to therapy. For this reason, FDG PET/CT was introduced for the early sequential monitoring of tumour response of breast cancer in 1993 [145].

FDG PET/CT can be used to assess therapy response to both early and late stages during treatment. From a clinical perspective, it is very important to identify non-responders early in the treatment course, particularly when multiple therapy cycles (e.g. chemotherapy or immunotherapy) are required, so that therapeutic strategies can be adjusted accordingly. The timing of PET scans is always dependent on the type of tumour and the treatment plan; however, standardised recommendations are often lacking due to the limited number of randomised, multicentre, prospective studies. However, a baseline scan is indispensable in any case, followed usually by a second scan after the first or second cycle of therapy. Changes in FDG uptake between the pre-therapeutic and early follow-up scan are used to predict histopathological response and patient outcome. The standardised uptake value (SUV) is the most widely used FDG PET parameter, and in most studies, relative changes (%) are calculated to quantify metabolic response.

Early therapy response, as assessed by FDG PET/CT, has shown promising results in single-centre studies and should be evaluated in randomised, prospective, multicentre trials in order to implement FDG PET/CT in clinical practice for this concern in the future. In this context, standardisation of patient preparation, data acquisition and processing and data interpretation are important issues. In order to establish criteria to assess therapy response with the help of PET/CT, for example, PERCIST criteria have been developed and implemented (PERCIST 1.0, PET Response Criteria in Solid Tumours) [144].

In this chapter, special emphasis will be on the use of FDG PET/CT for therapy response assessment, being discussed in separate paragraphs for almost all of the listed tumour entities.

21.2.1 Lung Cancer

Lung cancer is the most common cancer and the leading cause of cancer-related deaths worldwide [36]. Non-small cell lung cancer (NSCLC) is the main histologic type, accounting for 85% of all cases, which include adenocarcinoma, squamous cell carcinoma and large cell carcinoma as main subtypes. Small-cell lung cancer (SCLC) is another main histologic type of lung cancer with a poor prognosis compared to NSCLC.

21.2.1.1 Solitary Pulmonary Nodule

Solitary pulmonary nodules measuring ≥8 mm, when detected incidentally through conventional imaging, are metabolically characterised using FDG PET/CT, which offers high sensitivity (92–96%), but relatively low specificity (77–90%) [158]. False negativity may occur due to low spatial and contrast resolution of PET, the small size of subcentimeter nodules, a low number of hypermetabolic cells and certain histological subtypes that show low FDG avidity such as adenocarcinoma with a predominant lepidic pattern and carcinoid tumours. Conversely, inflammatory and infectious lesions are the main causes of false-positive findings [159].

21.2.1.2 Diagnosis, Staging and Radiation Treatment Planning in NSCLC Patients

Accurate diagnostic work-up and staging of NSCLC are mandatory, particularly regarding mediastinal lymph node involvement and distant metastases affecting therapy management and prognosis. In particular, it is crucial to differentiate patients with potentially curable and resectable disease at early stages from those, who are not suitable for radical surgery, following the currently used staging system based on the tumour–node–metastasis (TNM) classification system, which describes the primary tumour (T), lymph node involvement (N) and presence of distant metastases (M).

FDG PET/CT plays a key role in staging of NSCLC, showing high FDG avidity through upregulated hexokinase activity and increased expression of glucose transporter proteins. FDG PET/CT offers high diagnostic accuracy for TNM staging [6] and significantly improves staging as compared to CT alone, particularly in assessing lymph node involvement and detecting unsuspected distant metastases [38, 124] (Fig. 21.1). Multiple guidelines and professional societies strongly recommend the use of FDG PET/CT for diagnosis and staging (e.g. Interdisciplinary guideline of the German Respiratory Society/German Guidelines Programme Oncology, Cancer Care Ontario (CCO) and American Colleges of Chest Physicians and Radiologists (ACP/ACR)) [8, 9, 20, 121] as well as for detection of recurrence/restaging (e.g. Society of Nuclear Medicine and Molecular Imaging (SNMMI)) [66], particularly under specific conditions such as planned curatively intended treatment.

The use of PET in the Dutch randomised controlled PLUS trial allowed for the avoidance of futile thoracotomies in about 20% of patients with NSCLC (21% as compared to 41% of patients in the group with conventional work-up that did not undergo PET; relative risk reduction of 51% in favour of PET, $p = 0.003$) [139]. In another trial, Maziak et al. showed that in 337 patients with confirmed clinical stage I, II or IIIA NSCLC and being considered for surgery (170 assigned to PET/CT and

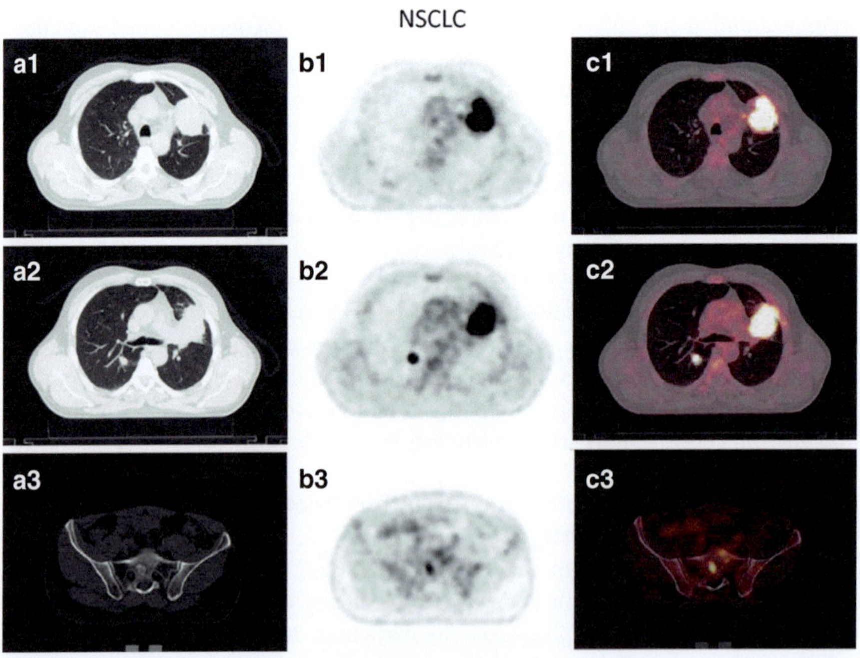

Fig. 21.1 A 47-year-old male patient with histopathologically proven non-small cell lung cancer of the left upper lung lobe, referred to FDG PET/CT for primary staging. FDG PET/CT confirmed FDG-positive primary tumour and an already suspected contralateral lung metastasis (cM1a); furthermore, PET/CT revealed an FDG-positive bone metastasis in the Os sacrum (cM1b); (A1-3) CT Scan, (B1-3) PET scan, (C1-3) PET/CT fused images

167 to conventional staging including CT of liver and adrenal glands as well as whole-body bone scan), disease was correctly up-staged in 23 of 167 PET/CT patients and in 11 of 162 conventional staging patients (13.8% vs. 6.8%), thereby sparing these patients from surgery. On the other hand, disease was incorrectly up-staged in eight PET/CT patients and one conventional staging patient (4.8% vs. 0.6%), and it was incorrectly under-staged in 25 PET/CT patients and 48 conventional staging patients, respectively (14.9% vs. 29.6%) [95]. In a recent retrospective study, Kung et al. included 186 potentially operable NSCLC patients who underwent whole-body FDG PET/CT examination in 2012. Due to disease up-staging, 34.9% (65 patients) became inoperable by the results of PET/CT; 102 of the remaining 121 patients received surgery—97 of those proceeded to surgery without further (neoadjuvant) treatment or investigation, four received neoadjuvant treatment and one had further investigations after PET/CT. As a consequence, changes in management plans occurred in 37.6% due to PET/CT—the authors concluded that PET/CT had great clinical impact with a significant reduction of futile surgery [78].

FDG PET/CT may also provide prognostic information in patients with NSCLC and SUVmax has been identified as a significant prognostic factor in preoperative early-stage NSCLC [3]. Histological subtypes of NSCLC demonstrated variable FDG uptake, which might aid in predicting histological subtype and inform treatment planning. SUVmax for adenocarcinoma is significantly lower than for squamous cell carcinoma [160].

Schreyögg et al. evaluated the diagnostic accuracy and cost-effectiveness of integrated PET/CT for the staging of NSCLC patients. The authors reported a diagnostic effectiveness in terms of correct TNM staging of 40% for CT alone and 60% for PET/CT. For the assessment of resectability, 84% of patients were staged correctly by PET/CT vs. 70% by CT alone. The cost-effectiveness analysis showed that costs for PET/CT were within the commonly accepted range for diagnostic tests or therapies [116].

With respect to the detection of mediastinal lymph node metastases several studies exist—although FDG PET/CT is more accurate than CT for the staging of mediastinal lymph nodes [124], it is still limited in its ability to differentiate between benign and metastatic lymph nodes. According to the results of prospective multicentrial trial, sensitivities and specificities of FDG PET/CT for detecting mediastinal lymph nodes were 72% and 91%, respectively [161]. There can be false-negative findings, for example, due to micrometastases, but false-positive findings seem to be the more decisive problem, for example, due to inflammation [81]. To solve this problem Rogasch et al. chose an approach similar to the Cheson/Deauville criteria for judging residual lymphoma tumour masses either as vital or not based on a visual scale [26]—after standardised windowing (threshold: 2 × liver SUV_{mean}) they used a 4-point scale as follows: [1] lymph node (LN) uptake ≤ mediastinal blood pool structures (MBPS); [2] MBPS < LN < liver; [3] liver ≤ LN < 'black'; [4] LN appears 'black'. As an optimal cut-off to differentiate benign vs. metastatic LNs they found a score >3, reaching high sensitivities (88.9–90.7%), high specificities (92.0–94.6%), high negative predictive values (NPV) (97.2–97.6%) and high accuracies (91.4–93.5%) for different readers with different levels of experience (positive predictive values (PPV) 72.7–80.0%) [113]. There are several other approaches, partly based on SUV_{max} [81] and on a ratio of lymph node SUV_{max} to primary tumour SUV_{max} [28], respectively, or even based on a decision tree model for predicting mediastinal lymph node metastases (including morphologic and functional criteria) [106]. Taken together, more studies applying this or similar decision tree models should be conducted to develop tools for FDG PET/CT readers and to make FDG PET/CT-based nodal staging more reliable.

Distant metastatic spread typically involves the adrenal glands, bones, brain or liver. Regarding a curative treatment intent, it is of particular interest whether there are distant metastases present or not, especially if they are unexpected, such as in a low tumour stage. However, the rate of unexpected distant metastases rises with the tumour stage as a prospective Australian trial by MacManus et al. [89] showed including tumour stage I–III patients: at tumour stage I the rate was 7.5%, at stage II 18% and at stage III 24%, which underlines the value of FDG PET/CT also in the staging of (locally) advanced patients, especially with respect to overall survival [131]. FDG PET/CT is suitable for the detection of metastases of the adrenal glands, bones and liver [6]. For bone metastases, it is superior to conventional bone scintigraphy (with sensitivity, specificity, NPV, PPV and accuracy > 90% each) [122], confirmed by similar results of Chang et al. [23]. In contrary, FDG PET/CT is not suitable for the detection of brain metastases due to the high glucose consumption of the normal surrounding brain tissue, resulting in an overall poor sensitivity [6]. Thus, additional magnetic resonance imaging (MRI) of the brain should be performed in all symptomatic patients and high-risk patients with curative intention (German S3 guideline, see AWMF [9].

False-negative findings on FDG PET/CT can arise from several factors, most commonly due to small lesion size (<5 mm, partial volume effect) and low-grade disease. Moreover, FDG PET sensitivity may be reduced in specific tumour types showing variable FDG uptake such as minimally invasive adenocarcinoma, bronchiolo-alveolar carcinoma, mucinous adenocarcinoma, well-differentiated carcinoid tumours and neuroendocrine tumours [6]. Conversely, false-positive findings are often attributable to infectious, inflammatory and granulomatous reasons, especially in patients with tuberculosis and sarcoidosis. Regarding the detection of distant metastasis, false positivity reasons included adrenal pathologies with high FDG uptakes such as adrenal hyperplasia and functioning adenoma.

FDG PET/CT has an important role in radiation therapy planning by allowing for more accurate delination of tumour volume, improving patient outcomes through high delivered doses to target lesions, while minimising exposure to surrounding healthy tissue. FDG PET/CT provides better inter- and intra-observer reproducilibility compared to CT, leads to reduction in estimated primary tumour volume, changing treatment intent and lowers the risk of locoregional progression without increasing toxicity [162]. Evidence from the multicentre, randomised, controlled PET-PLAN trial further supports these findings, demonstrating that PET-based planning allowed significantly more patients to receive higher mean total radiotherapy doses (≥68 Gy in 47% vs. 33% of cases), resulting in a reduced risk of locoregional progression compared to conventional planning (14% vs. 29%) [163].

21.2.1.3 Therapy Response Assessment in NSCLC Patients

Targeted treatment for advanced or metastatic NSCLC patients, which is determined by histologic subtype and molecular testing, included kinase inhibitors, antibody therapy and antibody-drug conjugate against specific genes (e.g. EGFR, KRAS, ALK and BRAF V600E). Positron Emission Tomography Response Criteria in Solid Tumors (PERCIST 1.0) has been introduced for treatment assessment, enabling earlier prediction of therapeutic efficacy and clinical outcomes. To reduce the risk of therapy-related false-positive results, response evaluation is typically recommended at 12 weeks postradiation therapy and 2 weeks after the initiation of chemotherapy.

In a meta-analysis conducted by Zhang et al., evaluating 13 studies with a total of 414 patients, a pooled sensitivity, specificity, PPV and NPV for PET-predicted response of 83%, 84%, 74% and 91%, respectively, were reported. All included studies had used pathological outcome as the gold standard. The predictive value of PET in NSCLC patients for evaluating pathological response was significantly higher than that of CT in this meta-analysis [154].

The NEOSCAN trial intended to assess the value of FDG PET/CT for an interim staging in the setting of neoadjuvant chemotherapy in order to guide further neoadjuvant treatment, dependent on response or non-response. 40 stage IB-IIIA lung cancer patients were included, receiving for two cycles either cisplatin/carboplatin plus pemetrexed (adenocarcinoma) or cisplatin/carboplatin plus gemcitabine (squamous cell carcinoma). A decrease by at least 35% in SUV_{peak} in the primary tumour was considered as response, along with continuation of the same therapy regimen for two more cycles, whereas therapy of non-responders was switched to vinorelbine plus docetaxel for two cycles. In all, 15 patients (38%) were non-responders, of which 10 patients (67%) reacted to vinorelbine plus docetaxel with partial or complete metabolic response as assessed by modified PERCIST criteria, one of those achieving major pathologic response. For all patients, response assessed by PET after 2 and 4 cycles of treatment correlated with major pathologic response (p = 0.016 and 0.034, respectively), whereas CT-based response assessment did not [22].

Treatment response following radiotherapy should be carefully evaluated due to the potential of radiation-induced effects, which carry a high risk of false-positive findings. These effects can be observed in early imaging including radiation-induced pneumonitis, and may persist for more than 12 months after treatment [7]. FDG PET/CT offers a distinct advantage over conventional imaging in accurately differentiating viable tumour tissue from postradiation inflammatory changes, thus enhancing the reliability of treatment response assessment [164].

21.2.1.4 Staging in SCLC Patients

SCLC is more aggressive than NSCLC and tends to spread rapidly with distant metastases. The staging of SCLC is based on a two-stage classification system introduced by the Veterans Administration Lung Group (VALSG) in the 1950s, which differentiates between limited disease (LD) and extensive disease (ED). Limited disease is defined as disease confined to one hemithorax, the mediastinum and the supraclavicular lymph nodes. All other cases, including those with malignant pleural effusion, are classified as ED [112].

Most of the spare literature concerning FDG PET/CT and SCLC analyse pre-therapeutic staging. In a systematic review and meta-analysis, Lu et al. showed that among 12 studies with a total of 369 patients, the pooled estimated sensitivity and specificity were 97.5% and 98.2%, respectively, for the detection of ED by FDG PET and FDG PET/CT. They regarded FDG PET/CT as a valuable imaging tool for the pre-therapeutic assessment of ED in patients with SCLC [88]. The results of patients with an up-staging after undergoing FDG PET/CT as compared to conventional imaging are similar among several studies; for example, Zer et al. found a change in the tumour stage up to extensive disease in 6/55 patients (10.9%) [154].

21.2.2 Thyroid Cancer

21.2.2.1 Differentiated Thyroid Cancer

Differentiated thyroid cancer (papillary or follicular, DTC) represents about 1% of all malignant tumours and is the most common endocrine cancer [14]. DTC is generally considered highly treatable and curable. However, approximately 30% of all patients with recurrence will develop local recurrence or metastases, which may not be detected by Iodine-131 whole-body scintigraphy due to a loss of the ability of the tumour cells to concentrate iodine as they undergo dedifferentiation [50]. The flip-flop phenomenon described by Feine et al. allows the identification of distinct uptake patterns of DTC. More aggressive tumours tend to show high FDG and low I-131 uptake, while more differentiated and less aggressive tumours exhibit low or no FDG uptake with high I-131 uptake [165].

According to the 2015 revised guidelines of the American Thyroid Association (ATA), ^{18}FDG PET/CT scanning should be considered in high-risk DTC [differentiated thyroid cancer] patients with elevated serum Tg [thyreoglobulin] (generally > 10 ng/mL) with negative RAI [radioiodine] imaging (strong recommendation, moderate-quality evidence)'. Furthermore, it 'may also be considered as […] a part of initial staging in poorly differentiated thyroid cancers and invasive Hürthle cell carcinomas […] (weak recommendation, low-quality evidence)' [57]. In the situation of suspected recurrence, elevated Tg levels and negative RAI scintigraphy, FDG PET/CT is also recommended by The Royal College of Radiologists (RCR) [129]. The European Society for Medical Oncology (ESMO) (working group 'thyroid cancer') emphasises the main indication of FDG PET/CT in metastatic patients who have lost radioiodine uptake [105]. According to the joint SNMMI and EANM practice guideline, FDG PET/CT is recommended preoperatively in more aggressive DTC histotypes and anaplastic thyroid cancer [166].

With respect to the Tg level 'cut-off' for the use of FDG PET/CT, studies have shown controversial results. However, a 'cut-off' of 10 ng/ml seems to be a reasonable value, maintaining high accuracy in terms of a good compromise between sensitivity and specificity [14]. The sensitivity depends on the histological subtype, and FDG PET is more sensitive in more aggressive subtypes such as poorly differentiated, tall cell and Hürthle cell thyroid cancer. Thus, the Tg 'cut-off' needs to be adapted and lowered in case of aggressive pathological variants of thyroid cancer that may produce low amounts of serum Tg [57]. The diagnostic accuracy of FDG PET/CT is generally high in patients with negative RAI scans and high Tg levels [14] (Fig. 21.2).

In a recent meta-analysis enrolling 20 studies with 958 thyroid cancer patients with a previous negative RAI scan, the combined sensitivity and specificity for conventional FDG PET were both found to be 84%; for FDG PET/CT, they were 93% and 81%, respectively, and the overall accuracies were 91% and 93%, respectively [18].

For detecting recurrence with FDG PET/CT Choi et al. reported a sensitivity, specificity, accuracy, PPV and NPV of 64%, 94%, 83%, 86% and 81%, respectively, including 84 papillary thyroid cancer patients with negative RAI scans and high Tg levels. They also investigated the effect of thyroid-stimulating hormone (TSH) stimulation in comparison with TSH suppression and could not find an added value for TSH stimulation [30].

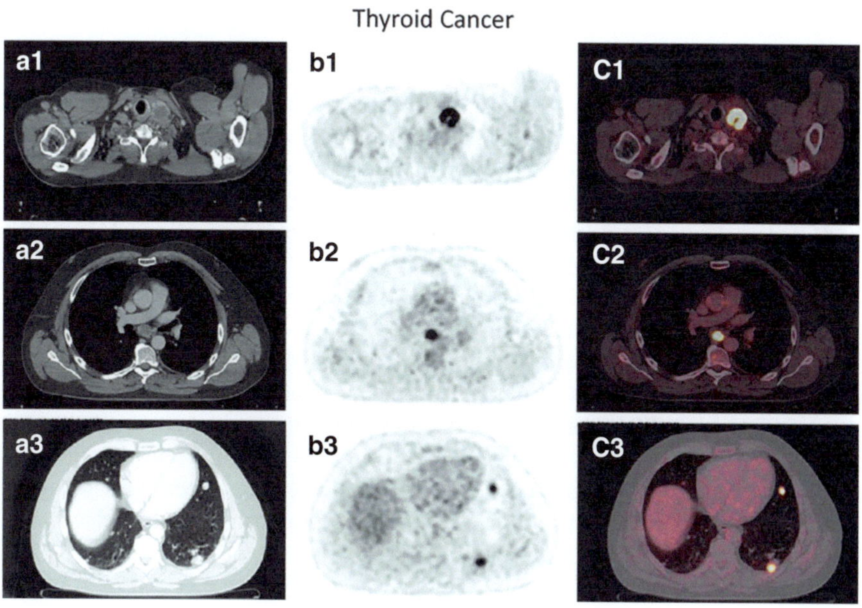

Fig. 21.2 A 53-year-old male patient with minimally invasive follicular thyroid cancer, referred to FDG PET/CT for restaging with known Iodine-131 positive local recurrence and a thyreoglobulin level of 319 μg/l under TSH suppression. Besides the local recurrence, FDG PET/CT showed an infracarinal FDG-positive lymph node metastasis and multiple FDG-positive pulmonary metastases; (A1-3) CT Scan, (B1-3) PET scan, (C1-3) PET/CT fused images

However, the impact of TSH on FDG PET/CT imaging is still an open issue, no consensus has been reached about the usefulness of high TSH levels. Levothyroxine withdrawal or alternatively the use of recombinant TSH might be preferable, especially in cases of relatively low Tg levels (<10 ng/ml), trying to improve the sensitivity of FDG PET [14]. According to ATA guidelines, 'To date, there is no evidence that TSH stimulation improves the prognostic value of ^{18}FDG-PET imaging' [57].

21.2.2.2 Medullary Thyroid Cancer

Medullary thyroid cancer (MTC) is a neuroendocrine tumour, accounting for 1–2% of thyroid malignancies. The role of FDG PET/CT in MTC is limited due to the heterogeneous biology of MTC, with a wide range of sensitivity (17–93%) and specificity (68–92%) results [167]. According to the meta-analysis, patient-based detection rate of FDG PET/CT differs from 59–69% in patients with recurrent MTC [168]. High FDG uptake is associated with more aggressive tumours and poor differentiation of MTC cells. Additionally, the sensitivity of FDG PET/CT increased in patients with shorter serum calcitonin and CEA doubling times [167].

21.2.3 Head and Neck Cancer

21.2.3.1 Diagnosis, Staging and Restaging

Head and neck cancers, the sixth most common cancer entities worldwide, originate from various anatomical sites, primarily arising from mucosal epithelium in the oral cavity. Smoking, alcohol use, smokeless tobacco use and human papillomavirus (HPV) infection are the major risk factors for oral cavity cancer, with smoking and alcohol having synergistic effects [133]. The incidence of HPV-associated head and neck cancer is increasing, most commonly arising from the oropharynx [94].

Histopathologically, squamous cell carcinomas account for the vast majority of head and neck cancers, with>90% [1, 27]. The most common involved site is the larynx, followed by the oral cavity including tongue, lips and salivary glands [1]. Less common histological subtypes include adenocarcinoma, adenoid cystic carcinoma and mucoepidermoid carcinoma.

A decisive prognostic factor is the metastatic involvement of cervical lymph nodes, crucial for an adequate therapeutic management [126]. Consequently, the role of FDG PET/CT in the initial staging of head and neck cancer patients was investigated in many studies. While FDG PET/CT is a highly sensitive imaging modality for detecting malignancy in this region, MRI remains superior for T-staging and physiological FDG uptake in head and neck region can limit the detection of small tumours due to background activity [169].

FDG PET/CT has been utilised in staging, especially for the detection of lymph node and distant metastases in clinically high-risk patients and for the detection of unknown primary tumours. Cacicedo et al. conducted a prospective study enrolling 84 patients with newly diagnosed, locally advanced head and neck squamous cell carcinoma (stage III–IV disease according to the American Joint Committee on Cancer (AJCC) classification (seventh edition), histologically confirmed. After a conventional work-up (physical examination and CT imaging of the head, neck and chest) each patient underwent FDG PET/CT and the results were separately discussed in multidisciplinary tumour boards—TNM stage was determined and afterwards validated by histopathological analysis. The authors found a discordance for 32/84 (38%) patients between the results of conventional work-up and FDG PET/CT with the highest impact on N stage (in 21/32, 65.7%), followed by a change in patient management in 22/84 patients (26%)—PET/CT TNM-classification was significantly more accurate (92.5% vs. 73.7%) than conventional staging with a p-value < 0.001 [17].

There is an ongoing debate, if FDG PET/CT should be implemented in the routine diagnostic work-up of locally advanced head and neck cancers—the National Comprehensive Cancer Network (NCCN) guidelines recommend consideration of FDG PET/CT in the assessment of the initial treatment strategy for loco-regionally advanced disease to evaluate for distant metastases [34]; also RCR recommends the use in this patient population or if initial imaging is inconclusive/with equivocal findings that would preclude radical treatment [129]. ESMO recommended FDG PET/CT as a preferred imaging modality to assess distant metastases in high-risk patients as well as to detect second lung primary in heavy smokers [170].

However, the main field of FDG PET/CT in head and neck cancer patients is the follow-up and treatment response assessment after chemoradiotherapy. According to ESMO, FDG PET/CT should be performed 10–12 weeks after completing treatment, or in cases of suspected recurrence [170].

In routine follow-up, FDG PET/CT is usually recommended after inconclusive conventional imaging to differentiate treatment effects from tumour residuals/recurrence [129] or if there is a high risk for distant metastases due to initial TNM stage, especially in patients considered for major salvage treatment [8]. Recurrence or relapse mostly occurs within the first 2–3 years after the first diagnosis [27, 58, 118]. FDG PET/CT has a significant advantage over MRI or CT in differentiation tumour recurrence from postradiogenic or postoperative inflammatory changes; however, it is recommended to perform FDG PET/CT 3 months after surgery due to false-positive results in early images [171].

In the management of local recurrence, direct laryngoscopic techniques and physical examination remain key aspects, followed by PET/CT or other imaging modalities as important adjuncts in detecting recurrence in lymph nodes and more distant sites [66] (Fig. 21.3).

A recent meta-analysis evaluating 23 studies (constituting 2247 PET/CT examinations) found a pooled sensitivity and specificity of 92% and 87%, respectively, for the detection of recurrence in general (local, regional and distant) in head and neck cancer patients by FDG PET/CT. The pooled sensitivity and specificity of scans performed 4–12 months after treatment were 95% and 78%, respectively, with similar sensitivity but higher specificity for scans performed $\geq$ 12 months after treatment, with 92% and 91%, respectively [118]. In order to differentiate between the primary site, the locoregional site and the distant site another meta-analysis including 27 studies (1195 patients) was conducted recently: the authors found a pooled sensitivity and specificity of 86.2% and 82.3%, respectively, for detecting

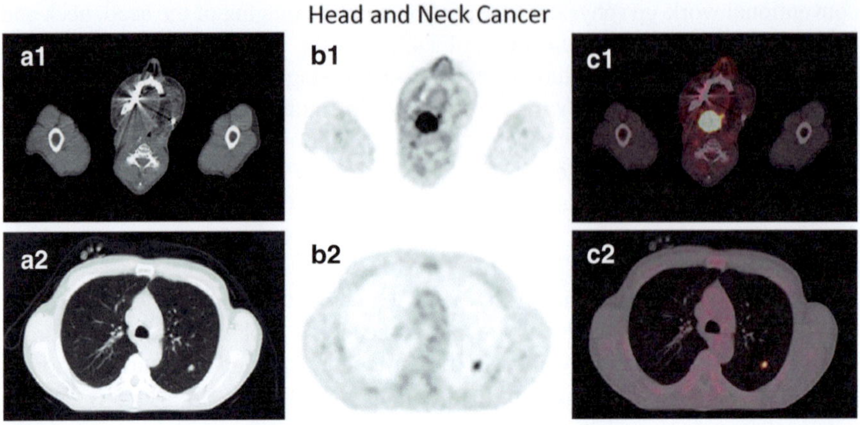

Fig. 21.3 A 55-year-old male patient with histopathologically proven second local recurrence of oropharyngeal carcinoma (initially TNM-classification pT2 pN0 L0 V0 R0 cM0, first recurrence rpT3 pN0 L0 V0 Pn1 cM0), referred to FDG PET/CT for restaging. FDG PET/CT confirmed FDG-positive recurrence in the right oropharynx; furthermore, PET/CT revealed an FDG-positive lung metastasis in the left upper lung lobe (cM1); (A1–2) CT Scan, (B1–2) PET scan, (C1–2) PET/CT fused images

recurrence at the primary site, of 72.3% and 88.3%, respectively, at the locoregional (neck) site and of 84.6% and 94.9%, respectively, for distant metastases [27].

21.2.3.2 Therapy Response Assessment

The American College of Radiology (ACR) proposed the Neck Imaging Reporting and Data System (NIRADS) for response assessment by different imaging modalities including CT, MRI or FDG PET/CT [172]. NIRADS classified primary tumour site, nodal and distant metastases into five categories. Category 0 indicates an incomplete evaluation due to an unavailable appropriate comparison examination; category 1 reflects no evidence of recurrence; category 2 indicates low suspicion; category 3 represents high suspicion; and category 4 confirms definite recurrence. According to meta-analyses, FDG PET/CT in head and neck cancer patients following treatment demonstrated that NIRADS ≥3 categories detected treatment failure or recurrence with a pooled sensitivity of 68% and a pooled specificity of 90% [173].

The prospective randomised PET-Neck trial investigated the role of FDG PET/CT performed 12 weeks after the end of chemoradiotherapy in 564 N2- or N3-patients to decide about the conduction of neck dissection, which was only employed if PET/CT showed an equivocal or incomplete response. PET/CT surveillance resulted in fewer neck dissections than did planned surgery (54 vs. 221), the 2-year overall survival rate was 84.9% in the surveillance group and 81.5% in the planned-surgery group—additionally, PET/CT surveillance was more cost-effective over the duration of the trial [96].

The use of FDG PET/CT in follow-up after chemoradiotherapy was also recommended by other authors. There is a broad consensus that a period of at least

12 weeks after the completion of treatment and the scan should be kept to avoid non-specific chemoradiotherapy-related inflammatory FDG uptake [118]. It is still unclear if HPV-positive patients should undergo FDG PET/CT at a later time after completion of primary treatment, since nodal disease might take longer to respond and regress in these patients [58, 63].

In an effort to standardise image interpretation, Marcus and colleagues proposed the so-called 'Hopkins criteria' in order to assess therapy response for head and neck cancers from the results of a post-therapy PET/CT scan by using a 5-point scale comparing the intensity (as compared to SUV values of the liver and the internal jugular vein) and pattern (focal or diffuse) of FDG PET uptake in primary tumour and neck nodes. This assessment was shown to be highly specific, with 92.2% and to carry a high NPV of 91.1% in an evaluated patient collective (57.5% HPV positive) [94].

21.2.4 Oesophageal Cancer

21.2.4.1 Diagnosis, Staging and Restaging

Oesophageal cancer is one of the most common cancers worldwide, being the eighth most common cancer and the sixth most common cause of cancer-related deaths [80]. There are two major histological subtypes of oesophageal cancer: squamous cell carcinoma and adenocarcinoma, the first being previously much more common than the second one. However, a marked increase in the incidence of oesophageal adenocarcinoma in Europe, North America and Australia has been observed during the past four decades, so the incidence of oesophageal adenocarcinoma has surpassed that of oesophageal squamous cell carcinoma in many western countries [80]. Oesophageal adenocarcinoma mostly originates in the lower third of the oesophagus, often involving the oesophago-gastric junction. The main pathophysiological pathway of oesophageal adenocarcinoma is likely to be chronic gastro-oesophageal reflux, causing a metaplasia known as 'Barrett's oesophagus'.

Relevant pre-therapeutic prognostic factors are local tumour invasion, locoregional lymph node and distant metastases. Endoscopic ultrasound and CT represent the most widely used imaging modalities for the assessment of local tumour invasion (T stage), locoregional lymph node involvement (N stage) and also distant metastases stage (M stage) [148].

Sensitivity and specificity of FDG PET/CT for staging oesophageal cancer have been investigated in many studies. Both squamous cell carcinoma and adenocarcinoma of oesophageal cancer have strong FDG affinity, offering high sensitivity and accuracy rates. For instance, Purandare et al. conducted a study enrolling 156 patients with potentially curable oesophageal adenocarcinoma and they found a change in the intent of treatment in 16% of the patients by detecting M1b disease with high sensitivity, specificity, PPV, NPV and accuracy (83.3%, 98.4%, 92.5%, 96.1% and 95.3%, respectively). The authors concluded that FDG PET/CT should be implemented in the initial staging work-up [109]. FDG PET/CT is recommended especially for patients with suspected metastatic disease, which also aids in distinguishing oligometastatic disease from polymetastatic disease.

In their systematic review and meta-analysis, Goense et al. assessed the performance of FDG PET/CT for the detection of recurrent oesophageal cancer after curatively intended treatment. Evaluating eight studies, they found a high sensitivity (96%) and moderate specificity (78%), concluding that histopathologic confirmation of PET/CT-suspected lesions remains necessary due to a considerable false-positive rate [53].

FDG PET/CT has been recommended in initial staging and risk assessment according to ESMO guideline, and they emphasised that FDG PET/CT should be carried out in patients who are candidates for oesophagectomy to identify unknown distant metastases and avoid futile surgery [174]. According to NCCN, possible distant metastases in staging are best assessed with FDG PET/CT, suggesting to perform FDG PET/CT in initial staging as routine clinical work-up if there is no evidence of M1 disease [175]. FDG PET/CT has high sensitivity for detecting primary lesions; however, it has limited performance for determining invasion of the mediastinum [175]. Another limitation of FDG PET/CT is the detection of locoregional metastatic nodes with a sensitivity of 51%, while EUS has a high sensitivity (85%). On the other hand, FDG PET/CT has significant sensitivity for the detection of distant metastases, which altered treatment management in 38% of cases.

21.2.4.2 Therapy Response Assessment

The MUNICON I trial was one of the first clinical trials to provide evidence that FDG PET can be used to individualise neoadjuvant therapy, in this trial, chemotherapy in patients with locally advanced oesophageal adenocarcinoma. Treatment was adapted based upon PET results conducted 2 weeks after chemotherapy induction in a way that metabolic responders (predefined as decreases of SUV values by 35% or more) received more cycles of chemotherapy for a maximum of 12 weeks, whereas metabolic non-responders underwent surgery immediately [86].

The prospective MUNICON II trial was designed to potentially improve the clinical outcome of metabolic non-responders by applying a salvage neoadjuvant chemoradiotherapy; the authors found an increased histopathologic response rate as compared to the results of the MUNICON I trial, but the primary endpoint of the study—to increase the R0-resection rate—was not met [157].

In contrast, if FDG PET/CT is used to assess therapy response in squamous cell carcinoma patients, it should be conducted after completion of the neoadjuvant therapy [103].

21.2.5 Gastric Cancer and Gastrointestinal Stromal Tumour (GIST)

21.2.5.1 Diagnosis, Staging and Restaging in Gastric Cancer Patients

Gastric cancer is the fifth most common cancer with decreased incidence rates and the fourth leading cause of cancer-related deaths worldwide [176]. Gastric adenocarcinoma accounts for about 95% of all types of gastric cancer. There are two major subtypes according to Lauren's classification: intestinal type, which often evolves from the distal stomach in association with chronic Helicobacter pylori infection, and diffuse or signet ring type (non-intestinal type), which commonly evolves from the proximal stomach and is more often found in Western patients combined with chronic reflux and obesity [74].

In the staging of gastric cancer, the role of FDG PET/CT is limited due to its reduced sensitivity. Only about 60% of locally advanced gastric cancers show FDG avidity [125]. According to ESMO guideline, FDG PET/CT is not routinely recommended for staging of gastric cancer, although FDG PET/CT may improve staging by detecting lymph nodes and distant metastases [177]. In particular, tumours such as signet ring cell carcinoma and mucinous adenocarcinoma tend to have low FDG avidity, which further limits the utility of FDG PET/CT. Furthermore, other reasons for low sensitivity are small tumour size, mucinous content and localisation in the distal third of the stomach [59]. The reported sensitivity of FDG PET for detecting gastric cancer ranges from 47 to 96% (mean sensitivity 77%, mean specificity 99%) [60]. For the detection of locoregional lymph nodes, FDG PET/CT seems to be more specific, but less sensitive as compared to CT alone. FDG PET/CT sensitivity, specificity and accuracy range from 41 to 74%, 75 to 100% and 51 to 76%, respectively, whereas these parameters for contrast-enhanced CT range from 70 to 83%, 62 to 92% and 67 to 80%, respectively [74].

Wu et al. conducted a systematic review and meta-analysis to evaluate the use of FDG PET for the detection of recurrent gastric cancer. Across nine studies involving 526 patients, the overall sensitivity of FDG PET was found to be 78% and the overall specificity 82% [149]. A more recent meta-analysis enrolling 14 studies with 828 patients reported a high sensitivity of 85% and a moderate specificity of 78% for FDG PET or FDG PET/CT for diagnosing recurrent gastric cancer—the authors concluded that FDG PET has a great value in the detection of recurrent gastric cancer after surgical resection, which might become more important in the future given the high recurrence rates of gastric cancer [84]. Another meta-analysis demonstrated similarly good sensitivity and specificity for FDG PET/CT for detecting recurrence of gastric cancer after curative resection, while emphasising the heterogeneity of the studies [178].

21.2.5.2 Diagnosis, Staging and Restaging in GIST Patients

Gastrointestinal stromal tumours (GISTs), most common mesenchymal malignancy of the gastrointestinal tract, mostly located in the stomach (60%), and small intestine [114]. The prevalence of GISTs is extremely rare, with an estimated prevalence of 15/100.000. Since GISTs often show a high FDG avidity, FDG PET/CT can be used to evaluate these tumours and their response to therapy [137]. FDG PET/CT has high sensitivity (89%) and specificity (97%) for restaging, which might significantly change treatment management [179]. A correlation between the FDG uptake and the malignant potential of GISTs presented by the Ki67 labelling index as a mitotic index has been reported by Kamiyama et al. [72].

FDG PET/CT is suitable for the initial staging of GIST patients, since at least half of the patients present with distant metastases at the time of diagnosis [92]. Most common sites for distant metastases are the liver and the peritoneum; locoregional lymph node metastases are very uncommon [114]. Nevertheless, there is a significant number of patients with GISTs of about 10% that do not show the typically strong FDG uptake on baseline PET scan—this might be related to a high degree of tumour necrosis and myxoid/zystoid degeneration [92, 114].

21.2.5.3 Therapy Response Assessment in GIST Patients

Metabolic response, as assessed by FDG PET/CT, is closely related to clinical outcome for GIST patients. Changes of FDG uptake occur early, whereas morphological changes occur late in the course of imatinib therapy [134]. In a systematic review and meta-analysis, Hassanzadeh-Rad et al. found that the accuracy of FDG PET/CT is higher in the detection of treatment failure (e.g. non-responders) than in the prediction of good response to therapy [56]. FDG PET/CT has been recommended by the ESMO guideline for early assessment of tumour response, providing early prediction of treatment response with high sensitivity, which is particularly useful in preoperative cytoreductive treatments [180].

21.2.6 Colorectal Cancer

21.2.6.1 Diagnosis, Staging and Restaging

Colorectal cancer is the third most common cancer worldwide, and the second leading cause of cancer-related deaths, with an increased incidence rate in young adults [181]. At an early stage, surgery is a curative treatment approach; however, for locally advanced cancers (pT3-4 or any T,N1) usually a multimodality treatment approach is chosen, which includes preoperative concomitant chemotherapy and radiotherapy [74].

In general, FDG PET/CT is considered not 'useful' in the initial staging of colorectal cancer patients, since the added value as compared to conventional imaging seems to be not significant [74]. However, in a retrospective study, Petersen et al. analysed the data from 67 patients, who underwent FDG PET/CT additionally to conventional imaging (CT, MRI and/or ultrasound) for initial staging—they found a change in treatment plans in 30% of the cases due to FDG PET/CT, another third of this 30% was either a change from intended curative to palliative therapy or vice versa [107]. Lee and Lee also conducted a retrospective study enrolling 266 colon cancer patients also undergoing both FDG PET/CT and conventional imaging. Multidetector CT and FDG PET/CT showed similar accuracy in detecting lymph node metastases in patients with clinical stage III (36.2% vs. 42%, $p = 0.822$) and stage IV (60.3% vs. 63.5%, $p = 0.509$) disease. However, FDG PET/CT results led to a change in management for 1 of 40 (2.5%) with clinical stage I, 0 of 25 (0%) with stage II, 9 of 138 (6.5%) with stage III and 8 of 63 patients (12.7%) with stage IV disease. The authors concluded that FDG PET/CT might be considered as a routine staging tool for clinical stage III and IV colon cancers [82]. FDG PET/CT might aid particularly in patients with increased tumour markers without evidence of metastatic disease, or to detect the extent of metastatic disease on potentially resectable metastases [23].

Considering the distant metastases, liver metastases are most common in colorectal cancer patients with an incidence of approximately 50–60%, of which about one-third are diagnosed at the same time as the primary tumour is detected [74]. A meta-analysis by Maffione et al. including a total of 1059 patients reported a high accuracy for FDG PET and FDG PET/CT for the detection and staging of liver lesions in colorectal cancer (pooled sensitivity and specificity of 93% in patient-based analysis, and 60% and 79%, respectively, in lesion-based analysis). PET showed a lower sensitivity as compared to MRI and CT in patient-based analysis (93%, 100% and 98%, respectively) and lesion-based analysis (66%, 89% and 79%, respectively); however, PET was more specific as compared to MRI and CT in both patient-based and lesion-based analysis (81%, 70% and 70%, respectively, and 86%, 81% and 67%, respectively). FDG PET and PET/CT results led to a change in management in an average of 24% of patients, entailing both exclusion from curative surgery and modification of the surgical approach. The mean incidence of extrahepatic disease shown by FDG PET or PET/CT, but not detected by conventional imaging, was 32% [90].

In the follow-up and detection of recurrent colorectal cancer, FDG PET/CT is regarded as a valuable tool. In a Danish study conducted by Engelmann et al. with a total of 66 prospectively included patients, FDG PET/CT detected all relapses occurring within the first 2 years. Cumulative relapse incidences for clinical stages I–III (n = 42 patients) at 6, 12, 18 and 24 months were 7.1%, 14.3%, 19% and 21.4% [43]. A recent meta-analysis including 26 studies (1794 patients) revealed a pooled sensitivity and specificity of 94% each for FDG PET and PET/CT in the detection of locally recurrent colorectal cancer [153]. Based on rising CEA levels (biochemical recurrence) many studies were conducted examining the usefulness of FDG PET/CT in this situation. In a systematic review and meta-analysis enrolling 11 studies with 510 patients Lu et al. found a pooled sensitivity and specificity of 90.3% and 80.0%, respectively, for FDG PET and a pooled sensitivity and specificity of 94.1% and 77.2%, respectively, for FDG PET/CT in the detection of recurrence in colorectal cancer patients with elevated CEA levels [87].

The use of FDG PET/CT in colorectal cancer patients is recommended by some professional societies such as RCR, seeing the usefulness in many indications, for example, initial staging of patients with synchronous metastases suitable for resection, restaging of patients with recurrence (suspected by rising tumour markers and/or clinical suspicion of recurrence with normal or equivocal findings on other imaging), especially if being considered for radical treatment and/or invasive targeted techniques, or assessment of treatment response in patients with rectal carcinoma post (chemo)radiotherapy with indeterminate findings on other imaging [129]. Also, SNMMI recommends the use of FDG PET/CT in restaging for local recurrence and (distant) metastases, especially in the case of rising tumour markers with negative or equivocal findings on conventional imaging [66]. Furthermore, in the initial staging, FDG PET/CT 'may be appropriate', if distant metastases are suspected in the pre-treatment staging of colorectal cancer according to the ACR Appropriateness Criteria® [49].

According to NCCN guidelines, FDG PET/CT is not indicated for preoperative staging of rectal cancer in general, and should only be used to evaluate an equivocal finding on a contrast-enhanced CT scan or in patients with a strong contraindication to intravenous contrast [13]. Following ESMO guidelines, PET/CT 'may be helpful' to characterise extrahepatic disease [136].

21.2.6.2 Therapy Response Assessment

For therapy response assessment in rectal cancer patients a meta-analysis conducted by Maffione et al. (34 studies, 1526 patients) found a high pooled accuracy for FDG PET and PET/CT to predict therapy response for the global cohort at the end of treatment (pooled sensitivity 73%, pooled specificity 77%), and especially for early interim PET performed between 1 and 2 weeks after the initiation of neoadjuvant chemoradiotherapy (pooled sensitivity 84%, pooled specificity 81%) [91].

21.2.7 Hepatocellular Carcinoma

Liver cancer, a fourth leading cause of cancer-related mortality, is the sixth most common cancer worldwide. Hepatocellular carcinoma (HCC) is the most common type of liver cancer, characterised by male preponderance and low overall survival rates. In staging and diagnosis of HCC, conventional imaging methods such as CT, USG and MRI, which is a preferred imaging modality, are most commonly employed.

Well-differentiated HCCs typically exhibit low FDG uptake due to low expression of GLUT activity and Glucose 6-phosphatase activity. In contrast, poorly differentiated HCC lesions often demonstrate high FDG uptake, which correlates with larger tumour size, elevated alpha-fetoprotein (AFP) levels, and the presence of microvascular invasion. FDG PET/CT plays a role in selected cases, but it is not recommended as a routine imaging modality for staging. The detection rate of FDG PET/CT is limited, with a reported sensitivity of 50–65%; however, FDG PET/CT demonstrated high sensitivity in identifying extrahepatic metastases with 77–100%. FDG PET/CT can provide valuable information in staging by reflecting the potential for tumour progression and metastases. Furthermore, metabolic parameters from FDG PET/CT may help predict microvascular invasion prior to liver transplantation, an important factor associated with tumour recurrence and overall survival. High FDG uptake is linked to an increased risk of recurrent disease, early tumour recurrence and poorer survival outcomes.

21.2.8 Pancreatic Cancer

21.2.8.1 Diagnosis, Staging and Restaging

Pancreatic cancer is one of the most lethal cancers with a very poor prognosis and poor overall survival (5-year survival rate of about 4% [141]). Curative therapy is limited to patients with localised disease who are eligible for surgical resection.

Commonly used imaging tools for the diagnosis of pancreatic cancer include ultrasound, endosonography, CT, MRI and magnetic resonance and endoscopic retrograde cholangiopancreatography (MRCP and ERCP). Since 70–90% of pancreatic cancers show a high FDG uptake, FDG PET/CT was introduced to potentially improve the detection of pancreatic adenocarcinomas.

Tang et al. assessed the diagnostic impact of FDG PET, FDG PET/CT and endoscopic ultrasonography in the diagnosis of patients with pancreatic carcinoma. The authors reported that FDG PET/CT had a high pooled sensitivity of 90.1%, while the specificity was moderate with 80.1% in comparison with endoscopic ultrasonography with a pooled sensitivity and specificity of 81.2% and 93.2%, respectively. They concluded that FDG PET/CT and endoscopic ultrasonography might have different (complementary) roles under different conditions in diagnosing pancreatic carcinoma [128].

Fletcher et al. reported that PET improved differentiation between benign and malignant pancreatic tissue in the diagnostic work-up of patients with suspected pancreatic lesions and might reduce the need for biopsy and surgery, influencing morbidity. They recommended FDG PET(/CT) as an additional tool in selected patients demonstrating inconclusive conventional imaging findings [47].

Royal College of Radiologists (RCR) suggested FDG PET/CT in diagnosis and staging of pancreas cancer to prevent futile resection. Another utility of FDG PET/CT according to RCR is to perform in selected patients with suspected recurrence but negative or equivocal results by other imaging methods.

Recently, several studies were conducted to investigate the usefulness of FDG PET/CT in the follow-up after curative surgery and in suspected recurrence, especially if tumour marker levels (CA 19-9) are high and conventional imaging is equivocal. Jung et al. investigated the usefulness of FDG PET/CT in the follow-up of curatively resected pancreatic cancer patients in comparison with CT alone: PET/CT showed a higher sensitivity (84.5% vs. 75.0%) and accuracy (84.5% vs. 74.5%) than CT alone, also in the detection of distant metastases (sensitivities 83.1% vs. 67.7%). In 19 out of 110 patients, recurrences were only seen on PET/CT [71].

In another study, the additional value of FDG PET/CT in unresectable pancreatic carcinoma patients prior to chemoradiotherapy was examined as compared to conventional imaging—in 19 out of 71 (26.8%), PET/CT staging showed distant metastases not detected by conventional staging, entailing a change in the conduction of chemoradiotherapy (or chemotherapy alone, respectively). The authors concluded that PET/CT-based staging might help to select the patients who are suitable for chemoradiotherapy, sparing those patients with metastases from futile radical protocols [132].

21.2.9 Melanoma

21.2.9.1 Diagnosis, Staging and Restaging

Malignant melanoma is one of the most common tumour entities in both sexes worldwide; but due to new efficient treatment options like immunotherapies, melanoma is not expected among the 10 cancer entities with the highest mortality rates [119]. Although malignant melanoma comprises only about 5% of all skin cancers, it is still the major cause of skin cancer deaths.

Since tumour stage is the most important predictive factor for survival rates, initial staging of the disease is crucial. According to AJCC, malignant melanoma is staged into localised disease (Stage I and II); lymph-node positive disease (Stage III); and advanced or metastatic disease (Stage IV) [182]. Surgery remains the gold standard in the treatment of locoregional disease, but even in stage IV patients (according to AJCC), survival rates have been improved by metastasectomy [111]. In general, FDG PET/CT has a higher sensitivity and specificity for detecting (distant) metastases as compared to conventional imaging. However, additional MRI of the head should be performed to exclude brain metastases, which might not be detected by PET/CT due to the high physiologic cerebral uptake and a resulting diminished sensitivity. Furthermore, by virtue of limited spatial resolution, FDG PET/CT is inferior to sentinel lymph node biopsy in the detection of clinically occult lymph node metastases.

According to NCCN guidelines, PET/CT is recommended in patients equal or higher than stage III with clinically suspicious lymph nodes or with in-transit metastases (IIIB or higher) [33]. ESMO guidelines state that 'before undertaking additional aggressive local surgical treatments, a detailed staging investigation, that includes high-resolution imaging techniques, such as PET, CT or magnetic resonance imaging is necessary to exclude distant metastases', and specify that 'in pT stages > pT3a [i.e. in patients equal or higher than stage IIA], CT or PET scans are recommended before surgical treatment and sentinel node biopsy' [41] (Fig. 21.4). The German S3 guideline is not in agreement with ESMO guidelines by stating PET/CT shall not be performed routinely as initial staging procedure up to stage

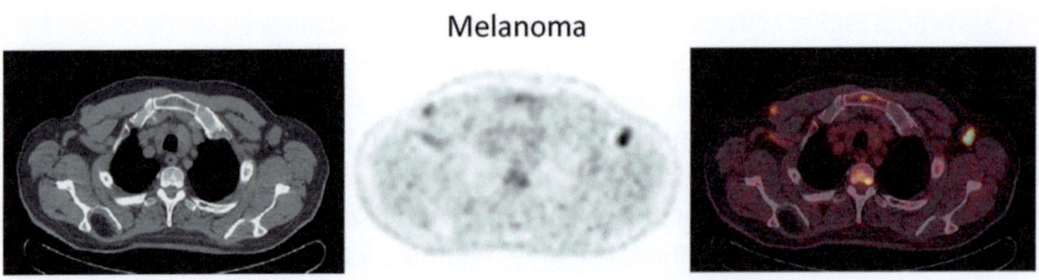

Fig. 21.4 A 78-year-old male patient with melanoma of the left shoulder, pT4b, corresponding to AJCC stage IIC, referred to FDG PET/CT for initial staging after primary resection without sentinel lymph node biopsy. FDG PET/CT showed an FDG-positive lymph node metastasis in the left axilla and revealed another suspicious FDG-positive nodule adjacent to the right musculus pectoralis major; (A1) CT Scan, (B1) PET scan and (C1) PET/CT fused images

IIA/IIB (suggesting to treat stage IIC patients like high-risk patients); however, in the primary staging of stage III patients and higher it has been shown that PET/CT is superior to the other methods in diagnostic accuracy [10].

A meta-analysis conducted by Xing et al., enrolling 10,528 patients (regardless of stage), investigated the utility of ultrasonography, CT, PET and PET/CT for staging and surveillance of melanoma patients. In the staging of distant metastases, the highest sensitivity of 80% was found for PET/CT, along with a moderate specificity of 87%. Similar results were found in the surveillance of patients with the help of PET/CT to exclude distant metastases [151]. A more recent meta-analysis aimed to review the utility of FDG PET in the detection of systemic metastases in patients with stage III melanoma, including 623 patients. The authors found a sensitivity and specificity of 89.42% and 88.78%, respectively; the area under the operating curve was 0.94. A change in stage and/or management was noted in 22% of patients [111].

In suspected recurrent disease, employment of FDG PET/CT is highly recommended by SNMMI [66], by CCO if just a solitary metastasis is identified at the time of recurrence prior to metastasectomy [20] and by NCCN in the case of nodal recurrence 'to evaluate specific signs or symptoms' [33].

A prospective multicentre PET registry study was conducted in Ontario (Canada) to assess the use of PET in advanced or high-risk melanoma as an adjunct to clinical and standard radiologic investigation. Approximately 319 patients with potentially resectable high-risk melanoma or recurrent disease under evaluation for isolated metastasis underwent PET/CT; 10 of those already presented with M1 stage (stage IV). A significant increase in stage to M1 was found after PET/CT in 17.6% of the patients, resulting in significantly more distant surgical interventions in this group as compared to the group without up-staging. None of the already assigned M1 patients was down-staged after PET/CT. The authors concluded that PET/CT has a significant impact on surgical management [123].

Usually, FDG PET/CT is not recommended for routine follow-up; however, according to ESMO guidelines and the German S3 guideline high-risk patients (starting from stage IIC onwards) should routinely undergo cross-sectional imaging, which may include cranial MRI and PET/CT, whole-body MRI or whole-body CT (German S3 guideline, AWMF [10] or 'ultrasound of lymph nodes, CT or whole-body PET or PET/CT scans' ESMO, see Dummer et al. [41].

In order to assess the value of FDG PET/CT for patient management of melanoma patients, Mena et al. carried out a retrospective study including 71 patients (regardless of stage) with four or more postoperative follow-up PET/CT scans (246 scans). Recurrence was found in 39.0% of the scans, and the examinations resulted in a change of the patient's management in approximately 16.7% of the scans. Change in management was significantly higher in patients with prior clinical suspicion of malignancy recurrence than in those without prior clinical suspicion. There was a statistically significant difference in the overall survival between patients with at least one positive scan and patients with four or more negative subsequent follow-up scans at the patient level [97]. More recently, a retrospective study analysed the data of 238 patients with 526 scans in Denmark—since 2015 PET/CT has been implemented in the Danish national follow-up programme as a routine examination at 6, 12 and 24 months after treatment for malignant melanoma of stage IIB or higher. However, in the analysis, melanoma patients were included regardless of stage (starting from stage IA onwards). The authors found a sensitivity, specificity, PPV and NPV of 89%, 92%, 78% and 97%, respectively. Here, there was no significant difference in the diagnostic accuracy of PET/CT between patients referred with or without clinical suspicion of relapse [140]. A prospective study including 170 postoperative stage III patients with a total of 502 scans and a median follow-up of 47 months found relapses in 38% of the patients, the majority of them being asymptomatic. Overall sensitivity and specificity of the approach of sub-stage specific (IIIA/B/C) PET surveillance were 70% and 87%, respectively. PPV and NPV were calculated sub-stage- and time point-dependent—a negative PET at 18 months implied NPVs of 80–84% for true non-recurrence in the follow-up period. The authors considered PET/CT to be suitable to detect (asymptomatic) resectable and potentially curable disease at relapse [83].

21.2.9.2 Therapy Response Assessment

The therapy of unresectable metastatic melanoma has changed significantly with the introduction of immune checkpoint inhibitor therapy—the first FDA-approved one was ipilimumab in 2011 for the treatment of malignant melanoma.

Sachpekidis et al. studied 41 patients with advanced melanoma prior to and after 2 cycles of ipilimumab treatment with FDG PET/CT (interim PET/CT). Earlier, the authors had found that the absolute number of new lesions is a better parameter for the prediction of immunotherapy response than changes in SUV and established the so-called PET Response Evaluation Criteria for Immunotherapy (PERCIMT). In this study, therapy response assessment was based on both the European Organization for Research and Treatment of Cancer (EORTC) criteria from 1999 and the proposed PERCIMT criteria. The patients were dichotomised into those with clinical benefit (CB, including stable disease (SD), partial response (PR) and complete response (CR)), accounting for 31 patients, and those without CB (no-CB) showing progressive disease (PD), affecting the remaining 10 patients. According to EORTC criteria interim PET/CT demonstrated PD (meaning no-CB) in 20 patients, according to PERCIMT criteria PD was seen in nine patients; SD and PR were seen in 19 patients according to EORTC criteria and in 30 patients according to PERCIMT criteria, and CR was seen in two patients according to both criteria, resulting in sensitivities (correctly predicting CB), specificities (correctly predicting no-CB), PPV, NPV and accuracies of 64.5%, 90.0%, 95.2%, 45.0% and 70.7%, respectively, for EORTC criteria, and 93.6%, 70.0%, 90.6%, 77.8% and 87.8%, respectively, for PERCIMT criteria [115].

21.2.10 Lymphoma

21.2.10.1 Diagnosis, Staging and Restaging

Lymphomas are a heterogeneous group of malignancies characterised by diverse morphologies, immunophenotypes and cytogenetics. The major subdivision into

Hodgkin's lymphoma (HL) and non-Hodgkin lymphoma (NHL) is based on histopathological criteria, with HL presenting 'Sternberg-Reed cells' microscopically. Although the World Health Organisation (WHO) does not recommend a 'grouping' of lymphomas, there is a further classification dividing NHLs into indolent (low-risk) and aggressive/highly aggressive (intermediate- and high-risk) NHLs, based on terms of biologic behaviour and the subsequently required aggressiveness of the treatment [67].

In international guidelines and recommendations by professional societies, FDG PET/CT is often recommended in the initial staging work-up of lymphoma patients, especially in HL patients, for example, RCR [129], NCCN [62] and ESMO [42]. While HL patients usually display a high FDG avidity on PET/CT scans, the FDG avidity of NHL patients differs. However, almost all histological (nodal) NHL subtypes were reported to be highly FDG avid with the exception of extra-nodal marginal zone lymphoma and small lymphocytic lymphoma [147], and lymphoplasmacytic lymphoma/Waldenström's macroglobulinemia and mycosis fungoides (unless there is a suspicion of aggressive transformation) [26].

Based on published data, a consensus statement of the Malignant Lymphomas Imaging Working Group (MLIWG) on International Conferences in 2011 and in 2013 (Lugano, Switzerland) recommended the use of PET/CT in the staging of all FDG-avid lymphomas, including indolent subtypes [26]. For patients with non-FDG avid lymphomas, diagnostic CT is recommended instead of FDG PET/CT, unless there is documented transformation. Baseline FDG PET/CT is also crucial, particularly for the assessment of lymphomas showing variable FDG avidity.

A prospective multicentre PET registry study published in 2017 was conducted to evaluate the clinical impact of pre-treatment FDG PET/CT on the staging and management of apparent limited-stage indolent lymphoma being considered for curative radiation therapy. Significantly, 47 patients (23.9%) of the included 197 patients were up-staged by the PET/CT result from the presumed limited-stage (stage I–II according to Cotswold-modified Ann Arbor classification) to advanced-stage disease (stage III–IV). Vice versa, 10 patients (5.1%) were down-staged, 4 of those patients from advanced-stage to limited-stage disease. After PET/CT (available data of 155 patients), 95 patients (61.3%) were planned to receive active treatment, of whom 59 patients were assigned to undergo the initially planned radiation therapy alone; finally, 34 patients of those received this treatment. The authors concluded that PET/CT should be implemented in the standard work-up of indolent lymphoma patients, as there was a significant impact on further clinical treatment in their study [98].

Instead of TNM staging, the staging of lymphoma patients follows the so-called 'Ann Arbor classification', lastly modified in Cotswold in 1988, which takes the site and the dissemination of involved lymphoid and extra-nodal tissue into account. The highest stage IV includes extra-nodal involvement other than contiguous/proximal lesions to the known nodal site, for example, bone marrow involvement. Since bone marrow biopsy is an invasive method and gives information only about a small part of the bone marrow, many studies were conducted to investigate the sensitivity and specificity of FDG PET/CT in the assessment of bone marrow involvement in lymphoma patients. Recently, in a retrospective analysis evaluating 832 HL patients from the German Hodgkin Study Group trials HD16, HD17 and HD18, the results of bone marrow biopsy and PET scans (either in combination with CT or MRT and in 31 patients (4%) PET alone) were compared. With bone marrow biopsy as the reference standard, PET showed a sensitivity, specificity, PPV, and NPV of 95.0%, 86.5%, 14.7% and 99.9%, respectively. Considering both bone marrow biopsy and PET as gold standard, sensitivity, specificity, PPV and NPV of PET were 99.2%, 100%, 100% and 99.9%, respectively. PET found 110 additional patients with suspect focal bone marrow lesions who would have been considered negative by biopsy. Regarding these results, bone marrow biopsy seems to be futile in PET-negative HL patients, and the authors recommended biopsies only in PET-positive patients who would undergo a changed treatment protocol as a result of the suspected bone marrow involvement [142].

Also in diffuse large B-cell lymphoma, the most common subtype with 30–35% of all NHL lymphomas, FDG PET/CT was reported to be more sensitive than bone marrow biopsy for the detection of bone marrow involvement [26]. In their systematic review and meta-analysis, Adams et al. included seven studies with a total of 654 patients. The pooled estimates for sensitivity and specificity of FDG PET/CT for detecting bone marrow involvement were 88.7% and 99.8%, respectively. The weighted summary proportion of FDG PET/CT negative patients with positive bone marrow biopsy was 3.1%. In conclusion, FDG PET/CT was considered as a complementary tool to bone marrow biopsy for detecting bone marrow involvement, since it cannot be ruled out by a negative FDG PET/CT scan [2]. However, even if positive PET findings were reported to be highly predictive and are considered usually sufficient to define advanced-stage disease [26], there is no consensus on whether diffuse FDG bone marrow uptake should be regarded as positive or negative for involvement [2]. Furthermore, the histological type of lymphomatous cells in the bone marrow (small or large cells, meaning discordant or concordant involvement) might have an influence on FDG avidity with FDG PET/CT being more sensitive in concordant bone marrow involvement [2].

Another retrospective study enrolling 185 patients with newly diagnosed lymphoma including indolent subtypes (47 patients, 30 follicular lymphomas and 17 marginal zone lymphomas) found a high concordance rate between bone marrow biopsy and PET/CT in the detection of bone marrow involvement for aggressive B-cell lymphoma (88.1%) and HL (93.8%), as well as high NPVs for PET/CT in the same histological subtypes (93.2% for aggressive B-cell lymphoma and 100% for HL). However, the concordance rate and NPV were much lower in indolent B-NHL with 66.0% and 66.7%, respectively—the authors considered bone marrow biopsy as an indispensable staging procedure in indolent lymphoma patients [29].

In follow-up, routine surveillance scans with FDG PET/CT are not recommended, since there is a high number of false-positive scans (>20%), leading to further unnecessary investigations, such as biopsies, and to increased patient anxiety. Therefore, follow-up scans should be based on clinical indications [26].

21.2.10.2 Therapy Response Assessment

According to the 'Lugano Classification' based on the results of the already mentioned two international conferences in Lugano, therapy response assessment is recommended to be performed by FDG PET/CT using the 5-point scale (Cheson/Deauville criteria), both for interim and end-of-treatment response for all FDG-avid lymphomas within clinical trials [26]. So far, therapy response should be assessed only visually, since there are not enough data for an SUV-based cut-off assessment. However, in NHL patients there are controversies about the interreader agreement after PET/CT applying the 5-point scale [11]. For end-of-treatment assessment, PET/CT is the standard of care for remission assessment in FDG-avid lymphoma (Fig. 21.5). However, for interim assessment, there are ongoing clinical trials evaluating and also questioning the usefulness of interim FDG PET/CT in therapy response assessment, especially during *immuno*chemotherapy in diffuse large B-cell lymphomas [11].

There are a lot of studies investigating the usefulness of FDG PET/CT in interim therapy response assessment in HL patients, also at advanced-stage disease. In an international prospective multicentre trial, 1119 patients with advanced-stage HL underwent interim PET/CT scans, of whom 937 patients showed negative scans. Those patients with negative PET findings after 2 cycles of ABVD (doxorubicin, bleomycin, vinblastine and dacarbazine) chemotherapy were randomly assigned to continue ABVD or omit bleomycin in the following four cycles. The 3-year progression-free survival rate and overall survival rate in the ABVD group were 85.7% and 97.2%, respectively; the corresponding rates in the AVD group were 84.4% and

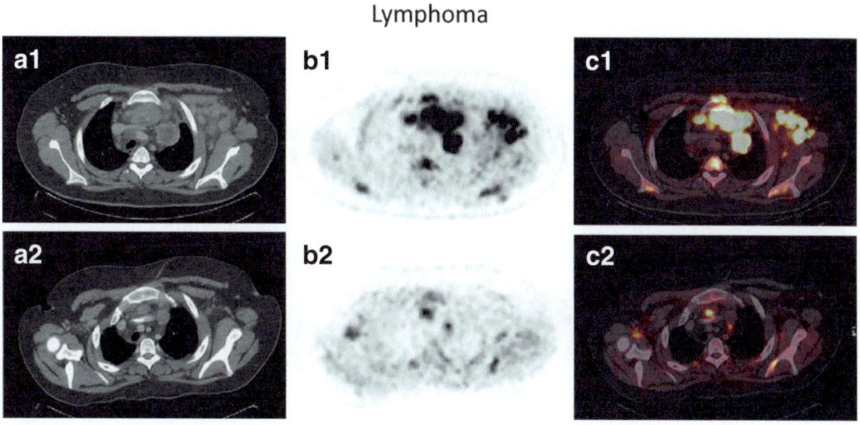

Fig. 21.5 A 19-year-old male patient with Hodgkin lymphoma, referred to FDG PET/CT for initial staging (August 2015; images A1/B1/C1) and for restaging (January 2016; images A2/B2/C2) after chemotherapy (6 cycles of BEACOPP August–December 2015). Initial FDG PET/CT showed manifestations of lymphoma on both sites of the diaphragm (Ann Arbor stage III). FDG PET/CT after chemotherapy showed vital lymphoma residuals in the mediastinum (visually Cheson/Deauville score 3–4, which means > mediastinal blood pool uptake, but ≤ liver uptake and moderately above liver uptake, respectively). As a consequence, the patient was referred to adjuvant radiotherapy; (A1-2) CT Scan, (B1-2) PET scan, (C1-2) PET/CT fused images

97.6%, respectively. In summary, the omission of bleomycin from the ABVD regimen after negative interim PET/CT resulted in a lower incidence of pulmonary toxic effects than with continued ABVD but not significantly lower efficacy [69].

Recently, in an open-label international phase 3 trial 1013 advanced-stage HL patients were randomised after negative interim FDG PET/CT (after 2 cycles of chemotherapy) to receive either standard eBEACOPP (in all 8 (before June 2011) or six cycles (after June 2011)) of bleomycin, etoposide, doxorubicin, cyclophosphamide, vincristine, procarbazine and prednisone in escalated doses) or de-escalated protocol with four cycles of eBEACOPP in all (experimental arm). In PET-negative patients, the 5-year progression-free survival rates in the standard and experimental arm were 90.8% and 92.2%, respectively. Furthermore, the application of only four cycles of eBEACOPP was associated with fewer severe infections (8% vs. 15% after 6/8 cycles) and organ toxicities (8% vs. 18% after 6/8 cycles). The authors concluded that interim PET negativity allows for a reduction to only four cycles of eBEACOPP without loss of tumour control [15].

21.2.11 Sarcoma

21.2.11.1 Diagnosis, Staging and Restaging

Sarcomas are a rare heterogeneous group of tumours composing about 1% of all malignancies [143], but carrying a high mortality rate, and presenting with varied radiologic appearances.

Primarily, sarcomas are divided into sarcomas originating from bone and cartilage, respectively, (such as osteosarcoma, Ewing's sarcoma or chondrosarcoma) or originating from soft tissue (such as liposarcoma, leiomyosarcoma and GIST).

With respect to the biologic potential, WHO has classified soft tissue tumours in four categories: benign, intermediate (locally aggressive), intermediate (rarely metastasising) and malignant [46]. The histological grade of soft tissue sarcomas and chondrosarcomas is supposed to be the most important prognostic factor in those cancer groups [31, 32].

A meta-analysis of FDG PET studies in patients with sarcoma concluded that FDG PET could discriminate between benign tumours and low-grade tumours and intermediate and high-grade tumours [12]. Also other authors found an accurate discrimination at least between low- and high-grade sarcomas employing FDG PET [24]. However, by use of FDG PET it remains difficult to distinguish low-grade tumours from benign tumours, as also confirmed by other studies, for example, Ioannidis and Lau found FDG PET to be positive in all intermediate and high-grade soft tissue tumours, in 74.4% of low-grade soft tissue tumours and still in 39.3% of benign lesions [65]. Czernin et al. investigated the baseline glucose metabolic phenotype of sarcoma in more than 100 patients with soft tissue sarcoma. The SUV differed considerably and significantly among the many histological subtypes. Liposarcomas, especially the myxoid variants, exhibited low FDG uptake. Sarcomas not otherwise specified (NOS), the most dedifferentiated variants, showed the highest FDG uptake. Overall, SUV_{max} was significantly higher in high-grade than in low-grade sarcomas (11.7 ± 9.1 g/ml vs. 3.7 ± 1.8 g/ml; $p < 0.001$) [35].

FDG PET/CT can be useful in the evaluation of soft tissue tumours for guiding biopsy, helping to sample in the area with the highest glucose utilisation [110]. ESMO guidelines also see a role for FDG PET/CT in defining the area a biopsy should be taken from [21]. Furthermore, according to the NCCN guidelines FDG PET/CT has a role in the staging, prognostication and therapy response assessment in patients with soft tissue sarcomas of the extremities, the superficial trunk or head and neck, but not in surveillance [143]. ESMO recommended FDG PET/CT in staging of the bone sarcomas as clinically indicated and preferred FDG PET/C over bone scan [183]. FDG PET/CT has a high negative predictive value for bone marrow metastases, and according to the ESMO guideline, bone marrow biopsies are not necessary in patients with localised disease and negative FDG PET/CT due to the very low incidence in this cohort [183].

A meta-analysis from 2012 enrolling 89 patients focused on the primary staging of high-grade bone and soft tissue sarcomas—the authors found a high sensitivity, specificity, PPV and NPV for the presence of distant metastases detected by FDG PET/CT with 95%, 96%, 87% and 98%, respectively. However, in the detection of lymph node metastases, the PPV was very low with 27%, but there were similarly high rates for sensitivity, specificity and NPV with 100%, 90% and 100%, respectively. The authors considered the use of FDG PET/CT to be 'feasible' in the initial assessment of patients with high-grade bone and soft tissue sarcoma. Furthermore, they found the SUV_{max} of the primary tumour to be a strong prognostic predictor of survival [51].

A more recent review and meta-analysis investigated the role of FDG PET and PET/CT in diagnosis, staging and recurrence assessment of bone sarcoma enrolling 42 trials with a total of 1530 patients; for discriminating primary bone sarcomas from benign lesions the authors found a pooled sensitivity of 96% and a pooled specificity of 79%, for detecting distant metastases the pooled results on a lesion-based level were 90% and 85% for sensitivity and specificity, respectively, and for detecting recurrence the pooled results on an examination-based level were 92% (sensitivity) and 93% (specificity), respectively (all values referring to PET/CT, even though, results for PET only were comparable) [85].

There are sarcomas that preferably occur in children and adolescents such as Ewing's sarcoma and rhabdomyosarcoma. In a study conducting 46 PET scans in 25 paediatric patients with Ewing's sarcoma or neuroectodermal sarcoma or rhabdomyosarcoma, a favourable accuracy was found for FDG PET (sensitivity, specificity, PPV and NPV were 86%, 80%, 89% and 67%, respectively) [99].

21.2.11.2 Therapy Response Assessment

Czernin et al. investigated the evaluation of therapy response in soft tissue sarcomas by determining the degree of FDG uptake decrease before and after treatment: In these studies, decreases of tumour FDG uptake by 35% after a single cycle and by > 60% at the end of treatment identified all pathological treatment responders, predicting the amount of necrotic tissue in excised tumour tissue (>95% necrosis) [35].

In osteosarcomas, Hongtao et al. carried out a meta-analysis examining the therapy response as assessed by FDG PET/CT—they showed that SUVs measured before and after treatment are valuable for predicting the histological response to chemotherapy [61].

21.2.12 Breast Cancer

21.2.12.1 Diagnosis, Staging and Restaging

Breast cancer is the most common type of cancer, and the leading cause of cancer-related death in women worldwide [108]. In 2022, breast cancer was the second most frequently diagnosed cancer, and fourth most common cancer-related mortality, when both sexes were included [119].

Invasive ductal carcinoma is the most common histopathological subtype of invasive breast cancer accounting for 50–70% of all cases, followed by invasive lobular carcinoma with 5–15%, and finally mucinous and tubular carcinoma representing 1–6% and 1–2% of the cases, respectively. Various factors can influence FDG avidity in breast cancer. In general, invasive ductal carcinoma tends to exhibit high FDG avidity, while invasive lobular carcinoma shows lower FDG uptake. Additionally, profileration rate, tumour grade, hormone receptor status may influence FDG avidity, potentially causing false-negative results. False-negative findings are often associated with specific histologic subtypes and smaller lesion sizes, while false-positive findings may occur due to postsurgical inflammation and granulomatous processes.

Mammography remains the principal imaging tool to screen for breast cancer. Small lesions cannot be characterised by FDG PET/CT due to the partial volume effect and limited spatial resolution—sensitivities of 59% in T1a–b (<10 mm) and 98% in T1c (11–20 mm) tumours have been reported [75]. According to NCCN guideline, FDG PET/CT is recommended in patients with advanced disease and invasive ductal histology; and FDG PET/CT could be useful in selected cases in earlier-stage disease with equivocal findings and suspected undetected nodal and distant disease. FDG PET/CT is also recommended in radiotherapy treatment planning, due to improved patient outcomes.

In a clinical trial, Koolen et al. enrolled 154 patients with primary stage II and III breast cancer to evaluate the role of FDG PET/CT in the staging work-up in comparison with conventional imaging techniques (bone scintigraphy, liver ultrasound and chest radiography) to exclude distant metastases prior to neoadjuvant chemotherapy. They found a sensitivity, specificity, PPV, NPV and accuracy of 100%, 96%, 80%, 100% and 97%, respectively; in 16 of 20 patients additional (distant) lesions, metastatic disease or new primary malignancy, were exclusively seen by PET/CT, leading to a change in treatment in 13 of 154 patients (8%). The authors concluded that FDG PET/CT is superior to conventional imaging techniques in the detection of distant metastases in untreated stage II and III breast cancer patients and may be of additional value prior to neoadjuvant chemotherapy [76]. For a recent retrospective study in a total of 234 stage I, II and III breast cancer patients FDG PET/CT was performed before (114 patients) or after surgery (120 patients)—hypermetabolic extra-axillary lymph nodes were detected in 42/234 patients (17.9%) and hypermetabolic distant metastases in 65/234 patients (27.7%), leading to a modification in the staging in 82/234 patients (35%) and in patient management in 69/234 patients (29.4%) [152]. Thus, FDG PET/seems to be of additional value in the staging starting already from stage II onwards (for more information also see Groheux [54]).

A meta-analysis conducted by Sun et al. including six studies comprising 609 patients at various disease stages and regardless of treatment status concluded that FDG PET/CT outperforms conventional imaging and demonstrates excellent diagnostic performance in staging of distant metastasis in breast cancer patients. The reported sensitivity and specificity were 99% and 95%, respectively compared to conventional imaging with a sensitivity of 57% and a specificity of 88% [127].

Since about 30–35% of all patients ultimately relapse after initial treatment [108, 150], surveillance is particularly important in those initially diagnosed with advanced tumour stages. Two-thirds of breast tumour recurrences are local and detection of local recurrence is a domain of mammography and/or ultrasound and, if inconclusive, MRI [108]. However, the 5-year survival rate in patients with distant metastases (mediastinal lymph nodes, bones, lungs, liver and brain) is markedly lower (25% vs. 80% in patients with locoregional recurrence) [150].

FDG PET/CT has no significant role in the routine follow-up of asymptomatic patients following curative-intent therapy; however, FDG PET/CT demonstrated superior accuracy over conventional imaging in the detection of breast cancer relapse. FDG PET/CT is an effective imaging modality in the assessment of locoregional relapse, primarily in chest wall, axillary and other lymph node metastases [184]. According to ESMO guideline, FDG PET/CT is recommended as a systemic imaging modality in the suspicion of oligometastatic disease [185].

In a recent meta-analysis and systematic review including 26 studies with 1752 patients with suspected recurrent breast cancer, FDG PET or PET/CT was shown to be a highly sensitive and moderately specific imaging modality for the detection of relapse with a sensitivity of 90% and a specificity of 81% [150]. A retrospective clinical study conducted by Jung et al. enrolling 1162 patients with 1819 examinations assessed the role of FDG PET/CT in the detection of locoregional recurrence or distant metastases as compared to conventional imaging (mammography, breast ultrasound, bone scintigraphy and chest radiography)—the authors found a sensitivity, specificity, PPV and NPV of 97.5%, 98.8%, 95.4% and 99.4%, respectively, for FDG PET/CT, the corresponding values for conventional imaging were 75.4%, 98.7%, 93.4% and 94.3%, respectively; thus, the sensitivity of FDG PET/CT was shown to be significantly higher as compared to conventional imaging. The authors considered FDG PET/CT as an acceptable diagnostic imaging modality for postoperative surveillance [70] (Fig. 21.6).

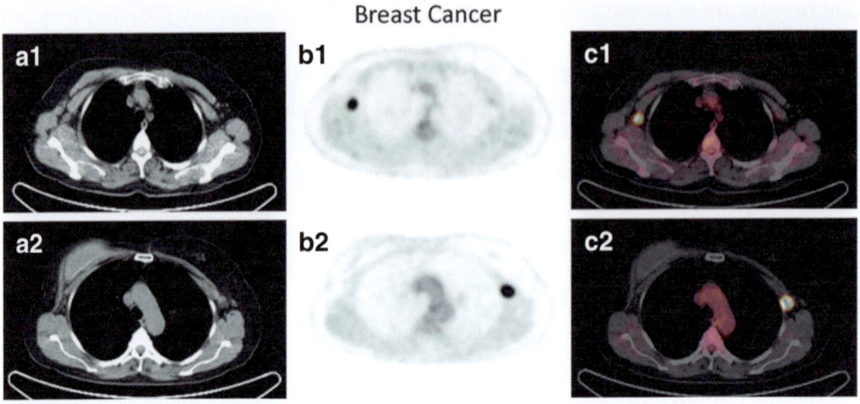

Fig. 21.6 A 56-year-old female patient with history of breast cancer of the right breast (initially TNM-classification pT1b pN0 L0 V0 R0 G3) after surgery and adjuvant radiation therapy, referred to FDG PET/CT for restaging; clinically already suspicious focal tumour in the right axilla. FDG PET/CT confirmed FDG-positive lymph node metastasis in the right axilla; furthermore, PET/CT revealed an FDG-positive node contralateral in the left axilla, either contralateral primary tumour or further lymph node metastasis; (A1-2) CT Scan, (B1-2) PET scan, (C1-2) PET/CT fused images

21.2.12.2 Therapy Response Assessment

For breast cancer, FDG PET/CT was examined in many studies in the setting of neoadjuvant chemotherapy to assess therapy response. A meta-analysis from 2012 enrolling 17 studies with 781 patients summarised a good pooled sensitivity of 84.0%, but only a moderate pooled specificity of 71.3%; however, the studies included were quite heterogeneous. For instance, only 11 studies had reported the receptor status (oestrogen, progesterone and human epidermal growth factor receptor (HER) 2). The authors recommended a combination of FDG PET/CT with other imaging modalities such as MRI, ultrasound and mammography to assess therapy response [25].

More recently, Tian et al. conducted a meta-analysis enrolling 22 studies with 1119 patients; the pathological response in both breast tissues and in the axillary lymph nodes and the accordance with FDG PET/CT results were evaluated. They found a pooled sensitivity of 81.9% and a better-pooled specificity of 79.3% as compared to the results of Cheng et al. the area under the curve being 0.87. Among the included studies there was also a high heterogeneity, the sensitivities in the different studies ranged from 63% to 100% and the specificities ranged from 38% to 97%—the authors suggested that only tumour subtypes with relevant FDG uptake at baseline can be assessed in the course of chemotherapy. In tumours with low initial FDG avidity change in glucose utilisation cannot reasonably be used for therapy response assessment in the course of chemotherapy, but obviously those tumour subtypes were also evaluated in the included studies [130].

FDG PET/CT allows for earlier assessment of treatment response compared to conventional imaging, as it can detect metabolic changes before anatomical alterations become evident. According to ESMO, FDG PET/CT plays a particularly significant role in patients with bone only or predominantly bone metastases. As metabolic response criteria, EANM-SNMMI guidelines recommended using standardised response criteria such as PERCIST or EORTC PET Response Criteria, especially for metastatic breast cancer. FDG PET/CT may help improve patient outcomes, particularly in specific subtypes, for example, HER2+ breast cancer and triple negative breast cancer, by enabling early detection of pathological complete response following primary systemic therapy.

21.2.13 Ovarian Cancer

21.2.13.1 Diagnosis, Staging and Restaging

Nearly 90% of ovarian cancers arise from the epithelium, the remaining 10% are germ cell and stromal tumours [117]. Ovarian cancer is the leading cause of death from gynaecologic cancer in the Western World [77]. The poor prognosis results from an advanced cancer stage, which affects about 70% of patients at the time of diagnosis [44]. Ovarian cancer spreads mainly by local extension, by early implantation on both the parietal and the visceral peritoneum, by lymphatic dissemination (involving the inguinal, pelvic, paraaortic and mediastinal lymph nodes) and rarely through the blood vessels [44]. The serum tumour marker CA-125 is widely used to assess the effectiveness of therapy and to detect tumour recurrence.

Unclear ovarian masses are evaluated with ultrasound, CT and/or MRI, usually followed by 'staging laparotomy'. Surgical exploration remains the standard reference for the initial staging of ovarian cancer [44, 117]. In the primary staging, FDG PET/CT has no definite role, but 'may be appropriate' according to the ACR Appropriateness Criteria® in the staging and follow-up of ovarian cancer [73]. FDG PET/CT was shown to be limited in the diagnosis of cancer of the ovaries due to physiologic FDG uptake observed in the ovaries of women at reproductive age; for this reason the examination should be conducted during the postmenstrual phase in premenopausal women. However, focal uptake in the region of the ovaries in postmenopausal women is suspicious of malignancy and should be further evaluated. False-positive results may also occur, for example, when physiologic bowel activity is mixed up with peritoneal spread [44]. On the other hand, FDG PET/CT may lead to false-negative results in borderline tumours, in lesions smaller than 5 mm (such as carcinomatosis), in women with cystic or necrotic lesions and in mucinous tumours. Still, FDG PET/CT is more sensitive than CT alone in detecting small peritoneal deposits [48, 77]. Furthermore, women with ovarian cancer confined to the pelvis may benefit from a preoperative FDG PET/CT in order to identify nodal metastases—in a prospective study enrolling 68 patients FDG PET/CT showed a high sensitivity, specificity, accuracy, PPV and NPV of 83.3%, 98.2%, 95.6%, 90.9% and 96.5%, respectively, in a patient-based analysis. The authors concluded that due to the high NPV, systematic pelvic and aortic lymphadenectomy could be avoided in many patients [120]. In addition, FDG PET/CT has the advantage of a whole-body examination ('one-stop shop'), hence it might also detect supradiaphragmatic involvement at the time of primary staging. Therefore, it is recommended in the guidelines of the European Society of Urogenital Radiology (ESUR) in suspected stage IV disease (advanced ovarian cancer) and in the presence of an indeterminate lymph node appearance [48].

The most important role of FDG PET/CT in ovarian cancer patients is the evaluation of tumour recurrence, especially when CA-125 levels are rising, and conventional imaging is inconclusive or negative [44, 48, 77, 117]. Referring to the ACR Appropriateness Criteria®, in this situation, FDG PET/CT is considered 'usually appropriate' [73] and is also recommended by RCR [129].

FDG PET/CT might provide prognostic value, which gives an insight into tumour biology and behaviour. There is a significant association between the primary tumour's SUVmax and the FIGO stage. FDG PET/CT can improve patient management through the detection of previously unknown metastatic lesions as well as evaluating the risk of residual cancer following surgical treatment.

21.2.13.2 Therapy Response Assessment

The role of FDG PET/CT for therapy response assessment has been investigated in several studies, showing promising results. CHIVA trial demonstrated that FDG PET/CT aids in evaluating early tumour response and predicting second-look surgery outcomes [186]. On the other hand, another prospective study demonstrated no additional value of FDG PET/CT over contrast-enhanced CT after neoadjuvant chemotherapy in advanced ovarian cancer patients. FDG PET/CT has been recommended as considered imaging modality by NCCN guidelines for treatment response assessment after primary or adjuvant chemotherapy [187].

21.2.14 Testicular Cancer

21.2.14.1 Diagnosis, Staging and Restaging

Testicular cancers are rare malignancies that primarily affect young and middle-aged men. They are classified into either germ cell tumours and non-germ cell tumours, the latter group including stromal tumours, lymphomas and metastases. The majority of testicular cancers are germ cell tumours, which are further subdivided into seminoma and non-seminomatous germ cell tumours (NSGCT) [102].

The NSGCT group consists of embryonal carcinoma, teratoma, yolk sac tumor, and choriocarcinoma showing varying aggressiveness. Mature teratomas typically do not show increased FDG uptake due to their low proliferation rate [5]. As mature teratoma is found in 30–45% of resected residual masses in NSGCT patients, this contributes significantly to false-negative results in PET scans prior to surgical resection. The presence of mature teratoma in residual lesions of seminoma patients is much lower (<5%). Therefore, FDG PET/CT plays a significant role in the evaluation of patients with residual seminoma as compared to those with residual NSGCT [37].

According to ESMO guideline, FDG PET/CT is not recommended as a routine imaging modality for the primary staging of germ cell tumours due to insufficient supporting evidence [188]. In contrast, FDG PET/CT is most helpful in the context of suspected tumour recurrence, particularly in cases where relapse is indicated by elevated tumour marker levels despite normal findings on conventional imaging and for the assessment of chemotherapy response. FDG PET/CT scan is recommended at least 6 weeks after completion of chemotherapy in patients who have residual tumours larger than 3 cm. Given its high negative predictive value of FDG PET/CT (>90%), patients with negative PET results might be followed without requiring any further immediate intervention.

21.2.14.2 Therapy Response Assessment

Therapy response has been extensively evaluated in seminoma patients with residual tumour masses following chemotherapy, particularly when viable tumour tissue is suspected. Treglia et al. published a systematic review and meta-analysis referring to this question—pooled sensitivity and specificity of FDG PET or PET/CT were 78% and 86%, respectively; FDG showed a high NPV of 94% with a moderate PPV of 58% and a high accuracy of 84%. In addition, they found a significantly higher sensitivity for patients with residual masses > 3 cm as compared to those < 3 cm (89% vs. 47%) [135].

Thus, the main indication of FDG PET/CT in testicular cancer is the differentiation of residual tumour from fibrosis in seminoma patients, in particular in lesions > 3 cm, as also recommended by CCO Cancer Care Ontario [20] and RCR [129]. In the assessment of residual tumour tissue after chemotherapy FDG PET/CT should be performed no earlier than 6 weeks after the completion of the treatment, as earlier imaging may lead to false-positive results due to inflammation following therapy. In cases with positive PET scan, the probability of residual seminoma is high and a biopsy should be considered before proceeding with additional treatment, such as radiotherapy or surgical resection [102].

There might be a future role for FDG PET/CT in the assessment of response to Cisplatin, Etoposide and Bleomycin (PEB) chemotherapy in metastatic seminoma patients, as Nechhi et al. pointed out: after 2 cycles of PEB 72.9% of the included 37 patients achieved a complete response (CR) and none of them relapsed (median follow-up of 18 months)—the authors concluded that patients showing CR on PET/CT scan do not need additional treatment after (according to risk stratification 3 or 4 cycles of) PEB [101]. GETUG SEMITEP Trial demonstrated the feasibility of omission of two additional cycles of chemotherapy in metastatic seminoma patients with negative FDG PET/CT after two cycles of chemotherapy [189].

21.2.15 Penile Cancer

21.2.15.1 Diagnosis, Staging and Restaging

Penile cancer is one of the rarest malignancies with a low incidence (≤1 per 100,000), which increases with age, with a peak during the sixth decade [55, 104]. The following section focuses on penile squamous cell carcinoma, which represents the vast majority of penile cancer subtypes (95%) [104].

As metastatic involvement of regional lymph nodes is a strong prognostic factor (excellent prognosis in N0-patients with cure in up to 90% [39, 104], invasive lymph node staging is required in patients at intermediate or high risk (intermediate risk: not well-differentiated pT1; high risk: pT2 or higher plus all G3 tumours) of lymphatic spread, that is, either modified radical inguinal lymphadenectomy (ILND) or dynamic sentinel node biopsy (DSNB) [55]. In enlarged palpable inguinal lymph nodes, the presence of metastases is more likely, but even in clinically unsuspicious lymph nodes, micrometastases occur with a frequency of about 20–25% [39, 55]. Despite its poorer prognosis, a cure is still possible in lymph node-positive disease—for this reason, improved imaging tools are needed to identify those patients. Due to low sensitivities for smaller metastases, FDG PET/CT is not recommended for cN0 patients [104]. Though there was an attempt by a Danish group to combine FDG PET/CT with sentinel node biopsy in cN0-patients and this combined approach showed a sensitivity of 94.4% [68]. In another prospective study, 41 cN0-patients underwent FDG PET/CT prior to bilateral modified or radical ILND—FDG PET/CT showed a high sensitivity but moderate specificity with 80% and 68%, respectively, as well as a high NPV of 91% (although low PPV of 44%). The authors concluded that FDG PET/CT cannot replace invasive nodal staging [40].

In clinically suspicious palpable lymph nodes FDG PET/CT can identify metastases and confirm lymph node involvement [55]. In nodal-positive patients, radical ILND with curative intention is indicated. FDG PET/CT might also help to identify pelvic lymph node metastases, if these are initially suspicious due to enlargement [138].

In follow-up, FDG PET/CT can improve the detection of early regional lymph node involvement and reveal more distant metastases, especially in patients with inguinal node-positive penile cancer (ESMO, see Van Poppel et al. [138]). In a recent study, Zhang et al. showed an overall sensitivity of 82% and specificity of 93% for the detection of distant metastases by FDG PET/CT in a patient-based analysis in 42 stage III- and IV-patients with advanced penile cancer, mostly in the clinical setting of restaging/evaluation of suspected recurrence (65% of the patients) [155].

21.2.16 Prostate Cancer

21.2.16.1 Diagnosis, Staging and Restaging

FDG PET/CT has demonstrated limited sensitivity for detecting differentiated prostate cancer and for imaging recurrent disease, as shown in various studies. However, incidental FDG uptake in the prostate gland warrants further investigation to rule out prostate cancer. Although the role of FDG PET/CT in prostate cancer is limited due to low glucose uptake of prostate cancer, recent studies highlighted an expanded role for FDG PET/CT, particularly in metastatic castrate resistant prostate cancer, which tends to exhibit high FDG avidity. In these cases, FDG PET/CT is an important tool to predict overall survival and treatment response rates of radionuclide treatments. Increased FDG uptake is most commonly observed in dedifferentiated and aggressive forms of prostate cancer, often associated with Gleason score >7, and the sensitivity for the detection of metastases increases in parallel with increasing serum PSA levels (for more information see the chapter concerning molecular imaging of prostate cancer in this book).

21.2.17 Bladder Cancer

21.2.17.1 Diagnosis/Detection and Staging

Bladder cancer is the tenth most common cancer type worldwide, with smoking being its most important risk factor. Most patients present with painless haematuria. The most crucial prognostic factor in bladder cancer is muscle invasiveness, which is strongly associated with nodal or distant metastases. Due to high physiological FDG uptake in the urinary tract and elevated background activity in the pelvis, the primary detection of bladder cancer and distinguishing small perivesical lymph nodes remain challenging.

In patients with muscle-invasive bladder cancer, FDG PET CT has not been recommended as a routine imaging modality according to the ESMO guideline; however, a high specificity rate of FDG PET/CT is highlighted for lymph node staging despite its equivocal sensitivity [190]. Conversely, according to a consensus statement by EAU and ESMO, FDG PET/CT should be performed in oligometastatic disease staging prior to planning radical treatment [191].

Recent studies have demonstrated the utility of FDG PET/CT in the detection of residual and recurrent disease. FDG PET/CT might influence the treatment strategy in post-treatment restaging aiding in early assessment of neoadjuvant chemotherapy. Zattoni et al. revealed superior diagnostic accuracy of FDG PET/CT over conventional imaging for the detection of recurrent disease. According to a retrospective, multicentre study (n = 287), sensitivity, specificity and accuracy of FDG PET/CT were 94%, 79% and 91%, respectively [192].

21.2.18 Cancer of Unknown Primary

21.2.18.1 Diagnosis/Detection and Staging

About 3–5% of all malignancies are classified as cancers of unknown primary (CUP) [45], mostly associated with a poor prognosis. By definition, CUPs present as histologically proven metastatic disease for which the site of origin cannot be identified at the time of diagnosis, despite extensive diagnostic work-up. The most common histological subtype of CUPs is adenocarcinoma, accounting for 70–80% of all cases, followed by undifferentiated carcinomas, squamous cell carcinomas and neuroendocrine carcinomas. The primary tumour often remains undetected on conventional imaging; thus, PET may improve the detection rate of CUPs and potentially improve patient outcome by optimising treatment planning. Recent meta-analyses has shown that lung tumours are the leading identified primary site in CUP cases, responsible for 29% of all cases, while 33% of patients remained classified as CUPs with no primary lesion detected on FDG PET/CT [193]. The detection rate of FDG PET/CT was 0.74 in patients with predominant brain metastases; 0.54 in patients with liver predominant disease, and the detection rate was low in patients with lymph node or soft-tissue predominant disease (0.35–0.37).

A distinct sub-group in the group within the heterogeneous group of malignancies includes patients with neck lymph node metastases from an occult primary tumour, accounting for up to 10% of all patients with CUP [19]. Since the most frequent histological subtype in neck lymph node metastases is squamous cell carcinoma, particularly when the upper neck is involved [19], and given that squamous cell carcinomas are typically FDG avid, there is a high probability of finding the primary tumour by virtue of FDG PET/CT, at least if the tumour size is not below the resolution limit. Zhu et al. conducted a meta-analysis including 246 patients and with 44, 97 and 68% for detection rate, sensitivity and specificity, respectively, they found a moderate detection rate, a high sensitivity and a low specificity [156].

Although FDG PET/CT is considered as optional imaging modality in the routine diagnostic work-up of CUP according to recent ESMO guideline, FDG PET/CT is specifically recommended in patients with single or oligometastatic disease to rule out additional metastases; and also in patients with cervical lymph node metastasis suspicious for head and neck cancer [194]. Currently, in patients with extra-cervical CUP, the evidence supporting routine use of FDG PET/CT remains limited. Consequently, most guidelines do not recommend its first-line use, except for the German Society of Haematology and Oncology, which advocates for FDG PET/CT as a preferred method for the primary tumour detection over conventional CT thorax or abdomen [64]. RCR recommends FDG PET/CT for the 'detection of the primary site when imaging and histopathology has failed to show a primary site, in cases where the primary site of tumour would impact chemotherapy decisions' [129].

A meta-analysis by Kwee et al. reported a primary tumour detection rate of 37%. Lung, oropharyngeal and pancreatic cancer were reported to represent the most frequently detected primary tumours [79]. Another meta-analysis was conducted by Moller et al., who found a detection rate of 39.5% for the primary site in patients with extra-cervical CUP. The pooled estimates for sensitivity, specificity and accuracy were 87%, 88% and 87.5%, respectively. The lungs were again the most commonly detected primary tumour site with 50% [100]. A more recent meta-analysis enrolling 1942 patients came to a similar result with an overall detection rate of 40.93%—the authors concluded that up-front application of FDG PET/CT might have a role in CUP patients by obviating many futile diagnostic procedures [16].

References

1. Abouzied MM, Fathala A, Alsugair A, Muhaideb AIA, Qahtani MHA (2017) Role of fluorodeoxyglucose-positron emission tomography/computed tomography in the evaluation of head and neck carcinoma. World J Nucl Med 16(4):257–265
2. Adams HJ, Kwee TC, de Keizer B, Fijnheer R, de Klerk JM, Nievelstein RA (2014) FDG PET/CT for the detection of bone marrow involvement in diffuse large B-cell lymphoma: systematic review and meta-analysis. Eur J Nucl Med Mol Imaging 41(3):565–574

3. Ajani JA, D'Amico TA, Almhanna K, Bentrem DJ, Besh S, Chao J et al (2015) Esophageal and esophagogastric junction cancers, version 1.2015. J Natl Compr Cancer Netw 13(2):194–227
4. Alavi A, Reivich M (2002) Guest editorial: the conception of FDG-PET imaging. Semin Nucl Med 32(1):2–5
5. Albers P, Bender H, Yilmaz H, Schoeneich G, Biersack HJ, Mueller SC (1999) Positron emission tomography in the clinical staging of patients with stage I and II testicular germ cell tumors. Urology 53(4):808–811
6. Ambrosini V, Nicolini S, Caroli P, Nanni C, Massaro A, Marzola MC et al (2012) PET/CT imaging in different types of lung cancer: an overview. Eur J Radiol 81(5):988–1001
7. Ambrosini V, Zucchini G, Nicolini S, Berselli A, Nanni C, Allegri V et al (2014) ^{18}F-FDG PET/CT impact on testicular tumours clinical management. Eur J Nucl Med Mol Imaging 41(4):668–673
8. American College of Radiology (ACR) Appropriateness Criteria® (2013). https://acsearch.acr.org/list. Accessed 12 Sept 2018
9. AWMF (2018) Leitlinienprogramm Onkologie (Deutsche Krebsgesellschaft, Deutsche Krebshilfe, AWMF): Prävention, Diagnostik, Therapie und Nachsorge des Lungenkarzinoms, Langversion 1.0, 2018, AWMF-Registernummer: 020/007OL, http://leitlinienprogramm-onkologie.de/Lungenkarzinom.98.0.html. Accessed 3 Jan 2019
10. AWMF (2018) Leitlinienprogramm Onkologie (Deutsche Krebsgesellschaft, Deutsche Krebshilfe, AWMF): Diagnostik, Therapie und Nachsorge des Melanoms, Langversion 3.1, 2018, AWMF Registernummer: 032/024OL, http://www.leitlinienprogramm-onkologie.de/leitlinien/melanom/. Accessed 3 Jan 2019
11. Barrington SF, Mikhaeel NG, Kostakoglu L, Meignan M, Hutchings M, Müeller SP et al (2014) Role of imaging in the staging and response assessment of lymphoma: consensus of the International Conference on Malignant Lymphomas Imaging Working Group. J Clin Oncol 32(27):3048–3058
12. Bastiaannet E, Groen H, Jager PL, Cobben DC, van der Graaf WT, Vaalburg W et al (2004) The value of FDG-PET in the detection, grading and response to therapy of soft tissue and bone sarcomas; a systematic review and meta-analysis. Cancer Treat Rev 30(1):83–101
13. Benson AB, Venook AP, Al-Hawary MM, Cederquist L, Chen YJ, Ciombor KK et al (2018) Rectal cancer, version 2.2018, NCCN clinical practice guidelines in oncology. J Natl Compr Cancer Netw 16(7):874–901
14. Bertagna F, Biasiotto G, Orlando E, Bosio G, Giubbini R (2010) Role of ^{18}F-fluorodeoxyglucose positron emission tomography/computed tomography in patients affected by differentiated thyroid carcinoma, high thyroglobulin level, and negative ^{131}I scan: review of the literature. Jpn J Radiol 28(9):629–636
15. Borchmann P, Goergen H, Kobe C, Lohri A, Greil R, Eichenauer DA et al (2018) PET-guided treatment in patients with advanced-stage Hodgkin's lymphoma (HD18): final results of an open-label, international, randomised phase 3 trial by the German Hodgkin Study Group. Lancet 390(10114):2790–2802
16. Burglin SA, Hess S, Høilund-Carlsen PF, Gerke O (2017) ^{18}F-FDG PET/CT for detection of the primary tumor in adults with extracervical metastases from cancer of unknown primary: a systematic review and meta-analysis. Medicine (Baltimore) 96(16):e6713
17. Cacicedo J, Fernandez I, Del Hoyo O, Dolado A, Gómez-Suarez J, Hortelano E et al (2015) Should PET/CT be implemented in the routine imaging work-up of locally advanced head and neck squamous cell carcinoma? A prospective analysis. Eur J Nucl Med Mol Imaging 42(9):1378–1389
18. Caetano R, Bastos CR, de Oliveira IA, da Silva RM, Fortes CP, Pepe VL et al (2016) Accuracy of positron emission tomography and positron emission tomography-CT in the detection of differentiated thyroid cancer recurrence with negative (131) I whole-body scan results: a meta-analysis. Head Neck 38(2):316–327
19. Calabrese L, Jereczek-Fossa BA, Jassem J, Rocca A, Bruschini R, Orecchia R et al (2005) Diagnosis and management of neck metastases from an unknown primary. Acta Otorhinolaryngol Ital 25(1):2–12

20. Cancer Care Ontario (2009) https://www.cancercareontario.ca/en/guidelines-advice/types-of-cancer. Accessed 12 Sept 2018
21. Casali PG, Abecassis N, Bauer S, Biagini R, Bielack S, Bonvalot S et al (2018) Soft tissue and visceral sarcomas: ESMO-EURACAN Clinical Practice Guidelines for diagnosis, treatment and follow-up. Ann Oncol 32(11):1348–1365
22. Chaft JE, Dunphy M, Naidoo J, Travis WD, Hellmann M, Woo K et al (2016) Adaptive neoadjuvant chemotherapy guided by (18)F-FDG PET in resectable non-small cell lung cancers: the NEOSCAN trial. J Thorac Oncol 11(4):537–544
23. Chang MC, Chen JH, Liang JA, Lin CC, Yang KT, Cheng KY et al (2012) Meta-analysis: comparison of F-18 fluorodeoxyglucose-positron emission tomography and bone scintigraphy in the detection of bone metastasis in patients with lung cancer. Acad Radiol 19(3):349–357
24. Charest M, Hickeson M, Lisbona R, Novales-Diaz JA, Derbekyan V, Turcotte RE (2009) FDG PET/CT imaging in primary osseous and soft tissue sarcomas: a retrospective review of 212 cases. Eur J Nucl Med Mol Imaging 36(12):1944–1951
25. Cheng X, Li Y, Liu B, Xu Z, Bao L, Wang J (2012) 18F-FDG PET/CT and PET for evaluation of pathological response to neoadjuvant chemotherapy in breast cancer: a meta-analysis. Acta Radiol 53(6):615–627
26. Cheson BD, Fisher RI, Barrington SF, Cavalli F, Schwartz LH, Zucca E et al (2014) Recommendations for initial evaluation, staging, and response assessment of Hodgkin and non-Hodgkin lymphoma: the Lugano classification. J Clin Oncol 32(27):3059–3068
27. Cheung PK, Chin RY, Eslick GD (2016) Detecting residual/recurrent head neck squamous cell carcinomas using PET or PET/CT: systematic review and meta-analysis. Otolaryngol Head Neck Surg 154(3):421–432
28. Cho J, Choe JG, Pahk K, Choi S, Kwon HR, Eo JS et al (2017) Ratio of mediastinal lymph node SUV to primary tumor SUV in ^{18}F-FDG PET/CT for nodal staging in non-small-cell lung cancer. Nucl Med Mol Imaging 51(2):140–146
29. Cho SF, Chang CC, Liu YC, Chang CS, Hsiao HH, Liu TC et al (2015) Utilization of ^{18}F-FDG PET/CT as a staging tool in patients with newly diagnosed lymphoma. Kaohsiung J Med Sci 31(3):130–137
30. Choi SJ, Jung KP, Lee SS, Park YS, Lee SM, Bae SK (2016) Clinical usefulness of F-18 FDG PET/CT in papillary thyroid cancer with negative radioiodine scan and elevated thyroglobulin level or positive anti-thyroglobulin antibody. Nucl Med Mol Imaging 50(2):130–136
31. Chow WA (2007) Update on chondrosarcomas. Curr Opin Oncol 19(4):371–376
32. Coindre JM, Terrier P, Guillou L, Le Doussal V, Collin F, Ranchère D et al (2001) Predictive value of grade for metastasis development in the main histologic types of adult soft tissue sarcomas: a study of 1240 patients from the French Federation of Cancer Centers Sarcoma Group. Cancer 91(10):1914–1926
33. Coit DG, Thompson JA, Algazi A, Andtbacka R, Bichakjian CK, Carson WE et al (2016) Melanoma, version 2.2016, NCCN clinical practice guidelines in oncology. J Natl Compr Cancer Netw 14(4):450–473
34. Colevas AD, Yom SS, Pfister DG, Spencer S, Adelstein D, Adkins D et al (2018) NCCN guidelines insights: head and neck cancers, version 1.2018. J Natl Compr Cancer Netw 16(5):479–490
35. Czernin J, Benz MR, Allen-Auerbach MS (2010) PET/CT imaging: the incremental value of assessing the glucose metabolic phenotype and the structure of cancers in a single examination. Eur J Radiol 73(3):470–480
36. de Groot PM, Wu CC, Carter BW, Munden RF (2018) The epidemiology of lung cancer. Transl Lung Cancer Res 7(3):220–233
37. De Santis M, Pont J (2004) The role of positron emission tomography in germ cell cancer. World J Urol 22(1):41–46
38. De Wever W, Ceyssens S, Mortelmans L, Stroobants S, Marchal G, Bogaert J et al (2007) Additional value of PET-CT in the staging of lung cancer: comparison with CT alone, PET alone and visual correlation of PET and CT. Eur Radiol 17(1):23–32

39. Djajadiningrat RS, Graafland NM, van Werkhoven E, Meinhardt W, Bex A, van der Poel HG et al (2014) Contemporary management of regional nodes in penile cancer—improvement of survival? J Urol 191(1):68–73
40. Dräger DL, Heuschkel M, Protzel C, Erbersdobler A, Krause BJ, Hakenberg OW et al (2018) [18F]FDG PET/CT for assessing inguinal lymph nodes in patients with penile cancer—correlation with histopathology after inguinal lymphadenectomy. Nuklearmedizin 57(1):26–30
41. Dummer R, Hauschild A, Lindenblatt N, Pentheroudakis G, Keilholz U, Committee EG (2015) Cutaneous melanoma: ESMO Clinical Practice Guidelines for diagnosis, treatment and follow-up. Ann Oncol 26(Suppl 5):v126–v132
42. Eichenauer DA, Aleman BMP, André M, Federico M, Hutchings M, Illidge T et al (2018) Hodgkin lymphoma: ESMO Clinical Practice Guidelines for diagnosis, treatment and follow-up. Ann Oncol 29(Supplement_4):iv19–iv29
43. Engelmann BE, Loft A, Kjær A, Nielsen HJ, Berthelsen AK, Binderup T et al (2014) Positron emission tomography/computed tomography for optimized colon cancer staging and follow up. Scand J Gastroenterol 49(2):191–201
44. Fischerova D, Burgetova A (2014) Imaging techniques for the evaluation of ovarian cancer. Best Pract Res Clin Obstet Gynaecol 28(5):697–720
45. Fizazi K, Greco FA, Pavlidis N, Daugaard G, Oien K, Pentheroudakis G et al (2015) Cancers of unknown primary site: ESMO Clinical Practice Guidelines for diagnosis, treatment and follow-up. Ann Oncol 26(Suppl 5):v133–v138
46. Fletcher C, Unni K, Mertens F (2002) WHO classification of tumours: pathology and genetics of tumours of soft tissue and bone. IARC Press, Lyon
47. Fletcher JW, Djulbegovic B, Soares HP, Siegel BA, Lowe VJ, Lyman GH et al (2008) Recommendations on the use of ^{18}F-FDG PET in oncology. J Nucl Med 49(3):480–508
48. Forstner R, Sala E, Kinkel K, Spencer JA, Radiology ESoU (2010) ESUR guidelines: ovarian cancer staging and follow-up. Eur Radiol 20(12):2773–2780
49. Fowler KJ, Kaur H, Cash BD, Feig BW, Gage KL, Garcia EM et al (2017) ACR appropriateness criteria® pretreatment staging of colorectal cancer. J Am Coll Radiol 14(5S):S234–S244
50. Frilling A, Görges R, Tecklenborg K, Gassmann P, Bockhorn M, Clausen M et al (2000) Value of preoperative diagnostic modalities in patients with recurrent thyroid carcinoma. Surgery 128(6):1067–1074
51. Fuglø HM, Jørgensen SM, Loft A, Hovgaard D, Petersen MM (2012) The diagnostic and prognostic value of ^{18}F-FDG PET/CT in the initial assessment of high-grade bone and soft tissue sarcoma. A retrospective study of 89 patients. Eur J Nucl Med Mol Imaging 39(9):1416–1424
52. Gallagher BM, Ansari A, Atkins H, Casella V, Christman DR, Fowler JS et al (1977) Radiopharmaceuticals XXVII. ^{18}F-labeled 2-deoxy-2-fluoro-d-glucose as a radiopharmaceutical for measuring regional myocardial glucose metabolism in vivo: tissue distribution and imaging studies in animals. J Nucl Med 18(10):990–996
53. Goense L, van Rossum PS, Reitsma JB, Lam MG, Meijer GJ, van Vulpen M et al (2015) Diagnostic performance of ^{18}F-FDG PET and PET/CT for the detection of recurrent esophageal cancer after treatment with curative intent: a systematic review and meta-analysis. J Nucl Med 56(7):995–1002
54. Groheux D (2017) FDG-PET/CT for systemic staging of patients with newly diagnosed breast cancer. Eur J Nucl Med Mol Imaging 44(9):1417–1419
55. Hakenberg OW, Compérat EM, Minhas S, Necchi A, Protzel C, Watkin N (2015) EAU guidelines on penile cancer: 2014 update. Eur Urol 67(1):142–150
56. Hassanzadeh-Rad A, Yousefifard M, Katal S, Asady H, Fard-Esfahani A, Moghadas Jafari A et al (2016) The value of (18) F-fluorodeoxyglucose positron emission tomography for prediction of treatment response in gastrointestinal stromal tumors: a systematic review and meta-analysis. J Gastroenterol Hepatol 31(5):929–935
57. Haugen BR, Alexander EK, Bible KC, Doherty GM, Mandel SJ, Nikiforov YE et al (2016) 2015 American Thyroid Association Management Guidelines for adult patients with thyroid nodules and differentiated thyroid cancer: the American thyroid association guidelines task force on thyroid nodules and differentiated thyroid cancer. Thyroid 26(1):1–133

58. Helsen N, Van den Wyngaert T, Carp L, Stroobants S (2018) FDG-PET/CT for treatment response assessment in head and neck squamous cell carcinoma: a systematic review and meta-analysis of diagnostic performance. Eur J Nucl Med Mol Imaging 45(6):1063–1071
59. Herrmann K, Benz MR, Krause BJ, Pomykala KL, Buck AK, Czernin J (2011) (18)F-FDG-PET/CT in evaluating response to therapy in solid tumors: where we are and where we can go. Q J Nucl Med Mol Imaging 55(6):620–632
60. Herrmann K, Ott K, Buck AK, Lordick F, Wilhelm D, Souvatzoglou M et al (2007) Imaging gastric cancer with PET and the radiotracers ^{18}F-FLT and ^{18}F-FDG: a comparative analysis. J Nucl Med 48(12):1945–1950
61. Hongtao L, Hui Z, Bingshun W, Xiaojin W, Zhiyu W, Shuier Z et al (2012) ^{18}F-FDG positron emission tomography for the assessment of histological response to neoadjuvant chemotherapy in osteosarcomas: a meta-analysis. Surg Oncol 21(4):e165–e170
62. Hoppe RT, Advani RH, Ai WZ, Ambinder RF, Aoun P, Bello CM et al (2017) Hodgkin lymphoma version 1.2017, NCCN clinical practice guidelines in oncology. J Natl Compr Cancer Netw 15(5):608–638
63. Huang SH, O'Sullivan B, Xu W, Zhao H, Chen DD, Ringash J et al (2013) Temporal nodal regression and regional control after primary radiation therapy for N2-N3 head-and-neck cancer stratified by HPV status. Int J Radiat Oncol Biol Phys 87(5):1078–1085
64. Hübner G, Borner M, Neben K, Stöger H (2018) CUP-Syndrom—Krebserkrankungen mit unbekanntem Primärtumor. DGHO (Deutsche Gesellschaft für Hämatologie und Onkologie), Onkopedia. https://www.onkopedia.com/de/onkopedia/guidelines/cup-syndrom-krebserkrankungen-mit-unbekanntem-primaertumor/@@view/html/index.html. Accessed 1 Sept 2018
65. Ioannidis JP, Lau J (2003) ^{18}F-FDG PET for the diagnosis and grading of soft-tissue sarcoma: a meta-analysis. J Nucl Med 44(5):717–724
66. Jadvar H, Colletti PM, Delgado-Bolton R, Esposito G, Krause BJ, Iagaru AH et al (2017) Appropriate use criteria for ^{18}F-FDG-PET/CT in restaging and treatment response assessment of malignant disease. J Nucl Med 58(12):2026–2037
67. Jakić-Razumović J, Aurer I (2002) The World Health Organization classification of lymphomas. Croat Med J 43(5):527–534
68. Jakobsen JK, Alslev L, Ipsen P, Costa JC, Krarup KP, Sommer P et al (2016) DaPeCa-3: promising results of sentinel node biopsy combined with (18) F-fluorodeoxyglucose positron emission tomography/computed tomography in clinically lymph node-negative patients with penile cancer—a national study from Denmark. BJU Int 118(1):102–111
69. Johnson P, Federico M, Kirkwood A, Fosså A, Berkahn L, Carella A et al (2016) Adapted treatment guided by interim PET-CT scan in advanced Hodgkin's lymphoma. N Engl J Med 374(25):2419–2429
70. Jung NY, Yoo IR, Kang BJ, Kim SH, Chae BJ, Seo YY (2016) Clinical significance of FDG-PET/CT at the postoperative surveillance in the breast cancer patients. Breast Cancer 23(1):141–148
71. Jung W, Jang JY, Kang MJ, Chang YR, Shin YC, Chang J et al (2016) The clinical usefulness of ^{18}F-fluorodeoxyglucose positron emission tomography-computed tomography (PET-CT) in follow-up of curatively resected pancreatic cancer patients. HPB (Oxford) 18(1):57–64
72. Kamiyama Y, Aihara R, Nakabayashi T, Mochiki E, Asao T, Kuwano H et al (2005) ^{18}F-fluorodeoxyglucose positron emission tomography: useful technique for predicting malignant potential of gastrointestinal stromal tumors. World J Surg 29(11):1429–1435
73. Kang SK, Reinhold C, Atri M, Benson CB, Bhosale PR, Jhingran A et al (2018) ACR Appropriateness Criteria® staging and follow-up of ovarian cancer. J Am Coll Radiol 15(5S):S198–S207
74. Kitajima K, Nakajo M, Kaida H, Minamimoto R, Hirata K, Tsurusaki M et al (2017) Present and future roles of FDG-PET/CT imaging in the management of gastrointestinal cancer: an update. Nagoya J Med Sci 79(4):527–543

75. Koolen BB, van der Leij F, Vogel WV, Rutgers EJ, Vrancken Peeters MJ, Elkhuizen PH et al (2014) Accuracy of ^{18}F-FDG PET/CT for primary tumor visualization and staging in T1 breast cancer. Acta Oncol 53(1):50–57
76. Koolen BB, Vrancken Peeters MJ, Aukema TS, Vogel WV, Oldenburg HS, van der Hage JA et al (2012) ^{18}F-FDG PET/CT as a staging procedure in primary stage II and III breast cancer: comparison with conventional imaging techniques. Breast Cancer Res Treat 131(1):117–126
77. Kumar Dhingra V, Kand P, Basu S (2012) Impact of FDG-PET and -PET/CT imaging in the clinical decision-making of ovarian carcinoma: an evidence-based approach. Womens Health (Lond) 8(2):191–203
78. Kung BT, Yong TK, Tong CM (2017) The pearl of FDG PET/CT in preoperative assessment of patients with potentially operable non-small-cell lung cancer and its clinical impact. World J Nucl Med 16(1):21–25
79. Kwee TC, Kwee RM (2009) Combined FDG-PET/CT for the detection of unknown primary tumors: systematic review and meta-analysis. Eur Radiol 19(3):731–744
80. Lagergren J, Smyth E, Cunningham D, Lagergren P (2017) Oesophageal cancer. Lancet 390(10110):2383–2396
81. Lee AY, Choi SJ, Jung KP, Park JS, Lee SM, Bae SK (2014) Characteristics of metastatic mediastinal lymph nodes of non-small cell lung cancer on preoperative F-18 FDG PET/CT. Nucl Med Mol Imaging 48(1):41–46
82. Lee JH, Lee MR (2014) Positron emission tomography/computed tomography in the staging of colon cancer. Ann Coloproctol 30(1):23–27
83. Lewin J, Sayers L, Kee D, Walpole I, Sanelli A, Te Marvelde L et al (2018) Surveillance imaging with FDG-PET/CT in the post-operative follow-up of stage 3 melanoma. Ann Oncol 29(7):1569–1574
84. Li P, Liu Q, Wang C, Wang T, Liu J, Huang G et al (2016) Fluorine-18-fluorodeoxyglucose positron emission tomography to evaluate recurrent gastric cancer after surgical resection: a systematic review and meta-analysis. Ann Nucl Med 30(3):179–187
85. Liu F, Zhang Q, Zhu D, Li Z, Li J, Wang B et al (2015) Performance of positron emission tomography and positron emission tomography/computed tomography using fluorine-18-fluorodeoxyglucose for the diagnosis, staging, and recurrence assessment of bone sarcoma: a systematic review and meta-analysis. Medicine (Baltimore) 94(36):e1462
86. Lordick F, Ott K, Krause BJ, Weber WA, Becker K, Stein HJ et al (2007) PET to assess early metabolic response and to guide treatment of adenocarcinoma of the oesophagogastric junction: the MUNICON phase II trial. Lancet Oncol 8(9):797–805
87. Lu YY, Chen JH, Chien CR, Chen WT, Tsai SC, Lin WY et al (2013) Use of FDG-PET or PET/CT to detect recurrent colorectal cancer in patients with elevated CEA: a systematic review and meta-analysis. Int J Color Dis 28(8):1039–1047
88. Lu YY, Chen JH, Liang JA, Chu S, Lin WY, Kao CH (2014) ^{18}F-FDG PET or PET/CT for detecting extensive disease in small-cell lung cancer: a systematic review and meta-analysis. Nucl Med Commun 35(7):697–703
89. MacManus MP, Hicks RJ, Matthews JP, Hogg A, McKenzie AF, Wirth A et al (2001) High rate of detection of unsuspected distant metastases by pet in apparent stage III non-small-cell lung cancer: implications for radical radiation therapy. Int J Radiat Oncol Biol Phys 50(2):287–293
90. Maffione AM, Lopci E, Bluemel C, Giammarile F, Herrmann K, Rubello D (2015) Diagnostic accuracy and impact on management of (18)F-FDG PET and PET/CT in colorectal liver metastasis: a meta-analysis and systematic review. Eur J Nucl Med Mol Imaging 42(1):152–163
91. Maffione AM, Marzola MC, Capirci C, Colletti PM, Rubello D (2015) Value of (18)F-FDG PET for predicting response to neoadjuvant therapy in rectal cancer: systematic review and meta-analysis. AJR Am J Roentgenol 204(6):1261–1268
92. Malle P, Sorschag M, Gallowitsch HJ (2012) FDG PET and FDG PET/CT in patients with gastrointestinal stromal tumours. Wien Med Wochenschr 162(19–20):423–429

93. Mamede M, Higashi T, Kitaichi M, Ishizu K, Ishimori T, Nakamoto Y et al (2005) [18F]FDG uptake and PCNA, Glut-1, and Hexokinase-II expressions in cancers and inflammatory lesions of the lung. Neoplasia 7(4):369–379
94. Marcus C, Ciarallo A, Tahari AK, Mena E, Koch W, Wahl RL et al (2014) Head and neck PET/CT: therapy response interpretation criteria (Hopkins Criteria)—interreader reliability, accuracy, and survival outcomes. J Nucl Med 55(9):1411–1416
95. Maziak DE, Darling GE, Inculet RI, Gulenchyn KY, Driedger AA, Ung YC et al (2009) Positron emission tomography in staging early lung cancer: a randomized trial. Ann Intern Med 151(4):221–228. W-48
96. Mehanna H, Wong WL, McConkey CC, Rahman JK, Robinson M, Hartley AG et al (2016) PET-CT surveillance versus neck dissection in advanced head and neck cancer. N Engl J Med 374(15):1444–1454
97. Mena E, Taghipour M, Sheikhbahaei S, Mirpour S, Xiao J, Subramaniam RM (2016) ^{18}F-FDG PET/CT and melanoma: value of fourth and subsequent posttherapy follow-up scans for patient management. Clin Nucl Med 41(9):e403–e409
98. Metser U, Dudebout J, Baetz T, Hodgson DC, Langer DL, MacCrostie P et al (2017) [18 F]-FDG PET/CT in the staging and management of indolent lymphoma: a prospective multicenter PET registry study. Cancer 123(15):2860–2866
99. Mody RJ, Bui C, Hutchinson RJ, Yanik GA, Castle VP, Frey KA et al (2010) FDG PET imaging of childhood sarcomas. Pediatr Blood Cancer 54(2):222–227
100. Moller AK, Loft A, Berthelsen AK, Damgaard Pedersen K, Graff J, Christensen CB et al (2011) ^{18}F-FDG PET/CT as a diagnostic tool in patients with extracervical carcinoma of unknown primary site: a literature review. Oncologist 16(4):445–451
101. Necchi A, Nicolai N, Alessi A, Miceli R, Giannatempo P, Raggi D et al (2016) Interim (18) F-Fluorodeoxyglucose positron emission tomography for early metabolic assessment of response to cisplatin, etoposide, and bleomycin chemotherapy for metastatic seminoma: clinical value and future directions. Clin Genitourin Cancer 14(3):249–254
102. Oldenburg J, Fosså SD, Nuver J, Heidenreich A, Schmoll HJ, Bokemeyer C et al (2013) Testicular seminoma and non-seminoma: ESMO Clinical Practice Guidelines for diagnosis, treatment and follow-up. Ann Oncol 24(Suppl 6):vi125–vi132
103. Ott K, Schmidt T, Lordick F, Herrmann K (2014) Importance of PET in surgery of esophageal cancer. Chirurg 85(6):505–512
104. Ottenhof SR, Leone AR, Horenblas S, Spiess PE, Vegt E (2017) Advancements in staging and imaging for penile cancer. Curr Opin Urol 27(6):612–620
105. Pacini F, Castagna MG, Brilli L, Pentheroudakis G, Group EGW (2012) Thyroid cancer: ESMO Clinical Practice Guidelines for diagnosis, treatment and follow-up. Ann Oncol 23(Suppl 7):vii110–vii119
106. Pak K, Kim K, Kim MH, Eom JS, Lee MK, Cho JS et al (2018) A decision tree model for predicting mediastinal lymph node metastasis in non-small cell lung cancer with F-18 FDG PET/CT. PLoS One 13(2):e0193403
107. Petersen RK, Hess S, Alavi A, Høilund-Carlsen PF (2014) Clinical impact of FDG-PET/CT on colorectal cancer staging and treatment strategy. Am J Nucl Med Mol Imaging 4(5):471–482
108. Piva R, Ticconi F, Ceriani V, Scalorbi F, Fiz F, Capitanio S et al (2017) Comparative diagnostic accuracy of ^{18}F-FDG PET/CT for breast cancer recurrence. Breast Cancer (Dove Med Press) 9:461–471
109. Purandare NC, Pramesh CS, Karimundackal G, Jiwnani S, Agrawal A, Shah S et al (2014) Incremental value of ^{18}F-FDG PET/CT in therapeutic decision-making of potentially curable esophageal adenocarcinoma. Nucl Med Commun 35(8):864–869
110. Rakheja R, Makis W, Skamene S, Nahal A, Brimo F, Azoulay L et al (2012) Correlating metabolic activity on ^{18}F-FDG PET/CT with histopathologic characteristics of osseous and soft-tissue sarcomas: a retrospective review of 136 patients. AJR Am J Roentgenol 198(6):1409–1416

111. Rodriguez Rivera AM, Alabbas H, Ramjaun A, Meguerditchian AN (2014) Value of positron emission tomography scan in stage III cutaneous melanoma: a systematic review and meta-analysis. Surg Oncol 23(1):11–16
112. Rodriguez E, Lilenbaum RC (2010) Small cell lung cancer: past, present, and future. Curr Oncol Rep 12(5):327–334
113. Rogasch JM, Apostolova I, Steffen IG, Steinkrüger FL, Genseke P, Riedel S et al (2016) Standardized visual reading of F18-FDG-PET in patients with non-small cell lung cancer scheduled for preoperative thoracic lymph node staging. Eur J Radiol 85(8):1345–1350
114. Ronellenfitsch U, Wängler B, Niedermoser S, Dimitrakopoulou-Strauss A, Hohenberger P (2014) Importance of PET for surgery of gastrointestinal stromal tumors. Chirurg 85(6):493–499
115. Sachpekidis C, Anwar H, Winkler J, Kopp-Schneider A, Larribere L, Haberkorn U et al (2018) The role of interim ^{18}F-FDG PET/CT in prediction of response to ipilimumab treatment in metastatic melanoma. Eur J Nucl Med Mol Imaging 45(8):1289–1296
116. Schreyögg J, Weller J, Stargardt T, Herrmann K, Bluemel C, Dechow T et al (2010) Cost-effectiveness of hybrid PET/CT for staging of non-small cell lung cancer. J Nucl Med 51(11):1668–1675
117. Schwarz JK, Grigsby PW, Dehdashti F, Delbeke D (2009) The role of ^{18}F-FDG PET in assessing therapy response in cancer of the cervix and ovaries. J Nucl Med 50(Suppl 1):64S–73S
118. Sheikhbahaei S, Taghipour M, Ahmad R, Fakhry C, Kiess AP, Chung CH et al (2015) Diagnostic accuracy of follow-up FDG PET or PET/CT in patients with head and neck cancer after definitive treatment: a systematic review and meta-analysis. AJR Am J Roentgenol 205(3):629–639
119. Siegel RL, Miller KD, Jemal A (2017) Cancer statistics, 2017. CA Cancer J Clin 67(1):7–30
120. Signorelli M, Guerra L, Pirovano C, Crivellaro C, Fruscio R, Buda A et al (2013) Detection of nodal metastases by ^{18}F-FDG PET/CT in apparent early stage ovarian cancer: a prospective study. Gynecol Oncol 131(2):395–399
121. Silvestri GA, Gonzalez AV, Jantz MA, Margolis ML, Gould MK, Tanoue LT et al (2013) Methods for staging non-small cell lung cancer: diagnosis and management of lung cancer, 3rd ed: American College of Chest Physicians evidence-based clinical practice guidelines. Chest 143(5 Suppl):e211S–ee50S
122. Silvestri GA, Gould MK, Margolis ML, Tanoue LT, McCrory D, Toloza E et al (2007) Noninvasive staging of non-small cell lung cancer: ACCP evidenced-based clinical practice guidelines (2nd edn). Chest 132(3 Suppl):178S–201S
123. Singnurkar A, Wang J, Joshua AM, Langer DL, Metser U (2016) ^{18}F-FDG-PET/CT in the staging and management of melanoma: a prospective multicenter Ontario PET registry study. Clin Nucl Med 41(3):189–193
124. Sobic-Saranovic D, Petrusic I, Artiko V, Pavlovic S, Subotic D, Saranovic D et al (2015) Comparison of ^{18}F-FDG PET/CT and MDCT for staging/restaging of non-small cell lung cancer. Neoplasma 62(2):295–301
125. Stahl A, Ott K, Weber WA, Becker K, Link T, Siewert JR et al (2003) FDG PET imaging of locally advanced gastric carcinomas: correlation with endoscopic and histopathological findings. Eur J Nucl Med Mol Imaging 30(2):288–295
126. Sun R, Tang X, Yang Y, Zhang C (2015) (18)FDG-PET/CT for the detection of regional nodal metastasis in patients with head and neck cancer: a meta-analysis. Oral Oncol 51(4):314–320
127. Sun Z, Yi YL, Liu Y, Xiong JP, He CZ (2015) Comparison of whole-body PET/PET-CT and conventional imaging procedures for distant metastasis staging in patients with breast cancer: a meta-analysis. Eur J Gynaecol Oncol 36(6):672–676
128. Tang S, Huang G, Liu J, Liu T, Treven L, Song S et al (2011) Usefulness of ^{18}F-FDG PET, combined FDG-PET/CT and EUS in diagnosing primary pancreatic carcinoma: a meta-analysis. Eur J Radiol 78(1):142–150
129. The Royal College Of Radiologists; Royal College Of Physicians Of London; Royal College Of Physicians And Surgeons Of Glasgow; Royal College Of Physicians Of Edinburgh; British Nuclear Medicine Society; Administration Of Radioactive Substances Advisory Committee

(2016) Evidence-based indications for the use of PET-CT in the United Kingdom 2016. Clin Radiol 71(7):e171–e188

130. Tian F, Shen G, Deng Y, Diao W, Jia Z (2017) The accuracy of ^{18}F-FDG PET/CT in predicting the pathological response to neoadjuvant chemotherapy in patients with breast cancer: a meta-analysis and systematic review. Eur Radiol 27(11):4786–4796
131. Tönnies S, Bauer TT, Misch D, Boch C, Blum T, Bittner RC et al (2012) Staging with ^{18}F-FDG-PET/CT influences stage-specific survival in advanced non-small cell lung cancer (NSCLC). Pneumologie 66(4):212–217
132. Topkan E, Parlak C, Yapar AF (2013) FDG-PET/CT-based restaging may alter initial management decisions and clinical outcomes in patients with locally advanced pancreatic carcinoma planned to undergo chemoradiotherapy. Cancer Imaging 13(3):423–428
133. Torre LA, Bray F, Siegel RL, Ferlay J, Lortet-Tieulent J, Jemal A (2015) Global cancer statistics, 2012. CA Cancer J Clin 65(2):87–108
134. Treglia G, Mirk P, Stefanelli A, Rufini V, Giordano A, Bonomo L (2012) ^{18}F-Fluorodeoxyglucose positron emission tomography in evaluating treatment response to imatinib or other drugs in gastrointestinal stromal tumors: a systematic review. Clin Imaging 36(3):167–175
135. Treglia G, Sadeghi R, Annunziata S, Caldarella C, Bertagna F, Giovanella L (2014) Diagnostic performance of fluorine-18-fluorodeoxyglucose positron emission tomography in the post-chemotherapy management of patients with seminoma: systematic review and meta-analysis. Biomed Res Int 2014:852681
136. Van Cutsem E, Cervantes A, Adam R, Sobrero A, Van Krieken JH, Aderka D et al (2016) ESMO consensus guidelines for the management of patients with metastatic colorectal cancer. Ann Oncol 27(8):1386–1422
137. Van den Abbeele AD (2008) The lessons of GIST—PET and PET/CT: a new paradigm for imaging. Oncologist 13(Suppl 2):8–13
138. Van Poppel H, Watkin NA, Osanto S, Moonen L, Horwich A, Kataja V et al (2013) Penile cancer: ESMO Clinical Practice Guidelines for diagnosis, treatment and follow-up. Ann Oncol 24(Suppl 6):vi115–vi124
139. van Tinteren H, Hoekstra OS, Smit EF, van den Bergh JH, Schreurs AJ, Stallaert RA et al (2002) Effectiveness of positron emission tomography in the preoperative assessment of patients with suspected non-small-cell lung cancer: the PLUS multicentre randomised trial. Lancet 359(9315):1388–1393
140. Vensby PH, Schmidt G, Kjær A, Fischer BM (2017) The value of FDG PET/CT for follow-up of patients with melanoma: a retrospective analysis. Am J Nucl Med Mol Imaging 7(6):255–262
141. Vincent A, Herman J, Schulick R, Hruban RH, Goggins M (2011) Pancreatic cancer. Lancet 378(9791):607–620
142. Voltin CA, Goergen H, Baues C, Fuchs M, Mettler J, Kreissl S et al (2018) Value of bone marrow biopsy in Hodgkin lymphoma patients staged by FDG PET: results from the German Hodgkin Study Group trials HD16, HD17, and HD18. Ann Oncol 29(9):1926–1931
143. von Mehren M, Randall RL, Benjamin RS, Boles S, Bui MM, Ganjoo KN et al (2018) Soft tissue sarcoma, version 2.2018, NCCN clinical practice guidelines in oncology. J Natl Compr Cancer Netw 16(5):536–563
144. Wahl RL, Jacene H, Kasamon Y, Lodge MA (2009) From RECIST to PERCIST: evolving considerations for PET response criteria in solid tumors. J Nucl Med 50(Suppl 1):122S–150S
145. Wahl RL, Zasadny K, Helvie M, Hutchins GD, Weber B, Cody R (1993) Metabolic monitoring of breast cancer chemohormonotherapy using positron emission tomography: initial evaluation. J Clin Oncol 11(11):2101–2111
146. Warburg O (1928) The chemical constitution of respiration ferment. Science 68(1767):437–443
147. Weiler-Sagie M, Bushelev O, Epelbaum R, Dann EJ, Haim N, Avivi I et al (2010) (18)F-FDG avidity in lymphoma readdressed: a study of 766 patients. J Nucl Med 51(1):25–30

148. Wong WL, Chambers RJ (2008) Role of PET/PET CT in the staging and restaging of thoracic oesophageal cancer and gastro-oesophageal cancer: a literature review. Abdom Imaging 33(2):183–190
149. Wu LM, Hu JN, Hua J, Gu HY, Zhu J, Xu JR (2012) ^{18}F-fluorodeoxyglucose positron emission tomography to evaluate recurrent gastric cancer: a systematic review and meta-analysis. J Gastroenterol Hepatol 27(3):472–480
150. Xiao Y, Wang L, Jiang X, She W, He L, Hu G (2016) Diagnostic efficacy of ^{18}F-FDG-PET or PET/CT in breast cancer with suspected recurrence: a systematic review and meta-analysis. Nucl Med Commun 37(11):1180–1188
151. Xing Y, Bronstein Y, Ross MI, Askew RL, Lee JE, Gershenwald JE et al (2011) Contemporary diagnostic imaging modalities for the staging and surveillance of melanoma patients: a meta-analysis. J Natl Cancer Inst 103(2):129–142
152. Yararbas U, Avci NC, Yeniay L, Argon AM (2018) The value of ^{18}F-FDG PET/CT imaging in breast cancer staging. Bosn J Basic Med Sci 18(1):72–79
153. Yu T, Meng N, Chi D, Zhao Y, Wang K, Luo Y (2015) Diagnostic value of (18)F-FDG PET/CT in detecting local recurrent colorectal cancer: a pooled analysis of 26 individual studies. Cell Biochem Biophys 72(2):443–451
154. Zhang C, Liu J, Tong J, Sun X, Song S, Huang G (2013) ^{18}F-FDG-PET evaluation of pathological tumour response to neoadjuvant therapy in patients with NSCLC. Nucl Med Commun 34(1):71–77
155. Zhang S, Li W, Liang F (2016) Clinical value of fluorine-18 2-fluoro-2-deoxy-D-glucose positron emission tomography/computed tomography in penile cancer. Oncotarget 7(30):48600–48606
156. Zhu L, Wang N (2013) ^{18}F-fluorodeoxyglucose positron emission tomography-computed tomography as a diagnostic tool in patients with cervical nodal metastases of unknown primary site: a meta-analysis. Surg Oncol 22(3):190–194
157. zum Büschenfelde CM, Herrmann K, Schuster T, Geinitz H, Langer R, Becker K et al (2011) (18)F-FDG PET-guided salvage neoadjuvant radiochemotherapy of adenocarcinoma of the esophagogastric junction: the MUNICON II trial. J Nucl Med 52(8):1189–1196
158. Groheux D, Quere G, Blanc E et al (2016) FDG PET-CT for solitary pulmonary nodule and lung cancer: literature review. Diagn Interv Imaging 97(10):1003–1017
159. Salaün PY, Abgral R, Malard O et al (2020) Good clinical practice recommendations for the use of PET/CT in oncology. Eur J Nucl Med Mol Imaging 47(1):28–50
160. Kaseda K (2020) Recent and current advances in FDG-PET imaging within the field of clinical oncology in NSCLC: a review of the literature. Diagnostics (Basel) 10(8):561
161. Kubota K, Matsuno S, Morioka N et al (2015) Impact of FDG-PET findings on decisions regarding patient management strategies: a multicenter trial in patients with lung cancer and other types of cancer. Ann Nucl Med 29(5):431–441
162. Vaz SC, Adam JA, Delgado Bolton RC et al (2022) Joint EANM/SNMMI/ESTRO practice recommendations for the use of 2-[(18)F]FDG PET/CT external beam radiation treatment planning in lung cancer V1.0. Eur J Nucl Med Mol Imaging 49(4):1386–1406
163. Nestle U, Schimek-Jasch T, Kremp S et al (2020) Imaging-based target volume reduction in chemoradiotherapy for locally advanced non-small-cell lung cancer (PET-Plan): a multicentre, open-label, randomised, controlled trial. Lancet Oncol 21(4):581–592
164. Ayeni A, Evbuomwan O, Vangu MW (2025) The role of [(18)F]FDG PET/CT in monitoring of therapy response in lung cancer. Semin Nucl Med 55(2):175–189
165. Feine U, Lietzenmayer R, Hanke JP et al (1996) Fluorine-18-FDG and iodine-131-iodide uptake in thyroid cancer. J Nucl Med 37(9):1468–1472
166. Avram AM, Giovanella L, Greenspan B et al (2022) SNMMI procedure standard/EANM practice guideline for nuclear medicine evaluation and therapy of differentiated thyroid cancer: abbreviated version. J Nucl Med 63(6):15n–35n
167. Giovanella L, Treglia G, Iakovou I et al (2020) EANM practice guideline for PET/CT imaging in medullary thyroid carcinoma. Eur J Nucl Med Mol Imaging 47(1):61–77

168. Cheng X, Bao L, Xu Z et al (2012) ^{18}F-FDG-PET and ^{18}F-FDG-PET/CT in the detection of recurrent or metastatic medullary thyroid carcinoma: a systematic review and meta-analysis. J Med Imaging Radiat Oncol 56(2):136–142
169. Szyszko TA, Cook GJR (2018) PET/CT and PET/MRI in head and neck malignancy. Clin Radiol 73(1):60–69
170. Machiels JP, René Leemans C, Golusinski W et al (2020) Squamous cell carcinoma of the oral cavity, larynx, oropharynx and hypopharynx: EHNS-ESMO-ESTRO Clinical Practice Guidelines for diagnosis, treatment and follow-up. Ann Oncol 31(11):1462–1475
171. Ebner R, Sheikh GT, Brendel M et al (2025) ESR essentials: staging and restaging with FDG-PET/CT in oncology-practice recommendations by the European Society for Hybrid, Molecular and Translational Imaging. Eur Radiol 35(4):1894–1902
172. Aiken AH, Rath TJ, Anzai Y et al (2018) ACR neck imaging reporting and data systems (NI-RADS): a white paper of the ACR NI-RADS Committee. J Am Coll Radiol 15(8):1097–1108
173. Datta D, Selvakumar B, Goel AD et al (2025) Diagnostic performance of NIRADS on F-18 FDG PET/CT in the post-treatment assessment of head and neck malignancies – a systematic review and meta-analysis. Eur J Nucl Med Mol Imaging 52:3846
174. Obermannová R, Alsina M, Cervantes A et al (2022) Oesophageal cancer: ESMO Clinical Practice Guideline for diagnosis, treatment and follow-up. Ann Oncol 33(10):992–1004
175. Ajani JA, D'Amico TA, Bentrem DJ et al (2023) Esophageal and Esophagogastric Junction Cancers, version 2.2023, NCCN Clinical Practice Guidelines in Oncology. J Natl Compr Cancer Netw 21(4):393–422
176. Yang WJ, Zhao HP, Yu Y et al (2023) Updates on global epidemiology, risk and prognostic factors of gastric cancer. World J Gastroenterol 29(16):2452–2468
177. Lordick F, Carneiro F, Cascinu S et al (2022) Gastric cancer: ESMO Clinical Practice Guideline for diagnosis, treatment and follow-up. Ann Oncol 33(10):1005–1020
178. Choi CI, Park JK, Jeon TY et al (2023) Diagnostic performance of F-18 FDG PET or PET/CT for detection of recurrent gastric cancer: a systematic review and meta-analysis. J Yeungnam Med Sci 40(Suppl):S37–S46
179. Inoue A, Ota S, Yamasaki M et al (2022) Gastrointestinal stromal tumors: a comprehensive radiological review. Jpn J Radiol 40(11):1105–1120
180. Casali PG, Blay JY, Abecassis N et al (2022) Gastrointestinal stromal tumours: ESMO-EURACAN-GENTURIS Clinical Practice Guidelines for diagnosis, treatment and follow-up. Ann Oncol 33(1):20–33
181. Siegel RL, Giaquinto AN, Jemal A (2024) Cancer statistics, 2024. CA Cancer J Clin 74(1):12–49
182. Gershenwald JE, Scolyer RA, Hess KR et al (2017) Melanoma staging: evidence-based changes in the American Joint Committee on Cancer eighth edition cancer staging manual. CA Cancer J Clin 67(6):472–492
183. Strauss SJ, Frezza AM, Abecassis N et al (2021) Bone sarcomas: ESMO-EURACAN-GENTURIS-ERN PaedCan Clinical Practice Guideline for diagnosis, treatment and follow-up. Ann Oncol 32(12):1520–1536
184. Groheux D, Vaz SC, Poortmans P et al (2024) Role of [(18)F]FDG PET/CT in patients with invasive breast carcinoma of no special type: literature review and comparison between guidelines. Breast 78:103806
185. Gennari A, André F, Barrios CH et al (2021) ESMO Clinical Practice Guideline for the diagnosis, staging and treatment of patients with metastatic breast cancer. Ann Oncol 32(12):1475–1495
186. Aide N, Fauchille P, Coquan E et al (2021) Predicting tumor response and outcome of second-look surgery with (18)F-FDG PET/CT: insights from the GINECO CHIVA phase II trial of neoadjuvant chemotherapy plus nintedanib in stage IIIc-IV FIGO ovarian cancer. Eur J Nucl Med Mol Imaging 48(6):1998–2008
187. Armstrong DK, Alvarez RD, Backes FJ et al (2022) NCCN guidelines® insights: ovarian cancer, version 3.2022. J Natl Compr Cancer Netw 20(9):972–980

188. Honecker F, Aparicio J, Berney D et al (2018) ESMO consensus conference on testicular germ cell cancer: diagnosis, treatment and follow-up. Ann Oncol 29(8):1658–1686
189. Loriot Y, Texier M, Culine S et al (2022) The GETUG SEMITEP trial: De-escalating chemotherapy in good-prognosis seminoma based on Fluorodeoxyglucose positron emission tomography/computed tomography. Eur Urol 82(2):172–179
190. Powles T, Bellmunt J, Comperat E et al (2022) Bladder cancer: ESMO Clinical Practice Guideline for diagnosis, treatment and follow-up. Ann Oncol 33(3):244–258
191. Voskuilen CS, van Gennep EJ, Einerhand SMH et al (2022) Staging (18)F-fluorodeoxyglucose positron emission tomography/computed tomography changes treatment recommendation in invasive bladder cancer. Eur Urol Oncol 5(3):366–369
192. Zattoni F, Incerti E, Colicchia M et al (2018) Comparison between the diagnostic accuracies of 18F-fluorodeoxyglucose positron emission tomography/computed tomography and conventional imaging in recurrent urothelial carcinomas: a retrospective, multicenter study. Abdom Radiol (NY) 43(9):2391–2399
193. Willemse JRJ, Lambregts DMJ, Balduzzi S et al (2024) Identifying the primary tumour in patients with cancer of unknown primary (CUP) using [(18)F]FDG PET/CT: a systematic review and individual patient data meta-analysis. Eur J Nucl Med Mol Imaging 52(1):225–236
194. Krämer A, Bochtler T, Pauli C et al (2023) Cancer of unknown primary: ESMO Clinical Practice Guideline for diagnosis, treatment and follow-up. Ann Oncol 34(3):228–246

Non-FDG PET/CT

22

Priscilla Guglielmo, Stefano Fanti, and Laura Evangelista

22.1 Introduction to Non-FDG PET Tracers

In recent years, molecular imaging has evolved into a cornerstone of precision oncology, propelled by the development and clinical integration of radiopharmaceuticals that transcend the traditional reliance on [^{18}F]fluorodeoxyglucose (FDG). Although FDG PET/CT remains the most widely utilized imaging modality in nuclear medicine, its limitations are increasingly recognized. Variable sensitivity in indolent tumors, lack of specificity due to uptake in inflammatory or infectious processes, and limited performance in certain anatomical districts (e.g., the brain, urinary tract, and prostate) underscore the need for alternative tracers with more specific biological targets.

This chapter is based on chapter Non-FDG PET/CT from the previous edition, written by Egesta Lopci.

P. Guglielmo (✉)
Department of Biomedical Sciences, Humanitas University, Pieve Emanuele, MI, Italy

Nuclear Medicine Unit, Humanitas Gavazzeni, Bergamo, BG, Italy
e-mail: priscilla.guglielmo@gavazzeni.it

S. Fanti
Metropolitan Nuclear Medicine, University Hospital S. Orsola-Malpighi, Alma Mater Studiorum, University of Bologna, Bologna, Italy
e-mail: stefano.fanti@aosp.bo.it

L. Evangelista
Department of Biomedical Sciences, Humanitas University, Pieve Emanuele, MI, Italy

Nuclear Medicine Department, Humanitas Clinical and Research Hospital – IRCCS, Rozzano, MI, Italy
e-mail: laura.evangelista@hunimed.eu

O. Schober et al. (eds.), *Molecular Imaging in Oncology - Volume 2*, Recent Results in Cancer Research 225, https://doi.org/10.1007/978-3-032-21415-7_4

This demand has catalyzed the development of a diverse repertoire of non-FDG radiopharmaceuticals, many of which are now entering routine clinical practice. These agents are designed to bind to tumor-specific molecular structures, such as overexpressed membrane receptors, metabolic pathways unique to malignant cells, or features of the tumor microenvironment. Examples include radiolabeled somatostatin analogs for neuroendocrine tumors, PSMA-targeting compounds for prostate cancer, choline and acetate derivatives for imaging lipid metabolism, and amino acid-based tracers for gliomas and other malignancies. By offering improved lesion detectability, more accurate disease characterization, and higher diagnostic confidence, these radiopharmaceuticals enhance the clinician's ability to tailor treatment strategies to individual patients.

Moreover, many of these agents possess theranostic properties, allowing for seamless transition from diagnosis to targeted radionuclide therapy using the same molecular scaffold. This paradigm shift supports the emergence of a more integrated, biology-driven approach to cancer care. The clinical impact of these innovations is particularly evident in tumor types where FDG has known limitations, such as well-differentiated neuroendocrine neoplasms, prostate cancer, and certain breast or brain tumors.

This chapter aims to provide a comprehensive overview of the most relevant non-FDG radiopharmaceuticals currently applied in oncology. Key aspects addressed include their molecular mechanisms and characteristics, and clinical indications, underscoring the growing importance of non-FDG agents in the broader context of individualized oncologic management.

22.2 DOTA-Based Radiopharmaceuticals

The chelating agent 1,4,7,10-tetraazacyclododecane-1,4,7,10-tetraacetic acid (DOTA) forms highly stable complexes with various radiometals, notably gallium-68 (^{68}Ga), making it an ideal scaffold for developing targeted PET tracers. By enabling the conjugation of biomolecules such as peptides, antibodies, and small molecules to PET radionuclides, DOTA-based compounds facilitate high-affinity targeting of specific cellular receptors and disease biomarkers. In clinical practice, DOTA-conjugated radiopharmaceuticals have achieved pivotal roles, particularly in the management of neuroendocrine tumors (NETs), meningiomas, and other malignancies characterized by receptor overexpression.

The most established application of DOTA-based PET imaging lies in the diagnosis and staging of neuroendocrine tumors (NETs). NETs often overexpress somatostatin receptors (SSTRs), particularly subtype 2 (SSTR2), which can be selectively targeted by somatostatin analogs conjugated to DOTA and labeled with gallium-68 (^{68}Ga). Three principal compounds dominate the field: [^{68}Ga]Ga-DOTA-TOC, [^{68}Ga]Ga-DOTA-TATE, and [^{68}Ga]Ga-DOTA-NOC. Each displays subtle differences in receptor affinity profiles, allowing for tailored imaging strategies depending on tumor subtype and patient characteristics.

The use of ^{68}Ga-DOTA-peptides has been shown to surpass traditional imaging techniques in sensitivity and specificity. In particular, comparative studies reveal that [^{68}Ga]Ga-DOTA-TATE PET/CT achieves detection rates of up to 90–95% for well-differentiated NETs, significantly outperforming conventional modalities such as octreotide scintigraphy (SRS) and anatomical imaging (CT, MRI) [1]. Importantly, PET imaging with DOTA-peptides enables visualization of both primary tumors and distant metastases, including in sites typically challenging to assess, such as bones and the mesentery.

Moreover, the introduction of DOTA-based PET imaging has reshaped clinical decision-making. In a substantial proportion of cases—reported in some series to exceed 40%—PET findings have led to changes in therapeutic plans, including surgery, systemic therapy, or enrollment into peptide receptor radionuclide therapy (PRRT) protocols (see Fig. 22.1). The high negative predictive value also offers reassurance in surveillance settings, potentially sparing patients from unnecessary invasive procedures.

Beyond neuroendocrine malignancies, DOTA-based PET tracers have demonstrated notable utility in imaging meningiomas. Meningiomas frequently express somatostatin receptors, making them amenable to visualization with [^{68}Ga]Ga-DOTA-peptides. Preoperative PET imaging provides critical information regarding tumor margins, skull base infiltration, and the involvement of eloquent brain regions, thus enhancing surgical planning. In cases of recurrent or residual disease, DOTA-PET can distinguish viable tumor tissue from postoperative changes with greater accuracy than MRI alone.

In addition, DOTA-based PET imaging is increasingly applied in the evaluation of paragangliomas and pheochromocytomas, rare neuroendocrine tumors that can pose diagnostic challenges. ^{68}Ga-DOTA-peptides have demonstrated high

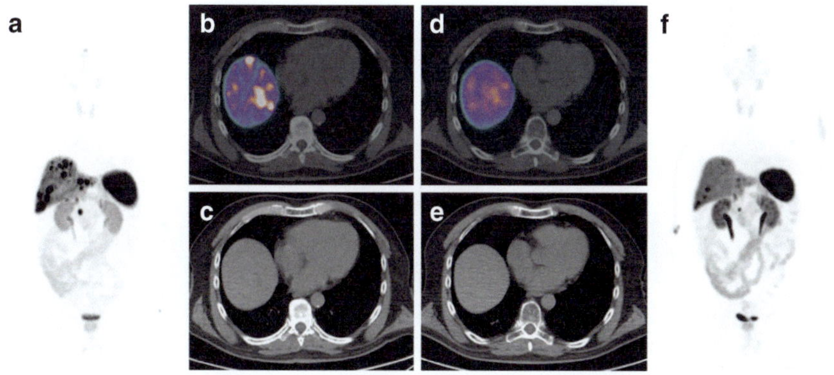

Fig. 22.1 A 65-year-old male patient diagnosed with a well-differentiated pancreatic neuroendocrine tumor (NET G2, Ki67 index: 15%) localized in the pancreatic tail underwent four cycles of peptide receptor radionuclide therapy (PRRT). Images (**a–c**) show baseline [^{68}Ga]Ga-DOTA-TOC PET/CT images obtained prior to therapy. Images (**d–f**) display follow-up PET/CT images acquired 6 months after completion of PRRT, demonstrating a partial response to treatment as evidenced by a marked reduction in radiotracer uptake and tumor burden in both liver and pancreatic lesions

sensitivity in detecting both hereditary and sporadic forms of these tumors, often outperforming metaiodobenzylguanidine (MIBG) scintigraphy, particularly in succinate dehydrogenase (SDH)-mutated disease [2].

Several technical aspects contribute to the success of DOTA-based PET imaging. Firstly, the availability of ^{68}Ge/^{68}Ga generators permits the onsite production of radiotracers without the need for a cyclotron, facilitating widespread clinical adoption even in centers with limited infrastructure. The physical characteristics of gallium-68, most notably its half-life of 68 min and positron emission properties, are well-suited for imaging peptides with rapid pharmacokinetics.

Radiolabeling with DOTA ensures high in vivo stability of the radiotracer, minimizing nonspecific binding and renal excretion artifacts. Furthermore, standardized production protocols and regulatory approvals have enhanced the reliability and reproducibility of DOTA-PET imaging across institutions.

The clinical impact of DOTA-based PET imaging extends well beyond initial diagnosis. In the context of NETs, DOTA-PET plays a crucial role in risk stratification, prognostication, and monitoring response to therapy. Semiquantitative parameters such as standardized uptake values (SUVs) provide insights into tumor biology and may correlate with proliferation indices like Ki67, guiding therapeutic intensity.

Moreover, dual-tracer strategies combining [^{68}Ga]Ga-DOTA-peptides with [^{18}F]FDG PET imaging allow for comprehensive assessment of tumor heterogeneity, particularly in high-grade NETs where dedifferentiation may result in loss of somatostatin receptor expression (see Fig. 22.2). This integrated imaging approach informs therapeutic selection, including the appropriateness of PRRT versus chemotherapy [3].

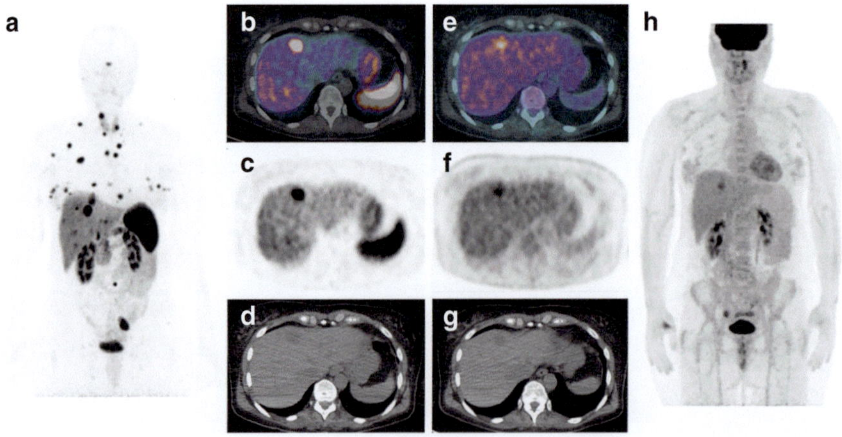

Fig. 22.2 A 47-year-old female patient with a metastatic, functioning, grade 3 neuroendocrine tumor (NET G3, Ki67 index: 22%) of unknown primary origin. The disease involves multiple metastatic sites, including the liver, peritoneum, lungs, bones, and breast. The imaging findings illustrate a marked heterogeneity in both somatostatin receptor expression and glucose metabolism. Images (**a–d**) show [^{68}Ga]Ga-DOTA-TOC PET/CT, revealing extensive multi-organ metastatic disease. In contrast, images (**e–h**) illustrate [^{18}F]FDG PET/CT images, in which metabolic activity is confined to a single hepatic lesion, indicating a mismatch pattern

Additionally, advances in imaging technology, such as digital PET systems and artificial intelligence-driven image analysis, promise to further enhance the sensitivity, resolution, and interpretative accuracy of DOTA-based imaging protocols [4, 5]. Through ongoing innovation in radiochemistry, tracer development, and imaging analysis, DOTA-based PET imaging is poised to play an increasingly central role in precision medicine.

22.2.1 Summary of Clinical Indications for [^{68}Ga]Ga-DOTA-Peptide PET/CT in NETs (Adapted from EANM 2017 Guidelines)

- *Staging at initial diagnosis*
- [^{68}Ga]Ga-DOTA-peptide PET/CT is recommended for the comprehensive assessment of disease extent at initial diagnosis, offering superior sensitivity for detecting both primary tumors and metastatic spread compared to conventional imaging modalities.
- *Restaging after therapy*
- Following surgical resection, systemic treatment, or peptide receptor radionuclide therapy (PRRT), DOTA-PET/CT is invaluable for evaluating residual disease, recurrence, or progression, with a high impact on subsequent management strategies.
- *Localization of unknown primary NETs*
- In patients presenting with metastatic disease and histopathological evidence of a neuroendocrine origin, but without an identifiable primary tumor, DOTA-PET/CT significantly enhances the likelihood of primary tumor detection.
- *Selection of candidates for PRRT*
- By accurately mapping SSTR expression, [^{68}Ga]Ga-DOTA-peptide PET/CT serves as an essential tool for identifying patients eligible for PRRT, ensuring that only SSTR-positive tumors are targeted with radionuclide therapy.
- *Prognostic stratification*
- The degree of radiotracer uptake on DOTA-PET/CT correlates with tumor differentiation and biological behavior, providing important prognostic information that complements histological grading and guides therapeutic decisions.
- *Assessment of suspected recurrence*
- In patients with biochemical relapse (e.g., rising chromogranin A levels) or clinical suspicion of recurrence, DOTA-PET/CT is the modality of choice for early detection, often revealing lesions occult on conventional imaging.
- *Evaluation of indeterminate lesions*
- When anatomical imaging (CT or MRI) identifies lesions of uncertain nature in patients with known or suspected NETs, DOTA-PET/CT assists in characterizing their neuroendocrine origin based on SSTR expression.

22.3 Choline-Based Radiopharmaceuticals

Choline-based radiopharmaceuticals, particularly [^{18}F]fluorocholine ([^{18}F]FCH) and [^{11}C]choline ([^{11}C]CH), have significantly broadened the applications of PET imaging in oncology. These tracers exploit the upregulated phospholipid metabolism characteristic of many malignancies, particularly prostate cancer, by targeting the increased synthesis of cell membrane components. Given their favorable kinetics and high tumor-to-background contrast, choline tracers have proven valuable for detecting tumor recurrence, staging, and evaluating treatment response [6].

Choline is a precursor molecule essential for the biosynthesis of phosphatidylcholine, a major constituent of cell membranes. In cancer cells, increased choline kinase activity and accelerated membrane turnover result in elevated choline uptake, providing a rationale for its use as a PET imaging biomarker.

[^{11}C]choline was the first choline-based radiotracer introduced into clinical practice. Its short half-life (20 min) necessitates an onsite cyclotron and radiochemistry infrastructure, limiting its availability. Conversely, [^{18}F]fluorocholine, with a longer half-life (110 min), allows broader clinical distribution and delayed imaging protocols without substantial compromise in image quality. Both tracers display rapid blood clearance, low urinary excretion (especially for [^{11}C]choline), and early peak uptake in target tissues, facilitating high-contrast images within a short post-injection window.

The principal and most extensively validated application of choline PET imaging lies in prostate cancer (PCa), particularly for detecting biochemical recurrence (BCR) following definitive therapy (see Fig. 22.3). Prostate-specific antigen (PSA) relapse remains a common clinical challenge, and early localization of recurrent disease is crucial for directing salvage therapy [7]. [^{18}F]fluorocholine and [^{11}C]choline PET/CT have demonstrated superior sensitivity compared to conventional imaging (CT, MRI, bone scan) in the detection of metastatic and locoregional recurrent lesions. Lesions identified by choline PET include pelvic lymph nodes, bone metastases, and local recurrences in the prostatic bed. The ability to differentiate oligometastatic from widespread disease holds substantial implications for patient management, influencing decisions regarding metastasis-directed therapy, systemic treatment initiation, or radiotherapy planning.

Although primarily utilized in the setting of recurrence, choline PET/CT has also been explored for initial staging in patients with high-risk PCa. Here, the modality can detect occult lymph node involvement or distant metastases that are not apparent on conventional imaging.

Beyond PCa, choline-based PET imaging has been investigated for several other malignancies. In hepatocellular carcinoma (HCC), [^{11}C]choline PET has demonstrated utility in detecting well-differentiated tumors, often missed by [^{18}F]FDG PET [8].

Moreover, brain tumors such as low-grade gliomas and meningiomas have shown increased uptake of choline tracers, assisting in the distinction between tumor recurrence and post-therapeutic changes [8].

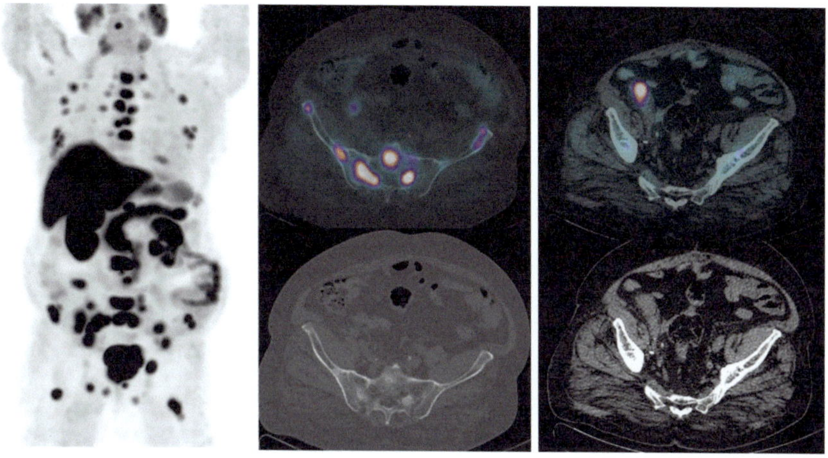

Fig. 22.3 A 73-year-old male patient with a history of prostate adenocarcinoma (Gleason Score 5 + 4), stage pT3bN0M0 with positive surgical margins (R1), and an initial PSA level of 223 ng/mL. The patient underwent radical prostatectomy followed by androgen deprivation therapy, achieving long-term disease control. Biochemical recurrence occurred 9 years after primary treatment, with a rising PSA reaching 369 ng/mL. The [^{18}F]Fluorocholine fused PET/CT images (upper row) reveal and the CT images alone (lower row), among others, nodal recurrence in the right external iliac region and skeletal metastases involving the pelvic bones

A particularly promising non-oncologic application is the use of [^{18}F]fluorocholine PET/CT in the localization of hyperfunctioning parathyroid glands in primary and secondary hyperparathyroidism (see Fig. 22.4). Traditional imaging modalities such as ultrasound and sestamibi scintigraphy may yield inconclusive results, especially in cases of multiglandular disease, small adenomas, or ectopic glands. Several studies have demonstrated that [^{18}F]fluorocholine PET/CT exhibits higher sensitivity and positive predictive value compared to conventional imaging [4, 5]. This approach facilitates precise surgical planning, particularly for minimally invasive parathyroidectomy, thereby reducing operative times and improving patient outcomes.

Standardized protocols for choline PET imaging involve early acquisition to capitalize on rapid tumor uptake and minimize background noise. Patient preparation is minimal compared to [^{18}F]FDG PET, with no fasting required and no significant impact from blood glucose levels. Quantitative parameters such as standardized uptake values (SUVs) provide semiquantitative assessments of tracer accumulation, although overlap between benign and malignant processes necessitates careful interpretation.

While both [^{18}F]FCH and [^{11}C]CH share similar mechanisms of uptake, certain practical and diagnostic differences warrant consideration. [^{11}C]choline offers advantages in reduced urinary excretion, potentially enhancing evaluation of pelvic lymph nodes and prostatic bed recurrences. However, the short half-life restricts its use to centers equipped with an on-site cyclotron. [^{18}F]fluorocholine, due to its longer half-life, is more accessible and allows centralized production and distribution.

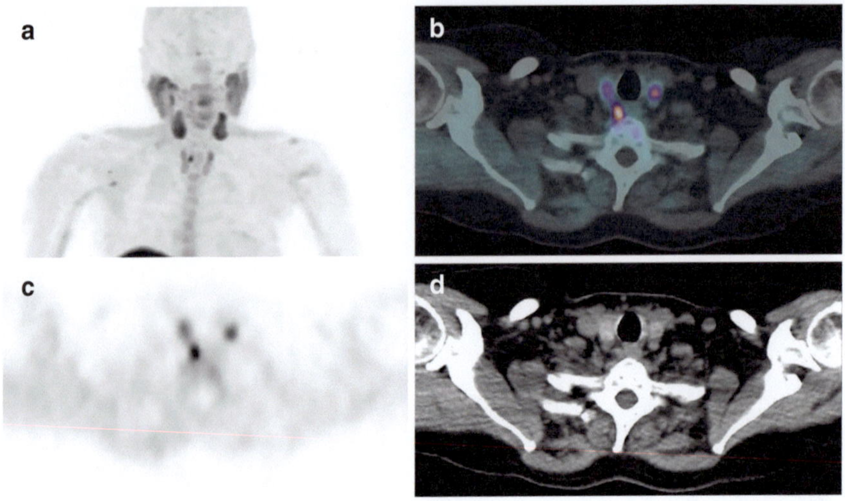

Fig. 22.4 62-year-old female patient with biochemically confirmed hyperparathyroidism (PTH level: 100 pg/mL). A subcentimetric, [^{18}F]fluorocholine-avid nodular lesion was identified posteromedially to the mid-to-upper third of the right thyroid lobe. (**a**) Maximum intensity projection; (**b**) fused [^{18}F]FCH PET/CT image; (**c**) PET image; (**d**) CT image

Despite slightly higher bladder activity, optimized imaging protocols (e.g., early voiding and hydration) can effectively mitigate this issue.

In conclusion, [^{18}F]fluorocholine and [^{11}C]choline PET imaging have profoundly impacted the diagnosis and management of prostate cancer and have shown promising potential in other malignancies such as hepatocellular carcinoma and brain tumors. Additionally, their emerging role in the precise localization of hyperfunctioning parathyroid glands represents an exciting diagnostic advance. Their ability to noninvasively detect disease recurrence, guide salvage therapy, inform staging, and facilitate surgical planning underscores their integral role in modern diagnostic imaging. Despite the rise of newer imaging biomarkers, choline PET remains a robust and valuable tool within the landscape of precision medicine.

22.4 Iodine-124 [^{124}I]

Iodine-124 ([^{124}I]) has emerged as a valuable radiopharmaceutical in nuclear medicine, particularly for its use in PET imaging. This radiolabeled isotope of iodine possesses a half-life of 4.18 days, which, when coupled with its favorable positron emission characteristics, makes it ideally suited for both diagnostic and theranostic applications. The relatively long half-life allows for extensive imaging studies, providing valuable insights into the biodistribution and pharmacokinetics of radiopharmaceuticals over several days. This characteristic has proven especially advantageous in the monitoring of targeted therapies, where longitudinal imaging can guide treatment decisions and assess therapeutic efficacy over time.

One of the most prominent clinical uses of [^{124}I] is in the imaging of thyroid cancer. [^{124}I]PET is a highly sensitive and specific technique for detecting recurrent (see Figs. 22.5 and 22.6) or metastatic thyroid cancer, especially in cases where conventional iodine-131 ([^{131}I]) scintigraphy fails to provide conclusive results. Unlike [^{131}I], which primarily relies on β-emission for treatment, [^{124}I] emits positrons, allowing for higher-resolution imaging with the added benefit of quantifying the tracer uptake. This capability has enabled clinicians to distinguish between benign and malignant lesions more effectively, thus facilitating the detection of distant metastases that may not be visible through other imaging modalities, such as CT or MRI. Furthermore, [^{124}I] PET imaging plays a crucial role in the assessment of thyroid cancer's response to treatment, particularly in the context of radioiodine therapy, where the precise identification of iodine-avid metastases is critical for determining the appropriate dosage of radioiodine therapy [9].

The use of extends beyond thyroid cancer and has been explored in the context of other malignancies, such as NETs and breast cancer. For neuroendocrine tumors, [^{124}I]-labeled somatostatin analogs, such as [^{124}I]DOTATATE, offer superior imaging capabilities when compared to traditional SRS. PET imaging with [^{124}I]DOTATATE allows for more precise delineation of tumor burden, providing valuable information regarding lesion localization, metastasis detection, and tumor progression. Similarly, in breast cancer, [^{124}I]-labeled trastuzumab (a monoclonal antibody targeting HER2/neu) has shown promising results for imaging HER2-positive tumors. The ability to monitor the spatial distribution of these targeted

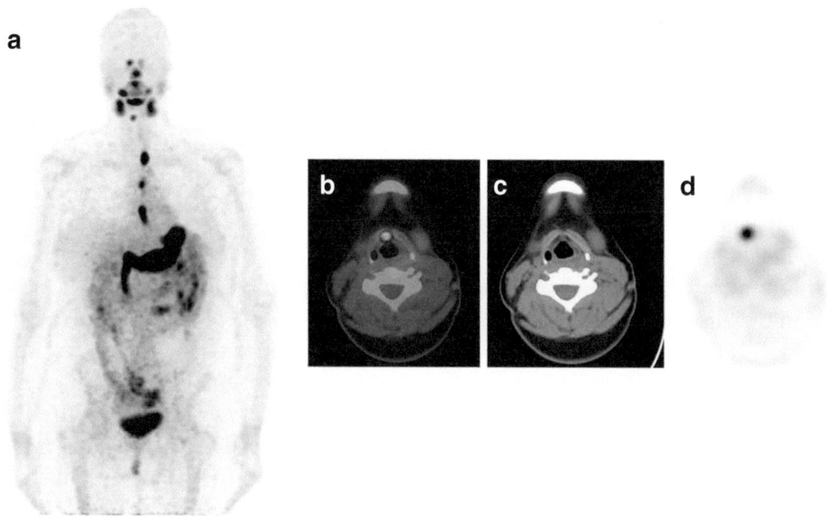

Fig. 22.5 43-year-old female patient with clinical suspicion of recurrent thyroid carcinoma. [^{124}I]iodine PET/CT imaging demonstrates a high uptake in correspondence of a nodule measuring approximately 1 cm located superior to the hyoid bone, consistent with disease recurrence. (**a**) Maximum intensity projection; (**b**) fused [^{124}I]iodine PET/CT image; (**c**) CT image; (**d**) PET image

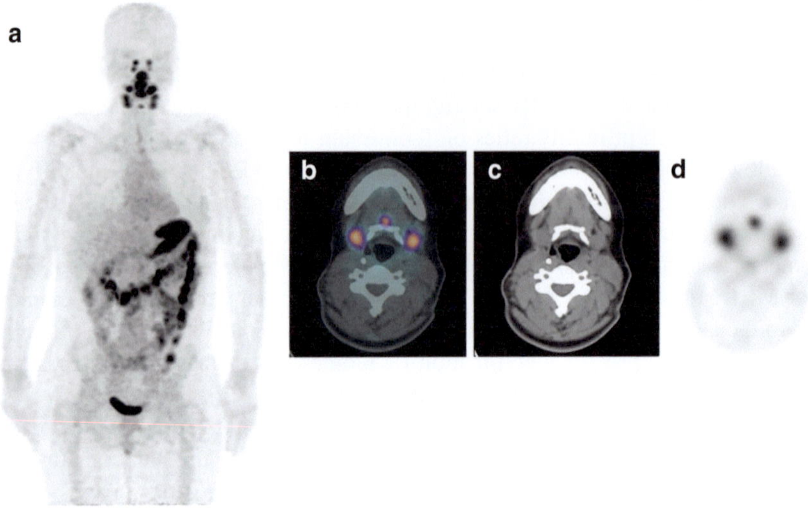

Fig. 22.6 A 26-year-old female patient with suspected recurrence of thyroid carcinoma. [^{124}I]iodine PET/CT images reveal a high uptake at a nodular lesion, approximately 1 cm in size, located adjacent to the right paramedian aspect of the thyroid cartilage, consistent with possible local recurrence. (**a**) Maximum intensity projection; (**b**) fused [^{124}I]iodine PET/CT image; (**c**) CT image; (**d**) PET image

agents enables clinicians to better assess tumor characteristics and guide personalized therapy based on receptor status and tumor heterogeneity.

Another important clinical application of [^{124}I] lies in its role in pre-therapeutic planning and treatment optimization. In patients undergoing therapies such as radioiodine ([^{131}I]) treatment for thyroid cancer, [^{124}I] PET imaging can be employed to assess the distribution and uptake of therapeutic radiopharmaceuticals. This imaging modality allows clinicians to evaluate whether a tumor is sufficiently targeted by the radiopharmaceutical and whether the lesion is likely to respond to therapy. By providing quantitative data on tracer uptake, [^{124}I] PET facilitates better selection of patients who are most likely to benefit from treatment and helps tailor therapy to individual tumor characteristics.

In terms of logistical advantages, [^{124}I] PET imaging offers a significant reduction in radiation exposure compared to conventional therapeutic isotopes like [^{131}I]. While [^{131}I] is primarily used for both diagnostic and therapeutic purposes, its use as a diagnostic tool is often limited by its lower imaging resolution and radiation burden. In contrast, [^{124}I] favorable imaging characteristics allow for high-quality PET imaging without the extensive radiation exposure associated with higher-energy isotopes. This makes [^{124}I] a safer alternative for repeated imaging, particularly in patients requiring serial scans for monitoring disease progression or response to therapy.

Despite its many advantages, the use of [^{124}I] remains constrained by several challenges. One notable limitation is the cost and availability of [^{124}I], as it requires specialized facilities for production and has limited commercial availability.

Furthermore, the relatively long half-life of [^{124}I] necessitates careful scheduling of imaging studies to avoid potential delays in treatment planning, especially when used in conjunction with other therapeutic agents. Additionally, while [^{124}I] PET imaging provides superior resolution compared to traditional iodine scintigraphy, its sensitivity may still be limited in certain clinical settings, particularly for detecting small lesions or assessing minimal residual disease. As such, ongoing advancements in radiopharmaceutical development, image processing techniques, and patient-specific modeling are essential to fully optimize the clinical utility of [^{124}I] in routine practice.

22.5 [^{18}F]NaF

[^{18}F]-fluoride (sodium fluoride, [^{18}F]NaF) is a highly effective radiopharmaceutical agent for skeletal imaging, with particular significance in oncological applications. [^{18}F]NaF PET/CT, by virtue of its unique pharmacokinetic properties and high-resolution imaging capabilities, has emerged as a superior alternative to conventional bone scintigraphy in several oncologic settings [10].

Upon administration, [^{18}F]NaF undergoes rapid blood clearance and exhibits intense uptake in areas of active osteoblastic remodeling, where metastatic deposits stimulate a reactive bone formation process. This biological behavior renders [^{18}F]NaF particularly sensitive to even small-volume or early metastatic skeletal disease, which may elude detection by traditional [^{99m}Tc]MDP bone scintigraphy. The half-life of ^{18}F (approximately 110 minutes) and its low positron energy enable high-quality PET imaging with optimal lesion contrast and precise anatomical localization when integrated with CT.

Several comparative studies have unequivocally demonstrated the superior diagnostic performance of [^{18}F]NaF PET/CT over planar bone scans and SPECT imaging. For instance, meta-analyses report that [^{18}F]NaF PET/CT achieves sensitivities and specificities exceeding 90% for detecting skeletal metastases, significantly outperforming ^{99m}Tc-labeled diphosphonates, which are limited by lower spatial resolution and reduced lesion detectability in complex anatomical regions [10].

In PCa, skeletal involvement represents the most common site of distant metastasis. Numerous investigations have confirmed that [^{18}F]NaF PET/CT outperforms conventional imaging, especially in patients with biochemical recurrence (rising PSA levels) and equivocal findings on standard bone scintigraphy. In this setting, [^{18}F]NaF PET/CT allows for early identification of oligometastatic disease, thereby informing curative-intent metastasis-directed therapies, such as stereotactic body radiotherapy.

In breast cancer, the skeletal system is similarly a frequent site of metastatic spread. The detection of bone-only disease has important therapeutic and prognostic implications. [^{18}F]NaF PET/CT enables sensitive visualization of both lytic and blastic lesions, providing a comprehensive skeletal survey and contributing to accurate staging and restaging (see Fig. 22.7).

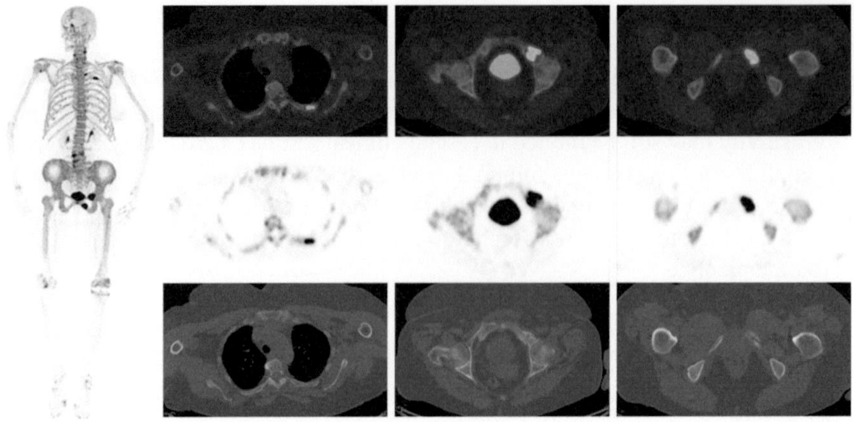

Fig. 22.7 A 64-year-old patient with metastatic breast cancer and concomitant fracture of the left hemipelvis. [18F]NaF PET/CT imaging was performed for skeletal assessment. Left: maximum intensity projection image. Top row: fused PET/CT images; middle row: PET images alone; bottom row: corresponding CT images

Moreover, in lung cancer and other malignancies with a predilection for osseous metastases—such as renal cell carcinoma, thyroid carcinoma, and multiple myeloma—[^{18}F]NaF PET/CT has demonstrated a high yield in uncovering skeletal disease, often altering patient management.

While [^{18}F]FDG PET/CT remains the standard for metabolic imaging in many cancers, its utility in pure bone imaging is limited by variable FDG uptake in skeletal lesions, particularly blastic metastases that may have low glycolytic activity. In contrast, ^{18}F-fluoride is not dependent on tumor metabolism but rather on osteoblastic response, offering complementary information to FDG.

Hybrid PET/MRI techniques, combining [^{18}F]NaF PET with high-resolution MRI, have further enhanced the diagnostic landscape, particularly in evaluating bone marrow infiltration and distinguishing viable metastases from post-therapy changes or benign degenerative disease.

Several expert panels and guidelines now recognize the value of [^{18}F]NaF PET/CT. The Society of Nuclear Medicine and Molecular Imaging (SNMMI) and the European Association of Nuclear Medicine (EANM) recommend its use in specific oncological contexts, particularly for staging high-risk prostate cancer, assessing suspected bone metastases with ambiguous findings on standard imaging, and in research protocols for novel therapeutic monitoring [10].

However, access to [^{18}F]NaF PET/CT remains variable, constrained by the availability of PET infrastructure, production requirements (cyclotron access), and healthcare cost considerations. In regions where PET/CT is readily accessible, [^{18}F]NaF imaging is increasingly incorporated into routine practice for selected patient cohorts.

Moreover, emerging artificial intelligence (AI) and radiomics approaches applied to [^{18}F]NaF PET datasets could offer quantitative, reproducible biomarkers of skeletal tumor burden, potentially refining prognostication and therapeutic monitoring [11].

22.6 [^{18}F]/[^{68}Ga]-Labeled PSMA

Prostate-specific membrane antigen (PSMA) PET/CT has revolutionized the imaging landscape of PCa, offering enhanced sensitivity and specificity compared to conventional modalities. Among the radiotracers developed for PSMA-targeted imaging, [^{68}Ga]Ga-PSMA-11 and [^{18}F]F-PSMA-1007 are prominently utilized, each possessing distinct pharmacokinetic properties that influence their clinical applications. While both tracers target PSMA, they possess distinct characteristics influencing their clinical utility. [^{68}Ga]Ga-PSMA-11 has a shorter half-life (~68 minutes) and is generator-produced, making it suitable for centers without cyclotron access. Conversely, [^{18}F]F-PSMA-1007 has a longer half-life (~110 min) and is cyclotron-produced, allowing for centralized production and distribution to distant sites. [^{18}F]F-PSMA-1007 also exhibits lower urinary excretion, potentially reducing interference in pelvic imaging. However, it may demonstrate higher nonspecific uptake in bones, necessitating careful interpretation to avoid false positives.

Accurate staging is crucial for optimal treatment planning in patients with intermediate- to high-risk PCa [12] (see Fig. 22.8). [^{68}Ga]Ga-PSMA-11 PET/CT has demonstrated superior diagnostic performance in detecting lymph node and bone metastases compared to conventional imaging modalities. For instance, a study [13] reported that [^{68}Ga]Ga-PSMA-11 PET/CT detected 95% of suspicious pelvic lymph nodes and 100% of extrapelvic lymph nodes, outperforming CT scans, which detected 75% in both categories. Additionally, [^{68}Ga]Ga-PSMA-11 PET/CT identified 100% of suspicious bone lesions, whereas bone scans detected only 63%. These findings underscore the modality's enhanced sensitivity in initial staging, leading to more accurate disease characterization and informed therapeutic decisions.

PSMA PET/CT has proven invaluable in detecting sites of recurrence in patients with rising PSA levels post-definitive therapy. [^{68}Ga]Ga-PSMA-11 PET/CT exhibits high detection rates even at low PSA levels, facilitating early identification of recurrent disease [14]. This early detection enables timely intervention, potentially improving patient outcomes.

In the context of metastatic castration-resistant prostate cancer (mCRPC), PSMA PET/CT plays a pivotal role in evaluating disease burden and guiding therapeutic strategies (see Fig. 22.9). [^{68}Ga]Ga-PSMA-11 PET/CT allows for precise localization of metastatic lesions, informing decisions regarding systemic therapies and eligibility for PSMA-targeted treatments [15]. Furthermore, PSMA PET/CT can assess treatment response, aiding in the optimization of therapeutic regimens.

The theranostic potential of PSMA-targeted agents has been exemplified by the use of [^{177}Lu]Lu-PSMA-617 for targeted radioligand therapy. [^{68}Ga]Ga-PSMA-11 PET/CT serves as a companion diagnostic tool, identifying patients who are likely to benefit from such therapies based on PSMA expression levels [16]. This approach enables personalized treatment, aligning therapeutic interventions with individual tumor biology.

The superior diagnostic accuracy of PSMA PET/CT has led to its incorporation into clinical guidelines for PCa management. Its applications span initial staging, detection of biochemical recurrence, assessment of metastatic disease, and selection

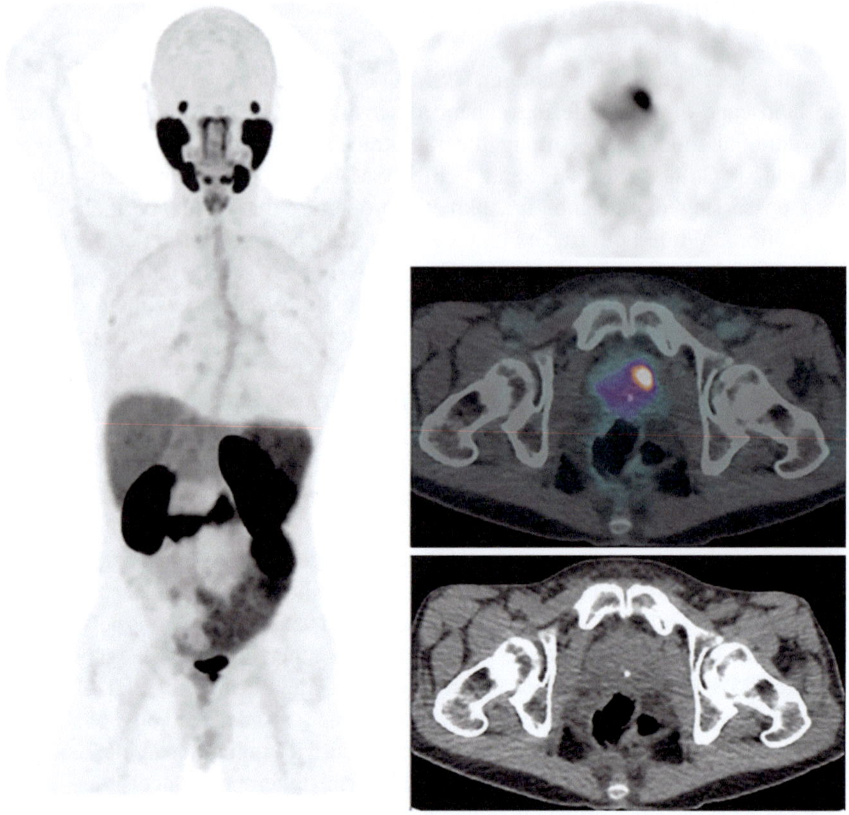

Fig. 22.8 A 67-year-old male patient with biopsy-proven prostate adenocarcinoma (Gleason Score 4 + 3) and an initial PSA level of 9.89 ng/mL. The [^{68}Ga]Ga-PSMA PET/CT performed for initial staging demonstrates radiotracer uptake confined to the left prostatic lobe, with no evidence of regional or distant metastatic disease, consistent with localized tumor involvement

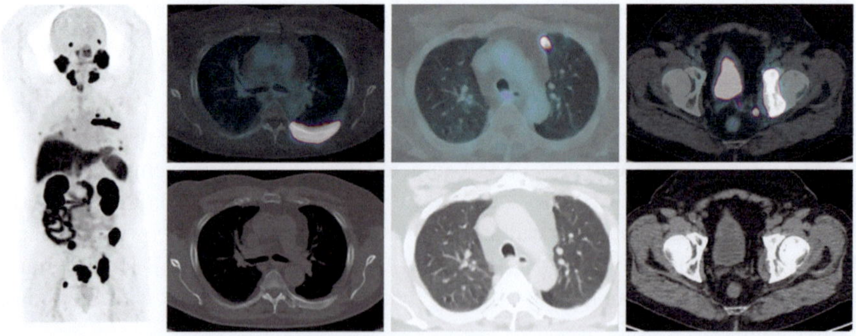

Fig. 22.9 78-year-old male patient with recurrent prostate adenocarcinoma, Gleason score 4 + 4, and a recent PSA level of 29.7 ng/mL. [^{68}Ga]Ga-PSMA-11 PET/CT imaging reveals multiple sites of disease recurrence involving the skeleton, lungs, and lymph nodes

for PSMA-targeted therapies [12, 17]. Ongoing research aims to further refine its role, optimize imaging protocols, and expand its utility across various clinical scenarios.

22.7 O-(2-[^{18}F]Fluoroethyl)-L-Tyrosine (FET)

The chapter discusses O-(2-[^{18}F]fluoroethyl)-L-tyrosine (FET) as a key PET radiotracer for brain tumor imaging. FET is a synthetic amino acid that mimics natural tyrosine but is modified with a fluoroethyl group, allowing it to be labeled with the positron-emitting isotope fluorine-18 (^{18}F). FET is synthesized via a nucleophilic substitution reaction where [^{18}F]fluoride replaces a leaving group (typically a tosylate or mesylate) on a precursor molecule. The process is efficient and amenable to automated synthesis modules (important for clinical production). The radiochemical yield is typically over 40%, and radiochemical purity exceeds 95%. Total synthesis time is around 40–60 minutes, allowing same-day use in PET centers. The final product is formulated in isotonic saline and must meet quality control standards.

FET is taken up by cells predominantly via the L-type amino acid transporter 1 (LAT1) and to a lesser extent LAT2. These transporters are overexpressed in tumor cells, particularly gliomas. It is not significantly incorporated into proteins or degraded intracellularly. This leads to stable tumor uptake over time, providing reproducible imaging results and simplifying interpretation. Its rapid blood clearance and stable tumor retention can significantly improve the signal-to-background ratio. FET is primarily used in patients with brain lesions, either primary or secondary. FET PET is extensively used in imaging of gliomas (WHO grades II–IV), because it can differentiate between neoplastic and non-neoplastic lesions and it is useful in identifying low-grade gliomas, which are often invisible on [^{18}F]FDG PET. Thanks to its pharmacokinetic behavior, dynamic PET imaging allows to distinguishing high-grade vs low-grade gliomas: high-grade tumors typically show early peak uptake followed by washout and low-grade tumors often show slow, steady uptake. FET PET aids in defining biological tumor volume, guiding biopsy or surgical resection margins more accurately than MRI alone; furthermore, it differentiates between tumor progression and treatment-induced changes (e.g., radiation necrosis or pseudoprogression). Moreover, FET PET has demonstrated the ability to detect the presence of secondary lesions in the brain, for example in patients with an history of lung cancer, breast cancer or others, thus increasing the sensitivity and letting to plan correct treatment planning (Figs. 22.10 and 22.11) [18, 19].

FET has some limitations and challenges, such as tumor specificity (some inflammatory or infectious lesions can also show mild uptake), it cannot be used for extracranial cancers and dynamic imaging complexity (while dynamic imaging adds diagnostic information, it increases acquisition and analysis complexity, which is a practical limitation for widespread use).

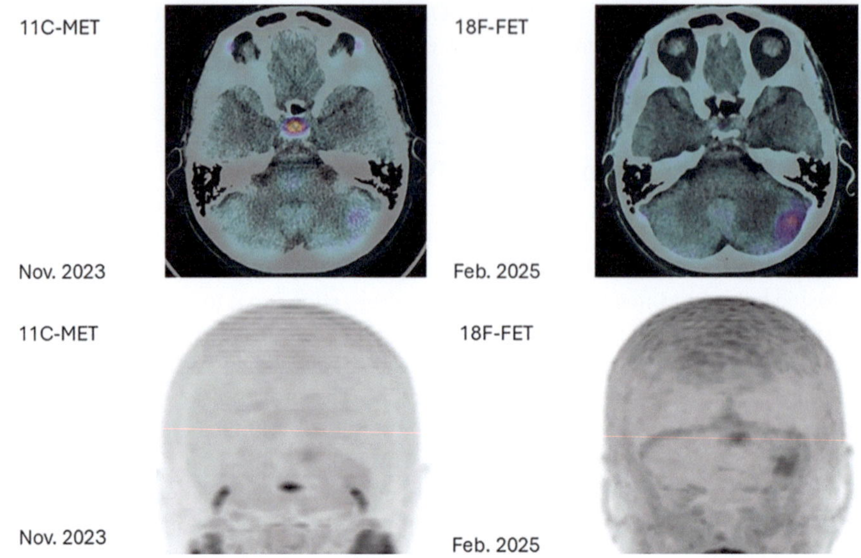

Fig. 22.10 Images in a patient with recurrent breast cancer. [^{11}C]MET PET/CT was considered negative in November 2023 (left). In February 2025, a follow-up imaging with [^{18}F]FET showed a moderate uptake in the left cerebellum lobe compatible with a brain recurrence of disease (right)

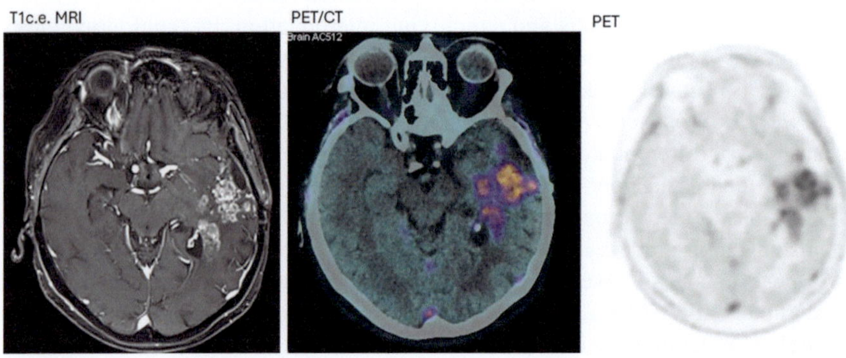

Fig. 22.11 (Left) MRI image showed a significant contrast enhancement (c.e.) in the left temporal lobe, suspected of a recurrent disease in a patient with glioblastoma, already surgically treated. (Middle and right) A moderate uptake of [^{18}F]FET was demonstrated in PET/CT images, affirming the presence of recurrent glioblastoma

22.8 [^{11}C]-Methionine

Methionine is an essential amino acid involved in protein synthesis and transmethylation reactions. When labeled with the positron-emitting radionuclide carbon-11 (^{11}C, half-life ≈ 20.4 minutes), methionine becomes a valuable tracer for visualizing increased amino acid transport and protein synthesis activity, which are often upregulated in tumor cells. ^{11}C-methionine is synthesized by incorporating ^{11}C into the methyl group of methionine, typically via a methylation reaction using [^{11}C]-methyl iodide or [^{11}C]-methyl triflate. The final product is administered intravenously, and due to its short half-life, its production must occur close to the PET imaging facility using an on-site cyclotron and automated synthesis module. It has high specificity for amino acid transporters such as LAT1, which are overexpressed in many tumors. It is rapidly taken up in metabolically active tissues with low background accumulation in normal brain parenchyma; it has a short half-life, enabling multiple scans in a day but requiring efficient logistics and radiochemistry infrastructure. The primary clinical applications of ^{11}C-methionine PET include (1) differentiation of tumor recurrence from post-treatment changes in gliomas and other brain tumors; (2) tumor delineation for radiotherapy planning, and (3) evaluation of amino acid metabolism in various cancers, including head and neck tumors, and multiple myeloma [20, 21] (see Figs. 22.10, 22.12, and 22.13). Compared to [^{18}F]FDG, [^{11}C]-methionine offers higher specificity in certain contexts, particularly in the brain, where FDG's high physiological uptake can obscure pathology. However, its limited availability due to the short half-life of ^{11}C and the need for an on-site cyclotron restricts its widespread clinical use.

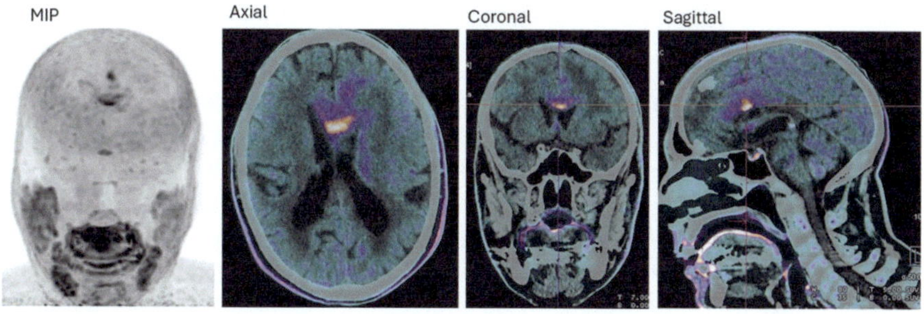

Fig. 22.12 Images of [^{11}C]MET PET/CT in a patient with multiple uptakes of tracer in a diverse brain region compatible with a diffuse gliomatosis

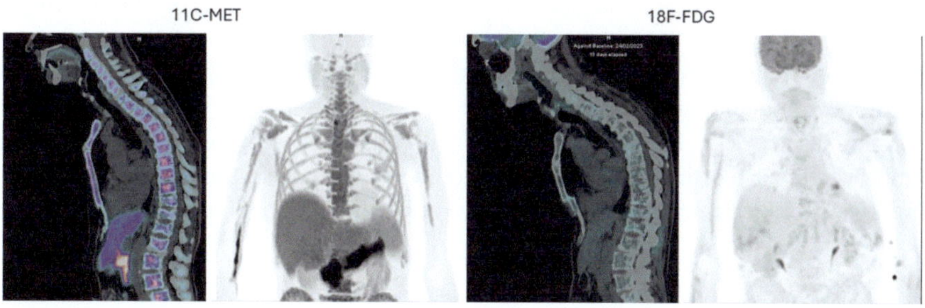

Fig. 22.13 Comparative images of a patient with a history of multiple myeloma. (left) [^{11}C]MET showed an intense uptake of the tracer in the bone marrow, while [^{18}F]FDG PET/CT (right) was slightly negative. The clinical messages provided by the images were different: widespread of disease vs. prognostic information

Table 22.1 Comparison between [^{18}F]FDG, [^{11}C]MET and [^{18}F]FET

Parameter	FET	MET	FDG
Target	LAT 1	LAT 1	Glucose metabolism
Uptake in normal brain	Low	Low	High
Tumor-to-background ratio	High	High	Moderate to low
Main clinical use	Brain tumors	Brain tumors, head and neck, multiple myeloma	Wide range of tumors
Half-life	110 min	20 min	110 min

In Table 22.1, the main differences between [^{18}F]FDG, [^{11}C]MET, and [^{18}F]FET are reported.

While [^{11}C]-methionine remains a gold standard in certain research and specialized clinical settings, the logistical challenges of [^{11}C] labeling are driving interest in alternative tracers labeled with longer-lived radionuclides, such as [^{18}F]-labeled amino acid analogs (e.g., [^{18}F]FET and [^{18}F]FDOPA). Nevertheless, [^{11}C]-methionine continues to provide critical insights into tumor biology and holds promise in the context of personalized oncology and therapy response monitoring.

^{18}F-fluoro-L-DOPA ([^{18}F]FDOPA) is a fluorinated analog of the amino acid L-3,4-dihydroxyphenylalanine (L-DOPA). Its dual role—neurological and oncological—makes FDOPA one of the most versatile PET radiotracers in clinical use today. L-DOPA is the precursor of dopamine and other catecholamines. FDOPA mimics L-DOPA in biochemical pathways and is taken up by large neutral amino acid transporters (LAT1/2) and subsequently decarboxylated by aromatic L-amino acid decarboxylase into ^{18}F-fluorodopamine in neurons or tumor cells. In neurology, FDOPA uptake reflects dopaminergic neuron integrity, while in oncology, it reflects amino acid transport and intracellular metabolism, often upregulated in neuroendocrine tumors and gliomas. Clinical applications are the following: neuro-oncology (1, tumor detection and delineation, particularly in low- and high-grade gliomas; 2, assessment of recurrence vs. post-treatment effects; and 3, therapy monitoring), movement disorders (1, parkinson's disease; 2, multiple system atrophy; and 3, progressive supranuclear palsy), neuroendocrine tumors (1, carcinoid tumors; 2, pheochromocytoma and paraganglioma—see Fig. 22.14—and 3, medullary thyroid carcinoma, see Fig. 22.15). In patients with medullary thyroid cancer is often employed in case of increase in the calcitonin levels. Indeed, the increase in tumor markers is often associated with a negative conventional imaging result; while also

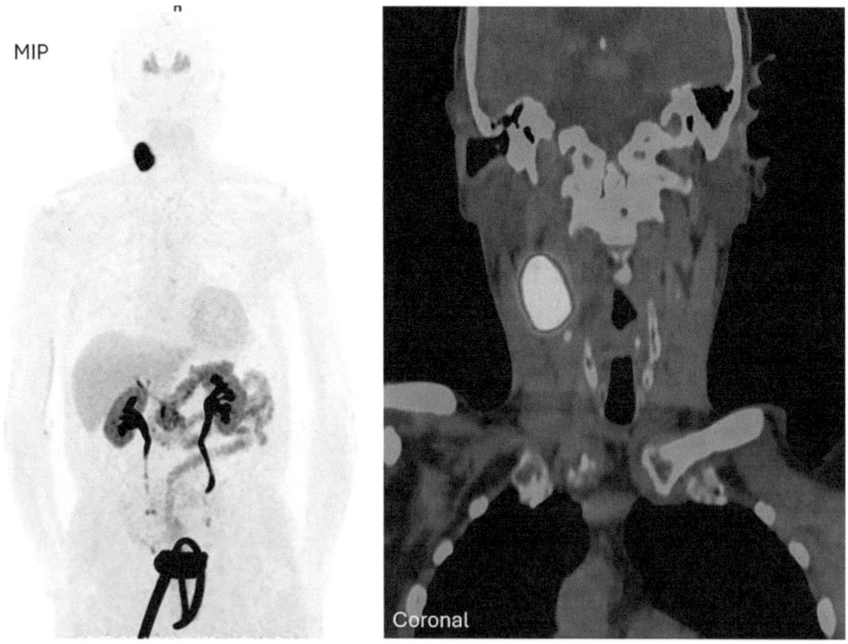

Fig. 22.14 A focal intense uptake of [^{18}F]DOPA in a patient with a diagnosis of paraganglioma

for lower levels, DOPA PET can detect the presence of a recurrence, thus increasing the success of the salvage treatments. In patients with pheochromocytoma, it can increase the detection rate, although the completeness can be obtained by including also [^{18}F]FDG PET/CT as additional imaging. In patients with brain disease, it can be used both in malignant and benign lesions. In the first subset of patients, it can be used as an alternative to [^{11}C]MET and [^{18}F]FET, although its accuracy is low. Indeed, it can be useful for patients with low-grade gliomas. In patients with neurodegenerative disease, it can be used as an alternative to ^{123}I-Ioflupane (see Fig. 22.16), although less data is now available in the literature, in terms of standardization [22, 23].

Despite its clinical advantages, FDOPA has some constraints, such as a synthesis more complex compared to other ^{18}F tracers, limited availability in some regions, though improving and nonspecific uptake in inflammatory or non-neoplastic conditions.

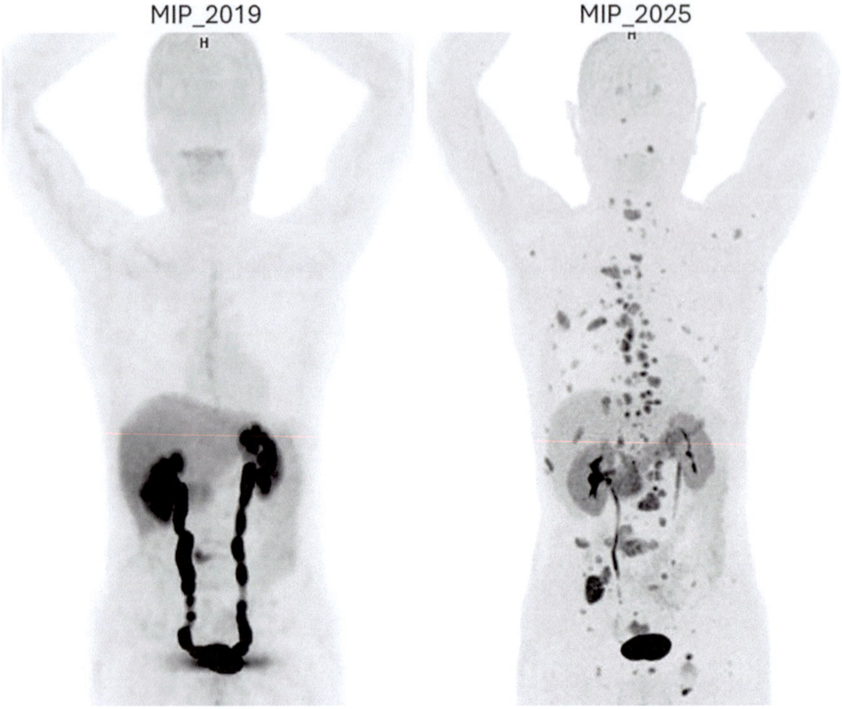

Fig. 22.15 Two MIP images in a patient with a history of medullary thyroid carcinoma. In 2019, for a small elevation of calcitonin level, the patient was submitted to DOPA PET/CT, which resulted in a negative. A second scan was performed after 5 years, due to a consistent elevation of calcitonin. PET/CT images showed intense multiple uptake of the radiopharmaceuticals in multiple sites of disease (bone and lymph nodes)

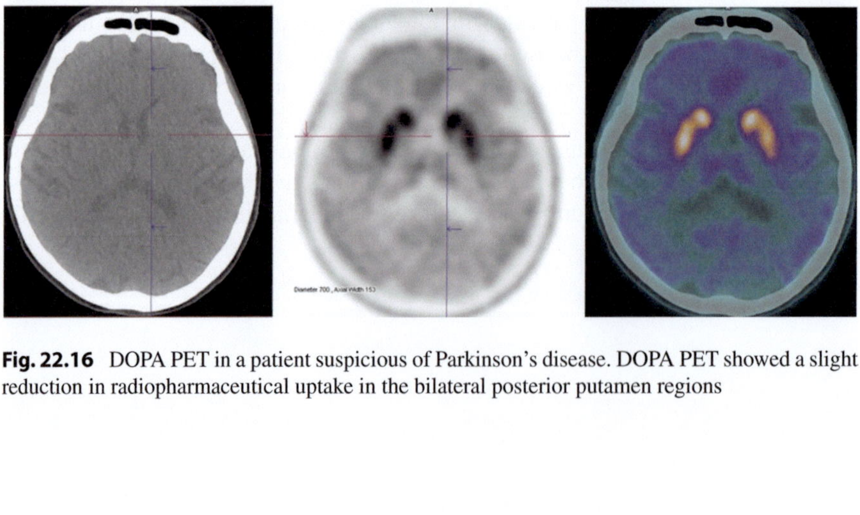

Fig. 22.16 DOPA PET in a patient suspicious of Parkinson's disease. DOPA PET showed a slight reduction in radiopharmaceutical uptake in the bilateral posterior putamen regions

22.9 [^{11}C]-Acetate

[^{11}C]-acetate is a radiolabeled small molecule used in PET to study oxidative metabolism and lipid synthesis. Originally investigated for myocardial perfusion and oxidative metabolism imaging, it has gained increasing use in oncology, particularly for imaging tumors with high lipid synthesis activity such as prostate cancer, hepatocellular carcinoma (HCC), and renal cell carcinoma. Unlike [^{18}F]FDG, which reflects glucose metabolism, ^{11}C-acetate provides complementary information about the tricarboxylic acid (TCA) cycle and de novo fatty acid synthesis, both of which are altered in many tumors.

Acetate is a key intermediate in cellular metabolism, entering the TCA cycle as acetyl-CoA and contributing to mitochondrial oxidative phosphorylation, fatty acid synthesis and cholesterol and phospholipid biosynthesis. In tumors, [^{11}C]-acetate uptake reflects both oxidative metabolism and lipogenesis. It is transported into cells and rapidly converted to acetyl-CoA by acetyl-CoA synthetase (ACSS2). In cancers with enhanced fatty acid metabolism—such as prostate or liver tumors—this pathway is markedly upregulated. [^{11}C]-acetate exhibits rapid uptake in tissues with high oxidative and lipogenic activity, with relatively low background in many non-target tissues. Usually, imaging starts 5–10 minutes post-injection and the physiologic uptake has been registered in myocardium, liver, pancreas, salivary glands, and kidneys. Unlike [^{18}F]FDG, it has low urinary excretion, making it ideal for pelvic imaging (e.g., prostate). ^{11}C-acetate is widely used in prostate cancer patients for primary tumor localization, especially in low-grade or FDG-negative disease, detection of local recurrence after prostatectomy or radiotherapy, staging of biochemical recurrence, particularly with low PSA levels and assessment of metastatic disease, often complementing ^{11}C- or ^{18}F-choline [24, 25].

It can also be used in HCC, because it can detect well-differentiated HCC, which may not show FDG uptake due to low glycolytic activity. Some studies have shown potential use in renal cell carcinoma, bladder cancer and gliomas and other brain tumors.

22.10 [^{18}F]-Fluorothymidine (FLT)

[^{18}F]-fluorothymidine ([^{18}F]FLT or FLT) is a non-invasive imaging biomarker of DNA synthesis via the thymidine salvage pathway. Its uptake correlates with the expression and activity of thymidine kinase-1 (TK1), a key enzyme upregulated during the S-phase of the cell cycle. FLT mimics natural thymidine but is not incorporated into DNA. Instead, it is taken up by nucleoside transporters and phosphorylated by TK1. Once phosphorylated, FLT becomes trapped intracellularly, allowing imaging of proliferative activity. TK1 expression is cell cycle–dependent and correlates with tumor aggressiveness. FLT uptake is considered a surrogate for Ki-67, a widely used histologic proliferation marker. This makes [^{18}F]FLT an attractive tracer for distinguishing between active tumor tissue and necrosis or post-therapy changes. FLT PET is used to grade tumors (higher uptake correlates with increased proliferation), differentiate recurrence vs. post-therapy effects, particularly in brain and lung cancers, monitor treatment response, especially in early-phase clinical trials of cytotoxic or targeted agents. Common indications include lung cancer (see Figs. 22.17 and 22.18), breast cancer, gliomas, lymphoma, colorectal and head & neck cancers [26–28].

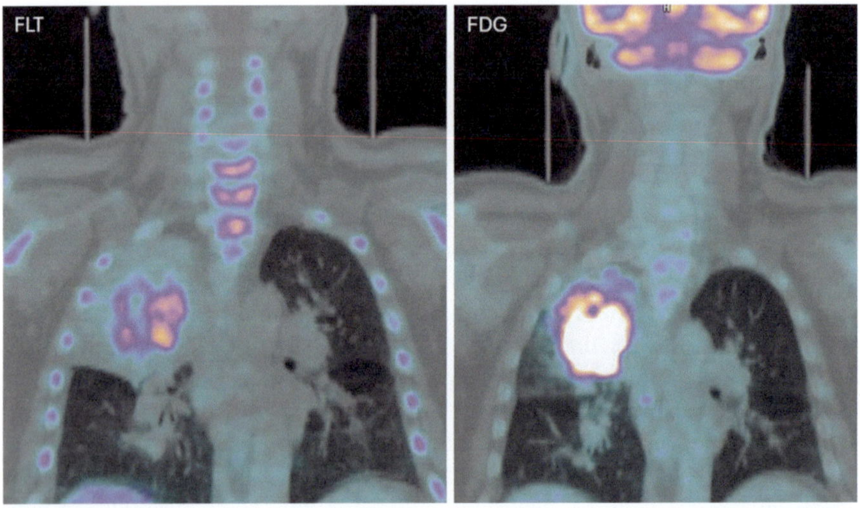

Fig. 22.17 Comparative images of [^{18}F]FLT and [^{18}F]FDG in a patient with lung cancer. FDG uptake was intense and homogeneous (right), while FLT uptake was inhomogeneous (left)

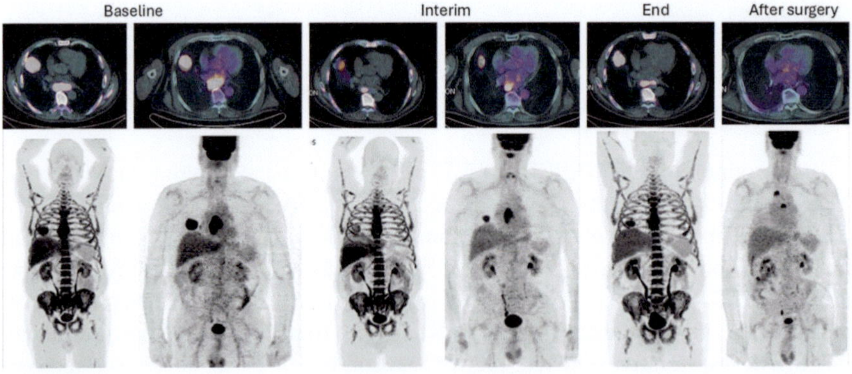

Fig. 22.18 Serial [^{18}F]FDG and [^{18}F]FLT PET/CT scan in a patient with lung cancer. The images were made at baseline, before starting any treatment, after 2 cycles of treatments and at the end or after the surgical approach

22.11 Tumor Hypoxia: [^{18}F]MISO, [^{18}F]FAZA, and [^{64}Cu]ATSM

Several PET radiotracers have been developed to visualize hypoxia in vivo, including [^{18}F]fluoromisonidazole ([^{18}F]MISO), [^{18}F]-fluoroazomycin arabinoside ([^{18}F]FAZA), and [^{64}Cu]-diacetyl-bis(N4-methylthiosemicarbazone) ([^{64}Cu]ATSM) (see Figs. 22.19, 22.20 and 22.21). These agents rely on bioreductive trapping in hypoxic cells, and each has unique pharmacokinetic properties. Most hypoxia tracers are nitroimidazole-based compounds, which undergo enzymatic one-electron reduction inside cells. Under normoxic conditions, these intermediates are rapidly reoxidized. However, in hypoxic conditions, further reduction leads to the

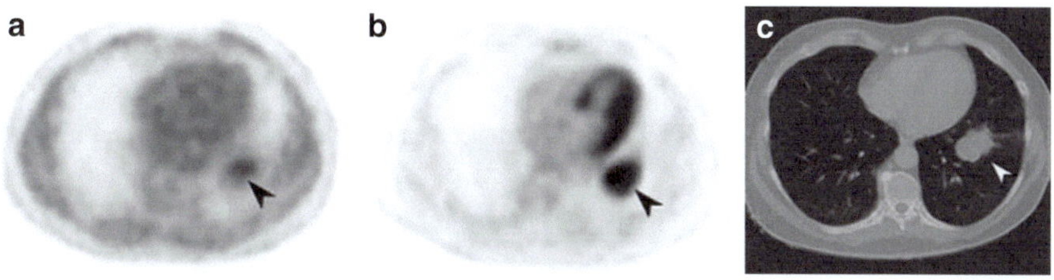

Fig. 22.19 (**a**) [^{18}F]FMISO uptake in non-small cell lung cancer (arrow). (**b**) Uptake of [^{18}F]FDG in the left lung tumor (black arrow). (**c**) Corresponding CT slice showing the left lung tumor (white arrow). (From Sze Ting Lee et al. [29])

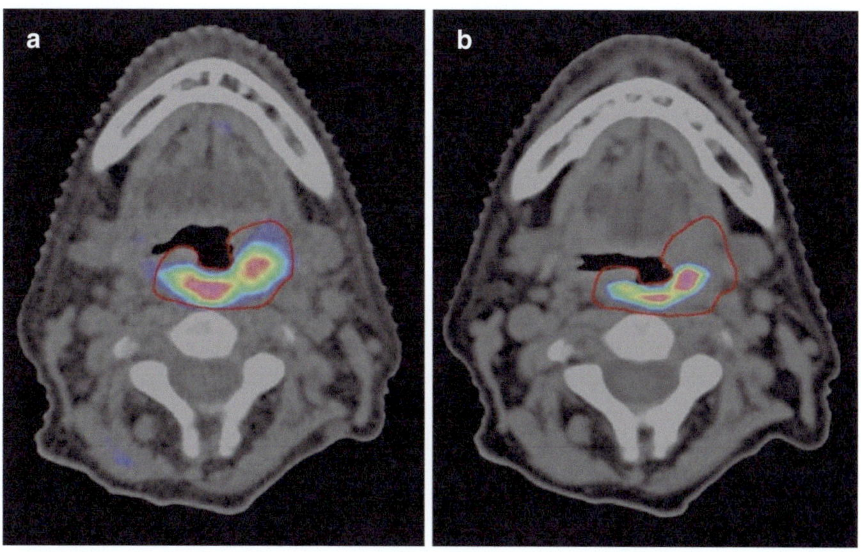

Fig. 22.20 [^{18}F]FAZA PET/CT images of a patient with an oropharyngeal p16-negative squamous cell carcinoma. The patient was imaged 2 h after injection of 10 mCi of [^{18}F]FAZA. a Baseline image: b image taken after a radiation dose of 12 Gy combined with daily nimorazole. The red line depicts the GTV delineated on the planning CT. (Courtesy of Lise Saxoe Mortensen. From Grégoire et al. [30])

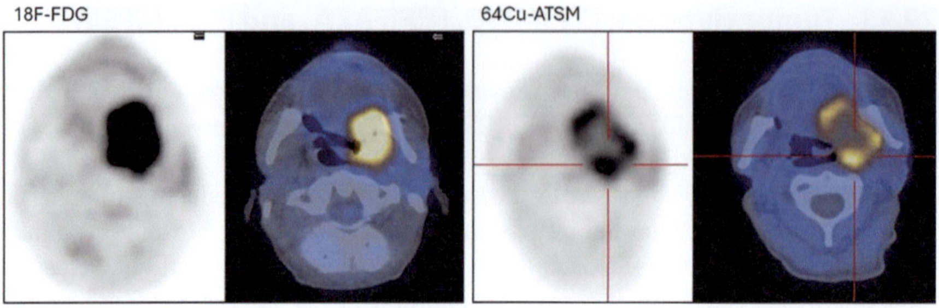

Fig. 22.21 Comparison between [^{18}F]FDG and [^{64}Cu]-ATSM PET in a patient with head and neck cancer. [^{18}F]FDG showed an intense and homogeneous uptake in the primary lesion, while [^{64}Cu]-ATSM showed an intense border of uptake and a low uptake in the center of the lesion. The hypoxia signal is useful to guide the painting radiotherapy

Table 22.2 Comparison among diverse radiopharmaceuticals against hypoxia mechanisms

Tracer	Uptake mechanism	Clearance	Imaging time (post-injection)	Notes
[^{18}F] MISO	Nitroimidazole, hypoxia-trapped	Slow	2–4 h	Extensive clinical validation
[^{18}F] FAZA	Nitroimidazole, more hydrophilic	Faster	1–2 h	Improved contrast vs. MISO
[^{64}Cu] ATSM	Redox-based trapping	Rapid	30 min–1 h	May reflect both hypoxia and metabolism

formation of reactive metabolites that bind intracellular macromolecules, leading to tracer retention in hypoxic regions. [^{64}Cu]ATSM, by contrast, follows a redox-based mechanism involving reduction of Cu(II) to Cu(I) under hypoxia, which results in selective cellular trapping.

In Table 22.2 are reported data about imaging Protocol and characteristics.

Hypoxia imaging helps to identify resistant tumor sub volumes for radiotherapy dose escalation, to predict treatment outcomes and to stratify patients for hypoxia-modifying therapies (e.g., tirapazamine, nimorazole). In patients with squamous cell carcinoma of the head and neck, hypoxia burden predicts poor radiotherapy response. In glioblastoma, it helps distinguish pseudoprogression from true recurrence, and in non-small cell lung cancer, it aids in planning intensity-modulated radiation therapy. For the monitoring of response to therapy, serial imaging with hypoxia tracers can show reoxygenation during treatment, identify non-responding hypoxic regions early and serve as a biomarker of therapeutic efficacy (e.g., anti-angiogenic agents) [31–33].

Property	[^{18}F]MISO	[^{18}F]FAZA	[^{64}Cu]ATSM
Chemical type	Nitroimidazole	Nitroimidazole	Metal complex
Hypoxia mechanism	Bioreductive trapping	Bioreductive trapping	Redox trapping
Tumor uptake	Moderate	Moderate	High (not always hypoxia-specific)

(continued)

Property	[^{18}F]MISO	[^{18}F]FAZA	[^{64}Cu]ATSM
Background signal	Moderate	Low	Variable
Imaging window	2–4 h	1–2 h	30–60 min
Half-life	~110 min	~110 min	~12.7 h

Some limitations and challenges are related to hypoxia tracers. For example, [^{18}F]MISO and [^{18}F]FAZA require delayed imaging due to slow clearance, [^{64}Cu]ATSM uptake can be influenced by redox state, not just oxygenation and tracer availability varies by region and cyclotron capabilities.

22.12 Next-Generation Theranostic Radiopharmaceuticals in Oncological PET Imaging

The future of oncological PET imaging lies in the rise of novel radiopharmaceuticals designed not only for detection but also for personalized radionuclide therapy—the cornerstone of theranostics. Moving beyond established agents like PSMA and somatostatin analogs, new molecular targets are emerging that promise broader cancer applicability and improved therapeutic outcomes. One of the most promising frontiers is the development of FAP-targeting tracers, such as [^{68}Ga]Ga-FAPI-46 and its therapeutic isotopologues (e.g., [^{177}Lu]FAPI, [^{225}Ac]FAPI). Unlike PSMA or DOTATATE, FAPI agents address the tumor stroma—particularly cancer-associated fibroblasts, which are abundant across many solid tumors. Early trials have shown rapid tumor uptake and low background activity, suggesting powerful potential for both imaging and treatment of otherwise hard-to-target malignancies like pancreatic, cholangiocarcinoma, and triple-negative breast cancer [34, 35].

Another compelling class includes CXCR4-targeted agents, such as [^{68}Ga]Pentixafor, designed to bind the chemokine receptor CXCR4, a key driver of tumor aggressiveness and metastatic behavior. Its therapeutic counterpart, [^{177}Lu]Pentixather, is showing early potential in hematologic malignancies and solid tumors, enabling the dual role of staging and treatment in diseases with limited therapeutic options [36].

Also gaining momentum are GRPR-targeted tracers, such as [^{68}Ga]RM2 and [^{177}Lu]NeoBOMB1, which aim at the gastrin-releasing peptide receptor, overexpressed in breast, prostate, and lung cancers. Their ability to noninvasively assess receptor status and deliver targeted radionuclide therapy could open new paths for managing hormone-sensitive malignancies.

Furthermore, integrin $\alpha v\beta 3$-targeted tracers like [^{68}Ga]Ga-NOTA-RGD derivatives are being studied for tumors with high angiogenic activity. While still in early-phase research, they offer both imaging of tumor neovascularization and therapeutic possibilities using isotopes like [^{177}Lu] or [^{90}Y] [37].

These agents represent a shift toward tumor biology-driven imaging and therapy, enabling a more universal and adaptable theranostic model. With ongoing preclinical refinement and expanding early-phase trials, such tracers may redefine cancer management by targeting mechanisms beyond classical receptors.

References

1. Sadowski SM, Neychev V, Millo C, Shih J, Nilubol N, Herscovitch P, Pacak K, Marx SJ, Kebebew E (2016) Prospective study of 68 Ga-DOTATATE positron emission tomography/computed tomography for detecting gastro-entero-pancreatic neuroendocrine tumors and unknown primary sites. J Clin Oncol 34(6):588–596. https://doi.org/10.1200/JCO.2015.64.0987
2. Hope TA, Allen-Auerbach M, Bodei L, Calais J, Dahlbom M, Dunnwald LK, Graham MM, Jacene HA, Heath CL, Mittra ES, Wright CL, Fendler WP, Herrmann K, Taïeb D, Kjaer A (2023) SNMMI procedure standard/EANM practice guideline for SSTR PET: imaging neuroendocrine tumors. J Nucl Med 64(2):204–210. https://doi.org/10.2967/jnumed.122.264860
3. Di Franco M, Fortunati E, Zanoni L, Fanti S, Ambrosini V (2025) The role of combined FDG and SST PET/CT in neuroendocrine tumors. J Neuroendocrinol 37(3). https://doi.org/10.1111/jne.13474
4. Quak E, Cavarec M, Ciappuccini R, Girault G, Rouzier R, Lequesne J (2023a) Detection, resection and cure: a systematic review and meta-analysis of 18F-choline PET in primary hyperparathyroidism. Q J Nucl Med Mol Imaging 67(2). https://doi.org/10.23736/S1824-4785.23.03512-4
5. Quak E, Weyts K, Jaudet C, Prigent A, Foucras G, Lasnon C (2023b) Artificial intelligence-based 68Ga-DOTATOC PET denoising for optimizing 68Ge/68Ga generator use throughout its lifetime. Front Med 10. https://doi.org/10.3389/fmed.2023.1137514
6. Yao N, Li W, Xu G, Duan N, Yu G, Qu J (2023) Choline metabolism and its implications in cancer. Front Oncol 13. https://doi.org/10.3389/fonc.2023.1234887
7. Wang R, Shen G, Huang M, Tian R (2021) The diagnostic role of 18F-choline, 18F-Fluciclovine and 18F-PSMA PET/CT in the detection of prostate cancer with biochemical recurrence: a meta-analysis. Front Oncol 11. https://doi.org/10.3389/fonc.2021.684629
8. Ghidaglia J, Golse N, Pascale A, Sebagh M, Besson FL (2022) 18F-FDG /18F-choline dual-tracer PET behavior and tumor differentiation in hepatocellular carcinoma. a systematic review. Front Med (Lausanne) 9. https://doi.org/10.3389/fmed.2022.924824
9. Roseland ME, Dewaraja YK, Wong KK (2022) Advanced imaging and theranostics in thyroid cancer. Curr Opin Endocrinol Diabetes Obes 29(5):456–465. https://doi.org/10.1097/MED.0000000000000740
10. Beheshti M, Mottaghy FM, Payche F, Behrendt FFF, Van den Wyngaert T, Fogelman I, Strobel K, Celli M, Fanti S, Giammarile F, Krause B, Langsteger W (2015) 18F-NaF PET/CT: EANM procedure guidelines for bone imaging. Eur J Nucl Med Mol Imaging 42(11):1767–1777. https://doi.org/10.1007/s00259-015-3138-y
11. Kairemo K, Kappadath SC, Joensuu T, Macapinlac HA (2020) A retrospective comparative study of sodium fluoride (NaF-18)-PET/CT and fluorocholine (F-18-CH) PET/CT in the evaluation of skeletal metastases in metastatic prostate cancer using a volumetric 3-D radiomics analysis. Diagnostics 11(1):17. https://doi.org/10.3390/diagnostics11010017
12. Fendler WP, Eiber M, Beheshti M, Bomanji J, Calais J, Ceci F, Cho SY, Fanti S, Giesel FL, Goffin K, Haberkorn U, Jacene H, Koo PJ, Kopka K, Krause BJ, Lindenberg L, Marcus C, Mottaghy FM, Oprea-Lager DE et al (2023) PSMA PET/CT: joint EANM procedure guideline/SNMMI procedure standard for prostate cancer imaging 2.0. Eur J Nucl Med Mol Imaging 50(5):1466–1486. https://doi.org/10.1007/s00259-022-06089-w
13. Rovera G, Grimaldi S, Oderda M, Marra G, Calleris G, Iorio GC, Falco M, Grossi C, Passera R, Campidonico G, Mangia ML, Deandreis D, Faletti R, Ricardi U, Gontero P, Morbelli S (2024) Comparative performance of 68Ga-PSMA-11 PET/CT and conventional imaging in the primary staging of high-risk prostate cancer patients who are candidates for radical prostatectomy. Diagnostics 14(17):1964. https://doi.org/10.3390/diagnostics14171964
14. Farolfi A, Calderoni L, Mattana F, Mei R, Telo S, Fanti S, Castellucci P (2021) Current and emerging clinical applications of PSMA PET diagnostic imaging for prostate cancer. J Nucl Med 62(5):596–604. https://doi.org/10.2967/jnumed.120.257238

15. Damjanovic J, Janssen J-C, Prasad V, Diederichs G, Walter T, Brenner W, Makowski MR (2019) 68Ga-PSMA-PET/CT for the evaluation of liver metastases in patients with prostate cancer. Cancer Imaging 19(1):37. https://doi.org/10.1186/s40644-019-0220-x
16. Shagera QA, Karfis I, Kristanto P, Spyridon S, Diamand R, Santapau A, Peltier A, Roumeguère T, Flamen P, Artigas C (2023) PSMA PET/CT for response assessment and overall survival prediction in patients with metastatic castration-resistant prostate cancer treated with androgen receptor pathway inhibitors. J Nucl Med 64(12):1869–1875. https://doi.org/10.2967/jnumed.123.265874
17. Ceci F, Oprea-Lager DE, Emmett L, Adam JA, Bomanji J, Czernin J, Eiber M, Haberkorn U, Hofman MS, Hope TA, Kumar R, Rowe SP, Schwarzenboeck SM, Fanti S, Herrmann K (2021) E-PSMA: the EANM standardized reporting guidelines v1.0 for PSMA-PET. Eur J Nucl Med Mol Imaging 48(5):1626–1638. https://doi.org/10.1007/s00259-021-05245-y
18. Lim W, Acker G, Hardt J, Kufeld M, Kluge A, Brenner W, Conti A, Budach V, Vajkoczy P, Senger C, Prasad V (2022) Dynamic 18F-FET PET/CT to differentiate recurrent primary brain tumor and brain metastases from radiation necrosis after single-session robotic radiosurgery. Cancer Treat Res Commun 32:100583. https://doi.org/10.1016/j.ctarc.2022.100583
19. Singnurkar A, Poon R, Detsky J (2023) 18F-FET-PET imaging in high-grade gliomas and brain metastases: a systematic review and meta-analysis. J Neurooncol 161(1):1–12. https://doi.org/10.1007/s11060-022-04201-6
20. Filippi L, Frantellizzi V, Bartoletti P, De Vincentis G, Schillaci O, Evangelista L (2023) Head-to-head Comparison between FDG and 11C-methionine in multiple myeloma: a systematic review. Diagnostics 13(12):2009. https://doi.org/10.3390/diagnostics13122009
21. Glaudemans AWJM, Enting RH, Heesters MAAM, Dierckx RAJO, van Rheenen RWJ, Walenkamp AME, Slart RHJA (2013) Value of 11C-methionine PET in imaging brain tumours and metastases. Eur J Nucl Med Mol Imaging 40(4):615–635. https://doi.org/10.1007/s00259-012-2295-5
22. Engler H, Damian A, Bentancourt C (2015) PET and the multitracer concept in the study of neurodegenerative diseases. Dement Neuropsychol 9(4):343–349. https://doi.org/10.1590/1980-57642015DN94000343
23. Li P, Zhang Y, Xu T, Zhu J, Wei T, Zhao W (2023) Sensitivities evaluation of five radiopharmaceuticals in four common medullary thyroid carcinoma metastatic sites on PET/CT: a network meta-analysis and systematic review. Nucl Med Commun 44(12):1114–1125. https://doi.org/10.1097/MNM.0000000000001773
24. Karanikas G, Beheshti M (2014) 11C-acetate PET/CT imaging. PET Clinics 9(3):339–344. https://doi.org/10.1016/j.cpet.2014.03.006
25. Spick C, Herrmann K, Czernin J (2016) Evaluation of prostate cancer with ^{11}C-Acetate PET/CT. J Nucl Med 57(Supplement 3):30S–37S. https://doi.org/10.2967/jnumed.115.169599
26. Been LB, Suurmeijer AJH, Cobben DCP, Jager PL, Hoekstra HJ, Elsinga PH (2004) [18F]FLT-PET in oncology: current status and opportunities. Eur J Nucl Med Mol Imaging 31(12):1659–1672. https://doi.org/10.1007/s00259-004-1687-6
27. Bollineni VR, Kramer GM, Jansma EP, Liu Y, Oyen WJG (2016) A systematic review on [18F]FLT-PET uptake as a measure of treatment response in cancer patients. Eur J Cancer 55:81–97. https://doi.org/10.1016/j.ejca.2015.11.018
28. Peck M, Pollack HA, Friesen A, Muzi M, Shoner SC, Shankland EG, Fink JR, Armstrong JO, Link JM, Krohn KA (2015) Applications of PET imaging with the proliferation marker [18F]-FLT. Q J Nucl Med Mol Imaging 59(1):95–104
29. Lee ST et al (2007) Hypoxia positron emission tomography imaging with ^{18}ffluoromisonidazole. Semin Nucl Med 37:451–461
30. Grégoire V et al (2017) Impact of hypoxia on head and neck cancer radiotherapy. Clin Transl Imaging 5:497–505
31. Colombié M, Gouard S, Frindel M, Vidal A, Chérel M, Kraeber-Bodéré F, Rousseau C, Bourgeois M (2015) Focus on the controversial aspects of 64Cu-ATSM in tumoral hypoxia mapping by PET imaging. Front Med (Lausanne) 2. https://doi.org/10.3389/fmed.2015.00058

32. Halmos GB, Bruine de Bruin L, Langendijk JA, van der Laan BFAM, Pruim J, Steenbakkers RJHM (2014) Head and neck tumor hypoxia imaging by 18F-fluoroazomycin-arabinoside (18F-FAZA)-PET. Clin Nucl Med 39(1):44–48. https://doi.org/10.1097/RLU.0000000000000286
33. Xu Z, Li X-F, Zou H, Sun X, Shen B (2017) 18F-Fluoromisonidazole in tumor hypoxia imaging. Oncotarget 8(55):94969–94979. https://doi.org/10.18632/oncotarget.21662
34. Guglielmo P, Alongi P, Baratto L, Abenavoli E, Buschiazzo A, Celesti G, Conte M, Filice R, Gorica J, Jonghi-Lavarini L, Lanzafame H, Laudicella R, Librando M, Linguanti F, Mattana F, Miceli A, Olivari L, Piscopo L, Romagnolo C et al (2023) Head-to-head comparison of FDG and radiolabeled FAPI PET: a systematic review of the literature. Life 13(9):1821. https://doi.org/10.3390/life13091821
35. Mori Y, Dendl K, Cardinale J, Kratochwil C, Giesel FL, Haberkorn U (2023) FAPI PET: fibroblast activation protein inhibitor use in oncologic and nononcologic disease. Radiology 306(2). https://doi.org/10.1148/radiol.220749
36. Lindenberg L, Ahlman M, Lin F, Mena E, Choyke P (2024) Advances in PET imaging of the CXCR4 receptor: [68Ga]Ga-PentixaFor. Semin Nucl Med 54(1):163–170. https://doi.org/10.1053/j.semnuclmed.2023.09.002
37. Ma Y, Gao F (2024) Advances of radiolabeled GRPR ligands for PET/CT imaging of cancers. Cancer Imaging 24(1):19. https://doi.org/10.1186/s40644-024-00658-y

Clinical MR Biomarkers

23

Daniel Paech, Sebastian Regnery, and Heinz-Peter Schlemmer

23.1 Diffusion-Weighted Imaging (DWI)

Diffusion-weighted imaging (DWI) sequences provide information on microstructural tissue correlates that are complementary to conventional MR techniques. Essentially, DWI provides a measure of diffusion motion of water molecules, which is assumed to be more restricted in malignant tumors than in benign lesions due to higher cellularity. Thus, DWI has emerged as a powerful method with a variety of clinical applications in oncologic imaging. In the following, applications in brain, prostate, and breast cancer are discussed.

23.1.1 Diffusion-Weighted Imaging in Brain Cancer Patients

DWI has become an essential part of most MRI protocols in neuroradiology, in particular to assess stroke and brain tumor patients. Among brain tumors, gliomas are the most common type of primary intra-axial neoplasms in adults. The World Health Organization (WHO) classification of brain tumors is commonly used to

D. Paech (✉)
Division of Radiology, German Cancer Research Center (DKFZ), Heidelberg, Germany

Department of Radiology, Mass General Brigham, Harvard Medical School, Boston, USA
e-mail: dpaech@bwh.harvard.edu

S. Regnery
Department of Radiation Oncology, University Hospital Heidelberg, Heidelberg, Germany
e-mail: Sebastian.regnery@med.uni-heidelberg.de

H.-P. Schlemmer
Division of Radiology, German Cancer Research Center (DKFZ), Heidelberg, Germany
e-mail: h.schlemmer@dkfz.de

O. Schober et al. (eds.), *Molecular Imaging in Oncology - Volume 2*, Recent Results in Cancer Research 225, https://doi.org/10.1007/978-3-032-21415-7_5

guide therapy and to assess overall prognosis. Patient prognosis and survival depend on the tumor grade and even more on molecular characteristics, particularly the isocitrate dehydrogenase (IDH) mutation status, and in glioblastoma also the O6-methylguanine-DNA-methyltransferase (MGMT) promoter methylation status. Several studies of DWI in glioma patients reported an association of overall survival (OS) and progression-free survival (PFS) with DWI parameters, particularly the apparent diffusion coefficient (ADC). The ADC is the most common DWI-derived imaging biomarker with broad clinical applications. The majority of studies published in the literature show an inverse correlation between the ADC and tumor cellularity [1–4]. Accordingly, many studies found decreased ADC values in brain tumors to be correlated with worse outcome (OS and/or PFS) [1, 5–7], higher WHO grade [4, 8], irrespective of contrast enhancement in T1w-MRI [9], and IDH mutation [10]. Regarding therapy response assessment, changes in ADC have been shown to be associated with treatment response in glioma patients early after radiation therapy [11, 12]. These changes have been hypothesized to be linked to cellular structure reflecting apoptosis and/or necrosis. However, reliable differentiation of radiation-induced contrast enhancement (often called "pseudoprogression") from tumor progression using the ADC alone is currently not possible.

Furthermore, DWI sequences can be used to measure the apparent diffusion tensor of water D in each voxel of an image. It has been reported that diffusion tensor imaging (DTI) can be used to differentiate normal white matter, edematous brain, and enhancing tumor margins [13]. Moreover, DTI has been applied in the perioperative assessment of glioma patients in order to identify possible pyramidal tract involvement. The authors concluded that DTI-based functional neuronavigation contributes to maximal safe resection of cerebral gliomas with pyramidal tract involvement, thereby decreasing postoperative motor deficits [14].

Diffusion kurtosis imaging (DKI), an extension of DTI, allows the simultaneous estimation of the ADC and the apparent excess kurtosis coefficient (AKC) on a direction-dependent basis. Investigations in glioma patients yielded significant differences in kurtosis parameters between high-grade and low-grade gliomas; hence, better separation was achieved with these parameters than with conventional diffusion imaging parameters [15].

23.1.2 Prostate MRI with Diffusion-Weighted Imaging

DWI represents one of the pillars of the standardized PI-RADS (Prostate Imaging Reporting and Data System) reading scheme (Fig. 23.1). One recent study even suggested that DWI alone might be sufficient to detect clinically significant prostate cancer [16], which underlines its diagnostic power. Multiple studies have shown that DWI, combined with various mathematical models, improves differentiation between malignant and benign tissue changes in the prostate [17–21]. Specifically, the ADC significantly correlates with the Gleason score (GS) of prostate cancer (PCa) [17, 18, 20]. Accordingly, some studies suggested that ADC is a prognostic marker for patients undergoing active surveillance or radical prostatectomy [22, 23]. Conflicting results have been reported about the potential use

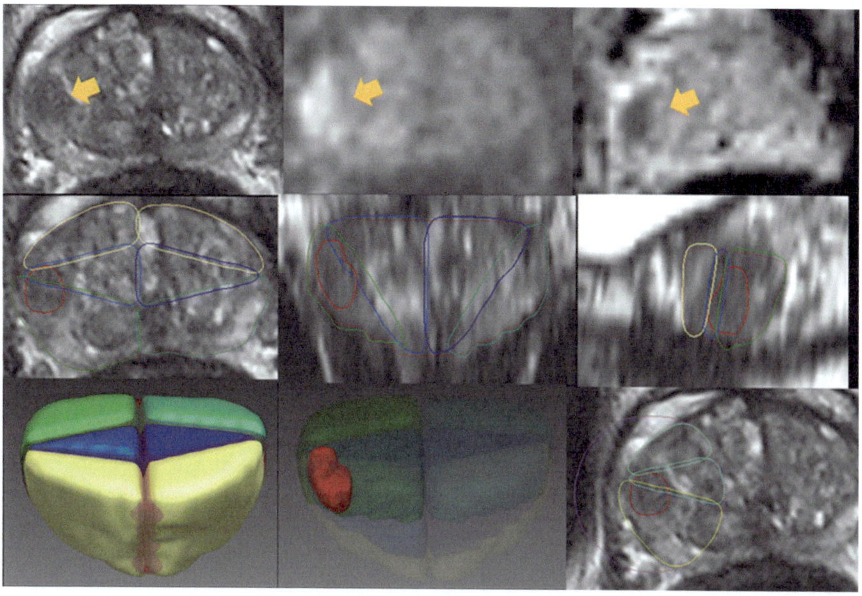

Fig. 23.1 Multiparametric MRI of the prostate. Top panel: axial T2-weighted image (left), DWI *b* value = 1500 s/mm^2 image (middle), and ADC map (right) demonstrate a suspicious lesion (arrows) with marked signal increase on *b* = 1500, a markedly decreased ADC value, and suspicious homogeneous hypointensity on the T2w image, PI-RADS 5. Middle panel: sextants are spatially defined for right and left anterior (yellow), middle (blue), and posterior (green) locations and shown together with the radiologically defined lesion (red) in axial (left), coronal (middle), and sagittal (right) planes. Bottom panel: volume renderings of the prostate segmentation seen from anteriorly superiorly with sextants shown (left) and lesion shown by decreasing the opacity of the sextant volumes (middle). (©*European Radiology*, Bonekamp et al. [35])

of ADC to detect small lymphatic metastases of prostate cancer [24, 25], while a recent report suggests a good correlation of PSMA-PET-signal and ADC in pelvic lymph nodes [26].

Also, histogram analysis of intravoxel incoherent motion (IVIM) is a feasible approach to stratification of prostate cancer according to the Gleason score. Recent investigations showed that D might perform better in distinguishing low-grade from high-grade carcinomas than the conventional ADC [27]. However, none of these approaches can currently replace lesion biopsy followed by histologic analysis. Therefore, the development of a reliable noninvasive tool to distinguish benign lesions, low-grade PCa, and high-grade PCa would be a major advance.

In 2021, a randomized controlled trial showed a significant improvement in biochemical recurrence-free survival after definitive radiotherapy (RT) when boosting the intraprostatic lesion visible on MRI [28]. Therefore, MRI techniques to reliably contour intraprostatic lesions have become an important topic. A multi-institutional study from 2023 suggested that radiation oncologists might miss intraprostatic lesions in 20% of cases, but a specific DWI-based map (Restriction Spectrum Imaging restriction score = RSIrs) could reduce this rate to merely 2% [29]. Moreover, MR-guided RT on hybrid machines, so-called MR-linacs, is an emerging technique [30, 31]. On the one hand, MR-linacs allow for highly precise treatment with online adaptation of the RT plan to changes in daily anatomy. On the other hand, sophisticated DWI becomes possible during treatment. Recent works suggested increases of D during radiotherapy [30] and of ADC during androgen deprivation [32], and early ADC changes could reflect radiotherapy response [33].

Finally, huge DWI datasets are now available to train AI models. Recently, a deep learning model based on T2w and T1w images, as well as DWI, detected clinically significant prostate cancers equally well as human radiologists and could also mostly localize the malignant lesion [34].

23.1.3 MR Mammography Using Diffusion-Weighted Imaging

DWI has extended the repertoire of noninvasive biomarkers in MR mammography. Especially in abbreviated, noncontrast-enhanced breast imaging protocols, DWI has become an integral part (Fig. 23.2). Decreased ADC has been shown to be associated with malignant breast tumors, which contributes to the differential diagnosis of unclarified lesions [36]. Furthermore, the ADC has been reported to correlate with pathologic biomarkers such as tumor cellularity, Ki67, and peritumoral lymphocytic infiltrate (PLI) in patients with estrogen receptor (ER)-positive breast cancer [37]. Consequently, DWI MRI is helpful for noninvasive characterization of suspicious breast masses and can increase the accuracy of conventional breast MRI assessment [38–40]. Besides the apparent diffusion coefficient (ADC), diffusion kurtosis imaging (DKI) parameters and fractional order calculus models (FROC) might provide insights into tissue heterogeneity [41–43]. Particularly, DKI, which quantifies the diffusion restriction, showed higher specificity than did conventional DWI for the assessment of benign and malignant breast lesions [42]. Intravoxel incoherent motion (IVIM) models use low b-values to calculate the perfusion fraction through bi-exponential fitting [44]. Diffusion tensor imaging (DTI) measures the direction of diffusion restriction and has been shown to correlate with the fibroglandular microarchitecture [45]. It should be discussed that DWI in breast tissue is challenging due to insufficient fat suppression and the heterogeneous tissue structure of the female breast [35, 46]. Additionally, there are differences in image acquisition protocols and post-processing methods that prevent a standardized clinical application so far [47].

A 2024 meta-analysis of more than 3500 patients suggests that noncontrast-enhanced DWI mammography yields modestly lower sensitivity at similar specificity to contrast-enhanced MR mammography. At the same time, noncontrast enhanced DWI MR mammography seems to offer higher diagnostic performance than standard mammography [48]. The authors discuss high study heterogeneity as an important limitation, which clearly reflects the lack of standardized protocols. Consequently, gadolinium contrast-enhanced MR mammography is currently considered the golden standard in MR mammography, but noncontrast-enhanced DWI mammography might be a promising future approach to mammography screening.

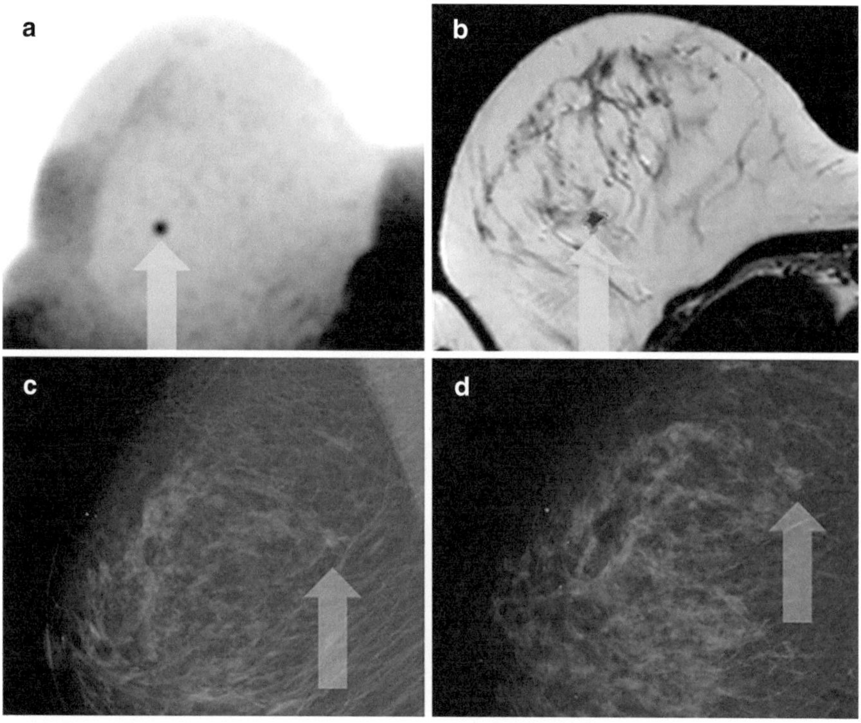

Fig. 23.2 Example of a female breast cancer screening participant with a suspicious lesion detected on X-ray mammography. (**a**) The MIBDI-MRI image (maximum intensity projection of diffusion-weighted imaging with background suppression, $b = 1500$ s/mm2, displayed with black-white-inversion) demonstrates a focal lesion within the breast parenchyma (as shown in the left image marked by the rose arrow). (**b**) Corresponding T2w-morphology (T2-TSE) that was evaluated in every patient with a lesion detected on the MIBDI-MRI, confirming the suspicious character of the lesion. Histopathology revealed an invasive ductal carcinoma (IDC, 4 mm). X-ray mammography depicting the suspicious lesion (arrows) in mediolateral oblique (**c**) and craniocaudal views (**d**). (©*Clinical Radiology*, Bickelhaupt et al. [49])

23.2 Perfusion MRI

Medical imaging techniques greatly benefit from the application of contrast agents. Gadolinium-based contrast agents (GBCAs) are most commonly used in MRI. Due to its paramagnetic properties, GBCA enhances the local nuclear relaxation rates of adjacent protons and thus modifies signal intensities in the images. Furthermore, the acquisition of time-resolved data, following the administration of a contrast agent, enables the derivation of quantitative parameters related to tissue perfusion and microvasculature. Major clinical applications of DCE MRI include brain, breast, prostate, and abdominal imaging in diagnostic oncology.

23.2.1 Perfusion MRI in the Brain

In the healthy brain, GBCAs are confined to the vascular spaces by the blood-brain barrier (BBB). Malignant gliomas often exhibit a disrupted BBB, causing further leakage of contrast agent into the extracellular-extravascular space (EES). Hence, T1w-GdCE MRI is used as the gold standard in clinical routine for diagnostics of brain tumors.

Dynamic susceptibility contrast (DSC) and dynamic contrast-enhanced (DCE) MRI have been widely applied to assess perfusion-related properties of brain tumors. DSC MRI is most commonly used in clinical routine to obtain semi-quantitative biomarkers such as the relative cerebral blood volume (rCBV) or the relative cerebral blood flow (rCBF) (Fig. 23.3). Quantitative MR-biomarkers can be determined

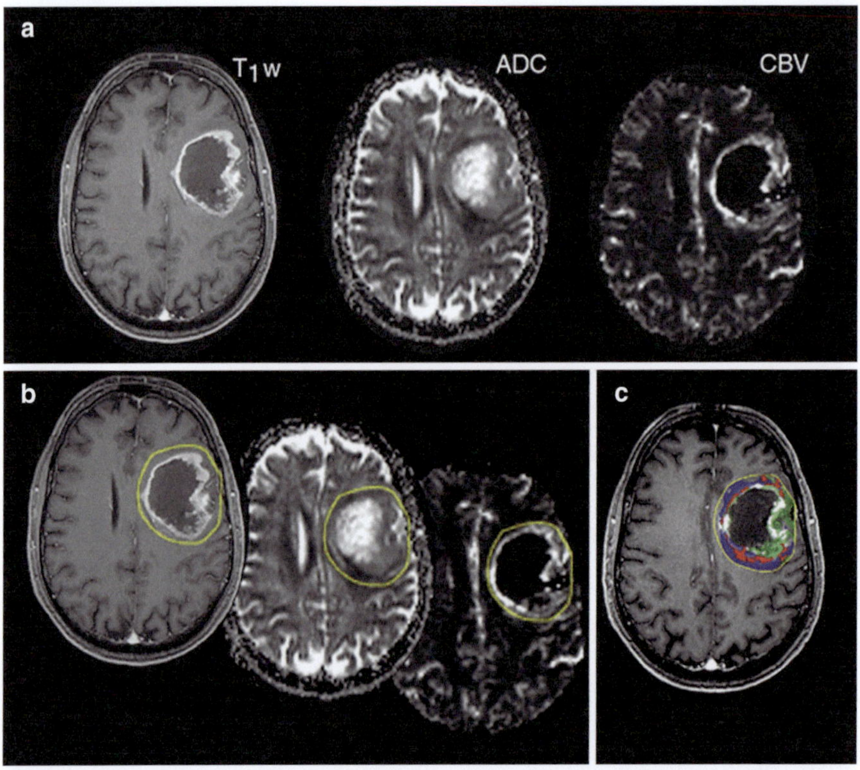

Fig. 23.3 Patient with a left frontal glioblastoma. (**a**) Gdce T1-w (left) image, ADC map (middle), and CBV map (right) shown. Decreased ADC values and increased CBV values can be observed, especially in the tumor rim, partially overlapping with the Gd contrast-enhancement. (**b**) Delineation of a region of interest (ROI) including the tumor and tumor periphery (yellow line). (**c**) Subsequently, an automatic identification algorithm has been applied to identify ADC hypointensities (ADC_{min} = 30th signal percentile blue) and CBV hyperintensities (CBV_{max} = 70th signal percentile = green) within the ROI. Red pixels represent regions where ADC_{min} and CBV_{max} match. (© *J Neurooncol*, Deike et al. [74])

through pharmacokinetic modeling analyses based on DCE-MRI data. Both approaches have been successfully applied for the assessment of parameters linked to blood volume, perfusion, and disruption of BBB in malignant gliomas [50–55].

rCBV is widely used to assess tumor vascularity and has been shown to be increased in WHO high-grade tumors compared to low-grade tumors [56, 57]. Additionally, peak height (PH) and the percentage of signal intensity recovery (PSR) derived from DSC perfusion MRI have enabled the differentiation of glioblastoma from brain metastases [58], while various cerebellar malignancies display different perfusion signatures [59]. Considering prognostic biomarkers, different investigators reported significantly increased rCBV in IDH-wt versus IDH-mut gliomas [52, 60]. Furthermore, increased rCBV and decreased PSR were reported in 1p/19q co-deleted (1p19q+) versus non-1p/19q co-deleted tumors (1p19q-) [61, 62]. Finally, higher rCBV values were reported in nonenhancing regions of IDH-mut astrocytoma versus IDH-wt glioblastoma [63]. Therefore, the DSC-based estimation of rCBV may enable the characterization of histologic and genetic subtypes in glioma patients prior to invasive procedures. Accordingly, increased rCBV values in the tumor region of glioma patients were reported to be associated with worse outcome (OS and/or PFS) [64–66]. Recently, it was suggested that vessel architectural imaging, which combines DSC and DCE-MRI, can characterize how brain metastases are vascularized, and that brain metastases with particularly large-caliber vessels are more resistant to immune-checkpoint therapy [67]. However, rCBV did not enable the prediction of chemosensitivity prior to treatment [65].

The degree of endothelial permeability is typically represented by the endothelial permeability surface area product or the transfer coefficient transfer constant (K^{trans}) [68]. K^{trans} is commonly determined on DCE MRI data using the Tofts and Kermode model. Besides permeability, K^{trans} also depends on several other factors, including vascular surface area and flow [68]. It has been reported to be significantly correlated with the tumor grade of gliomas [68, 69]. This correlation reflects a more pronounced BBB disruption in high-grade gliomas compared to low-grade tumors.

The volume fraction of extravascular extracellular space (v_e) is given by the leakage volume due to contrast extravasation outside the vascular space. It is considered as an index of tumor necrosis and an inverse index of tumor cellularity [70]. Few studies demonstrated that v_e may be useful to distinguish intra- from extra-axial masses and may also be positively correlated with tumor grade [71–73].

23.2.2 Arterial Spin Labeling (ASL) in Brain Tumors

A promising alternative for gadolinium-dependent perfusion MRI is given by non-contrast arterial spin labeling (ASL). Here, magnetically labeled blood water is used as an endogenous flow tracer to provide CBF quantification without the need for contrast media administration.

The label is usually performed by saturating or inverting the magnetization of the blood water molecules. After inversion delay (TI), a so-called tagged image is acquired and compared with a reference image without inverted or saturated blood water magnetization. The signal difference between these two images is proportional to the amount of magnetization delivered to the tissue and reflects local perfusion [75]. Thus, ASL represents a promising technique for noncontrast perfusion MRI [76]. Even though we are not there yet, the clinical application of ASL in malignant brain tumors may be useful as an adjunctive modality. Several studies have already shown the possibility of discriminating low- and high-grade gliomas using ASL [77]. Recently, a systematic review suggested that ASL-derived CBF might outperform DSC-derived CBF in differentiating HGGs from BMs [78]. Moreover, ASL identifies the cortical high-flow sign, a hallmark of IDH-mut oligodendrogliomas, more effectively than DSC-based maps [79].

23.2.3 Breast Perfusion Imaging

Gadolinium contrast-enhanced sequences are commonly used in breast MRI for the detection of abnormalities. Increased contrast enhancement of lesions is a central imaging finding of malignant breast tumors, which is caused by physiologically increased perfusion and leakage of the blood-tissue barrier.

Contrast-enhanced breast MRI enables fast and robust image acquisition with high spatial and temporal resolution. Using abbreviated contrast-enhanced MR protocols for breast cancer detection, high diagnostic sensitivities of up to 100% and a high negative predictive value (NPV) of up to 99.8% have been reported [80]. Using maximum intensity projections (MIPs), generated from only one pre- and one postcontrast acquisition and their derived images (first postcontrast subtracted [FAST] and maximum-intensity projection [MIP] images), has been shown to yield diagnostic accuracy equivalent to that of the regular full diagnostic protocol, and resulted in an additional cancer detection of 18.2 per 1000 [80]. Besides the identification of suspicious lesions, a positive correlation of initial contrast enhancement ratios with tumor grade has been reported [81]. However, this method has its limits in breast tissues with a high degree of background parenchymal enhancement (BPE), since high BPE might mask focal suspicious contrast enhancement [82]. Additional hemodynamic properties of malignant lesions can also be acquired and quantified using advanced imaging techniques such as time-resolved angiography with interleaved stochastic trajectories (TWIST), which may help to further increase the diagnostic accuracy of breast DCE MRI [83].

23.2.4 Prostate Perfusion Imaging

Even though malignant prostate lesions usually demonstrate high uptake of contrast agent, nonmalignant diseases such as prostatitis or benign prostatic hyperplasia are also known to enhance avidly with an enhancement pattern similar to prostate cancer [84]. Therefore, prostate DCE MRI alone has limited specificity and should only be interpreted together with other sequences such as T2-w imaging and ADC (derived from DWI), as recommended by the Prostate Imaging Reporting and Data System (PI-RADS). One investigation has even raised the question whether lesions with equivocal appearance on DWI, but strong dynamics on DCE MRI, should be upgraded from PIRADS 3–4 at all, due to the low specificity of DCE MRI [85].

Besides primary diagnosis, DCE-MRI assessment of patients with prostate cancer during and after primary proton and carbon ion irradiation revealed increased transfer constant (K^{trans}) and leakage space volume (v_e) in antihormonal therapy (AHT) naïve patients with persistent PSA elevation compared to those with PSA suppression. Consequently, these quantitative biomarkers may aid in the assessment of treatment response in prostate cancer [86].

23.2.5 Abdominal Perfusion MRI

Main applications in abdominal DCE-MRI, both nonquantitative and quantitative parameters, include renal, hepatic, and pancreatic lesion characterization. MRI can classify different liver lesions more accurately than multi-detector CT [87, 88]. The majority of incidental liver findings can be easily depicted and correctly identified by a combination of the information from the comprehensive liver magnetic resonance examination. These include malignant tumors, cysts, haemangiomas, focal nodular hyperplasia, adenomas, and other benign hepatic diseases [87]. Typically, three phases of contrast enhancement are clinically assessed to characterize liver tumors: (1) arterial phase images, (2) portal venous phase images, and (3) delayed equilibrium phase images. These three sequences take advantage of the dual blood supply to the liver via the hepatic artery and the portal vein to visualize the different phases of liver and tumour enhancement [87]. Thereby, perfusion data provide information on the tumor microvasculature and alterations in tumor perfusion that can be used to evaluate response to chemotherapy, antiangiogenic treatment, or percutaneous ablation of liver tumours [89–91]. Besides liver imaging, DCE-MRI has proven its utility in predicting and monitoring the effects of a variety of oncologic treatments in bone sarcomas and renal, bladder, and pancreatic cancers [92–95]. For instance, quantitative measures of K^{trans} in pancreatic tumors have been shown to enable the prediction of response to combined chemotherapy and antiangiogenic therapy [95]. The ability to detect and visualize tumor perfusion yields a more accurate diagnosis and improves the assessment of tumor treatment response [87]. Consequently, DCE MRI provides crucial complementary information to morphological sequences in the assessment of tumors.

23.3 Susceptibility-Weighted Imaging (SWI)

Susceptibility-weighted imaging (SWI) is a magnetic resonance imaging (MRI) technique that detects susceptibility differences between tissues by combining magnitude and phase information in gradient echo data [96]. SWI is sensitive to both paramagnetic and diamagnetic substances, particularly to deoxygenated blood and intracranial calcifications. SWI has therefore been applied to various pathologies, including intracranial hemorrhage, traumatic brain injury, stroke, neoplasm, and multiple sclerosis [96]. However, SWI does not provide quantitative measures of magnetic susceptibility, since phase information is nonlocal and orientation-dependent. This major limitation can be overcome using quantitative susceptibility mapping (QSM) approaches that yield susceptibility values of each voxel as a scalar quantity [96]. Furthermore, QSM can remove so-called blooming artifacts (as observed in conventional T2*w images), thus providing an accurate definition of the distribution of magnetic biomaterials in MRI.

Clinical applications of QSM are currently being probed mainly in neurodegenerative and inflammatory diseases to assess hemorrhage and to measure metabolic consumption of oxygen. QSM can detect calcifications in tumors with high sensitivity and has been demonstrated to be superior to phase imaging for the detection of intracranial hemorrhage and calcification [97]. QSM is suggested to correlate with different types of tumor-infiltrating macrophages in glioblastoma [98]. Moreover, QSM and T2*-mapping have gained interest during the experimental treatment of glioblastoma with pharmacological ascorbate [99, 100]. Ascorbate exploits specific differences in tumor iron metabolism. The aim is to increase cytotoxic intracellular radicals via the reduction of Fe^{3+} to Fe^{2+}. A recent phase II clinical trial reported promising results when combining ascorbate with radiotherapy and temozolomide. Furthermore, this trial employed QSM and T2*-mapping as noninvasive biomarkers of iron metabolism and established their correlation with progression-free survival [99, 100].

23.4 Magnetic Resonance Spectroscopy (MRS)

MR spectroscopy (MRS) allows to noninvasively detect metabolic features of tumor tissue in vivo. Proton MRS is essentially applied in clinical practice either as a single voxel or a multivoxel method because protons have the highest MR sensitivity, therefore enabling higher spatial resolution than MR spectroscopy of x-nuclei (nuclei other than protons).

Generally, proliferative tumor tissue shows intense resonances of choline-containing compounds (Cho) in proton MR spectra, and the technique can easily be performed on clinical 1.5 T MR scanners using routine receiver coils, sequence protocols, and evaluation software [101] (Fig. 23.4). MRS has to be considered as part of a combined diagnostic approach, including morphologic and functional MR imaging (MRI), e.g., for detecting areas of increased tumor vascularization by dynamic contrast enhanced MRI. The metabolic information can then be used to (1) differentiate malignant from benign mass lesions; (2) grade the aggressiveness of malignant tumors; (3) guide biopsy in heterogeneous mass lesions; (4) aid treatment planning in radiotherapy, chemotherapy, and surgery; and (5) monitor treatment effects of different chemo- and/or radiotherapy regimes [102–105]. However, MRS is not as robust as MRI, and the spectral quality strongly depends on the magnetic field homogeneity, which is influenced by the examined anatomic region and tissue

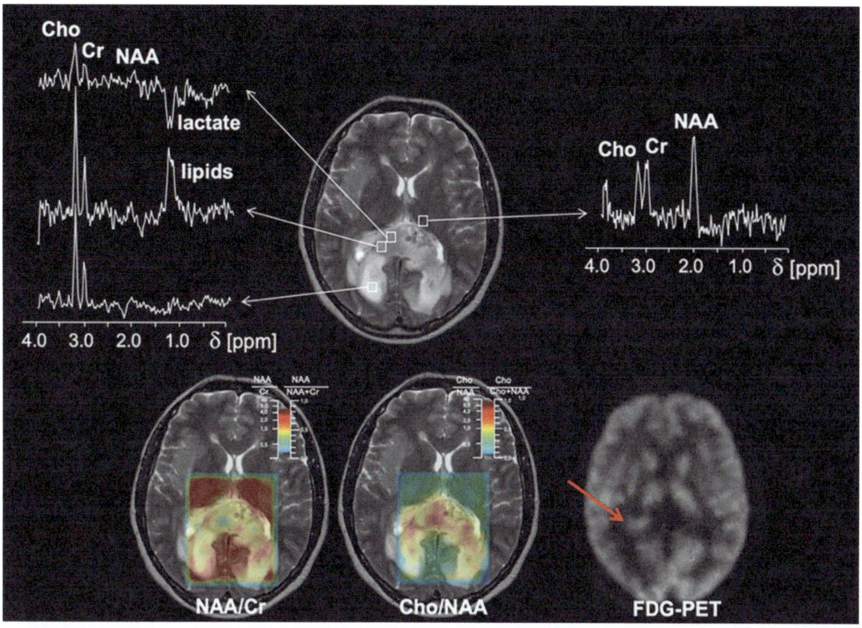

Fig. 23.4 A 39-year-old patient with a recurrent grade II astrocytoma after stereotactic irradiation with 54 Gy. Axial T2-weighted MRI 8 months after irradiation reveals a posterior mass with surrounding edema. The white grid on the T2w MRI marks the area of 1H-CSI examined (PRESS, TE = 135 ms). The 1H MR spectra measured in the mass (voxels 1, 2) show markedly increased signal intensity ratios from Cho to Cr and Cho to NAA. At the tumor margin (voxel 3), a lower relative signal intensity of the Cho resonance, but an additional lactate peak. Voxel 4 shows the spectrum of a normal appearing brain region. The recurrent tumor has high Cho or Cho/NAA and Cho/(Cho + NAA) values as well as low NAA and NAA/Cr and NAA/(NAA + Cr) values. However, the absolute signal intensity of the Cho resonance varies considerably in the tumor region (e.g., different SNR spectra 1 and 2 and the inhomogeneous color distribution of the Cho image in the tumor)

characteristics. Additionally, the specificity of MRS is limited because increased Cho levels are also observed in benign disorders, e.g., in inflammation. In brain tumors and prostate cancer, however, MRS has been proven to be a valuable diagnostic tool for staging and therapy monitoring in large clinical trials. It is well known from the literature that various cancer cells have increased lactate and lipid production associated with altered pH values in the tumor microenvironment [106]. These metabolic changes cause an acidification of the extracellular compartment (pHe) and an alkalization of the intracellular space (pHi) [107]. Decreased pH_e values were shown to enhance tumor invasiveness and angiogenesis. Increased pH_i values have been reported to increase cancer resistance to radiation and chemotherapy, as well as to contribute to enhanced proliferation and reduced apoptosis [108–110]. In this context, in vitro 1H MRS studies of astrocytoma biopsies have shown that lipid levels correlate with tumor necrosis [111]. Mobile lipids have also been shown to arise in some tumor cells under hypoxic stress prior to necrosis [112,

113]. Therefore, such insights into metabolic features could further our understanding of the pathophysiologically altered metabolism in tumors with impact on therapy planning and prognostication [110, 114]. Recently, this was underlined by a report of stronger correlation between MRS and IDH mutation status than traditional histopathological grading in astrocytoma [115].

23.5 Protein-Weighted MRI Using Chemical Exchange Saturation Transfer (CEST)

Chemical exchange saturation transfer (CEST) magnetic resonance imaging (MRI) represents a novel technique that enables large signal amplification of low-concentration molecules in vivo. CEST contrasts make use of the spontaneous chemical exchange between solute-bound protons and protons of free bulk water that to a large extent depends on the concentration of cellular proteins. Therefore, CEST MRI may add valuable information in diagnostic oncology prior to invasive procedures as well as in the follow-up setting for therapy monitoring.

Proteins and peptides have amide groups, which resonate around +3.5 parts per million (ppm) relative to the water proton signal. The majority of CEST studies published in the literature aimed at quantifying the amide proton transfer (APT) effect, most commonly assessed using the magnetization transfer ratio asymmetry (MTR_{asym}) approach proposed by Zhou et al. [116]. The resulting contrast is usually referred to as APT-weighted APT-w MRI in the literature.

Besides APT, relayed nuclear Overhauser effects (rNOE) and amine resonances can be observed in the so-called Z-Spectrum (Fig. 23.5), which is commonly acquired in CEST MRI through selective radiofrequency (RF) saturation [117]. Recently, more sophisticated approaches have been proposed, enabling simultaneous quantification of multiple CEST pools by using Lorentzian fit analysis on data with high spectral resolution obtained at 7.0 T [Fig. 23.1] [118–122]. CEST MRI significantly extends the currently available repertoire of MR biomarkers in diagnostic oncology and has recently been investigated in numerous clinical studies, with a large majority applied to neuro-oncologic diseases.

23.5.1 Brain Tumors

Preoperative assessment of glioma with APT(-w) CEST MRI has been shown to correlate with WHO tumor grade [123, 124] and has the potential to distinguish high- and low-grade glioma also for nonenhancing lesions [125] (Fig. 23.6). For rNOE-mediated CEST effects, correlation with tumor grade [126] and cellularity have also been reported [127]. While increased APT effects are observed in high-grade glioma, decreased rNOE signals were reported in both high-grade and low-grade glioma (Fig. 23.6) [118, 121, 124, 126, 127]. Interestingly, first experiences in pediatric patients also suggest a clear contrast between tumors and white matter with different APT signals in different brain tumor entities. But pilocytic astrocytoma, which is considered rather benign, presents

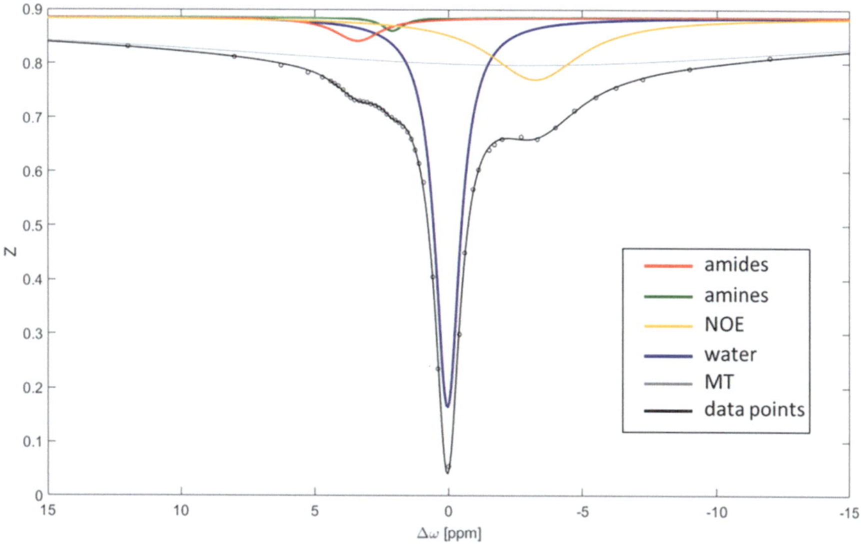

Fig. 23.5 CEST effects in the Z-spectrum at 7.0 Tesla. The most prominent resonances downfield from the water resonance can be assigned to the amide protons ($\Delta\omega = +3.5$ ppm) and fast-exchanging amines ($\Delta\omega = +2.7$ ppm). Upfield ($\Delta\omega = -2.0$ ppm to -5.0 ppm), a broader resonance can be observed, which is due to relayed nuclear Overhauser effects (rNOE). *Z*-spectrum acquired in the brain of a healthy volunteer at a 7 T whole body MRI scanner. [Parameters: 120 Gaussian-shaped pulses à 15 ms; B1 = 0.9 μT; 60 offsets, read out: FoV 195 × 170, matrix 128 × 112, slice 5 mm, TE = 3.61 ms, TR = 7.4 ms, flip angle 10°]

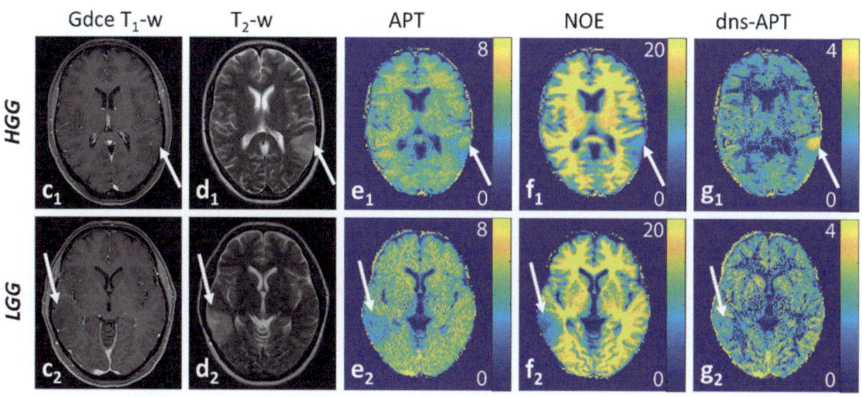

Fig. 23.6 Association of CEST MRI and WHO tumor grade (HGG vs. LGG) in newly diagnosed, untreated glioma patients. Two exemplary patients with high-grade glioma (HGG: glioblastoma, c_1 –g_1) and low-grade glioma (LGG: Oligodendroglioma II, c_2 –g_2) are shown: c_i: Gdce T1-w, di: T2-w (TSE), relaxation-compensated multi-pool CEST MRI at 7 T with separated APT (e_i), NOE (f_i), and downfield NOE-suppressed (dns)-APT (g_i) effects [unit: %]. Increased APT signals can be observed in the HGG tumor, especially at dns-APT imaging, whereas the LGG tumor displays hypo–/isointense to the surrounding normal appearing tissue. The glioblastoma patient shows only a small spot-like contrast enhancement in the tumor region (c_1), while a clear hyperintensity is displayed within the tumor at dns APT imaging (g_1, white arrow). (©*Neuro-Oncology*, Oxford Academic, Paech et al. [124])

significantly higher APT signal than other astrocytoma WHO grade I-II [128]. In general, different approaches of APT-mediated CEST MRI were shown to be associated with the IDH-mutation status in newly diagnosed gliomas [124, 129]. This finding is plausible since mutations in IDH gene-encoded enzymes cause widespread alterations of amino acid concentrations with a global downregulation of protein expression. Therefore, APT CEST MRI may represent an alternative MR biomarker that may help to determine IDH mutation status noninvasively.

Prognostication and early response assessment are major challenges in daily clinical decision-making in glioma patients [130]. Several studies reported increased APT-w signals in progressive tumors compared with treatment-related changes [131, 132] and to be associated with survival and progression-free survival (PFS) in glioma patients [133]. Furthermore, investigations of early treatment response in glioblastoma patients enabled the distinction of treatment responders from nonresponders at a time point as early as 2 weeks after the start of radiochemotherapy based on APT and rNOE imaging [134]. Similarly, early follow-up CEST-MRI 6–8 weeks after radiochemotherapy seems to differentiate tumor progression from treatment-related changes and correlates with both PFS and OS [135, 136]. APT and rNOE-mediated CEST contrasts were additionally shown to enable prognostication of response to first-line chemo-radiation therapy prior to treatment [133, 134, 137]. A recent systematic review and meta-analysis conclude that APT-imaging improves the noninvasive discrimination of treatment-related changes from tumor progression in glioma patients, but these promising results need to be confirmed in larger prospective study cohorts [138].

23.5.2 Applications of CEST MRI in Other Organs

CEST MRI has also been demonstrated to be feasible in other oncologic diseases. In 2011, CEST MRI was applied for the first time in 12 patients with biopsy-proven prostate cancer [139]. The study showed that APT-mediated CEST effects were significantly increased in the tumor region compared with the benign tissue of the peripheral zone [139]. These results are corroborated by a significant correlation between the APT signal in prostate tumors and the Gleason score, even though the relatively young field of CEST imaging does not reach the power of established DWI biomarkers so far [140, 141]. Investigations in breast cancer patients showed a positive correlation between APT CEST signal intensity and proliferation rates [142, 143]. Apart from that, the APT CEST contrast was recently also used to distinguish benign and malignant pulmonary lesions [144] as well as benign and malignant head and neck tumors [145]. All these recent studies indicate the high potential of CEST MRI as an additional, noninvasive tool in diagnostic oncology. However, further methodological research and technical improvements are required to enable robust clinical trials in larger cohorts.

23.6 Dynamic Glucose-Enhanced (DGE) MRI

Most common MRI contrast agents are based on the paramagnetic metal gadolinium (Gd), which enhances the nuclear relaxation rates of adjacent protons, thereby modifying signal intensities in the acquired images. Recently, Gd-based contrast agents (GBCA) have been subject to criticism, since several studies reported the accumulation of gadolinium in deep gray matter nuclei after serial application [146–151]. Besides, there is a known risk of developing nephrogenic systemic fibrosis for patients with renal failure [152]. Consequently, the development of novel MRI techniques using biodegradable contrast agents is highly desirable. A promising substance for such a new type of contrast agent is natural D-glucose, since it can be detected through chemical exchange saturation transfer (CEST) [153–155] or chemical exchange sensitive spin-lock (CESL) [156, 157]. The basic idea of these approaches is to measure signal changes after intravenous glucose administration with sufficiently high temporal and spatial resolution. The feasibility of dynamic glucose-enhanced DGE-MRI in humans has recently been proven in independent studies employing both CEST and CESL-based techniques [157–160]. Figure 23.7 shows glucose-enhanced images of a patient with newly diagnosed right-frontal glioblastoma [158]. The tumor regions of patients with glioblastoma showed increased glucose concentrations partially overlapping with the corresponding gadolinium-enhancement and relative cerebral blood volume (rCBV) maps, which are routinely acquired in diagnostic neuro-oncology [158]. However, also beyond disrupted blood-brain barrier regions, increased signal intensities can be observed at glucose-enhanced images (Fig. 23.7). Origins of signal changes in DGE-MRI are still under debate. Generally, glucose signal can result from concentration changes in three different compartments: (1) the intravascular space, (2) the extravascular and extracellular space (EES), and (3) the intracellular space. Latest results indicate major contributions of tissue perfusion and blood-brain barrier (BBB) leakage [158, 160, 161]. Besides, DGE-MRI contrasts may be additionally altered by local pH, since an acidic tumor microenvironment enhances DGE signals through the modulation of the proton exchange rate.

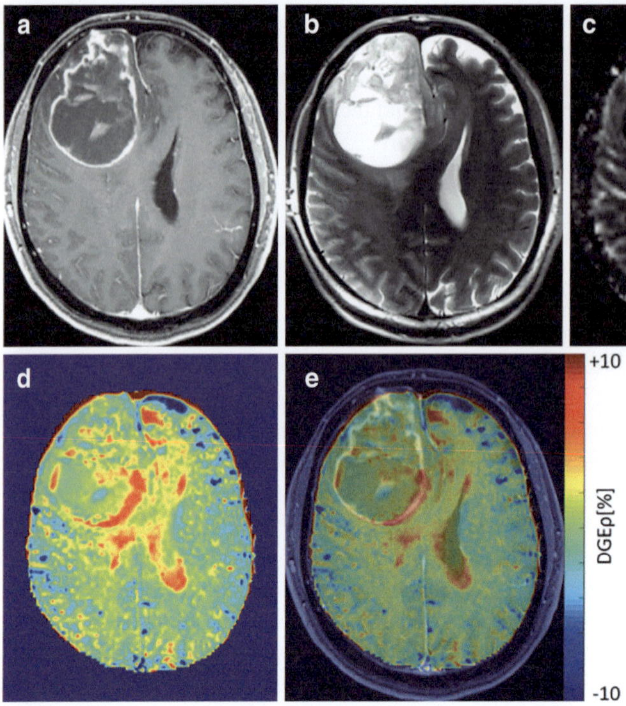

Fig. 23.7 T1ρ-weighted dynamic glucose-enhances (DGE_ρ) MRI at 7 T in a patient with newly diagnosed glioblastoma, compared with GdCE T1-w, T2-w, and perfusion imaging. (**a**) GdCE T1-w images, (**b**) T2-w images, and (**c**) rCBV maps are displayed. T2-w and (**d**) DGE_ρ images obtained at 7 T. (**e**) Fusion images of GdCE T1-w and DGE_ρ images. The DGE_ρ contrast displays regions of increased signal intensity, particularly in the dorsomedial tumor region (overlapping with the ring enhancement on GdCE-T1), and beyond the borders of BBB disruption (**e**). Some regions of increased glucose uptake cannot be delineated on the GdCE T1-w, T2-w, and perfusion images. Partial overlap can be observed between DGE_ρ and rCBV images. (Original figure from Paech et al. [158] with reprint permission from RSNA)

23.7 MR Fingerprinting for Quantitative Relaxometry (T1 and T2 Mapping)

Magnetic resonance fingerprinting (MRF) is an imaging approach to quantitatively measure multiple tissue properties simultaneously. This technique has been shown to enable rapid acquisition of T1 and T2 maps that correlate well with conventional T1 and T2 mapping methods [162, 163]. Initial clinical studies employing MRF-based techniques have reported promising results in brain, breast, and prostate cancer [164, 165]. Moreover, the application of four-dimensional MRF, i.e., reconstruction of multiple breathing phases, has been feasible in a small patient cohort with liver tumors. The authors have reported both good geometric accuracy and good tumor contrast, so that 4D-MRF could be useful for radiation treatment planning for moving targets in the body as well [166].

23.7.1 Prostate Relaxometry

A study performed by Yu and colleagues employed an MRF-based T1, T2, and standard apparent diffusion coefficient (ADC) mapping approach to differentiate cancer lesions in the peripheral zone from normal prostate tissue [167]. They reported that T1, T2, and ADC were all significant univariate predictors in the differentiation between histologically proven prostate cancer and normal-appearing peripheral zone (NPZ). Moreover, MRF-derived T2 and ADC helped to separate high- or intermediate-grade prostate cancer from low-grade cancer. Ultimately, T1, T2, and ADC were all significant predictors in the differentiation between histologically proven prostatitis and NPZ, while the combination of T1 and ADC yielded the best discrimination.

23.7.2 Brain Relaxometry

MR fingerprinting allows rapid simultaneous T1 and T2 measurement in brain tumors and surrounding tissues (Fig. 23.8). First clinical application in a study cohort of 31 patients with untreated intra-axial brain tumors showed that MRF-derived T1 and T2 maps have the potential to distinguish between gliomas and brain metastases [168]. Broader applications and investigations in larger study cohorts are needed to assess the full diagnostic potential of MRF-derived biomarkers.

23.7.3 Breast Relaxometry

Synthetic relaxometry has recently been applied to a cohort of approximately 100 women with breast cancer during neoadjuvant chemotherapy (NAC) [165]. The authors concluded that synthetic relaxometry decreased after NAC, and that the extent of this decrease correlated with the degree of pathological remission. A joint model, including cancer subtype, ADC, changes in T1, and tumor size, yielded the

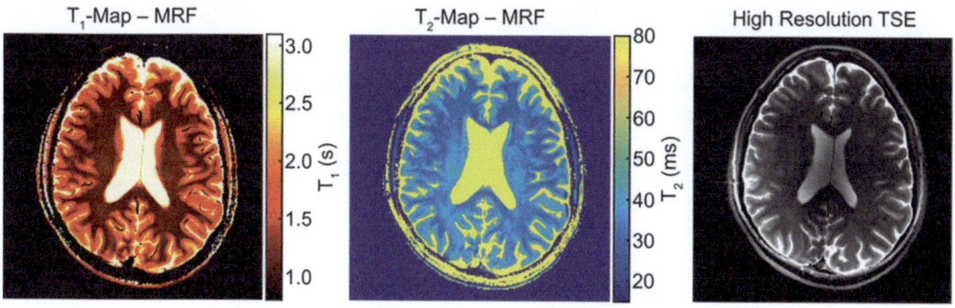

Fig. 23.8 Brain relaxometry: quantitative T1 and T2 maps derived from MR fingerprinting in a healthy volunteer at 7 T using fast imaging with steady-state precession (FISP)-based sequence. (Figure courtesy of Sebastian Flassbeck, MSc, German Cancer Research Center, Division of Medical Physics in Radiology)

highest predictive performance. Moreover, early clinical applications of magnetic resonance spectroscopic fingerprinting (MRSF) have been reported in breast cancer patients [169].

23.8 Challenges to Implement Clinical MR Biomarkers in Multicenter Trials

Application of MR biomarkers on a larger scale for tumor staging and therapy response assessment is still challenging. Both multicenter clinical studies as well as an effective clinical routine require the standardization of examination protocols, data evaluation algorithms, documentation procedures, and quality assurance measures. To develop imaging biomarkers for different human body regions and for particular clinical questions, information platforms are needed that include centers of excellence, ongoing imaging biomarker research projects, clinical studies, and educational activities. International collaborative organizations tackle key issues by coordinating research activities on quantitative imaging biomarkers and by providing recommendations. The goal of the Quantitative Imaging Biomarkers Alliance (QIBA) of the Radiologic Society of North America (RSNA) is to provide technical performance standards and tools for producing reliable quantitative imaging biomarkers for use in the clinical imaging community, e.g., for improved precision of DWI and DCE-MRI-derived biomarkers in multicenter oncology trials [170]. The QIBA accredits centers suitable for multicenter trials based on certain quality criteria. The European Imaging Biomarker Alliance (EIBALL) is a subcommittee of the European Society for Radiology (ESR) supported for its operational activities by the European Institute for Biomedical Imaging Research (EIBIR). EIBALL collaborates with QIBA and other European imaging societies, e.g., European Society of Molecular and Functional Imaging (ESMOFIR) and the European Society of Magnetic Resonance in Medicine and Biology (ESMRMB), to exploit synergies. Thus, EIBALL lists, for example, core institutions and networks of collaborating institutions in Europe involved in imaging biomarker development and publishes white papers and recommendations [171–173]. Potential imaging sites can be identified that qualify for multicenter clinical trials concerning biological validation as well as application, e.g., by the European Organization of Research and Treatment of Cancer (EORTC). New clinical trials can include early advanced imaging tools, in particular when imaging is used as the primary endpoint.

References

1. Ellingson BM, Malkin MG, Rand SD, Connelly JM, Quinsey C, LaViolette PS et al (2010) Validation of functional diffusion maps (fDMs) as a biomarker for human glioma cellularity. J Magn Reson Imaging 31(3):538–548. https://doi.org/10.1002/jmri.22068. PubMed PMID: 20187195; PubMed Central PMCID: PMCPMC2903058
2. Gupta RK, Cloughesy TF, Sinha U, Garakian J, Lazareff J, Rubino G et al (2000) Relationships between choline magnetic resonance spectroscopy, apparent diffusion coefficient and quanti-

tative histopathology in human glioma. J Neurooncol 50(3):215–226. https://doi.org/10.1023/a:1006431120031. PubMed PMID: 11263501
3. Kono K, Inoue Y, Nakayama K, Shakudo M, Morino M, Ohata K et al (2001) The role of diffusion-weighted imaging in patients with brain tumors. AJNR Am J Neuroradiol 22(6):1081–1088. PubMed PMID: 11415902; PubMed Central PMCID: PMCPMC7974804
4. Sugahara T, Korogi Y, Kochi M, Ikushima I, Shigematu Y, Hirai T et al (1999) Usefulness of diffusion-weighted MRI with echo-planar technique in the evaluation of cellularity in gliomas. J Magn Reson Imaging 9(1):53–60. https://doi.org/10.1002/(sici)1522-2586(199901)9:1<53::aid-jmri7>3.0.co;2-2. PubMed PMID: 10030650
5. Hamstra DA, Chenevert TL, Moffat BA, Johnson TD, Meyer CR, Mukherji SK et al (2005) Evaluation of the functional diffusion map as an early biomarker of time-to-progression and overall survival in high-grade glioma. Proc Natl Acad Sci USA 102(46):16759–16764. https://doi.org/10.1073/pnas.0508347102. Epub 20051102. PubMed PMID: 16267128; PubMed Central PMCID: PMCPMC1276616
6. Higano S, Yun X, Kumabe T, Watanabe M, Mugikura S, Umetsu A et al (2006) Malignant astrocytic tumors: clinical importance of apparent diffusion coefficient in prediction of grade and prognosis. Radiology 241(3):839–846. https://doi.org/10.1148/radiol.2413051276. Epub 20061010. PubMed PMID: 17032910
7. Murakami R, Sugahara T, Nakamura H, Hirai T, Kitajima M, Hayashida Y et al (2007) Malignant supratentorial astrocytoma treated with postoperative radiation therapy: prognostic value of pretreatment quantitative diffusion-weighted MR imaging. Radiology 243(2):493–499. https://doi.org/10.1148/radiol.2432060450. Epub 20070313. PubMed PMID: 17356177
8. Yang D, Korogi Y, Sugahara T, Kitajima M, Shigematsu Y, Liang L et al (2002) Cerebral gliomas: prospective comparison of multivoxel 2D chemical-shift imaging proton MR spectroscopy, echoplanar perfusion and diffusion-weighted MRI. Neuroradiology 44(8):656–666. https://doi.org/10.1007/s00234-002-0816-9. Epub 20020629. PubMed PMID: 12185543
9. Lee EJ, Lee SK, Agid R, Bae JM, Keller A, Terbrugge K (2008) Preoperative grading of presumptive low-grade astrocytomas on MR imaging: diagnostic value of minimum apparent diffusion coefficient. AJNR Am J Neuroradiol 29(10):1872–1877. https://doi.org/10.3174/ajnr.A1254. Epub 20080821. PubMed PMID: 18719036; PubMed Central PMCID: PMCPMC8118927
10. Leu K, Ott GA, Lai A, Nghiemphu PL, Pope WB, Yong WH et al (2017) Perfusion and diffusion MRI signatures in histologic and genetic subtypes of WHO grade II-III diffuse gliomas. J Neurooncol 134(1):177–188. https://doi.org/10.1007/s11060-017-2506-9. Epub 20170525. PubMed PMID: 28547590; PubMed Central PMCID: PMCPMC7927357
11. Chenevert TL, Stegman LD, Taylor JM, Robertson PL, Greenberg HS, Rehemtulla A, Ross BD (2000) Diffusion magnetic resonance imaging: an early surrogate marker of therapeutic efficacy in brain tumors. J Natl Cancer Inst 92(24):2029–2036. https://doi.org/10.1093/jnci/92.24.2029. PubMed PMID: 11121466
12. Moffat BA, Chenevert TL, Lawrence TS, Meyer CR, Johnson TD, Dong Q et al (2005) Functional diffusion map: a noninvasive MRI biomarker for early stratification of clinical brain tumor response. Proc Natl Acad Sci U S A 102(15):5524–5529. https://doi.org/10.1073/pnas.0501532102. Epub 20050401. PubMed PMID: 15805192; PubMed Central PMCID: PMCPMC555936
13. Sinha S, Bastin ME, Whittle IR, Wardlaw JM (2002) Diffusion tensor MR imaging of high-grade cerebral gliomas. AJNR Am J Neuroradiol 23(4):520–527. PubMed PMID: 11950638; PubMed Central PMCID: PMCPMC7975109
14. Wu JS, Zhou LF, Tang WJ, Mao Y, Hu J, Song YY et al (2007) Clinical evaluation and follow-up outcome of diffusion tensor imaging-based functional neuronavigation: a prospective, controlled study in patients with gliomas involving pyramidal tracts. Neurosurgery 61(5):935–948; discussion 48-9. https://doi.org/10.1227/01.neu.0000303189.80049.ab. PubMed PMID: 18091270

15. Van Cauter S, Veraart J, Sijbers J, Peeters RR, Himmelreich U, De Keyzer F et al (2012) Gliomas: diffusion kurtosis MR imaging in grading. Radiology 263(2):492–501. https://doi.org/10.1148/radiol.12110927. Epub 20120308. PubMed PMID: 22403168
16. Park SH, Choi MH, Lee YJ, Jung SE (2024) Rationale for adopting a combination of monoparametric MRI with the prostate-specific antigen in detecting clinically significant prostate cancer: comparison with standard biparametric and multiparametric MRI. Br J Radiol. https://doi.org/10.1093/bjr/tqae134. Epub 20240830. PubMed PMID: 39212614
17. Vargas HA, Akin O, Franiel T, Mazaheri Y, Zheng J, Moskowitz C et al (2011) Diffusion-weighted endorectal MR imaging at 3 T for prostate cancer: tumor detection and assessment of aggressiveness. Radiology 259(3):775–784. https://doi.org/10.1148/radiol.11102066. Epub 20110324. PubMed PMID: 21436085; PubMed Central PMCID: PMCPMC3099046
18. Langer DL, van der Kwast TH, Evans AJ, Plotkin A, Trachtenberg J, Wilson BC, Haider MA (2010) Prostate tissue composition and MR measurements: investigating the relationships between ADC, T2, K(trans), v(e), and corresponding histologic features. Radiology 255(2):485–494. https://doi.org/10.1148/radiol.10091343. PubMed PMID: 20413761
19. Bonekamp D, Kohl S, Wiesenfarth M, Schelb P, Radtke JP, Götz M et al (2018) Radiomic machine learning for characterization of prostate lesions with MRI: comparison to ADC values. Radiology 289(1):128–137. https://doi.org/10.1148/radiol.2018173064. Epub 20180731. PubMed PMID: 30063191
20. Hambrock T, Somford DM, Huisman HJ, van Oort IM, Witjes JA, van de Kaa Hulsbergen-CA et al (2011) Relationship between apparent diffusion coefficients at 3.0-T MR imaging and Gleason grade in peripheral zone prostate cancer. Radiology 259(2):453–461. https://doi.org/10.1148/radiol.11091409. PubMed PMID: 21502392
21. Jung SI, Donati OF, Vargas HA, Goldman D, Hricak H, Akin O (2013) Transition zone prostate cancer: incremental value of diffusion-weighted endorectal MR imaging in tumor detection and assessment of aggressiveness. Radiology 269(2):493–503. https://doi.org/10.1148/radiology.13130029. Epub 20130722. PubMed PMID: 23878284
22. Morgan VA, Riches SF, Thomas K, Vanas N, Parker C, Giles S, Desouza NM (2011) Diffusion-weighted magnetic resonance imaging for monitoring prostate cancer progression in patients managed by active surveillance. Br J Radiol 84(997):31–37. https://doi.org/10.1259/bjr/14556365. PubMed PMID: 21172965; PubMed Central PMCID: PMCPMC3473800
23. Park SY, Kim CK, Park BK, Lee HM, Lee KS (2011) Prediction of biochemical recurrence following radical prostatectomy in men with prostate cancer by diffusion-weighted magnetic resonance imaging: initial results. Eur Radiol 21(5):1111–1118. https://doi.org/10.1007/s00330-010-1999-9. Epub 20101103. PubMed PMID: 21046403
24. Roy C, Bierry G, Matau A, Bazille G, Pasquali R (2010) Value of diffusion-weighted imaging to detect small malignant pelvic lymph nodes at 3 T. Eur Radiol 20(8):1803–1811. https://doi.org/10.1007/s00330-010-1736-4. Epub 20100224. PubMed PMID: 20182732
25. Thoeny HC, Froehlich JM, Triantafyllou M, Huesler J, Bains LJ, Vermathen P et al (2014) Metastases in normal-sized pelvic lymph nodes: detection with diffusion-weighted MR imaging. Radiology 273(1):125–135. https://doi.org/10.1148/radiol.14132921. Epub 20140602. PubMed PMID: 24893049
26. Noto B, Eveslage M, Auf der Springe K, Exler A, Faldum A, Heindel W et al (2024) Robustness of apparent diffusion coefficient-based lymph node classification for diagnosis of prostate cancer metastasis. Eur Radiol 34(7):4504–4515. https://doi.org/10.1007/s00330-023-10406-8. Epub 20231215. PubMed PMID: 38099965; PubMed Central PMCID: PMCPMC11213742
27. Zhang YD, Wang Q, Wu CJ, Wang XN, Zhang J, Liu H et al (2015) The histogram analysis of diffusion-weighted intravoxel incoherent motion (IVIM) imaging for differentiating the gleason grade of prostate cancer. Eur Radiol 25(4):994–1004. https://doi.org/10.1007/s00330-014-3511-4. Epub 20141128. PubMed PMID: 25430007
28. Kerkmeijer LGW, Groen VH, Pos FJ, Haustermans K, Monninkhof EM, Smeenk RJ et al (2021) Focal boost to the intraprostatic tumor in external beam radiotherapy for patients with

localized prostate cancer: results from the FLAME randomized phase III trial. J Clin Oncol 39(7):787–796. https://doi.org/10.1200/jco.20.02873. Epub 20210120. PubMed PMID: 33471548

29. Lui AJ, Kallis K, Zhong AY, Hussain TS, Conlin C, Digma LA et al (2023) ReIGNITE radiation therapy boost: a prospective, international study of radiation oncologists' accuracy in contouring prostate tumors for focal radiation therapy boost on conventional magnetic resonance imaging alone or with assistance of restriction spectrum imaging. Int J Radiat Oncol Biol Phys 117(5):1145–1152. https://doi.org/10.1016/j.ijrobp.2023.07.004. Epub 20230714. PubMed PMID: 37453559; PubMed Central PMCID: PMCPMC11088932
30. Kooreman ES, van Houdt PJ, Keesman R, van Pelt VWJ, Nowee ME, Pos F et al (2021) Daily Intravoxel Incoherent Motion (IVIM) in prostate cancer patients during mr-guided radiotherapy-a multicenter study. Front Oncol 11:705964. https://doi.org/10.3389/fonc.2021.705964. Epub 20210813. PubMed PMID: 34485138; PubMed Central PMCID: PMCPMC8415108
31. Ristau J, Hörner-Rieber J, Buchele C, Klüter S, Jäkel C, Baumann L et al (2022) Stereotactic MRI-guided radiation therapy for localized prostate cancer (SMILE): a prospective, multicentric phase-II-trial. Radiat Oncol 17(1):75. https://doi.org/10.1186/s13014-022-02047-w. Epub 20220415. PubMed PMID: 35428327; PubMed Central PMCID: PMCPMC9011377
32. Franco FB, Leeman JE, Fedorov A, Vangel M, Fennessy FM (2024) Early change in apparent diffusion coefficient as a predictor of response to neoadjuvant androgen deprivation and external beam radiation therapy for intermediate- to high-risk prostate cancer. Clin Radiol 79(4):e607–ee15. https://doi.org/10.1016/j.crad.2023.12.022. Epub 20240119. PubMed PMID: 38302377; PubMed Central PMCID: PMCPMC11348292
33. Onal C, Erbay G, Oymak E, Guler OC (2023) The impact of the apparent diffusion coefficient for the early prediction of the treatment response after definitive radiotherapy in prostate cancer patients. Radiother Oncol 184:109677. https://doi.org/10.1016/j.radonc.2023.109677. Epub 20230420. PubMed PMID: 37084886
34. Cai JC, Nakai H, Kuanar S, Froemming AT, Bolan CW, Kawashima A et al (2024) Fully automated deep learning model to detect clinically significant prostate cancer at MRI. Radiology 312(2):e232635. https://doi.org/10.1148/radiol.232635. PubMed PMID: 39105640; PubMed Central PMCID: PMCPMC11366675
35. Bonekamp D, Schelb P, Wiesenfarth M, Kuder TA, Deister F, Stenzinger A et al (2019) Histopathological to multiparametric MRI spatial mapping of extended systematic sextant and MR/TRUS-fusion-targeted biopsy of the prostate. Eur Radiol 29(4):1820–1830. https://doi.org/10.1007/s00330-018-5751-1. Epub 20181016. PubMed PMID: 30327861
36. Deike-Hofmann K, Koenig F, Paech D, Dreher C, Delorme S, Schlemmer HP, Bickelhaupt S (2019) Abbreviated MRI protocols in breast cancer diagnostics. J Magn Reson Imaging 49(3):647–658. https://doi.org/10.1002/jmri.26525. Epub 20181016. PubMed PMID: 30328180
37. Marini C, Iacconi C, Giannelli M, Cilotti A, Moretti M, Bartolozzi C (2007) Quantitative diffusion-weighted MR imaging in the differential diagnosis of breast lesion. Eur Radiol 17(10):2646–2655. https://doi.org/10.1007/s00330-007-0621-2. Epub 20070314. PubMed PMID: 17356840
38. Bickelhaupt S, Tesdorff J, Laun FB, Kuder TA, Lederer W, Teiner S et al (2017) Independent value of image fusion in unenhanced breast MRI using diffusion-weighted and morphological T2-weighted images for lesion characterization in patients with recently detected BI-RADS 4/5 x-ray mammography findings. Eur Radiol 27(2):562–569. https://doi.org/10.1007/s00330-016-4400-9. Epub 20160518. PubMed PMID: 27193776
39. Shin HJ, Kim SH, Lee HJ, Gong G, Baek S, Chae EY et al (2016) Tumor apparent diffusion coefficient as an imaging biomarker to predict tumor aggressiveness in patients with estrogen-receptor-positive breast cancer. NMR Biomed 29(8):1070–1078. https://doi.org/10.1002/nbm.3571. Epub 20160622. PubMed PMID: 27332719
40. Yabuuchi H, Matsuo Y, Sunami S, Kamitani T, Kawanami S, Setoguchi T et al (2011) Detection of non-palpable breast cancer in asymptomatic women by using unenhanced

diffusion-weighted and T2-weighted MR imaging: comparison with mammography and dynamic contrast-enhanced MR imaging. Eur Radiol 21(1):11–17. https://doi.org/10.1007/s00330-010-1890-8. Epub 20100718. PubMed PMID: 20640898

41. Ei Khouli RH, Jacobs MA, Mezban SD, Huang P, Kamel IR, Macura KJ, Bluemke DA (2010) Diffusion-weighted imaging improves the diagnostic accuracy of conventional 3.0-T breast MR imaging. Radiology 256(1):64–73. https://doi.org/10.1148/radiol.10091367. PubMed PMID: 20574085; PubMed Central PMCID: PMCPMC2897691
42. Jensen JH, Helpern JA, Ramani A, Lu H, Kaczynski K (2005) Diffusional kurtosis imaging: the quantification of non-gaussian water diffusion by means of magnetic resonance imaging. Magn Reson Med 53(6):1432–1440. https://doi.org/10.1002/mrm.20508. PubMed PMID: 15906300
43. Sun K, Chen X, Chai W, Fei X, Fu C, Yan X et al (2015) Breast cancer: diffusion kurtosis mr imaging-diagnostic accuracy and correlation with clinical-pathologic factors. Radiology 277(1):46–55. https://doi.org/10.1148/radiol.15141625. Epub 20150504. PubMed PMID: 25938679
44. Bickelhaupt S, Steudle F, Paech D, Mlynarska A, Kuder TA, Lederer W et al (2017) On a fractional order calculus model in diffusion weighted breast imaging to differentiate between malignant and benign breast lesions detected on X-ray screening mammography. PLoS One 12(4):e0176077. https://doi.org/10.1371/journal.pone.0176077. Epub 20170428. PubMed PMID: 28453516; PubMed Central PMCID: PMCPMC5409173
45. Liu C, Liang C, Liu Z, Zhang S, Huang B (2013) Intravoxel incoherent motion (IVIM) in evaluation of breast lesions: comparison with conventional DWI. Eur J Radiol 82(12):e782–e789. https://doi.org/10.1016/j.ejrad.2013.08.006. Epub 20130813. PubMed PMID: 24034833
46. Eyal E, Shapiro-Feinberg M, Furman-Haran E, Grobgeld D, Golan T, Itzchak Y et al (2012) Parametric diffusion tensor imaging of the breast. Invest Radiol 47(5):284–291. https://doi.org/10.1097/RLI.0b013e3182438e5d. PubMed PMID: 22472798
47. Partridge SC, McDonald ES (2013) Diffusion weighted magnetic resonance imaging of the breast: protocol optimization, interpretation, and clinical applications. Magn Reson Imaging Clin N Am 21(3):601–624. https://doi.org/10.1016/j.mric.2013.04.007. Epub 20130610. PubMed PMID: 23928248; PubMed Central PMCID: PMCPMC3740446
48. Pötsch N, Sodano C, Baltzer PAT (2024) Performance of diffusion-weighted imaging-based noncontrast mri protocols for diagnosis of breast cancer: a systematic review and meta-analysis. Radiology 311(2):e232508. https://doi.org/10.1148/radiol.232508. PubMed PMID: 38771179
49. Bickelhaupt S, Paech D, Laun FB, Steudle F, Kuder TA, Mlynarska A et al (2017) Maximum intensity breast diffusion MRI for BI-RADS 4 lesions detected on X-ray mammography. Clin Radiol 72(10):900.e1-.e8. https://doi.org/10.1016/j.crad.2017.05.017. Epub 20170704. PubMed PMID: 28687167
50. Tofts PS, Kermode AG (1991) Measurement of the blood-brain barrier permeability and leakage space using dynamic MR imaging. 1. fundamental concepts. Magn Reson Med 17(2):357–367. https://doi.org/10.1002/mrm.1910170208
51. Sourbron S, Ingrisch M, Siefert A, Reiser M, Herrmann K (2009) Quantification of cerebral blood flow, cerebral blood volume, and blood–brain-barrier leakage with DCE-MRI. Magn Reson Med 62(1):205–217. https://doi.org/10.1002/mrm.22005
52. Leu K, Ott GA, Lai A, Nghiemphu PL, Pope WB, Yong WH et al (2017) Perfusion and diffusion MRI signatures in histologic and genetic subtypes of WHO grade II–III diffuse gliomas. J Neuro-Oncol 134(1):177–188. https://doi.org/10.1007/s11060-017-2506-9
53. Lacerda S, Law M (2009) Magnetic resonance perfusion and permeability imaging in brain tumors. Neuroimaging Clin N Am 19(4):527–557. https://doi.org/10.1016/j.nic.2009.08.007
54. Thompson G, Mills SJ, Stivaros SM, Jackson A (2010) Imaging of brain tumors: perfusion/permeability. Neuroimaging Clin N Am 20(3):337–353. https://doi.org/10.1016/j.nic.2010.04.008

55. Cha S, Yang L, Johnson G, Lai A, Chen M-H, Tihan T et al (2006) Comparison of microvascular permeability measurements, ktrans, determined with conventional steady-state T1-weighted and first-pass T2*-weighted mr imaging methods in gliomas and meningiomas. Am J Neuroradiol 27(2):409–417
56. Boxerman J, Schmainda K, Weisskoff R (2006) Relative cerebral blood volume maps corrected for contrast agent extravasation significantly correlate with glioma tumor grade, whereas uncorrected maps do not. Am J Neuroradiol 27(4):859–867
57. Aronen HJ, Gazit IE, Louis DN, Buchbinder BR, Pardo FS, Weisskoff RM et al (1994) Cerebral blood volume maps of gliomas: comparison with tumor grade and histologic findings. Radiology 191(1):41–51
58. Cha S, Lupo JM, Chen M-H, Lamborn KR, McDermott MW, Berger MS et al (2007) Differentiation of glioblastoma multiforme and single brain metastasis by peak height and percentage of signal intensity recovery derived from dynamic susceptibility-weighted contrast-enhanced perfusion MR imaging. Am J Neuroradiol 28(6):1078–1084. https://doi.org/10.3174/ajnr.A0484
59. Pons-Escoda A, Garcia-Ruiz A, Garcia-Hidalgo C, Gil-Solsona R, Naval-Baudin P, Martin-Noguerol T et al (2023) MR dynamic-susceptibility-contrast perfusion metrics in the presurgical discrimination of adult solitary intra-axial cerebellar tumors. Eur Radiol 33(12):9120–9129. https://doi.org/10.1007/s00330-023-09892-7. Epub 20230713. PubMed PMID: 37439938
60. Tan W, Xiong J, Huang W, Wu J, Zhan S, Geng D (2017) Noninvasively detecting Isocitrate dehydrogenase 1 gene status in astrocytoma by dynamic susceptibility contrast MRI. J Magn Reson Imaging 45(2):492–499. https://doi.org/10.1002/jmri.25358
61. Jenkinson MD, Smith TS, Joyce KA, Fildes D, Broome J, du Plessis DG et al (2006) Cerebral blood volume, genotype and chemosensitivity in oligodendroglial tumours. Neuroradiology 48(10):703–713. https://doi.org/10.1007/s00234-006-0122-z. Epub 2006/08/26. PubMed PMID: 16937145
62. Pons-Escoda A, Garcia-Ruiz A, Naval-Baudin P, Martinez-Zalacain I, Castell J, Camins A et al (2024) Differentiating IDH-mutant astrocytomas and 1p19q-codeleted oligodendrogliomas using DSC-PWI: high performance through cerebral blood volume and percentage of signal recovery percentiles. Eur Radiol 34(8):5320–5330. https://doi.org/10.1007/s00330-024-10611-z. Epub 20240129. PubMed PMID: 38282078; PubMed Central PMCID: PMCPMC11255054
63. Pons-Escoda A, Naval-Baudin P, Viveros M, Flores-Casaperalta S, Martinez-Zalacaín I, Plans G et al (2024) DSC-PWI presurgical differentiation of grade 4 astrocytoma and glioblastoma in young adults: rCBV percentile analysis across enhancing and non-enhancing regions. Neuroradiology 66(8):1267–1277. https://doi.org/10.1007/s00234-024-03385-0. Epub 20240605. PubMed PMID: 38834877; PubMed Central PMCID: PMCPMC11246293
64. Bonekamp D, Deike K, Wiestler B, Wick W, Bendszus M, Radbruch A, Heiland S (2015) Association of overall survival in patients with newly diagnosed glioblastoma with contrast-enhanced perfusion MRI: Comparison of intraindividually matched T1 – and T2 (*) -based bolus techniques. J Magn Reson Imaging 42(1):87–96. https://doi.org/10.1002/jmri.24756. Epub 20140922. PubMed PMID: 25244574
65. Jenkinson MD, Smith TS, Joyce KA, Fildes D, Broome J, du Plessis DG et al (2006) Cerebral blood volume, genotype and chemosensitivity in oligodendroglial tumours. Neuroradiology 48(10):703–713. https://doi.org/10.1007/s00234-006-0122-z. Epub 20060826. PubMed PMID: 16937145; PubMed Central PMCID: PMCPMC1592467
66. Law M, Young RJ, Babb JS, Peccerelli N, Chheang S, Gruber ML et al (2008) Gliomas: predicting time to progression or survival with cerebral blood volume measurements at dynamic susceptibility-weighted contrast-enhanced perfusion MR imaging. Radiology 247(2):490–498. https://doi.org/10.1148/radiol.2472070898. Epub 20080318. PubMed PMID: 18349315; PubMed Central PMCID: PMCPMC3774106
67. Kim AE, Lou KW, Giobbie-Hurder A, Chang K, Gidwani M, Hoebel K et al (2024) Abnormal vascular structure and function within brain metastases is linked to pembrolizumab resis-

tance. Neuro Oncol 26(5):965–974. https://doi.org/10.1093/neuonc/noad236. PubMed PMID: 38070147; PubMed Central PMCID: PMCPMC11066943

68. Cha S, Yang L, Johnson G, Lai A, Chen MH, Tihan T et al (2006) Comparison of microvascular permeability measurements, K(trans), determined with conventional steady-state T1-weighted and first-pass T2*-weighted MR imaging methods in gliomas and meningiomas. AJNR Am J Neuroradiol 27(2):409–417. PubMed PMID: 16484420; PubMed Central PMCID: PMCPMC8148770
69. Thompson G, Mills SJ, Stivaros SM, Jackson A (2010) Imaging of brain tumors: perfusion/permeability. Neuroimaging Clin N Am 20(3):337–353. https://doi.org/10.1016/j.nic.2010.04.008. PubMed PMID: 20708550
70. Mills SJ, Soh C, Rose CJ, Cheung S, Zhao S, Parker GJM, Jackson A (2010) Candidate biomarkers of extravascular extracellular space: a direct comparison of apparent diffusion coefficient and dynamic contrast-enhanced MR imaging—derived measurement of the volume of the extravascular extracellular space in glioblastoma multiforme. Am J Neuroradiol 31(3):549–553. https://doi.org/10.3174/ajnr.A1844
71. Lüdemann L, Grieger W, Wurm R, Budzisch M, Hamm B, Zimmer C (2001) Comparison of dynamic contrast-enhanced MRI with WHO tumor grading for gliomas. Eur Radiol 11(7):1231–1241. https://doi.org/10.1007/s003300000748. PubMed PMID: 11471617
72. Lüdemann L, Grieger W, Wurm R, Wust P, Zimmer C (2005) Quantitative measurement of leakage volume and permeability in gliomas, meningiomas and brain metastases with dynamic contrast-enhanced MRI. Magn Reson Imaging 23(8):833–841. https://doi.org/10.1016/j.mri.2005.06.007. Epub 20050909. PubMed PMID: 16275421
73. Zhu XP, Li KL, Kamaly-Asl ID, Checkley DR, Tessier JJ, Waterton JC, Jackson A (2000) Quantification of endothelial permeability, leakage space, and blood volume in brain tumors using combined T1 and T2* contrast-enhanced dynamic MR imaging. J Magn Reson Imaging 11(6):575–585. https://doi.org/10.1002/1522-2586(200006)11:6<575::aid-jmri2>3.0.co;2-1. PubMed PMID: 10862055
74. Deike K, Wiestler B, Graf M, Reimer C, Floca RO, Bäumer P et al (2016) Prognostic value of combined visualization of MR diffusion and perfusion maps in glioblastoma. J Neurooncol 126(3):463–472. https://doi.org/10.1007/s11060-015-1982-z. Epub 20151030. PubMed PMID: 26518541
75. Telischak NA, Detre JA, Zaharchuk G (2015) Arterial spin labeling MRI: clinical applications in the brain. J Magn Reson Imaging 41(5):1165–1180. https://doi.org/10.1002/jmri.24751. Epub 20140919. PubMed PMID: 25236477
76. Wamelink I, Azizova A, Booth TC, Mutsaerts H, Ogunleye A, Mankad K et al (2024) Brain tumor imaging without gadolinium-based contrast agents: feasible or fantasy? Radiology 310(2):e230793. https://doi.org/10.1148/radiol.230793. PubMed PMID: 38319162; PubMed Central PMCID: PMCPMC10902600
77. Kong L, Chen H, Yang Y, Chen L (2017) A meta-analysis of arterial spin labelling perfusion values for the prediction of glioma grade. Clin Radiol 72(3):255–261. https://doi.org/10.1016/j.crad.2016.10.016. Epub 20161206. PubMed PMID: 27932251
78. Mohammadi S, Ghaderi S, Jouzdani AF, Azinkhah I, Alibabaei S, Azami M, Omrani V (2024) Differentiation between high-grade glioma and brain metastasis using cerebral perfusion-related parameters (cerebral blood volume and cerebral blood flow): a systematic review and meta-analysis of perfusion-weighted MRI techniques. J Magn Reson Imaging. https://doi.org/10.1002/jmri.29473. Epub 20240620. PubMed PMID: 38899965
79. Yamashita K, Togao O, Kikuchi K, Kuga D, Sangatsuda Y, Fujioka Y et al (2024) The cortical high-flow sign of oligodendroglioma, IDH-mutant and 1p/19q-codeleted: comparison between arterial spin labeling and dynamic susceptibility contrast methods. Neuroradiology 66(2):187–192. https://doi.org/10.1007/s00234-023-03267-x. Epub 20231221. PubMed PMID: 38127124
80. Kuhl CK, Schrading S, Strobel K, Schild HH, Hilgers RD, Bieling HB (2014) Abbreviated breast magnetic resonance imaging (MRI): first postcontrast subtracted images and maximum-intensity projection-a novel approach to breast cancer screening with MRI. J Clin

Oncol 32(22):2304–2310. https://doi.org/10.1200/jco.2013.52.5386. Epub 20140623. PubMed PMID: 24958821
81. Heacock L, Melsaether AN, Heller SL, Gao Y, Pysarenko KM, Babb JS et al (2016) Evaluation of a known breast cancer using an abbreviated breast MRI protocol: correlation of imaging characteristics and pathology with lesion detection and conspicuity. Eur J Radiol 85(4):815–823. https://doi.org/10.1016/j.ejrad.2016.01.005. Epub 20160119. PubMed PMID: 26971429
82. Klifa C, Suzuki S, Aliu S, Singer L, Wilmes L, Newitt D et al (2011) Quantification of background enhancement in breast magnetic resonance imaging. J Magn Reson Imaging 33(5):1229–1234. https://doi.org/10.1002/jmri.22545. PubMed PMID: 21509883; PubMed Central PMCID: PMCPMC3081108
83. Mann RM, Mus RD, van Zelst J, Geppert C, Karssemeijer N, Platel B (2014) A novel approach to contrast-enhanced breast magnetic resonance imaging for screening: high-resolution ultrafast dynamic imaging. Invest Radiol 49(9):579–585. https://doi.org/10.1097/rli.0000000000000057. PubMed PMID: 24691143
84. Padhani AR, Gapinski CJ, Macvicar DA, Parker GJ, Suckling J, Revell PB et al (2000) Dynamic contrast enhanced MRI of prostate cancer: correlation with morphology and tumour stage, histological grade and PSA. Clin Radiol 55(2):99–109. https://doi.org/10.1053/crad.1999.0327. PubMed PMID: 10657154
85. Messina E, Pecoraro M, Laschena L, Bicchetti M, Proietti F, Ciardi A et al (2023) Low cancer yield in PI-RADS 3 upgraded to 4 by dynamic contrast-enhanced MRI: is it time to reconsider scoring categorization? Eur Radiol 33(8):5828–5839. https://doi.org/10.1007/s00330-023-09605-0. Epub 20230413. PubMed PMID: 37045981; PubMed Central PMCID: PMCPMC10326099
86. Bonekamp D, Wolf MB, Edler C, Katayama S, Schlemmer HP, Herfarth K, Röthke M (2016) Dynamic contrast enhanced MRI monitoring of primary proton and carbon ion irradiation of prostate cancer using a novel hypofractionated raster scan technique. Radiother Oncol 120(2):313–319. https://doi.org/10.1016/j.radonc.2016.05.012. Epub 20160526. PubMed PMID: 27237059
87. Low RN (2007) Abdominal MRI advances in the detection of liver tumours and characterisation. Lancet Oncol 8(6):525–535. https://doi.org/10.1016/s1470-2045(07)70170-5. PubMed PMID: 17540304
88. Semelka RC, Martin DR, Balci C, Lance T (2001) Focal liver lesions: comparison of dual-phase CT and multisequence multiplanar MR imaging including dynamic gadolinium enhancement. J Magn Reson Imaging 13(3):397–401. https://doi.org/10.1002/jmri.1057. PubMed PMID: 11241813
89. Cuenod C, Leconte I, Siauve N, Resten A, Dromain C, Poulet B et al (2001) Early changes in liver perfusion caused by occult metastases in rats: detection with quantitative CT. Radiology 218(2):556–561. https://doi.org/10.1148/radiology.218.2.r01fe10556. PubMed PMID: 11161178
90. Ichikawa T, Haradome H, Hachiya J, Nitatori T, Araki T (1998) Characterization of hepatic lesions by perfusion-weighted MR imaging with an echoplanar sequence. AJR Am J Roentgenol 170(4):1029–1034. https://doi.org/10.2214/ajr.170.4.9530054. PubMed PMID: 9530054
91. Pandharipande PV, Krinsky GA, Rusinek H, Lee VS (2005) Perfusion imaging of the liver: current challenges and future goals. Radiology 234(3):661–673. https://doi.org/10.1148/radiol.2343031362. PubMed PMID: 15734925
92. Akisik MF, Sandrasegaran K, Bu G, Lin C, Hutchins GD, Chiorean EG (2010) Pancreatic cancer: utility of dynamic contrast-enhanced MR imaging in assessment of antiangiogenic therapy. Radiology 256(2):441–449. https://doi.org/10.1148/radiol.10091733. Epub 20100601. PubMed PMID: 20515976
93. Barentsz JO, Berger-Hartog O, Witjes JA, Hulsbergen-van der Kaa C, Oosterhof GO, VanderLaak JA et al (1998) Evaluation of chemotherapy in advanced urinary bladder cancer

with fast dynamic contrast-enhanced MR imaging. Radiology 207(3):791–797. https://doi.org/10.1148/radiology.207.3.9609906. PubMed PMID: 9609906

94. Reddick WE, Taylor JS, Fletcher BD (1999) Dynamic MR imaging (DEMRI) of microcirculation in bone sarcoma. J Magn Reson Imaging 10(3):277–285. https://doi.org/10.1002/(sici)1522-2586(199909)10:3<277::aid-jmri8>3.0.co;2-s. PubMed PMID: 10508287
95. Rosen MA, Schnall MD (2007) Dynamic contrast-enhanced magnetic resonance imaging for assessing tumor vascularity and vascular effects of targeted therapies in renal cell carcinoma. Clin Cancer Res 13(2 Pt 2):770s–776s. https://doi.org/10.1158/1078-0432.Ccr-06-1921. PubMed PMID: 17255308
96. Liu C, Li W, Tong KA, Yeom KW, Kuzminski S (2015) Susceptibility-weighted imaging and quantitative susceptibility mapping in the brain. J Magn Reson Imaging 42(1):23–41. https://doi.org/10.1002/jmri.24768. Epub 20141001. PubMed PMID: 25270052; PubMed Central PMCID: PMCPMC4406874
97. Chen W, Zhu W, Kovanlikaya I, Kovanlikaya A, Liu T, Wang S et al (2014) Intracranial calcifications and hemorrhages: characterization with quantitative susceptibility mapping. Radiology 270(2):496–505. https://doi.org/10.1148/radiol.13122640. Epub 20131028. PubMed PMID: 24126366; PubMed Central PMCID: PMCPMC4228745
98. Nazem A, Guiry SC, Pourfathi M, Ware JB, Anderson H, Iyer SK et al (2022) MR susceptibility imaging for detection of tumor-associated macrophages in glioblastoma. J Neurooncol 156(3):645–653. https://doi.org/10.1007/s11060-022-03947-3. Epub 20220119. PubMed PMID: 35043276
99. Petronek MS, Bodeker KL, Lee CY, Teferi N, Eschbacher KL, Jones KA et al (2024) Iron-based biomarkers for personalizing pharmacological ascorbate therapy in glioblastoma: insights from a phase 2 clinical trial. J Neurooncol 166(3):493–501. https://doi.org/10.1007/s11060-024-04571-z. Epub 20240129. PubMed PMID: 38285244
100. Petronek MS, Monga V, Bodeker KL, Kwofie M, Lee CY, Mapuskar KA et al (2024) Magnetic resonance imaging of iron metabolism with T2* mapping predicts an enhanced clinical response to pharmacologic ascorbate in patients with GBM. Clin Cancer Res 30(2):283–293. https://doi.org/10.1158/1078-0432.Ccr-22-3952. PubMed PMID: 37773633; PubMed Central PMCID: PMCPMC10841843
101. Horská A, Barker PB (2010) Imaging of brain tumors: MR spectroscopy and metabolic imaging. Neuroimaging Clin N Am 20(3):293–310. https://doi.org/10.1016/j.nic.2010.04.003. PubMed PMID: 20708548; PubMed Central PMCID: PMCPMC2927327
102. Castillo M, Smith JK, Kwock L (2000) Correlation of myo-inositol levels and grading of cerebral astrocytomas. AJNR Am J Neuroradiol 21(9):1645–1649. PubMed PMID: 11039343; PubMed Central PMCID: PMCPMC8174883
103. Preul MC, Caramanos Z, Collins DL, Villemure JG, Leblanc R, Olivier A et al (1996) Accurate, noninvasive diagnosis of human brain tumors by using proton magnetic resonance spectroscopy. Nat Med 2(3):323–325. https://doi.org/10.1038/nm0396-323. PubMed PMID: 8612232
104. Schlemmer HP, Bachert P, Henze M, Buslei R, Herfarth KK, Debus J, van Kaick G (2002) Differentiation of radiation necrosis from tumor progression using proton magnetic resonance spectroscopy. Neuroradiology 44(3):216–222. https://doi.org/10.1007/s002340100703. PubMed PMID: 11942375
105. Schlemmer HP, Bachert P, Herfarth KK, Zuna I, Debus J, van Kaick G (2001) Proton MR spectroscopic evaluation of suspicious brain lesions after stereotactic radiotherapy. AJNR Am J Neuroradiol 22(7):1316–1324. PubMed PMID: 11498420; PubMed Central PMCID: PMCPMC7975210
106. Gatenby RA, Gillies RJ (2004) Why do cancers have high aerobic glycolysis? Nat Rev Cancer 4(11):891–899. https://doi.org/10.1038/nrc1478. PubMed PMID: 15516961
107. Webb BA, Chimenti M, Jacobson MP, Barber DL (2011) Dysregulated pH: a perfect storm for cancer progression. Nat Rev Cancer 11(9):671–677. https://doi.org/10.1038/nrc3110. Epub 20110811. PubMed PMID: 21833026

108. Fukumura D, Xu L, Chen Y, Gohongi T, Seed B, Jain RK (2001) Hypoxia and acidosis independently up-regulate vascular endothelial growth factor transcription in brain tumors in vivo. Cancer Res 61(16):6020–6024. PubMed PMID: 11507045
109. Reichert M, Steinbach JP, Supra P, Weller M (2002) Modulation of growth and radiochemosensitivity of human malignant glioma cells by acidosis. Cancer 95(5):1113–1119. https://doi.org/10.1002/cncr.10767. PubMed PMID: 12209698
110. Wenger KJ, Hattingen E, Franz K, Steinbach JP, Bähr O, Pilatus U (2017) Intracellular pH measured by (31) P-MR-spectroscopy might predict site of progression in recurrent glioblastoma under antiangiogenic therapy. J Magn Reson Imaging 46(4):1200–1208. https://doi.org/10.1002/jmri.25619. Epub 20170206. PubMed PMID: 28165649
111. Kuesel AC, Sutherland GR, Halliday W, Smith IC (1994) 1H MRS of high grade astrocytomas: mobile lipid accumulation in necrotic tissue. NMR Biomed 7(3):149–155. https://doi.org/10.1002/nbm.1940070308. PubMed PMID: 8080717
112. Barba I, Cabañas ME, Arús C (1999) The relationship between nuclear magnetic resonance-visible lipids, lipid droplets, and cell proliferation in cultured C6 cells. Cancer Res 59(8):1861–1868. PubMed PMID: 10213493
113. Howe FA, Barton SJ, Cudlip SA, Stubbs M, Saunders DE, Murphy M et al (2003) Metabolic profiles of human brain tumors using quantitative in vivo 1H magnetic resonance spectroscopy. Magn Reson Med 49(2):223–232. https://doi.org/10.1002/mrm.10367. PubMed PMID: 12541241
114. Maintz D, Heindel W, Kugel H, Jaeger R, Lackner KJ (2002) Phosphorus-31 MR spectroscopy of normal adult human brain and brain tumours. NMR Biomed 15(1):18–27. https://doi.org/10.1002/nbm.735. PubMed PMID: 11840549
115. Majós C, Pons-Escoda A, Naval P, Güell A, Lucas A, Vidal N et al (2024) Proton MR spectroscopy shows improved performance to segregate high-grade astrocytoma subgroups when defined with the new 2021 World Health Organization classification of central nervous system tumors. Eur Radiol 34(4):2174–2182. https://doi.org/10.1007/s00330-023-10138-9. Epub 20230923. PubMed PMID: 37740778
116. Zhou J, Payen JF, Wilson DA, Traystman RJ, van Zijl PC (2003) Using the amide proton signals of intracellular proteins and peptides to detect pH effects in MRI. Nat Med 9(8):1085–1090. https://doi.org/10.1038/nm907. Epub 2003/07/23. PubMed PMID: 12872167.
117. Ward KM, Aletras AH, Balaban RS (2000) A new class of contrast agents for MRI based on proton chemical exchange dependent saturation transfer (CEST). J Magn Reson (San Diego, Calif : 1997) 143(1):79–87. https://doi.org/10.1006/jmre.1999.1956. Epub 2000/03/04. PubMed PMID: 10698648
118. Jones CK, Huang A, Xu J, Edden RA, Schar M, Hua J et al (2013) Nuclear overhauser enhancement (NOE) imaging in the human brain at 7T. Neuroimage 77:114–124. https://doi.org/10.1016/j.neuroimage.2013.03.047. PubMed PMID: 23567889; PubMed Central PMCID: PMCPMC3848060
119. Zaiss M, Schmitt B, Bachert P (2011) Quantitative separation of CEST effect from magnetization transfer and spillover effects by lorentzian-line-fit analysis of z-spectra. J Magn Reson (San Diego, Calif : 1997) 211(2):149–155. https://doi.org/10.1016/j.jmr.2011.05.001. Epub 2011/06/07. PubMed PMID: 21641247
120. Zaiss M, Windschuh J, Goerke S, Paech D, Meissner JE, Burth S et al (2017) Downfield-NOE-suppressed amide-CEST-MRI at 7 tesla provides a unique contrast in human glioblastoma. Magn Reson Med 77(1):196–208. https://doi.org/10.1002/mrm.26100. PubMed PMID: 26845067
121. Zaiss M, Windschuh J, Paech D, Meissner JE, Burth S, Schmitt B et al (2015) Relaxation-compensated CEST-MRI of the human brain at 7T: unbiased insight into NOE and amide signal changes in human glioblastoma. Neuroimage 112:180–188. https://doi.org/10.1016/j.neuroimage.2015.02.040. PubMed PMID: 25727379
122. Zaiss M, Xu J, Goerke S, Khan IS, Singer RJ, Gore JC et al (2014) Inverse Z-spectrum analysis for spillover-, MT-, and T1 -corrected steady-state pulsed CEST-MRI--application to pH-weighted MRI of acute stroke. NMR Biomed 27(3):240–252. https://doi.org/10.1002/

nbm.3054. Epub 2014/01/08. PubMed PMID: 24395553; PubMed Central PMCID: PMCPMC4520220
123. Togao O, Yoshiura T, Keupp J, Hiwatashi A, Yamashita K, Kikuchi K et al (2014) Amide proton transfer imaging of adult diffuse gliomas: correlation with histopathological grades. Neuro Oncol 16(3):441–448. https://doi.org/10.1093/neuonc/not158. PubMed PMID: 24305718; PubMed Central PMCID: PMCPMC3922507
124. Paech D, Windschuh J, Oberhollenzer J, Dreher C, Sahm F, Meissner J-E et al (2018) Assessing the predictability of IDH mutation and MGMT methylation status in glioma patients using relaxation-compensated multi-pool CEST MRI at 7.0 Tesla. Neuro Oncol:noy073-noy. https://doi.org/10.1093/neuonc/noy073
125. Togao O, Hiwatashi A, Yamashita K, Kikuchi K, Keupp J, Yoshimoto K et al (2017) Grading diffuse gliomas without intense contrast enhancement by amide proton transfer MR imaging: comparisons with diffusion – and perfusion-weighted imaging. Eur Radiol 27(2):578–588. https://doi.org/10.1007/s00330-016-4328-0. PubMed PMID: 27003139
126. Heo HY, Jones CK, Hua J, Yadav N, Agarwal S, Zhou J et al (2016) Whole-brain amide proton transfer (APT) and nuclear overhauser enhancement (NOE) imaging in glioma patients using low-power steady-state pulsed chemical exchange saturation transfer (CEST) imaging at 7T. J Magn Reson Imaging 44(1):41–50. https://doi.org/10.1002/jmri.25108. PubMed PMID: 26663561; PubMed Central PMCID: PMCPMC4902781
127. Paech D, Zaiss M, Meissner J-E, Windschuh J, Wiestler B, Bachert P et al (2014) Nuclear overhauser enhancement mediated chemical exchange saturation transfer imaging at 7 Tesla in glioblastoma patients. PLoS One 9(8):e104181. https://doi.org/10.1371/journal.pone.0104181
128. Obdeijn IV, Wiegers EC, Alic L, Plasschaert SLA, Kranendonk MEG, Hoogduin HM et al (2024) Amide proton transfer weighted imaging in pediatric neuro-oncology: initial experience. NMR Biomed 37(6):e5122. https://doi.org/10.1002/nbm.5122. Epub 20240218. PubMed PMID: 38369653
129. Jiang S, Zou T, Eberhart CG, Villalobos MAV, Heo HY, Zhang Y et al (2017) Predicting IDH mutation status in grade II gliomas using amide proton transfer-weighted (APTw) MRI. Magn Reson Med 78(3):1100–1109. https://doi.org/10.1002/mrm.26820. Epub 2017/07/18. PubMed PMID: 28714279; PubMed Central PMCID: PMCPMC5561497
130. Wen PY, van den Bent M, Youssef G, Cloughesy TF, Ellingson BM, Weller M et al (2023) RANO 2.0: update to the response assessment in neuro-oncology criteria for high- and low-grade gliomas in adults. J Clin Oncol 41(33):5187–5199. https://doi.org/10.1200/jco.23.01059. Epub 20230929. PubMed PMID: 37774317; PubMed Central PMCID: PMCPMC10860967
131. Park JE, Kim HS, Park KJ, Kim SJ, Kim JH, Smith SA (2016) Pre – and posttreatment glioma: comparison of amide proton transfer imaging with MR spectroscopy for biomarkers of tumor proliferation. Radiology 278(2):514–523. https://doi.org/10.1148/radiol.2015142979. Epub 2015/10/23. PubMed PMID: 26491847.
132. Park KJ, Kim HS, Park JE, Shim WH, Kim SJ, Smith SA (2016) Added value of amide proton transfer imaging to conventional and perfusion MR imaging for evaluating the treatment response of newly diagnosed glioblastoma. Eur Radiol 26(12):4390–4403. https://doi.org/10.1007/s00330-016-4261-2. Epub 2016/02/18. PubMed PMID: 26883333.
133. Paech D, Dreher C, Regnery S, Meissner JE, Goerke S, Windschuh J et al (2019) Relaxation-compensated amide proton transfer (APT) MRI signal intensity is associated with survival and progression in high-grade glioma patients. Eur Radiol. https://doi.org/10.1007/s00330-019-06066-2. Epub 2019/02/28. PubMed PMID: 30809720
134. Mehrabian H, Myrehaug S, Soliman H, Sahgal A, Stanisz GJ (2018) Evaluation of glioblastoma response to therapy with chemical exchange saturation transfer. Int J Radiat Oncol Biol Phys 101(3):713–723. https://doi.org/10.1016/j.ijrobp.2018.03.057
135. Kroh F, von Knebel Doeberitz N, Breitling J, Maksimovic S, König L, Adeberg S et al (2023) Semi-solid MT and APTw CEST-MRI predict clinical outcome of patients with glioma early

after radiotherapy. Magn Reson Med 90(4):1569–1581. https://doi.org/10.1002/mrm.29746. Epub 20230615. PubMed PMID: 37317562

136. von Knebel Doeberitz N, Kroh F, Breitling J, König L, Maksimovic S, Graß S et al (2023) CEST imaging of the APT and ssMT predict the overall survival of patients with glioma at the first follow-up after completion of radiotherapy at 3T. Radiother Oncol 184:109694. https://doi.org/10.1016/j.radonc.2023.109694. Epub 20230506. PubMed PMID: 37150450
137. Regnery S, Adeberg S, Dreher C, Oberhollenzer J, Meissner JE, Goerke S et al (2018) Chemical exchange saturation transfer MRI serves as predictor of early progression in glioblastoma patients. Oncotarget 9(47):28772–28783. https://doi.org/10.18632/oncotarget.25594. Epub 2018/07/10. PubMed PMID: 29983895; PubMed Central PMCID: PMCPMC6033360
138. Essed RA, Prysiazhniuk Y, Wamelink IJ, Azizova A, Keil VC (2024) Performance of amide proton transfer imaging to differentiate true progression from therapy-related changes in gliomas and metastases. Eur Radiol. https://doi.org/10.1007/s00330-024-11004-y. Epub 20240812. PubMed PMID: 39134744
139. Jia G, Abaza R, Williams JD, Zynger DL, Zhou J, Shah ZK et al (2011) Amide proton transfer MR imaging of prostate cancer: a preliminary study. J Magn Reson Imaging 33(3):647–654. https://doi.org/10.1002/jmri.22480. PubMed PMID: 21563248; PubMed Central PMCID: PMCPMC4287206
140. Takayama Y, Nishie A, Sugimoto M, Togao O, Asayama Y, Ishigami K et al (2016) Amide proton transfer (APT) magnetic resonance imaging of prostate cancer: comparison with Gleason scores. Magma 29(4):671–679. https://doi.org/10.1007/s10334-016-0537-4. Epub 20160310. PubMed PMID: 26965511
141. Yin H, Wang D, Yan R, Jin X, Hu Y, Zhai Z et al (2021) Comparison of diffusion kurtosis imaging and amide proton transfer imaging in the diagnosis and risk assessment of prostate cancer. Front Oncol 11:640906. https://doi.org/10.3389/fonc.2021.640906. Epub 20210415. PubMed PMID: 33937041; PubMed Central PMCID: PMCPMC8082407
142. Zhang S, Seiler S, Wang X, Madhuranthakam AJ, Keupp J, Knippa EE et al (2018) CEST-Dixon for human breast lesion characterization at 3 T: a preliminary study. Magn Reson Med 80(3):895–903. https://doi.org/10.1002/mrm.27079. Epub 20180110. PubMed PMID: 29322559; PubMed Central PMCID: PMCPMC5980671
143. Loi L, Zimmermann F, Goerke S, Korzowski A, Meissner JE, Deike-Hofmann K et al (2020) Relaxation-compensated CEST (chemical exchange saturation transfer) imaging in breast cancer diagnostics at 7T. Eur J Radiol 129:109068. https://doi.org/10.1016/j.ejrad.2020.109068. Epub 20200524. PubMed PMID: 32574936
144. Ohno Y, Kishida Y, Seki S, Yui M, Miyazaki M, Koyama H, Yoshikawa T (2018) Amide proton transfer-weighted imaging to differentiate malignant from benign pulmonary lesions: Comparison with diffusion-weighted imaging and FDG-PET/CT. J Magn Reson Imaging 47(4):1013–1021. https://doi.org/10.1002/jmri.25832. Epub 20170811. PubMed PMID: 28799280
145. Choi SH (2018) Can amide proton transfer MRI distinguish benign and malignant head and neck tumors? Radiology 288(3):791–792. https://doi.org/10.1148/radiol.2018180914. Epub 20180612. PubMed PMID: 29893644
146. Radbruch A, Weberling LD, Kieslich PJ, Eidel O, Burth S, Kickingereder P et al (2015) gadolinium retention in the dentate nucleus and globus pallidus is dependent on the class of contrast agent. Radiology 275(3):783–791. https://doi.org/10.1148/radiol.2015150337. PubMed PMID: 25848905
147. Kanda T, Ishii K, Kawaguchi H, Kitajima K, Takenaka D (2014) High signal intensity in the dentate nucleus and globus pallidus on unenhanced T1-weighted MR images: relationship with increasing cumulative dose of a gadolinium-based contrast material. Radiology 270(3):834–841. https://doi.org/10.1148/radiol.13131669. PubMed PMID: 24475844
148. Kanda T, Osawa M, Oba H, Toyoda K, Kotoku J, Haruyama T et al (2015) High signal intensity in dentate nucleus on unenhanced T1-weighted MR images: association with linear

versus macrocyclic gadolinium chelate administration. Radiology 275(3):803–809. https://doi.org/10.1148/radiol.14140364. PubMed PMID: 25633504
149. McDonald RJ, McDonald JS, Kallmes DF, Jentoft ME, Murray DL, Thielen KR et al (2015) Intracranial gadolinium deposition after contrast-enhanced MR imaging. Radiology 275(3):772–782. https://doi.org/10.1148/radiol.15150025. PubMed PMID: 25742194
150. Radbruch A, Haase R, Kickingereder P, Bäumer P, Bickelhaupt S, Paech D et al (2017) Pediatric brain: no increased signal intensity in the dentate nucleus on unenhanced T1-weighted MR images after consecutive exposure to a macrocyclic gadolinium-based contrast agent. Radiology 283(3):828–836. https://doi.org/10.1148/radiol.2017162980. PubMed PMID: 28273007
151. Radbruch A (2016) Are some agents less likely to deposit gadolinium in the brain? Magn Reson Imaging 34(10):1351–1354. https://doi.org/10.1016/j.mri.2016.09.001
152. Thomsen HS, Morcos SK, Almén T, Bellin M-F, Bertolotto M, Bongartz G et al (2012) Nephrogenic systemic fibrosis and gadolinium-based contrast media: updated ESUR contrast medium safety committee guidelines. Eur Radiol 23(2):307–318. https://doi.org/10.1007/s00330-012-2597-9
153. Chan KWY, McMahon MT, Kato Y, Liu G, Bulte JWM, Bhujwalla ZM et al (2012) Natural D-glucose as a biodegradable MRI contrast agent for detecting cancer. Magn Reson Med 68(6):1764–1773. https://doi.org/10.1002/mrm.24520
154. Rivlin M, Horev J, Tsarfaty I, Navon G (2013) Molecular imaging of tumors and metastases using chemical exchange saturation transfer (CEST) MRI. Sci Rep 3. https://doi.org/10.1038/srep03045
155. Walker-Samuel S, Ramasawmy R, Torrealdea F, Rega M, Rajkumar V, Johnson SP et al (2013) In vivo imaging of glucose uptake and metabolism in tumors. Nat Med 19(8):1067–1072. https://doi.org/10.1038/nm.3252. http://www.nature.com/nm/journal/v19/n8/abs/nm.3252.html#supplementary-information
156. Jin T, Mehrens H, Hendrich KS, Kim S-G (2014) Mapping brain glucose uptake with chemical exchange-sensitive spin-lock magnetic resonance imaging. J Cereb Blood Flow Metab 34(8):1402–1410. https://doi.org/10.1038/jcbfm.2014.97. PubMed PMID: PMC4126103
157. Schuenke P, Koehler C, Korzowski A, Windschuh J, Bachert P, Ladd ME et al (2017) Adiabatically prepared spin-lock approach for T1ρ-based dynamic glucose enhanced MRI at ultrahigh fields. Magn Reson Med 78(1):215–225. https://doi.org/10.1002/mrm.26370
158. Paech D, Schuenke P, Koehler C, Windschuh J, Mundiyanapurath S, Bickelhaupt S et al (2017) T1ρ-weighted dynamic glucose-enhanced MR imaging in the human brain. Radiology 285(3):914–922. https://doi.org/10.1148/radiol.2017162351. PubMed PMID: 28628422
159. Schuenke P, Paech D, Koehler C, Windschuh J, Bachert P, Ladd M et al (2017) Fast and quantitative t1ρ-weighted dynamic glucose enhanced MRI. Sci Rep 7:42093. https://doi.org/10.1038/srep42093
160. Xu X, Yadav NN, Knutsson L, Hua J, Kalyani R, Hall E et al (2015) Dynamic glucose-enhanced (DGE) MRI: translation to human scanning and first results in glioma patients. Tomography 1(2):105
161. Tao J, Bistra I, Kevin HT, Michel M, Ping W, Hunter M, Seong-Gi K (2018) Chemical exchange–sensitive spin-lock (CESL) MRI of glucose and analogs in brain tumors. Magn Reson Med 80(2):488–495. https://doi.org/10.1002/mrm.27183
162. Chen Y, Jiang Y, Pahwa S, Ma D, Lu L, Twieg MD et al (2016) MR fingerprinting for rapid quantitative abdominal imaging. Radiology 279(1):278–286. https://doi.org/10.1148/radiol.2016152037. Epub 20160121. PubMed PMID: 26794935; PubMed Central PMCID: PMCPMC4819902
163. Jiang Y, Ma D, Seiberlich N, Gulani V, Griswold MA (2015) MR fingerprinting using fast imaging with steady state precession (FISP) with spiral readout. Magn Reson Med 74(6):1621–1631. https://doi.org/10.1002/mrm.25559. Epub 20141209. PubMed PMID: 25491018; PubMed Central PMCID: PMCPMC4461545
164. Panda A, Mehta BB, Coppo S, Jiang Y, Ma D, Seiberlich N et al (2017) Magnetic resonance fingerprinting-an overview. Curr Opin Biomed Eng 3:56–66. https://doi.

org/10.1016/j.cobme.2017.11.001. PubMed PMID: 29868647; PubMed Central PMCID: PMCPMC5984038
165. Du S, Gao S, Zhao R, Liu H, Wang Y, Qi X et al (2022) Contrast-free MRI quantitative parameters for early prediction of pathological response to neoadjuvant chemotherapy in breast cancer. Eur Radiol 32(8):5759–5772. https://doi.org/10.1007/s00330-022-08667-w. Epub 20220310. PubMed PMID: 35267091
166. Liu C, Li T, Cao P, Hui ES, Wong YL, Wang Z et al (2023) Respiratory-correlated 4-dimensional magnetic resonance fingerprinting for liver cancer radiation therapy motion management. Int J Radiat Oncol Biol Phys 117(2):493–504. https://doi.org/10.1016/j.ijrobp.2023.04.015. Epub 20230426. PubMed PMID: 37116591
167. Yu AC, Badve C, Ponsky LE, Pahwa S, Dastmalchian S, Rogers M et al (2017) Development of a combined MR fingerprinting and diffusion examination for prostate cancer. Radiology 283(3):729–738. https://doi.org/10.1148/radiol.2017161599. Epub 20170210. PubMed PMID: 28187264; PubMed Central PMCID: PMCPMC5452885
168. Badve C, A Y, Dastmalchian S, Rogers M, Ma D, Jiang Y et al (2017) MR fingerprinting of adult brain tumors: initial experience. AJNR Am J Neuroradiol 38(3):492–499. https://doi.org/10.3174/ajnr.A5035. Epub 20161229. PubMed PMID: 28034994; PubMed Central PMCID: PMCPMC5352493
169. Nissan N, Kulpanovich A, Agassi R, Allweis T, Haas I, Carmon E et al (2023) Probing lipids relaxation times in breast cancer using magnetic resonance spectroscopic fingerprinting. Eur Radiol 33(5):3744–3753. https://doi.org/10.1007/s00330-023-09560-w. Epub 20230328. PubMed PMID: 36976338
170. Shukla-Dave A, Obuchowski NA, Chenevert TL, Jambawalikar S, Schwartz LH, Malyarenko D et al (2019) Quantitative imaging biomarkers alliance (QIBA) recommendations for improved precision of DWI and DCE-MRI derived biomarkers in multicenter oncology trials. J Magn Reson Imaging 49(7):e101–ee21. https://doi.org/10.1002/jmri.26518. Epub 20181119. PubMed PMID: 30451345; PubMed Central PMCID: PMCPMC6526078
171. European Society of Radiology (ESR) (2010) White paper on imaging biomarkers. Insights Imaging 1(2):42–45. https://doi.org/10.1007/s13244-010-0025-8. Epub 20100527. PubMed PMID: 22347903; PubMed Central PMCID: PMCPMC3259342
172. European Society of Radiology (ESR) (2013) ESR statement on the stepwise development of imaging biomarkers. Insights Imaging 4(2):147–152. https://doi.org/10.1007/s13244-013-0220-5. Epub 20130209. PubMed PMID: 23397519; PubMed Central PMCID: PMCPMC3609959
173. European Society of Radiology (ESR) (2015) Magnetic Resonance Fingerprinting – a promising new approach to obtain standardized imaging biomarkers from MRI. Insights Imaging 6(2):163–165. https://doi.org/10.1007/s13244-015-0403-3. Epub 20150324. PubMed PMID: 25800993; PubMed Central PMCID: PMCPMC4376817

Potential Clinical Applications of Hyperpolarized ^{13}C and ^{2}H MRI

24

Richard Hesketh and Kevin Brindle

24.1 Introduction

24.1.1 Clinical MRI

Many will be familiar with the use of ^{1}H MRI to image tissue anatomy. The relatively high sensitivity of the proton to NMR detection, combined with the abundance of tissue water protons (~80 M), makes it possible to image anatomy in the clinic at millimetre resolution. The relaxation properties of water protons in different tissues can be used to provide image contrast, in contrast to x-ray computed tomography (CT), which provides very little soft tissue contrast. MRI has a long history of use in oncology, where the differing relaxation properties of tumour water protons can aid tumour detection and also response to treatment, where a positive response can be detected as a reduction in tumour volume [1].

The use of cross-sectional anatomical imaging with CT and MRI has exploded in the last 40 years, and there are now over 120 million exams performed annually in the United States compared to <5 million in 1980. The imaging techniques have advanced significantly over this period, particularly in terms of image acquisition speed, contrast and spatial resolution. Computer advances, particularly picture archiving and communication systems (PACS) replacing printed films, have also contributed significantly to improving the diagnostic accuracy of imaging. More than half of all imaging exams are performed for oncology, where these are for

R. Hesketh
Centre for Medical Imaging, University College London, London, UK
e-mail: r.hesketh@ucl.ac.uk

K. Brindle (✉)
Cancer Research UK Cambridge Institute, University of Cambridge, Cambridge, UK
e-mail: kmb1001@cam.ac.uk

O. Schober et al. (eds.), *Molecular Imaging in Oncology - Volume 2*, Recent Results in Cancer Research 225, https://doi.org/10.1007/978-3-032-21415-7_6

detection, staging and re-staging. We discuss here the opportunities for metabolic imaging with MRI.

24.1.2 Cancer and Metabolism

Cancer is a heterogeneous group of diseases characterized by dysregulated cell proliferation and an invasive phenotype that confers the ability to invade local tissues and metastasize to distant sites. The underlying cause of cancers is mutations, and an accumulation of "driver" mutations is typically required to initiate tumourigenesis and circumvent mechanisms involved in DNA repair, senescence and apoptosis. In addition to tumour cells, a range of normal host cells are recruited and exploited to develop the tumour microenvironment into a self-regulating tissue capable of promoting proliferation, cellular immortality, immune evasion and angiogenesis [2]. To support tumorigenesis, numerous metabolic pathways are upregulated in response to the increased demands for energy, proteins, fatty acids and other macromolecules [3]. Aerobic glycolysis, in which glucose is metabolized to lactate preferentially, even in the presence of oxygen, was first observed in cancer cells by Otto Warburg in 1924. We now know that a switch from oxidative metabolism to glycolysis is a simplistic description of cancer metabolism and although the Warburg effect is regularly observed in vitro and in vivo, in reality, aberrations are observed across metabolic pathways with complex temporal and spatial variations. Furthermore, abnormal metabolism is not limited to tumour cells, but there is a complex interplay between different cells in the tumour microenvironment.

For decades, cancers have been categorized clinically by their tissue of origin and histological appearance. Increasingly, molecular subcategorization is performed, facilitated by immunohistochemistry, fluorescence in situ hybridization, and a range of "omic" technologies including whole genome sequencing. Thus, tumour subcategories have increased from a few different subtypes to tens of molecular subcategories, with each subcategory having its own risk factors, pattern of disease and prognosis, and with increasingly different treatment options. The growing understanding of the complexity of cancer biology is a challenge for current clinical imaging but opens up multiple opportunities for more sophisticated diagnostics, including molecular and metabolic imaging.

24.1.3 MR Spectroscopy

From the very earliest applications of MRI to biological systems, it was recognized that the technique could also detect signals from small molecule metabolites. This exploits a key feature of magnetic resonance, which is "chemical shift", where the frequency of a signal is a function of the chemical environment of the nucleus giving rise to it. The technique can thus detect not only the presence of a signal but also identify which molecule is giving rise to that signal. Localized proton (^{1}H) NMR spectra of human brain tumours are shown in Fig. 24.1. Signals from the lactate

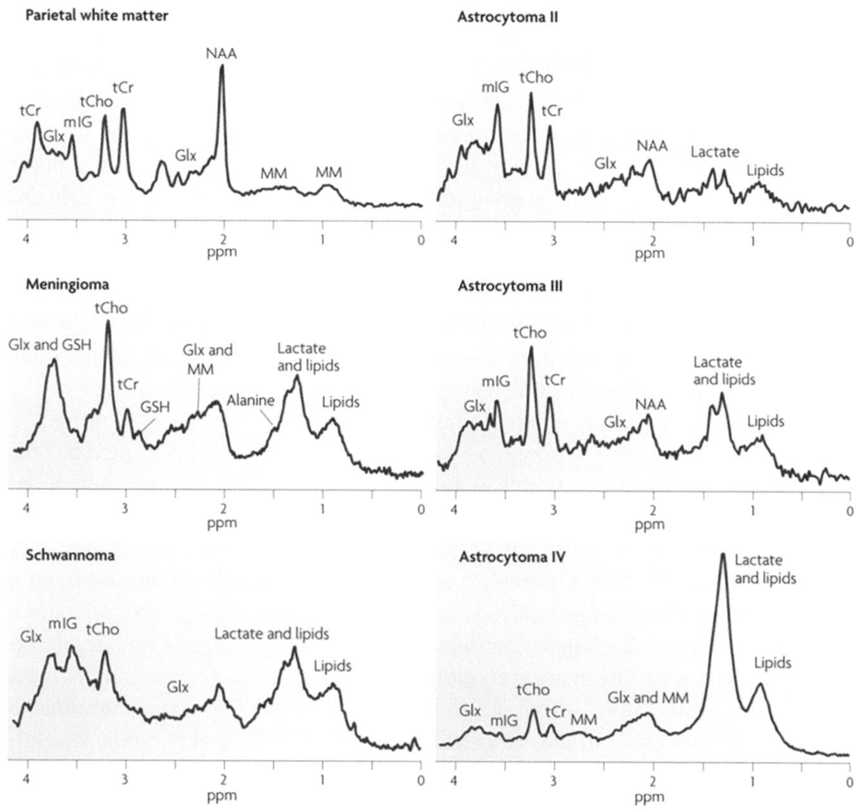

Fig. 24.1 ^{1}H spectra from normal human brain and adult brain tumours. Abbreviations: Glx glutamate and glutamine, GSH glutathione, mIG myo-inositol and glycine, MM macromolecules, NAA N-acetyl aspartate, tCho total cholines, tCr total creatines. (Spectra courtesy of F. Howe, St. George's Hospital Medical School, London, UK. Reproduced, with permission, from [4])

methyl group, the methyl and methylene protons of lipids, N-acetyl aspartate (NAA, a neuronal cell marker), unresolved resonances from glutamate and glutamine (Glx), total creatine (creatine plus phosphocreatine), total choline (which includes contributions from various choline-containing compounds, including phosphocholine) and glutathione (GSH) are observable. The tumours show elevated concentrations of lipids, which are predominantly in cytoplasmic lipid droplets, and lactate and choline-containing compounds when compared to normal brain (in this example, parietal white matter). The intense water resonance at 4.7 ppm (not shown) had to be suppressed in order to detect the signals from the metabolites, which are present in only mM concentrations. Although the proton nucleus is relatively sensitive to detection when compared to other NMR-active nuclei, such as ^{13}C, ^{15}N and ^{31}P, the spectra are more poorly resolved, reflecting the relatively narrow chemical shift range of ^{1}H. For example, the signal from lactate is frequently masked by lipid signals, as observed in the astrocytoma IV spectrum. These spectra show that different types of brain tumour have different metabolism and therefore ^{1}H spectra can be used to determine the type of tumour present, without the need for biopsy, which can provide prognostic information.

Proton spectra have been used with various tumour types in addition to brain tumours, including prostate and breast, to assess tumour grade and to detect treatment response. In brain tumours, a higher lipid signal is associated with a higher grade and poorer survival, and in low-grade gliomas, mutations in isocitrate dehydrogenases (IDH) 1 and 2 can be detected through the resultant accumulation of 2-hydroxyglutarate (2-HG). In prostate cancer, higher total choline (tCho) signal indicates the presence of disease, and the tCho/creatine ratio can correlate with tumour grade. A higher tCho signal and water/fat signal ratio in breast cancer can be used to distinguish benign from malignant lesions, with a decrease in tCho signal providing an early indication of treatment response. However, proton spectroscopy has not yet become a routine tool in the clinic. In prostate cancer, it was considered difficult to apply in a routine clinical setting, and in breast cancer, it has been limited by long signal acquisition times and chest wall motion. The technique has shown more promise in the brain because of a lack of motion and better detection sensitivity, as more of the tumour can fill the detector coil when compared to tumours in other tissues.

^{1}H spectra, such as these, provide a metabolite profile of the tissue at a point in time. Since metabolism in general, and tumour metabolism in particular, operates in a steady state, where the rate of production of a metabolite equals its rate of consumption, there is no information about metabolic flux. However, measurements of flux are frequently more informative. For example, the high concentrations of tumour lactate observed in the ^{1}H spectra shown in Fig. 24.1 may be the result of increased glycolytic flux, but they could also be the result of decreased lactate washout in a poorly perfused tumour. If we want to measure metabolic flux using magnetic resonance, then we need to introduce an isotopically labelled substrate, where this label is typically ^{13}C, ^{15}N or ^{2}H. The presence of high lactate concentrations observed in ^{1}H MRS spectra of stroke lesions was shown, in a very early study, to be due to increased glycolytic flux by infusing the patients with [1-^{13}C]glucose [5]. This resulted in ^{13}C-labelling of the lactate methyl group, which split the methyl proton resonance into a doublet due to $^{13}C - {}^{1}H$ spin-spin coupling, demonstrating that the increased lactate concentration in the lesion was due to increased glycolytic flux. ^{13}C is much less sensitive to MRS detection than the proton and detecting the ^{13}C label indirectly in the ^{1}H spectrum significantly enhanced the sensitivity of its detection. Nevertheless, despite this lack of sensitivity, the direct detection of ^{13}C-labelled substrates and their metabolites has been used in a variety of systems. For example, in human breast cancer xenografts in mice, infusion of the animals with [1-^{13}C]glucose resulted in tumour signals from the labelled glucose and from lactate [6]. A value for glycolytic flux could be obtained by acquiring a series of spectra and fitting the glucose and lactate ^{13}C signal intensities to a kinetic model of glycolysis. However, the signal intensities were insufficient for imaging and were localized by placing the detector coil directly over the subcutaneous tumour. Imaging of ^{13}C-labelled metabolites required a massive gain in sensitivity. This has been obtained using nuclear spin hyperpolarization techniques.

24.1.4 Nuclear Spin Hyperpolarization

When a spin ½ nucleus, such as ^{1}H or ^{13}C, is placed in a strong magnetic field, the spins adopt one of two energy levels, corresponding to spins aligned with (lower energy level) and against the applied magnetic field (higher energy level). It is the difference in these spin populations that gives rise to the signal in the NMR experiment. However, the interaction is so weak that the two energy levels are nearly equally populated, with a slight excess of spins in the lower energy level, which explains why NMR is such an insensitive spectroscopic technique. The conventional approach to increasing sensitivity is to build higher field magnets, increasing the population difference and hence the signal. A much more effective alternative to increasing the difference in spin populations is to use nuclear spin hyperpolarization techniques.

Dynamic nuclear polarization (DNP) has been the most widely used technique to hyperpolarize ^{13}C-labelled substrates for use in vitro and in vivo and is currently being tested in early-phase clinical trials. The ^{13}C labelled substrate is mixed with a stable radical, usually a trityl radical, and rapidly frozen to form a glass. The sample is then cooled to ~1.2 K in a high magnetic field (current clinical devices operate at 5 T (the earth's magnetic field is ~50 μT)) at which temperature the unpaired electron spin on the radical becomes completely polarized, i.e. the electron spins are all aligned with the magnetic field. The electron spins are then excited with microwave radiation, which transfers the electron spin polarization to the nuclear spins. The breakthrough in transferring this technique to a liquid state experiment came with the realization and demonstration that this frozen sample could be warmed rapidly to room temperature with substantial retention of this nuclear spin polarization [7] and a greater than 10,000x increase in the sensitivity of detection. This meant that it was now possible to hyperpolarize the ^{13}C spins in a ^{13}C-labelled substrate and then inject this hyperpolarized ^{13}C-labelled substrate intravenously and image its location in the body and, because of chemical shift, its conversion into other cellular metabolites. The most widely used substrate thus far has been [1-^{13}C]pyruvate, which, when injected in vivo, exchanges its hyperpolarized ^{13}C label with the endogenous lactate pool. Since the lactate concentration is frequently elevated in tumours, they can be quite conspicuous in ^{13}C spectroscopic images (Fig. 24.2).

A fundamental limitation of the technique is the short lifetime of the spin polarization, which in pyruvate decays in vivo with a time constant of 20–30 s. This means that injection and imaging must be accomplished within 2–3 min, and limits the application of the technique to substrates that are taken up into cells very quickly and undergo subsequent fast metabolism. For example, pyruvate is taken up rapidly into cells on the monocarboxylate transporters (MCTs) and undergoes fast interconversion with lactate in the reaction catalysed by lactate dehydrogenase (LDH). Pyruvate also undergoes slower oxidation in the reaction catalysed by the mitochondrial pyruvate dehydrogenase (PDH) complex to produce, in the case of [1-^{13}C]pyruvate, $^{13}CO_2$, which then undergoes rapid interconversion with bicarbonate ($H^{13}CO_3^-$) (Fig. 24.3). Labelled CO_2 and HCO_3^- are observed in oxidative tissues such as the heart and the brain, but are rarely observed in tumours, as PDH activity in most

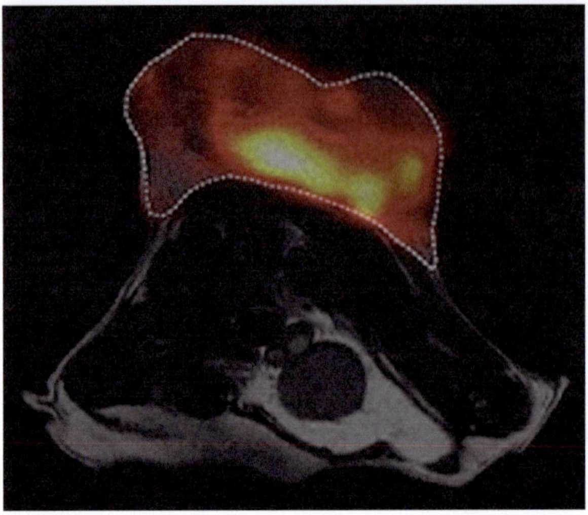

Fig. 24.2 Injection of hyperpolarized [1-^{13}C]pyruvate results in the labelling of lactate in a murine lymphoma model. Labelled lactate is represented by the colour image, which is overlaid on a ^{1}H MR image of tissue anatomy, which is shown in grey scale. The tumour is outlined with a dotted white line. Note that lactate labelling is restricted largely to one area of the tumour. (Reproduced with permission from [8])

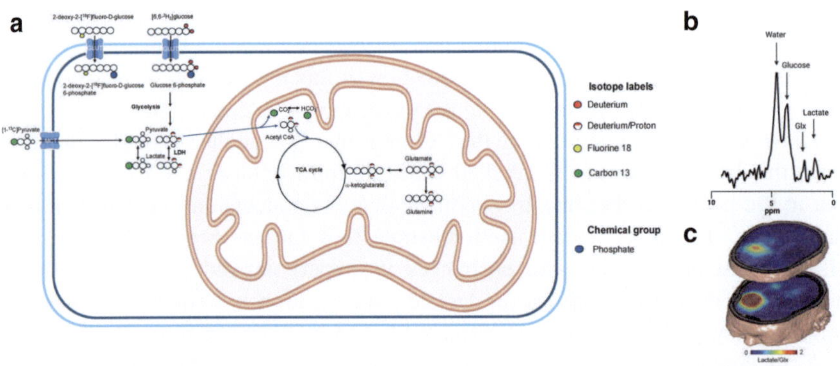

Fig. 24.3 Metabolic imaging with hyperpolarized [1-^{13}C]pyruvate, [6,6-$^{2}H_2$]glucose and 2-deoxy-2-[^{18}F]fluoro-D-glucose ([^{18}F]FDG). (**a**) The fate of the hyperpolarized ^{13}C, ^{2}H and ^{18}F labels is shown. (Created in BioRender. Brindle, K. (2026) https://BioRender.com/d8bnivs) (**b**) ^{2}H spectrum acquired from the brain of a mouse with an orthotopically implanted patient-derived glioblastoma xenograft following the injection of [6,6′-$^{2}H_2$]glucose (unpublished data). (**c**) Maps of the labelled lactate/Glx ratio in a glioblastoma patient following oral administration of [6,6′-$^{2}H_2$] glucose. The tumour shows a higher ratio reflecting increased glycolytic and decreased TCA cycle activity when compared to the normal brain. (Image reproduced with permission from [12])

tumours is relatively low. The polarization lifetime can be extended by placing the ^{13}C label in a position where spin-spin coupling with protons in the molecule is small (e.g. the carboxyl group in the case of [1-^{13}C]pyruvate) or by replacing spin-coupled protons with deuterium. Protons in solvent water can also relax the polarization, which can be reduced during the dissolution process by replacing water with D_2O.

DNP hyperpolarizers have a number of drawbacks. The cryogenic systems needed to reach 1.2K are expensive and bulky, and initially were difficult to operate, and clinical systems require pharmacy facilities to formulate and package the sterile sample for subsequent polarization, which adds to the already substantial cost. Efforts are being made to reduce costs and simplify the process. For example, it may be possible to polarize substrates in a central facility and then ship the polarized samples to the imaging facility at low temperature and high magnetic field, conditions under which the polarization relaxation time constant may be several hours. An alternative approach to polarizing the ^{13}C nucleus is to transfer spin order from parahydrogen (parahydrogen-induced polarization (PHIP)), either by binding the parahydrogen and ^{13}C-labelled molecule to the surface of an iridium metal catalyst [9] or by chemically reacting the parahydrogen with the ^{13}C-labelled molecule [10]. These techniques allow for the rapid transfer of spin polarization to the target ^{13}C-labelled molecule at room temperature and within seconds, as opposed to the tens of minutes required for the DNP process. A challenge for the clinical application of these PHIP techniques has been the requirement for the rapid removal of the metal catalysts and solvents used in the process; nevertheless, it seems likely that a PHIP-based polarizer will enter the clinic in the next 1–2 years. Since these polarizers do not require the complex cryogenics required for the DNP process, they are inherently cheaper and the possibility for providing pre-packaged materials for polarization avoids the need for on-site pharmacy facilities, which will also reduce costs.

24.1.5 Deuterium Metabolic Imaging (DMI)

The NMR properties of deuterium would appear to make it a very unpromising nucleus for isotope labelling studies of metabolism. The nucleus is relatively insensitive to detection, and its quadrupolar nature results in broad resonances. This coupled with its low resonance frequency and narrow chemical shift range result in crowded and poorly resolved spectra. However, the nucleus, depending on its chemical environment, frequently has a very short spin lattice relaxation time (T_1), which means that the relative insensitivity of detection can be compensated by rapid signal averaging, which, because of the short T_1, can be accomplished with little signal saturation. The low natural abundance of the isotope (0.0115%) means that there is very little background signal, for example, tissue water signal (HOD) corresponds to ~10 mM ^{2}H. Contrast this with ^{1}H spectroscopy, which requires very effective suppression of the intense solvent resonance, which results from ~80 M tissue water protons. The HOD signal in DMI also provides a convenient in-built intensity standard that allows the ^2H signal intensities from labelled metabolites to be converted into concentrations. Nevertheless, the low sensitivity of detection and poor spectral resolution make it advantageous to work at higher magnetic fields (>7 T), which potentially could limit clinical application, although clinical studies have been performed at 3 T.

The current interest in DMI can be traced back to two papers published in 2017 [11] and 2018 [12] that investigated brain metabolism by infusing [6,6-$^2H_2$]glucose. The latter showed in an orthotopically implanted glioma model in the rat, increased lactate labelling and decreased glutamate/glutamine (Glx) labelling in the tumour when compared to the surrounding brain, indicating increased glycolytic activity and decreased TCA cycle activity in the tumour (Fig. 24.3). This was a landmark study since they showed a similar result in a glioma patient in which the labelled glucose was administered orally (Fig. 24.3c).

24.1.6 Metabolic Imaging with Hyperpolarized ^{13}C and ^2H-Labelled Substrates

Since the first publication describing the solution state DNP experiment in 2003 [7], there have been numerous publications describing the use of [1-^{13}C]pyruvate for investigating tumour metabolism in vivo. Despite the requirement for the ^{13}C label to be located at a position in the labelled molecule where the polarization lifetime is relatively long and where the delivery, cell uptake and subsequent metabolism of the labelled substrate must be very rapid, numerous labelled metabolites have shown utility for investigating metabolism in vivo [13]. The first clinical study with hyperpolarized [1-^{13}C]pyruvate, which was in prostate cancer, was published in 2013 [14], and there are now numerous ongoing clinical studies with this substrate. Although a later development, DMI has now also been used with numerous other ^2H-labelled substrates [15] and there have been further clinical studies. In discussing the potential clinical applications in oncology of hyperpolarized ^{13}C and ^2H MRI, we will limit our discussion to those substrates that are in clinical trials, including hyperpolarized [1-^{13}C]pyruvate, [6,6-$^2H_2$]glucose, [1-^{13}C]α-ketoglutarate, [^{13}C]bicarbonate and [^{13}C, ^{15}N]urea (https://clinicaltrials.gov/) and fumarate (^{13}C and ^2H labelled), which are about to go into clinical trials.

24.1.6.1 Hyperpolarized [1-^{13}C]Pyruvate and [6,6-$^2H_2$]Glucose

Among the first papers describing the use of hyperpolarized [1-^{13}C]pyruvate in oncology were two, one that described how it could be used to grade tumours [16] and another how it could be used to detect early responses to treatment [17]. In a mouse model of prostate cancer, lactate labelling increased with tumour grade, and in a murine lymphoma model, lactate labelling showed a marked decrease within 24 h of starting chemotherapy. DMI with [6,6′-$^2H_2$]glucose can be used in much the same way. Glioblastoma shows different metabolic subtypes that have differing prognoses and therapeutic vulnerabilities. In mice implanted orthotopically with patient-derived xenografts and injected with [6,6′-$^2H_2$]glucose, there were differences in lactate and Glx labelling that correlated with metabolic subtype, with a mesenchymal glycolytic subtype showing higher levels of lactate and lower levels of Glx labelling when compared to a more oxidative subtype [18] that was more sensitive to radiotherapy [19]. The glycolytic subtype also showed higher levels of lactate labelling from hyperpolarized [1-^{13}C]pyruvate than the oxidative subtype [20]. In the same murine lymphoma model used with hyperpolarized [1-^{13}C]pyruvate described above, chemotherapy resulted in a profound decrease in ^{2}H-labelled lactate production in animals injected with [6,6′-$^{2}H_2$]glucose within 24 h of starting treatment [21].

Tumour glycolytic activity can also be assessed using PET measurements of the uptake of 2-deoxy-2-[^{18}F]fluoro-D-glucose ([^{18}F]FDG), which is an analogue of glucose that enters cells via the glucose transporters (GLUTs) and is trapped in the cell via phosphorylation by the first enzyme in the glycolytic pathway, hexokinase (Fig. 24.3). Both [1-^{13}C]pyruvate and [^{18}F]FDG interrogate glycolysis and the overall aim of using both agents is to image upregulation of this pathway as a surrogate for disease. But even in the clinical setting, it is an oversimplification to consider both agents as measures of "hypermetabolic" tissue: both experiments measure an independent set of reactions at opposite ends of the glycolytic pathway. [^{18}F]FDG-PET measures perfusion, cell uptake and the intracellular trapping that follows phosphorylation by hexokinase, while imaging with [1-^{13}C]pyruvate is affected by perfusion and cellular uptake (and efflux) via the monocarboxylate transporters, and by exchange of hyperpolarized ^{13}C label with the endogenous lactate pool in the reaction catalysed by LDH (Fig. 24.3). The glycolysis link between [1-^{13}C]pyruvate and [^{18}F]FDG means that under many circumstances there are likely to be similar changes in the metabolism of both agents, but there have been several preclinical examples where this relationship is lost, particularly following chemotherapy. In the preclinical experimental setting, it is usually possible to explain this via the specific chemotherapeutic effects on enzyme and transporter expression and activity [22]. In clinical practice, the initial focus has been directed towards using hyperpolarized [1-^{13}C]pyruvate in organs where [^{18}F]FDG is limited by high or variable background uptake or accumulation, particularly in the brain, heart and urinary tract. We anticipate that tumour grading and treatment monitoring will be the main clinical applications of imaging with hyperpolarized [1-^{13}C]pyruvate and [6,6′-$^{2}H_2$]glucose in the future.

An important distinction between hyperpolarized [1-^{13}C]pyruvate and [^{18}F]FDG on the one hand and [6,6′-$^{2}H_2$]glucose on the other is that the former measures aspects of glycolytic activity, whereas [6,6′-$^{2}H_2$]glucose can be used to measure flux through the entire pathway and also flux into the TCA cycle. For example, in the murine lymphoma model discussed above, fitting of the [6,6′-$^{2}H_2$]glucose and ^{2}H-lactate image intensities to a model of the glycolytic pathway allowed the estimation of maps of glycolytic flux in the tumour (in mM/min) [21].

24.1.6.2 Hyperpolarized [^{13}C,^{15}N]Urea

Hyperpolarized ^{13}C-urea is not taken up by most tissues and has been shown to provide an accurate measure of blood perfusion in animal tumour models [23]. The agent shows good contrast and can be combined with hyperpolarized [1-^{13}C] pyruvate for simultaneous imaging of both tumour perfusion and metabolism. The attractiveness of the agent as a tool for imaging perfusion has been enhanced by concerns over the potential toxicity of gadolinium-based contrast media. The substitution of ^{15}N for the naturally abundant ^{14}N removes a strong source of relaxation of the polarization and thus improves the sensitivity of detection.

24.1.6.3 Hyperpolarized [1,4-$^{13}C_2$]Fumarate and [2,3-$^{2}H_2$]Fumarate

Imaging the metabolism of hyperpolarized [1-^{13}C]pyruvate, [6,6′-$^{2}H_2$]glucose or [^{18}F]FDG can give an early indication of whether a drug has hit its target, but does not necessarily provide an unequivocal indication of subsequent tumour cell death. There has been considerable interest in the development of imaging methods that can detect tumour cell death post treatment, including targeted PET agents [24] and MRI methods, such as diffusion-weighted MRI, which can be used to detect changes in tumour cellularity. However, there are currently no imaging methods in routine use in the clinic that can reliably detect cell death. Early studies with hyperpolarized [1,4-$^{13}C_2$]fumarate showed that it could be used to detect necrotic cells in posttreatment tumours [25]. Fumarase is an intracellular enzyme with a very high turnover number that catalyses the hydration of fumarate to produce malate. In most viable cell types, fumarate enters the cells very slowly. However, in necrotic cells, fumarate can rapidly enter the cell, or fumarase can leak out of the cell into the tumour interstitial space, resulting in the rapid production of malate. Using the malate/fumarate signal intensity ratio compensates for any differences in perfusion, and the fact that fumarase has no coenzyme requirement means that the enzyme can remain active in a necrotic cell or in the extracellular space. The short half-life of the polarization means that malate build-up can only be detected over the first few minutes following fumarate injection, and therefore, although the sensitivity of signal detection is high, the contrast that is generated (malate/fumarate signal ratio) is limited. This is not the case for [2,3-$^{2}H_2$]fumarate, where in murine tumour models, the malate concentration continues to build up over more than 60 min and in favourable cases can give a malate/fumarate ratio (contrast) >10 [26]. [2,3-$^{2}H_2$]fumarate can also be administered orally and can give contrast as high as that observed after intravenous administration, which should facilitate clinical translation. Since the malate/fumarate ratio provides positive contrast, the acquisition of relatively low-resolution images integrates all the cell death present in the voxel, and thus the technique can be used to detect relatively low levels of diffuse necrosis. This is in contrast to diffusion-weighted MRI, which, for the detection of low levels of diffuse necrosis, requires the acquisition of relatively high-resolution images. Imaging with both hyperpolarized [1,4-$^{13}C_2$]fumarate and [2,3-$^{2}H_2$]fumarate has been shown to be more sensitive at detecting posttreatment tumour cell death than DW-MRI [19, 27].

24.1.6.4 Hyperpolarized [^{13}C]Bicarbonate

Tumours frequently show a low extracellular pH, which can be detected using hyperpolarized $H^{13}CO_3^-$. The ^{13}C label in the injected bicarbonate rapidly equilibrates with the endogenous CO_2 pool, in both a spontaneous reaction and in one catalyzed by the enzyme carbonic anhydrase. The $H^{13}CO_3^-/^{13}CO_2$ signal intensity ratio, when substituted into the Henderson-Hasselbach equation and using the pKa for bicarbonate, can be used to create images of pH [28]. The hyperpolarized $^{13}CO_2$ released through the oxidation of [1-^{13}C]pyruvate, following equilibration with endogenous bicarbonate, can be used to estimate intracellular pH. A limitation of the technique is that it relies on the $H^{13}CO_3^-$ and $^{13}CO_2$ signal intensities, which can be differentially affected by their polarization lifetimes. An alternative pH probe that has been used to investigate extracellular pH in tumours is [1,5-$^{13}C_2$]zymonic acid [29], in which pH is estimated from the chemical shift of its resonances. This can provide a more reliable estimate of pH than one based on resonance intensities.

24.1.6.5 Hyperpolarized [1-^{13}C]α-Ketoglutarate

Gain-of-function mutations in isocitrate dehydrogenase (IDH) 1 and 2 are observed in approximately 80% of gliomas, particularly those of lower grade, and result in a neomorphic activity in which the enzyme produces 2-hydroxyglutarate (2-HG) from α-ketoglutarate. This oncometabolite drives tumour development by inhibiting cellular dioxygenases, resulting in changes in DNA and histone methylation, and the mutant enzyme is a target for drug treatment. Recently, it has been shown, for example, that vorasidenib, an inhibitor of mutant IDH1 and 2, more than doubled progression-free survival in patients with IDH-mutant grade II glioma [30]. Increases in the rate of 2-HG synthesis in IDH mutant tumours and decreases resulting from the use of inhibitors of mutant IDH have been detected in tumour models of IDH-mutant gliomas using ^{13}C MRSI following the injection of hyperpolarized [1-^{13}C]α-ketoglutarate [31]. The technique could be used in the clinic to detect IDH mutations, to determine eligibility for IDH inhibitor treatment, and subsequently to detect response to treatment. However, it should be noted that increases in the steady-state concentration of 2-HG in IDH mutant tumours have already been detected in the clinic using ^{1}H MRS. Hyperpolarized [1-^{13}C]α-ketoglutarate has recently entered phase-one trials in healthy volunteers.

24.2 Clinical Niche for Metabolic MRI

24.2.1 Cancer Detection

Current imaging technologies are able to detect gross anatomical abnormalities. Depending on the imaging modality and tissue of interest, the lower limit of size detection for masses ranges from a few millimetres to a few centimetres. However, imaging is poor at indicating whether these growths are benign or cancerous. Therefore, few cancers are diagnosed and treated based solely on radiological appearances, a notable exception being some hepatocellular carcinomas in patients with liver cirrhosis. In the majority of cases, a tissue sample is required for pathological diagnosis, where the diagnostic accuracy of a core biopsy for cancer versus benign disease approaches 99% in most tissues. Furthermore, tissue samples permit, with increasing frequency, treatment decisions to be tailored based on the specific gene expression pattern within the tumour. In a minority of tumours with specific molecular markers, radionuclide-labelled SPECT/PET tracers can be highly sensitive and specific, for example gallium-68-DOTATATE for the PET diagnosis of neuroendocrine tumours. As our understanding of tumour biology expands, new radionuclide tracers are being developed which target these molecular aberrations and have considerable clinical potential, for example [^{89}Zr]-girentuximab, which binds carbonic anhydrase IX (CAIX), for the diagnosis of clear cell renal carcinoma [32]. However, many of these have a significant limitation, for example, poorly differentiated and more aggressive cancers often tend to lose their defining molecular characteristics. Loss of cell surface CAIX in clear cell renal carcinoma, for example, which is a feature of poor prognosis, may mean that the most aggressive tumours will be falsely negative on [^{89}Zr]-girentuximab PET. This need not be a limitation for metabolic imaging since aggressive tumours frequently show more marked alterations in metabolism.

The frequently upregulated glycolytic activity of tumours results in elevated [^{18}F]FDG uptake and is widely used in cancer imaging, but similar to anatomical imaging, it has limited specificity for the differentiation of benign and malignant diseases, particularly when inflammatory processes can also take up [^{18}F]FDG and appear mass-like (Fig. 24.4).

24.2.2 Tumour Grading and Detection of Subtypes

Detecting early-stage cancers is becoming increasingly common through a combination of increased awareness, screening programmes and the wider use of cross-sectional imaging. For some cancers, this has created a new predicament, for example, in the case of renal and prostate cancer, the majority of small renal masses and localized prostate cancers have lifetime rates of metastasis of only a few percent and probably do not require treatment. However, the probability of metastasis positively correlates with increasing tumour grade and therefore using imaging to infer grade and to differentiate clinically significant cancers becomes of utmost importance. In renal cancer, there is currently no way of grading tumours on imaging. In prostate cancer, metrics based on diffusion-weighted (DWI) MRI, most commonly

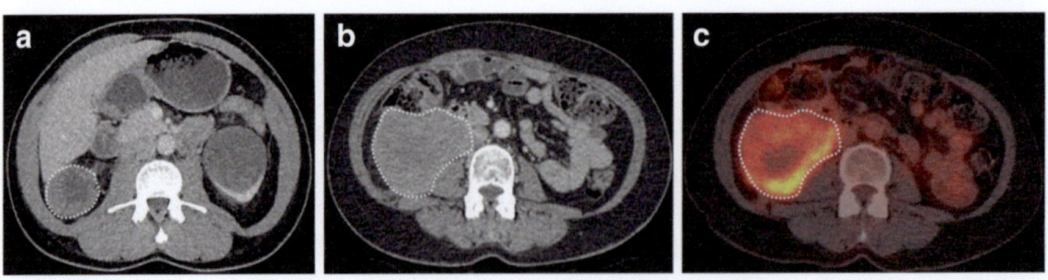

Fig. 24.4 CT scan and an [^{18}F]FDG-PET/CT scan showing a poorly differentiated carcinoma versus IgG4-related disease (white dashed outlines). (**a**) Poorly differentiated carcinoma; (**b**) IgG4-related disease (a benign inflammatory condition) showing (**c**) high [^{18}F]FDG uptake in the inflammatory lesion. The IgG4 mass enlarged over 10 years, in which time the patient had multiple biopsies to re-confirm the absence of malignancy (RLH, unpublished data)

the apparent diffusion coefficient (ADC), correlate moderately with Gleason grading and subjective interpretation of DWI and ADC sequences are now the cornerstone of prostate MRI [33].

The global targeted therapy market was valued at $170 billion per year in 2023 and is expected to grow by a further 10% by 2030. Currently, decisions to treat with targeted therapy are either empirical or based on molecular expression determined in a biopsy or surgical specimen. The latter is inherently flawed by inter- and intra-tumoural heterogeneity, and numerous studies have demonstrated both temporal variation and a lack of concordance between different biopsy sites. In time, liquid biopsy (sampling the plasma for tumour DNA) may prove to be more representative of whole tumours than single-site biopsies; however, imaging will remain the only way to sample whole tumours and their metastases non-invasively. While imaging cannot perform a comprehensive molecular analysis, it is conceivable that imaging biomarkers could infer individual gene expression patterns that will determine treatment. As already mentioned, [^{89}Zr]Zr-girentuximab is being used to detect CAIX expression in renal cancer, and the enzyme is being investigated as a potential therapeutic target. In breast and gastric cancers, HER-2 expression determines eligibility for HER-2 targeted therapy. [^{89}Zr]Zr-trastuzumab, which binds to the HER-2 receptor, has demonstrated the ability to detect HER-2 positive metastases in patients where the primary tumour was negative for HER-2, and clinical trials of efficacy are ongoing [34].

24.2.3 Detecting Treatment Response

Routine radiological reporting relies heavily on single-diameter measurements of lesions, backed by the RECIST guidelines [1], which were introduced for clinical trial reporting. The main source of inaccuracy in this method is the limited repeatability and reproducibility of lesion measurement. An inability to detect small changes in tumour size means that response assessment is delayed following treatment for a minimum of 1 month, usually longer. An accurate early marker of response would reduce the side effects and costs of ineffective treatment, as well as potentially facilitating switching of treatment regimens.

Additionally, response is becoming more nuanced, and a "one size fits all" approach to all tumours and treatments is no longer appropriate. The difficulty of differentiating pseudoprogression and true progression on early anatomical and [^{18}F]FDG-PET imaging following immunotherapy has been well documented and even led to a revision in RECIST guidelines. However, there are other frequent sources of confusion in imaging. Radiotherapy is commonly used with curative and palliative intent. Traditional radiotherapy often results in fibrosis and inflammation within the treatment zone, which can be present for years and is challenging to differentiate from tumour recurrence or incomplete treatment on [^{18}F]FDG-PET. Newer targeted radiotherapy treatments, including proton beam therapy, stereotactic ablative radiotherapy (SABR) and selective internal radiotherapy (SIRT), also result in variable imaging findings. In the case of SABR, tumours can continue to show MRI contrast agent enhancement and may remain stable in size for years following treatment. Even the presence of viable tumour cells in post-SABR biopsies does not necessarily correlate with long-term response, potentially due to radiation-induced senescence predominating over cell death (Fig. 24.5).

24.2.4 Clinical Translation of Imaging Biomarkers

For a new imaging biomarker to translate into routine clinical practice, it must provide novel information that is not already available via standard of care imaging or other tests, answer a clinically relevant question, and thus have the power to change clinical management. This needs to be coupled with sufficient test accuracy, repeatability and reproducibility. These criteria do not have fixed values but vary for each test and application. The test also needs to be acceptable to patients in terms of safety, time and invasiveness, and be practical and cost-effective to deliver. There is no doubt that hyperpolarized substrates can provide novel metabolic information, but whether this will translate beyond a research tool remains to be determined. Early efforts to perform human hyperpolarized experiments have been challenging due to the aforementioned issues of first-generation clinical DNP systems, limiting the evidence base to feasibility case reports and series. Nevertheless, the studies delivered so far have clearly demonstrated an excellent safety profile for hyperpolarized [1-^{13}C]pyruvate with no severe adverse events reported globally following over one thousand injections, and the vast majority of patients experiencing no side effects. As an initial step towards clinical test validation, acceptable cross-site

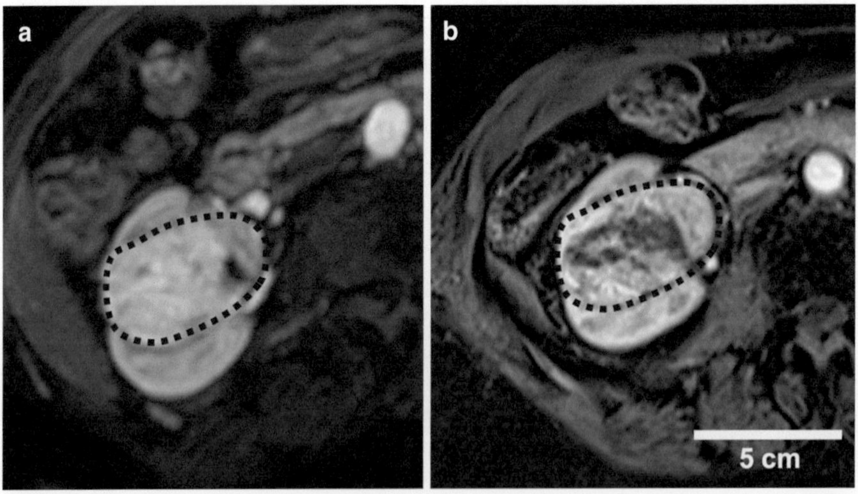

Fig. 24.5 Post-contrast fat-saturated T1W MRI of a clear cell renal carcinoma (black dashed outline) in the right kidney, imaged: (**a**) before treatment with SABR. (**b**) Eight months after treatment. The tumour is unchanged in volume and still demonstrates avid peripheral contrast agent-mediated enhancement, although there is an increased central zone of necrosis

reproducibility and single-site repeatability have been reported for brain and renal imaging [35, 36].

24.3 Clinical Studies with Hyperpolarized ^{13}C- and ^{2}H-Labelled Substrates

24.3.1 Imaging with Hyperpolarized [1-^{13}C]Pyruvate

In 2013, just 10 years after the publication of the dissolution DNP method, hyperpolarized [1-^{13}C]pyruvate became the first hyperpolarized substrate to be trialled in humans [14] and has continued to be the most intensively investigated.

24.3.1.1 Tumour Detection and Grading

Higher metabolic rates and increased aerobic lactate production are features associated with multiple types of high-grade tumours. Serum lactate and LDH often correlate with high-grade tumours arising in multiple different tissues, but are limited by their lack of specificity. Therefore, imaging and quantifying this shift to aerobic glycolysis has been proposed as a method of grading tumours. There is yet to be a clinically validated method of grading tumours using imaging. In prostate cancer, ADC has a moderate correlation with Gleason grading, but the difference between grades, particularly the indolent Gleason 3+3 lesions and the clinically significant Gleason 3+4 lesions, is small, reducing the specificity for detecting clinically significant disease to <50%. More advanced modelling of diffusion-weighted imaging may be able to improve this and reduce the number of biopsies that are needed, but there is still significant scope for improvement, particularly as biopsy-derived Gleason score is prone to error, often correlating poorly with the Gleason score of the surgically resected tumour.

Several studies in prostate cancer patients have demonstrated increased lactate signals in tumour regions compared to healthy tissue [37, 38], while a study of 12 patients found a trend towards increased lactate signal in higher grades of tumour (Figs. 24.6 and 24.7). Furthermore, in a single patient, an occult site of disease was detected with an elevated lactate/pyruvate ratio that was not visible on standard-of-care MRI [14].

As in prostate cancer, a significant proportion of primary renal cancers (RCC) have little to no metastatic potential. For tumours less than 4 cm in diameter, the overall metastatic rate is <5%. However, the risk of metastasis increases with grade to approximately 30% for those with sarcomatoid change [39]. Unlike prostate cancer, an additional complexity is that there are multiple primary renal tumour subtypes, both benign and malignant, which have variable histological patterns. On standard-of-care imaging (MRI or CT), there is substantial overlap in appearance between these different types and grades.

The most common and aggressive renal tumour subtype, clear cell renal cell carcinoma (RCC), has a loss of function of the von-Hippel-Lindau tumour suppressor gene in approximately 90% of patients. Loss of VHL leads to stabilization of

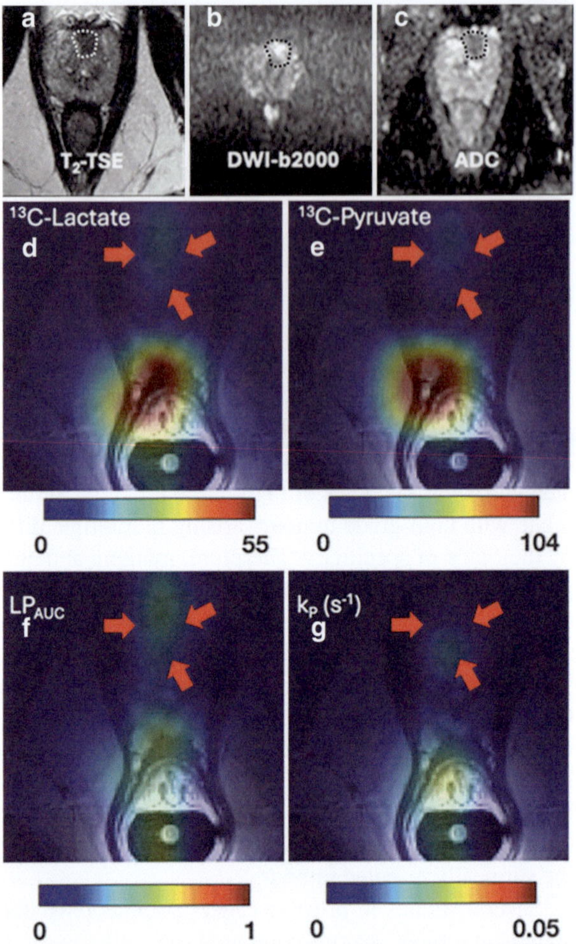

Fig. 24.6 Prostate MRI with Gleason 3+4 tumour in the anterior transitional zone (outline and red arrows). (**a**) T_2-weighted image; (**b**) diffusion-weighted image; (**c**) apparent diffusion coefficient image; (**d**) [1-^{13}C]lactate image; (**e**) [1-^{13}C]pyruvate image; (**f**) lactate/pyruvate area under the curve (AUC) ratio map and (**g**) k_{PL} rate constant map (first-order rate constant describing flux of hyperpolarized ^{13}C label between pyruvate and lactate). (Images courtesy of Professor Shonit Punwani, University College London)

hypoxia-inducible factors (particularly HIF1α), one of the effects of which is to upregulate glycolysis. With a combined total of twenty patients, two studies [36, 40] have separately demonstrated a trend towards increasing lactate signal in higher grades of clear cell RCC and variable signal across different tumour types (Fig. 24.7).

24.3.1.2 Imaging Tumour Treatment Response

Extensive pre-clinical literature has demonstrated that a change in lactate-pyruvate exchange, usually a reduction in exchange rate, is a sensitive method for detecting a response to chemotherapy, which can precede a detectable decrease in tumour volume. Moreover, there are preclinical examples where hyperpolarized [1-^{13}C]pyruvate can detect a response but not [^{18}F]FDG-PET [22]. Initial case series and reports in patients have produced promising results. In seven breast cancer patients treated with chemotherapy (including a PARP inhibitor), a change in the lactate/pyruvate ratio at 1–2 weeks after the initiation of chemotherapy was associated with a

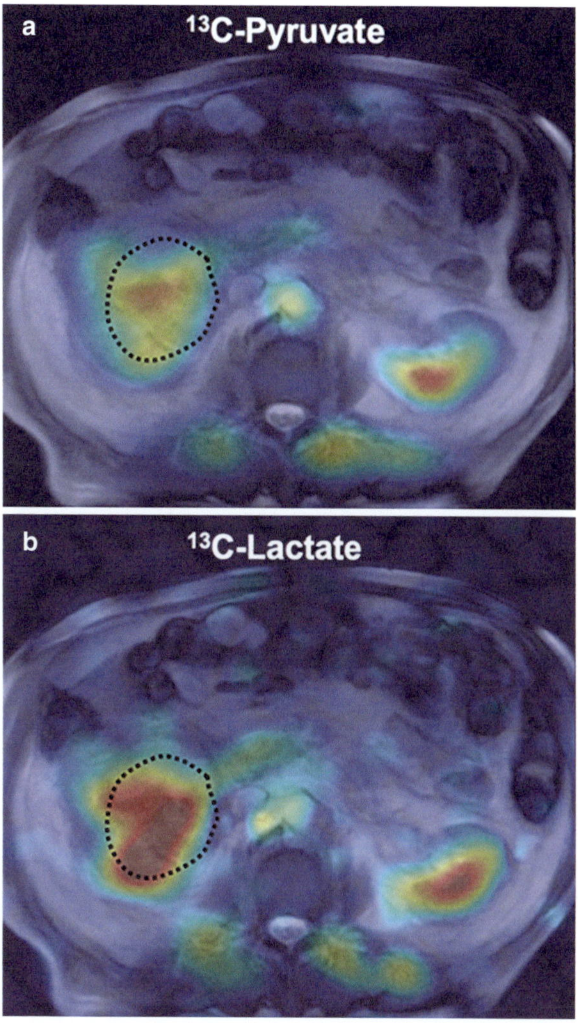

Fig. 24.7 ^{13}C MRI with hyperpolarized [1-^{13}C]pyruvate of a WHO/ISUP grade 2 clear cell RCC (dashed outline) of the right kidney, demonstrating an increased lactate/pyruvate ratio in the tumour relative to the normal contralateral kidney. (Images courtesy of Professor Shonit Punwani and Dr Rafat Chowdhury, University College London)

pathological complete response, although in this case, there was a >20% increase in the ratio as opposed to a decrease [41]. In a patient with metastatic prostate cancer imaged before and after 2 months after the start of chemotherapy, the lactate/pyruvate ratio was reduced approximately in proportion to the decrease in tumour volume and the levels of prostate-specific antigen in the circulation [42]. In a study containing four patients with pancreatic cancer who underwent hyperpolarized [1-^{13}C]pyruvate MRI at baseline and 4 weeks after starting variable chemotherapy regimens, changes in the alanine/pyruvate and lactate/pyruvate ratios were detected at 4 weeks after therapy initiation, which preceded anatomical changes [43].

These initial proof-of-principle studies, albeit limited by small cohort sizes, clearly demonstrate that post-treatment imaging with hyperpolarized [1-^{13}C]

pyruvate can detect early evidence of treatment response. To progress the field, subsequent clinical trials require careful design and should target the areas where current treatment response monitoring is most challenging.

24.3.2 [6,6′-$^2H_2$]glucose

^{2}H MRI with [6,6′-$^2H_2$]glucose shares potential applications with hyperpolarized ^{13}C-labelled pyruvate, and further human trials focussed on protocol optimization have commenced at several sites globally. With the potentially lower costs, experimental simplicity and the potential for oral contrast administration, the technique has some important advantages for translation when compared to hyperpolarized ^{13}C-labelled substrates. ^{2}H MRI with [6,6-$^2H_2$]glucose has entered into proof-of-concept human studies at several sites, with studies investigating monitoring treatment response in glioblastoma multiforme and grading and differentiation of renal cell carcinoma.

24.4 Future for Clinical Studies

Over 60 hyperpolarized substrates have been used in pre-clinical studies and shown to be sensitive to a wide range of biological processes. In addition to the applications mentioned above, in vivo imaging capable of detecting the metabolic dysregulation associated with infection and inflammation, inborn errors of metabolism, redox state, pH, perfusion and immune cell activation has provided a novel insight into tumour biology. Furthermore, a large amount of work has been performed in both pre-clinical and clinical studies to optimize substrate preparation, imaging protocols and pulse sequences and to investigate different metrics that could facilitate clinical translation of hyperpolarized ^{13}C and deuterium metabolic imaging. The next steps are to progress the studies performed from the feasibility and proof-of-principle stage towards delivery of trials designed to determine the impact of hyperpolarized and deuterium imaging on clinical decision making. It is likely that the first significant phase-II trial of hyperpolarized MRI in humans will investigate its role in the grading of tumours. This is likely to be initiated as a multi-site study in prostate cancer, specifically to investigate whether hyperpolarized [1-^{13}C]pyruvate adds value to ^{1}H MRI for differentiating clinically significant (Gleason 3+4) disease.

While challenges exist, it must be remembered that since the invention of dissolution DNP in 2003 both techniques have accelerated towards clinical translation faster than was the case for [^{18}F]FDG-PET, where there was 30 years between the invention of the cyclotron and the synthesis of [^{18}F]FDG and a further 20 years before its establishment as a clinical technique in the 1990s. If a clinical application can be demonstrated, there is little doubt that the technical challenges will be overcome, and hyperpolarized ^{13}C and deuterium metabolic imaging can become established clinical imaging techniques.

References

1. Schwartz LH et al (2016) RECIST 1.1-update and clarification: from the RECIST committee. Eur J Cancer 62:132–137. https://doi.org/10.1016/j.ejca.2016.03.081
2. Hanahan D (2022) Hallmarks of cancer: new dimensions. Cancer Discov 12:31–46. https://doi.org/10.1158/2159-8290.Cd-21-1059
3. Martínez-Reyes I, Chandel NS (2021) Cancer metabolism: looking forward. Nat Rev Cancer 21:669–680. https://doi.org/10.1038/s41568-021-00378-6
4. Brindle K (2008) New approaches for imaging tumour responses to treatment. Nat Rev Cancer 8:94–107. https://doi.org/10.1038/nrc2289
5. Rothman DL et al (1991) Localized proton NMR observation of [3-^{13}C]lactate in stroke after [1-^{13}C]glucose infusion. Magn Reson Med 21:302–307. https://doi.org/10.1002/mrm.1910210215
6. Rivenzon-Segal D, Margalit R, Degani H (2002) Glycolysis as a metabolic marker in orthotopic breast cancer, monitored by in vivo ^{13}C MRS. Am J Physiol Endocrinol Metab 283:E623–E630. https://doi.org/10.1152/ajpendo.00050.2002
7. Ardenkjær-Larsen JH et al (2003) Increase in signal-to-noise ratio of > 10,000 times in liquid-state NMR. Proc Natl Acad Sci 100:10158–10163. https://doi.org/10.1073/pnas.1733835100
8. Fala M et al (2021) Comparison of ^{13}C MRI of hyperpolarized [1-^{13}C]pyruvate and lactate with the corresponding mass spectrometry images in a murine lymphoma model. Magn Reson Med 85:3027–3035. https://doi.org/10.1002/mrm.28652
9. Adams RW et al (2009) Reversible interactions with para-hydrogen enhance NMR sensitivity by polarization transfer. Science 323:1708–1711. https://doi.org/10.1126/science.1168877
10. Reineri F, Boi T, Aime S (2015) ParaHydrogen induced polarization of ^{13}C carboxylate resonance in acetate and pyruvate. Nat Commun 6:5858. https://doi.org/10.1038/ncomms6858
11. Lu M, Zhu XH, Zhang Y, Mateescu G, Chen W (2017) Quantitative assessment of brain glucose metabolic rates using in vivo deuterium magnetic resonance spectroscopy. J Cereb Blood Flow Metab 37:3518–3530. https://doi.org/10.1177/0271678x17706444
12. De Feyter HM et al (2018) Deuterium metabolic imaging (DMI) for MRI-based 3D mapping of metabolism in vivo. Sci Adv 4:eaat7314. https://doi.org/10.1126/sciadv.aat7314
13. Kurhanewicz J et al (2019) Hyperpolarized ^{13}C MRI: path to clinical translation in oncology. Neoplasia 21:1–16. https://doi.org/10.1016/j.neo.2018.09.006
14. Nelson SJ et al (2013) Metabolic imaging of patients with prostate cancer using hyperpolarized [1-^{13}C]pyruvate. Sci Transl Med 5:198ra108. https://doi.org/10.1126/scitranslmed.3006070
15. Chen Ming Low J, Wright AJ, Hesse F, Cao J, Brindle KM (2023) Metabolic imaging with deuterium labeled substrates. Prog Nucl Magn Reson Spectrosc 134-135:39–51. https://doi.org/10.1016/j.pnmrs.2023.02.002
16. Albers MJ et al (2008) Hyperpolarized ^{13}C lactate, pyruvate, and alanine: noninvasive biomarkers for prostate cancer detection and grading. Cancer Res 68:8607–8615. https://doi.org/10.1158/0008-5472.Can-08-0749
17. Day SE et al (2007) Detecting tumor response to treatment using hyperpolarized ^{13}C magnetic resonance imaging and spectroscopy. Nat Med 13:1382–1387. https://doi.org/10.1038/nm1650
18. Low JCM et al (2024) Deuterium metabolic imaging differentiates glioblastoma metabolic subtypes and detects early response to chemoradiotherapy. Cancer Res 84:1996–2008. https://doi.org/10.1158/0008-5472.Can-23-2552
19. Hesse F et al (2022) Imaging glioblastoma response to radiotherapy using ^{2}H magnetic resonance spectroscopy measurements of fumarate metabolism. Cancer Res 82:3622–3633. https://doi.org/10.1158/0008-5472.Can-22-0101
20. Mair R et al (2018) Metabolic imaging detects low levels of glycolytic activity that vary with levels of c-Myc expression in patient-derived xenograft models of glioblastoma. Cancer Res 78:5408–5418. https://doi.org/10.1158/0008-5472.Can-18-0759
21. Kreis F et al (2020) Measuring tumor glycolytic flux in vivo by using fast deuterium MRI. Radiology 294:289–296. https://doi.org/10.1148/radiol.2019191242

22. Ros S et al (2020) Metabolic imaging detects resistance to PI3Kα inhibition mediated by persistent FOXM1 expression in ER(+) breast cancer. Cancer Cell 38:516–533.e519. https://doi.org/10.1016/j.ccell.2020.08.016
23. von Morze C et al (2011) Imaging of blood flow using hyperpolarized [^{13}C]Urea in preclinical cancer models. J Magn Reson Imaging 33:692–697. https://doi.org/10.1002/jmri.22484
24. Neves AA, Brindle KM (2014) Imaging cell death. J Nucl Med 55:1–4. https://doi.org/10.2967/jnumed.112.114264
25. Gallagher FA et al (2009) Production of hyperpolarized [1,4-$^{13}C_2$]malate from [1,4-$^{13}C_2$]fumarate is a marker of cell necrosis and treatment response in tumors. Proc Natl Acad Sci USA 106:19801–19806. https://doi.org/10.1073/pnas.0911447106
26. Hesse F et al (2021) Monitoring tumor cell death in murine tumor models using deuterium magnetic resonance spectroscopy and spectroscopic imaging. Proc Natl Acad Sci 118:e2014631118. https://doi.org/10.1073/pnas.2014631118
27. Bohndiek SE et al (2010) Detection of tumor response to a vascular disrupting agent by hyperpolarized ^{1}3C magnetic resonance spectroscopy. Mol Cancer Ther 9:3278–3288. https://doi.org/10.1158/1535-7163.Mct-10-0706
28. Gallagher FA et al (2008) Magnetic resonance imaging of pH in vivo using hyperpolarized ^{13}C-labelled bicarbonate. Nature 453:940–943. https://doi.org/10.1038/nature07017
29. Düwel S et al (2017) Imaging of pH in vivo using hyperpolarized ^{13}C-labelled zymonic acid. Nat Commun 8:15126. https://doi.org/10.1038/ncomms15126
30. Mellinghoff IK et al (2023) Vorasidenib in IDH1- or IDH2-mutant low-grade glioma. N Engl J Med 389:589–601. https://doi.org/10.1056/NEJMoa2304194
31. Hong D et al (2023) Monitoring response to a clinically relevant IDH inhibitor in glioma-Hyperpolarized ^{13}C magnetic resonance spectroscopy approaches. Neurooncol Adv 5:vdad143. https://doi.org/10.1093/noajnl/vdad143
32. Verhoeff SR et al (2019) Lesion detection by [^{89}Zr]Zr-DFO-girentuximab and [^{18}F]FDG-PET/CT in patients with newly diagnosed metastatic renal cell carcinoma. Eur J Nucl Med Mol Imaging 46:1931–1939. https://doi.org/10.1007/s00259-019-04358-9
33. Surov A, Meyer HJ, Wienke A (2020) Correlations between apparent diffusion coefficient and Gleason Score in prostate cancer: a systematic review. Eur Urol Oncol 3:489–497. https://doi.org/10.1016/j.euo.2018.12.006
34. Ulaner GA, Hyman DM, Lyashchenko SK, Lewis JS, Carrasquillo JA (2017) ^{89}Zr-Trastuzumab PET/CT for detection of human epidermal growth factor receptor 2–positive metastases in patients with human epidermal growth factor receptor 2–negative primary breast cancer. Clin Nucl Med 42:912–917. https://doi.org/10.1097/rlu.0000000000001820
35. Bøgh N et al (2022) Initial experience on hyperpolarized [1-^{13}C]Pyruvate MRI multicenter reproducibility-are multicenter trials feasible? Tomography 8:585–595. https://doi.org/10.3390/tomography8020048
36. Tang S et al (2021) Metabolic imaging with hyperpolarized ^{13}C pyruvate magnetic resonance imaging in patients with renal tumors—initial experience. Cancer 127:2693–2704. https://doi.org/10.1002/cncr.33554
37. Chowdhury R et al (2023) Quantification of prostate cancer metabolism using 3D multiecho bSSFP and hyperpolarized [1-^{13}C] pyruvate: metabolism differs between tumors of the same Gleason Grade. J Magn Reson Imaging 57:1865–1875. https://doi.org/10.1002/jmri.28467
38. Granlund KL et al (2020) Hyperpolarized MRI of human prostate cancer reveals increased lactate with tumor grade driven by Monocarboxylate Transporter 1. Cell Metab 31:105–114.e103. https://doi.org/10.1016/j.cmet.2019.08.024
39. Monda SM et al (2023) The metastatic risk of renal cell carcinoma by primary tumor size and subtype. Eur Urol Open Sci 52:137–144. https://doi.org/10.1016/j.euros.2023.04.015
40. Ursprung S et al (2022) Hyperpolarized ^{13}C-Pyruvate metabolism as a surrogate for tumor grade and poor outcome in renal cell carcinoma—a proof of principle study. Cancer 14:335
41. Woitek R et al (2021) Hyperpolarized Carbon-13 MRI for early response assessment of Neoadjuvant chemotherapy in breast cancer patients. Cancer Res 81:6004–6017. https://doi.org/10.1158/0008-5472.Can-21-1499

42. Chen H-Y et al (2020) Hyperpolarized ^{13}C-pyruvate MRI detects real-time metabolic flux in prostate cancer metastases to bone and liver: a clinical feasibility study. Prostate Cancer Prostatic Dis 23:269–276. https://doi.org/10.1038/s41391-019-0180-z
43. Gordon JW et al (2024) Hyperpolarized ^{13}C metabolic MRI of patients with pancreatic ductal adenocarcinoma. J Magn Reson Imaging 60:741–749. https://doi.org/10.1002/jmri.29162

Clinical PET/MR

25

Wolfgang Weber

The introduction of clinical PET/CT in 2000 has led to a dramatic increase in PET imaging in clinical research and patient management (Fig. 25.1). When integrated PET/MR systems entered the clinic about 10 years later, it was expected that PET/MR would have a similar impact. However, research activity as well as clinical acceptance of PET/MR have been much slower. The number of published research studies on PET/MR remains significantly lower than that on PET/CT (Fig. 25.1). MR imaging provides several advantages when compared to CT, including a lack of ionizing radiation, high soft tissue contrast, and the ability to measure physiologic parameters as well as multiparametric imaging. Therefore, there were good reasons to believe that PET/MR would improve staging accuracy, treatment monitoring, and biological characterization of the tumor tissue. Combining the molecular information of PET with MR in one examination was thus anticipated to spark clinical research and result in new clinical indications for imaging in oncologic patients.

W. Weber (✉)
School of Medicine and Health, Department of Nuclear Medicine, Technical University Munich, Munich, Germany

O. Schober et al. (eds.), *Molecular Imaging in Oncology - Volume 2*, Recent Results in Cancer Research 225, https://doi.org/10.1007/978-3-032-21415-7_7

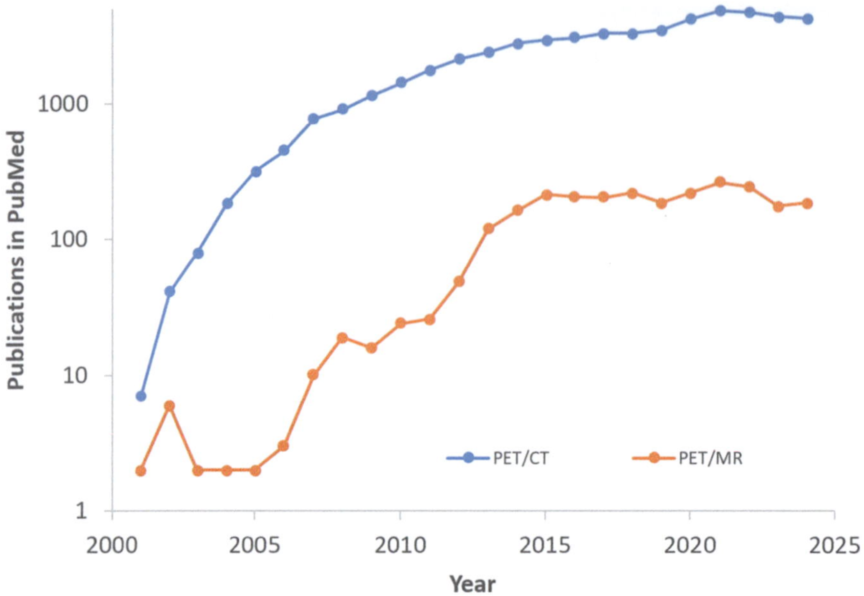

Fig. 25.1 Number of publications in the database Medline including the term PET/CT or PET/MR

25.1 Fundamental Differences Between PET/MR and PET/CT Imaging in Oncology

In retrospect, there are several reasons why oncologic research and clinical applications of PET/MR developed more slowly compared to PET/CT. First, accurate attenuation correction proved more difficult to establish than expected. Therefore, PET/MR research focused for several years on methodological aspects instead of studies of tumor biology or the development of new clinical applications [1, 2]. Accurate attenuation correction is a prerequisite for research applications of PET/MR, which require quantitative data. It is also a prerequisite for some clinical applications of PET/MR, such as treatment monitoring. Attenuation correction is particularly challenging for oncologic PET, which typically involves whole-body imaging, and attenuation correction needs to be accurate for different body regions. Furthermore, the normal anatomy is frequently distorted by previous treatments, treatment-related complications, or tumor progression. For example, air-filled lung tissue may be replaced by pleural effusions, or bone structures may be replaced by a metal implant. Therefore, atlas-based approaches that “convert” an MR image into a “synthetic” CT for attenuation correction are more difficult to implement than for brain imaging studies. While some inaccuracies compared to PET/CT remain, the problem of attenuation correction has probably been solved with reasonable accuracy for many research and clinical applications, i.e., errors due to attenuation correction are reasonably small when compared to the expected biological signals.

Second, many whole PET/MR protocols were typically lengthy because they acquired a combination of a dedicated MR of one body region with a whole-body MRI. For whole-body MRI, several MR sequences were acquired as it is standard for standalone whole-body MR (e.g., T1 VIBE Dixon, diffusion-weighted EPI, T2-weighted TIRM, T2-weighted HASTE, T1 weighted VIBE post-contrast) [3]. Each of these imaging sequences may show specific artifacts, e.g., due to patient motion. This made whole-body PET/MR not only time consuming to acquire (45–60 min per scan), but also challenging to interpret because of the enormous number of images to be reviewed. Typical scan times for PET/MR are 2–3 times longer than for a PET/CT with contrast-enhanced CT. In contrast to PET/CT—which had drastically reduced acquisition times of PET due to the fast CT-based attenuation correction—integrated PET/MR has considerably increased the duration of a PET scan. Combined with the high costs of PET/MR installation and maintenance, this has limited clinical interest in replacing PET/CT with PET/MR for whole-body staging.

However, for specific applications, imaging times have been reduced to less than 30 min for PET/MR, which will likely improve clinical acceptance [3–6]. Long acquisition times may therefore become less of an issue in the future.

Third, and probably most importantly, the introduction of PET/CT provides for the first time spatially well-matched anatomical information for findings on PET. With PET/CT, the anatomical location of abnormal findings on PET could be precisely described, and focal hypermetabolic lesions on PET could be matched with subtle abnormalities on the corresponding CT scan. Conversely, a malignant lesion can frequently be ruled out based on the lack of a corresponding finding on CT. This allowed for a much more specific interpretation of PET and has greatly increased the confidence of clinicians in PET findings. The ability to precisely correlate PET and CT findings has also led to some new scientific discoveries. For example, the existence of substantial amounts of metabolically active brown adipose tissue in adults was not known until PET/CT scans showed that linear FDG uptake in the neck was not located in cervical muscles, but in fatty tissue.

With respect to anatomic correlation and precise localization of PET findings, the introduction of PET/MR was a less significant step than the advent of PET/CT. Standalone PET provided (almost) no anatomical information, and the anatomical data provided by combining PET with CT were entirely new. Especially when performed as a combination of PET and contrast-enhanced CT, PET/CT already provided quite detailed information, which was only incrementally improved by PET/MR. Thus, PET/CT very quickly stimulated research and clinical applications, whereas the impact of PET/MR is more subtle.

Lastly, CT is the standard imaging modality for staging many of the cancers for which FDG PET has been found to be most clinically useful. These include, for example, lung cancer, melanoma, and lymphoma. Instead of performing separate CT and PET scans, it was obvious to image these tumors with an integrated PET/CT system. Subsequently, clinical studies quickly showed that integrated PET/CT is not only logistically easier to perform and read than two separate studies, but also provides increased staging accuracy due to the exact co-localization of CT and PET findings. Of course, MR is also used clinically for imaging of many malignancies, but often not as the primary staging modality, rather as a "problem-solving modality" if uncertainties remain on CT. CT remains the preferred primary imaging modality because of its robustness, speed, and higher sensitivity for the detection of lung metastases. Since whole-body imaging for staging and re-staging is by far the most common application of FDG PET in oncology, there were obvious indications for PET/CT imaging. This was less the case for PET/MR, because MR is much less commonly used for whole-body imaging than CT. For the same reason, it is not too surprising that for many cancers, PET/MR has not shown superior staging accuracy when compared to PET with contrast-enhanced CT (see the following section).

Against this backdrop, this chapter provides an overview of the use of FDG PET/MR for whole-body staging while focusing on applications where PET/MR with FDG or PSMA (prostate-specific membrane antigen) ligands is used for tumor staging.

25.2 Clinical Studies Evaluating PET/MR in Different Oncological Diseases

Spick et al. have summarized the results of studies comparing PET/CT and PET/MR imaging published until 2016 [7]. Their review includes 46 comparative studies in a total of 2340 patients. MR was mostly used for anatomical localization of abnormal findings on PET. There were 7 studies in head and neck cancer, 6 studies in lung cancer, 7 in gastrointestinal cancers and neuroendocrine, 5 in gastrointestinal and neuroendocrine tumors, 5 in gynecological cancers and breast cancer, 3 in prostate cancer, 5 in lymphoma, and 13 in mixed populations. Except for three studies in prostate cancer and two studies in neuroendocrine tumors, all studies used FDG as the imaging agent. In the following sections, the results from the analysis by Spicks et al. [7], combined with results from more recent papers, will be presented.

Spicks et al. [7] focused on the question if PET/MR is superior to PET/CT. A different way to look at the available clinical studies is to ask if PET/MR is superior to standalone MR. This perspective will also be included in the following summary of the clinical literature.

25.2.1 Head and Neck Cancers

Although FDG PET/MR has shown advantages compared to FDG PET/CT for soft criteria such as "lesion conspicuity" [8], studies have so far failed to prospectively show a statistically significant difference between PET/MR and PET/CT with respect to the detection of lymph node and distant metastases (Table 25.1). Considering that PET/MR imaging is substantially more complex and expensive than PET/CT, this can be seen as a negative result. Nevertheless, PET/MR facilitates the interpretation of images by head and neck surgeons due to the typical high

Table 25.1 Detection of lymph node metastases in newly diagnosed patients with squamous cell carcinomas of the head and neck by FDG PET/MR

				Reference	FDG PET/MR				
Authors	year	Cancer types	N	Positive LN regions/total	Sensitivity	Specificity	Comparator	Sensitivity	Specificity
Platzeck et al. [9]	2014	Floor of the mouth (10), tongue (9), mandible (7), maxilla (3), larynx (2), piriform sinus (2), other (5)	38	38/391	90%	95%	MR neck	66%	97%
Schaarschmidt et al. [10]	2016	Tonsil (3), base of tongue (3), tongue (2), CUP (2), hypopharynx (1), larynx (1)	12	NR	81%	99%	MR neck	78%	99%
Chan [11]	2018	Nasopharynx	113	NR	100%	99%	MR neck	94%	100%
Huang	2020	Hypopharynx	11	17/54	88%	98%	PET/CT	93%	94%

Results are presented for neck lymph node regions. *N* Number of patients. *NR* not reported. PET/CT was performed with IV contrast in all studies contrast between tumor and surrounding normal tissues [12]. Several studies also report that PET/MR improves the detection of tumor infiltration in neighboring structures, which is essential for planning of surgical procedures and radiotherapy [8, 10, 13–16]. With the existing data, this potential improvement of T staging is difficult to analyze statistically because patient populations are quite heterogeneous (Table 25.1), and different anatomical structures are involved depending on the exact tumor location. This aspect of tumor staging should therefore be studied systematically for different tumor locations.

25.2.2 Nonsmall Cell Lung Cancer

For the use of PET/MR in nonsmall cell lung cancer (NSCLS), Spicks et al. analyzed 6 studies including a total of 194 patients. No statistically significant differences between PET/CT and PET/MR with respect to T and N staging were observed [7]. However, PET/MR was less sensitive than PET/CT for the detection of small pulmonary metastases or second primary tumors (e.g., multifocal adenocarcinomas). This is not an unexpected finding, considering artifacts from respiratory motion on whole-body MRI that limit the detection of small pulmonary nodules as well as the limited sensitivity of current PET systems for detection of hypermetabolic pulmonary lesions with a diameter of less than 1 cm. On a patient level, however, these differences between PET/CT and PET/MRI did not affect management in a statistically significant way [7]. As CT is the primary imaging modality for NSCLS and MR is only used in selected cases with unclear findings on CT, it is unlikely that FDG PET/MR will become an alternative to FDG PET/CT in NSCLC.

25.2.3 Gastrointestinal Cancers and Neuroendocrine Tumors

Most studies on the use of PET/MR in gastrointestinal cancers are small pilot studies that lack the statistical power to reliably detect differences in sensitivity and specificity between PET/MR and PET/CT. Among the 7 studies including 201 patients reviewed by Spicks et al. [7], only one study reported a superior diagnostic accuracy of PET/MR as compared to PET/CT. However, one potential advantage of PET/MR is the high sensitivity of MRI for the detection of liver metastases. Thus, several studies have reported that PET/MR can detect small liver metastases that are not found on PET or CT [17, 18].

Conversely, however, it is not clear if PET can detect a substantial number of liver metastases that are negative on MRI. In a group of 18 patients with neuroendocrine tumors, DOTANOC PET combined with diffusion-weighted MRI of the liver had the same diagnostic accuracy for the detection of liver metastases as liver MRI with the MR contrast agent gadoxetate [19]. Lee et al. [20] compared contrast-enhanced multidetector CT, FDG PET/MR, and MR with liver-specific contrast agents in 55 patients with colorectal cancer and suspected liver metastases. The diagnostic performance of PET/MR was significantly higher than that of CT, but there was no significant difference between MR with liver-specific contrast agents and PET/MR. Eighteen patients underwent neoadjuvant chemotherapy. Residual FDG uptake after therapy was associated with a markedly worse prognosis following surgical resection. The one-year recurrence-free survival of patients with no hypermetabolic metastases after neoadjuvant therapy ($n = 6$) was 80% as compared to only 14% for patients with hypermetabolic liver lesions after therapy [20]. This suggests that PET/MR may be helpful to assess response to neoadjuvant therapy. However, this needs to be further studied in a larger series of patients.

The advantages of PET/MR over PET/CT for the detection of liver metastases are, of course, highly dependent on the MR and CT protocol used. For example, FDG PET/MR with only T1- and T2-weighted images had a similar diagnostic accuracy as FDG PET combined with contrast-enhanced CT in a study of 55 patients with suspected liver metastases from gastrointestinal cancers [21]. In this study, 120 liver lesions were analyzed, of which 79 were considered to be metastases. In contrast, 25% of the liver metastases seen on PET/MR were false negatives on FDG PET combined with low-dose CT [21]. In a similar study, Beiderwellen et al. [22] compared FDG PET/CT (with IV contrast) and liver MRI, including T1wFLASH before and after contrast, T1w dynamic VIBE, T2wHASTE, T2wTSEIn, and DWI. A total of 32 patients were included, and 113 lesions were analyzed. In this patient population, the sensitivity of PET/MR (92%) was significantly higher than that of PET/CT (68%) at similar specificities (100% vs. 97%).

In addition, the criteria for interpretation will also affect the reported sensitivity and specificity. For example, are lesions without FDG uptake above liver background considered suspicious for metastases when they meet criteria for malignancy on CT or MR? Finally, it is often not feasible to use histology as the reference standard in studies of the diagnostic accuracy of imaging tests to detect liver metastases. Lesions are often too small for biopsies, and in patients with multifocal disease, not all lesions can be validated by histology. Therefore, a combination of histology and follow-up imaging is commonly used as a reference standard. However, follow-up may be incomplete, particularly in retrospective studies; growth of metastases may be inhibited by effective therapies; the criteria for "significant growth" of metastases may differ between studies, etc. Therefore, comparisons of the diagnostic accuracy of imaging technologies for the detection of liver metastases need to be interpreted with caution. Overall, the detection of liver metastases by PET/MR needs further evaluation in prospective clinical studies with rigorous endpoints that define the diagnostic accuracy and prognostic value of PET/MR in this setting.

25.2.4 Gynecologic Malignancies

MR is commonly used for the staging of pelvic malignancies due to its high soft tissue contrast that allows better definition of tumor extension and therefore more accurate staging. In the review by Spicks et al., the results of 5 studies, including a total of 154 patients, were analyzed. In these studies, FDG PET/CT and FDG PET/

MR had been compared for the detection and staging of primary and recurrent gynecologic cancers. As seen for several other tumor types, FDG PET/MR increased interpreter confidence when compared to FDG PET/CT, but there was no statistically significant difference in staging accuracy or patient management (Tables 25.2 and 25.3). However, in recurrent gynecological cancers, a recently published study in 71 patients has indicated [24] that FDG PET/MR significantly improves the detection of recurrent tumors on the patient level, as well as staging accuracy on a lesion level (Table 25.2). A clear limitation of this and other studies (Tables 25.2 and 25.3) is the heterogeneous patient populations that are frequently a mix of several gynecologic tumor types. These tumors differ markedly in the frequency of metastases, the site of metastases, and the metabolic activity of the tumor tissue. Therefore, future prospective studies in well-defined patient populations are necessary to determine if PET/MR should be used instead of standalone MR in certain patient populations.

25.2.5 Breast Cancer

MR plays a central part in the initial diagnosis and staging of breast cancer as well as in the restaging of recurrent breast cancer. Therefore, there are multiple possible applications of FDG PET/MR in breast cancer, ranging from more accurate cancer detection in patients with suspected breast cancer to monitoring response to systemic therapy in patients with advanced disease. In their review, Spicks et al. [7] identified only two studies on the use of FDG PET/MR in breast cancer, which only described the feasibility of FDG PET/MR for staging and restaging of breast cancer patients [32, 33]. Since then, a few additional studies have investigated the potential clinical utility of FDG PET/MR in breast cancer. Botsikas et al. evaluated in a retrospective study the sensitivity of breast MR and FDG PET/MR for the detection of primary breast cancers, lymph node, and distant metastases in 58 patients who were imaged prior to surgery. FDG PET/MR did not improve the sensitivity for the detection of primary tumors or lymph node metastases [34]. The same group also compared FDG PET/MR and FDG PET/CT in patients with newly diagnosed or recurrent breast cancer. FDG PET/MR was more sensitive than FDG PET/CT for the detection of osseous metastases on a lesion basis. However, this had no effect on M staging on a per-patient basis. There was also no significant difference in the accuracy of N staging [29]. Wang et al. [35] used FDG PET/MR to monitor tumor response to neoadjuvant chemotherapy in a small group of 14 patients with newly diagnosed invasive breast cancer. FDG PET was performed before neoadjuvant therapy and after the first or second chemotherapy cycle. Standardized uptake values of the tumor tissue and total lesion glycolysis were measured on PET; choline signal to noise ratios, peak enhancement ratios from dynamic contrast enhanced MRI, and ADC coefficients were measured on MRI. A combination of PET and MR parameters, the ratio of change in SUV divided by change in ADC, showed the closest correlation with histologic response to therapy. While these findings need to be confirmed in larger patient populations, they are promising and one of the few

Table 25.2 Detection and staging of primary and recurrent malignancies of the female pelvis by PET/MR on a patient basis

				Diagnosis by reference standard		FDG PET/MR				
First author	year	Cancer types	N	yes	no	Sensitivity	Specificity	Comparator	Sensitivity	Specificity
Grueneisen [3]	2015	Ovarian (13), cervical (7), endometrial cancer (4)[a]	24	21	3	95%	NR	PET/CT	95%	NR
Beiderwellen [23]	2015	Ovarian (11), cervical (8)[a]	19	16	3	100%	NR	PET/CT	100%	NR
Kirchner [6]	2017	Ovarian (23), cervical (12), endometrial (3), vulvar (3), vaginal (1) cancer[a]	43	38	5	95%	80%	PET/CT	97%	80%
Sawicki [24]	2018	Cervical (32), ovarian (26), endometrial (7), vulvar (4), vaginal (2) cancer[a]	71	55	16	100%	94%	MRI	86%	94%
Steiner [25]	2021	Cervical cancer	33	17	16	59%	88%	MRI	71%	75%
Tsuyoshi [26]	2020	Endometrical cancer[b]	23	2	21	100%	91%	MRI/CT	50%	95%
		Endometrical cancer[c]	11	3	8	33%	67%	MRI/CT	67%	88%
Tsuyoshi [27]	2020	Ovarian cancer[b]	27	6	21	100%	100%	MRI/CT	33%	100%
		Ovarian cancer[c]	13	12	1	100%	100%	MRI/CT	25%	100%

NR not reported. *N* number of patients.
[a]Detection of recurrence
[b]N-Staging
[c]M-Staging

Table 25.3 Detection and staging of primary and recurrent breast cancer by PET/MR on a patient basis

			Diagnosis by reference standard		FDG PET/MR				
First author	year	N	yes	no	Sensitivity	Specificity	Comparator	Sensitivity	Specificity
Melsaether[a] [28]	2016	51[b]	30	32	100%	86%	PET/CT	97%	77%
		51[c]	8	43	100%	95%	PET/CT	88%	95%
Botsikas [29]	2019	80[b]	13	67	85%	97%	PET/CT	69%	100%
		80[c]	46	34	87%	68%	PET/CT	83%	76%
Bruckmann [30]	2021	154[b]	7	147	100%[d]	100%[d]	MRI	100%	100%
							CT	71%	99%
							Bone scan	27%	99%
Morawitz [31]	2022	182[c]	73	109	82%	86%	MRI	70%	95%
							CT	63%	96%

N, number of patients
[a]Detection of primary or recurrent breast cancer and metastases
[b]M-Staging
[c]N-Staging (axillary lymph nodes)
[d]Bone metastases only

examples where a true multimodal and multiparametric combination of PET and MR parameters is used to address a clinical question [35]. A summary of the diagnostic accuracy of FDG-PET/MR in comparison to other imaging modalities is shown in Table 25.3.

25.2.6 Lymphoma

FDG PET/CT is the imaging modality of choice in FDG avid lymphomas. Most of the diagnostic information is derived from the PET part of the PET/CT study, and CT imaging mostly serves to provide anatomical correlation and exclude nonmalignant causes of increased FDG uptake, such as FDG uptake by activated brown adipose tissue. It is therefore not surprising that FDG PET/MR has been found to be superior to FDG PET/MR for imaging of lymphoma patients [7].

25.2.7 Prostate Cancer

Multiparametric MR of the prostate (MP-MRI) is now a central part of the initial staging and restaging of patients with prostate cancer. MP-MRI involves T2-weighted, diffusion-weighted, and dynamic contrast-enhanced MR of the prostate. MP-MRI has been shown to improve the diagnosis of prostate cancer in a randomized controlled trial [36, 37] and is now widely adopted to evaluate patients with elevated PSA in order to decide if a prostate biopsy should be performed [38].

However, MP-MRI of the prostate is far from perfect, and the cancer detection rate of MP-MRI-guided targeted biopsy is in the range of 11–54% [38] clearly indicating that MR findings are not specific for prostate cancer. There is therefore a significant potential to improve the diagnostic accuracy of MP-MRI by PET/MR. MP-MRI has also limitations in sensitivity, especially in the transition zone. Reporting of MP-MRI has been standardized by the Prostate Imaging Reporting and Data System (PIRADS), but the reproducibility of the image interpretation is only modest even among experienced radiologists [39, 40].

Conversely, MP-MRI can improve the diagnostic accuracy of PET imaging in two ways. First, it can identify tumors that are negative for molecular markers detected by PET imaging. For example, about 10% of primary prostate cancers do not express PSMA and cannot be detected by PSMA PET/CT [41]. These are typically rather poorly differentiated tumors that can be well detected by MP-MRI. In addition, there are typical MP-MRI characteristics of benign prostatic nodules caused by prostate hyperplasia (BPH). Thus, MP-MRI can decrease the number of false-positive PET studies.

A meta-analysis by Li et al. [40] has identified 9 studies that have compared prostate MR with PET/MR [41–49]. In all these studies, a MP-MRI and a PET/MR were performed in the same patient. Two studies used F-18-fluorocholine as the radiotracer, and one used the amino acid analog F-18-FACBC as the radiotracer. The other 6 PET/MR studies were performed with the PSMA ligand

Ga-68-PSMA-11. Overall, the studies included a total of 353 patients. The studies used different reference standards and different statistical approaches to determine sensitivity and specificity (on a lesion basis or various numbers of prostate regions ranging from 2 to 30, Table 25.4). Despite this heterogeneity, PSMA PET/MR improved sensitivity in 5 of the 6 studies. Specificity was higher for PET/MR in 3 studies, identical in one, and lower in one study (Table 25.4). Choline PET/MR also demonstrated higher sensitivity than MP-MRI, albeit at lower specificity. In the one study with F-18-FACBC, the sensitivity of PET/MR was slightly higher than of MP-MRI, and the specificity was slightly lower (Table 25.4). Figures 25.2 and 25.3 give examples for PSMA PET/MR studies in patients with prostate cancer.

In the meta-analysis of all nine studies, the pooled sensitivity and specificity of PET/MR were 78% and 90%, as compared to 60% and 88% for MP-MRI. In a ROC (receiver operator characteristic curve) analysis, the area under the curve of PET/MR (0.93) was significantly larger than that of MP-MRI (0.84), indicating a higher diagnostic accuracy of PET/MR as compared to MP-MRI [40].

The potential of PSMA PET/MR is underlined by the prospective PRIMARY study, which enrolled 296 men with suspected prostate cancer [50]. Sensitivity, specificity, positive, and negative predictive value for clinically significant prostate cancer were determined for MRI, PSMA PET, and the combination of PSMA PET and MP-MRI. The combination PSMA PET and MRI was defined as negative for clinically significant prostate cancer, when there was no PSMAM positive lesion in the prostate, and the PIRAD score was less than 4. Conversely, the combination of PSMA PET and MRI was classified as positive when there was either a lesion on MRI with a PIRADS score of more than 3, or if there was PSMA positive lesion with a PIRADS score of 2 or 3. Clinically significant prostate cancer (csPCa) was defined as an International Society of Urological Pathology (ISUP) grade group > = 2 malignancy. In the total patient population, 56% had csPCa, 67% had a PIRADS 3–5 lesion, 73% were PSMA positive, and 81% were positive on the combined PSMA-PET/MRI analysis. The combination of PSMA-PET and MRI improved NPV compared with MRI alone (91% vs 72%, $p < 0.001$). Of all men studied, 19% were negative on PSMA-PET/MR and could potentially have avoided biopsy, at the risk of delayed csPCa detection in 1.7% of them [50].

The ongoing randomized PRIMARY-2 trial will prospectively test if the number of prostate biopsies can be safely reduced by the combination of PSMA-PET and multiparametric MRI [51]. In addition, there is very early evidence that biopsy may also be avoided in patient that have typical findings for csPCa on PSMA PET and MP-MRI [52]. These patients may directly undergo prostatectomy without a prostate biopsy for confirmation of malignancy. However, such a strategy still needs to be evaluated in adequately powered prospective studies.

Table 25.4 Detection of prostate cancer on PET/MRI as compared to MP-MRI

Authors	Year	N patients	Tracer	Analysis approach	Positive/total	PET/MR		MP-MRI		Reference standard
						Sensitivity	Specificity	Sensitivity	Specificity	
Eiber et al. [41]	2016	53	Ga-68-PSMA-11	6 segments	202/318	76%	97%	58%	82%	Step sections
Al-Bayati et al. [42]	2018	22	Ga-68-PSMA-11	Lesions	32/41	88%	100%	59%	67%	Biopsy
Taneja et al. [43]	2018	35	Ga-68-PSMA-11	Lesions	6/35	93%	83%	97%	67%	Biopsy
Hicks et al. [44]	2018	32	Ga-68-PSMA-11	30 regions	412/960	74%	88%	50%	90%	Step sections
Jena et al. [45]	2018	82	Ga-68-PSMA-11	Lesions	63/84	90%	86%	76%	86%	Biopsy
Park et al. [48]	2018	33	Ga-68-PSMA-11	Lobes	57/66	86%	88%	53%	100%	Step sections
Jambor et al. [45]	2018	26	F-18-FACBC	12 regions	164/313	88%	93%	77%	99%	Step sections

N Number of patients. Analysis approach: Number of analyzed regions per prostate or analysis on a lesion basis. *NA* Not available

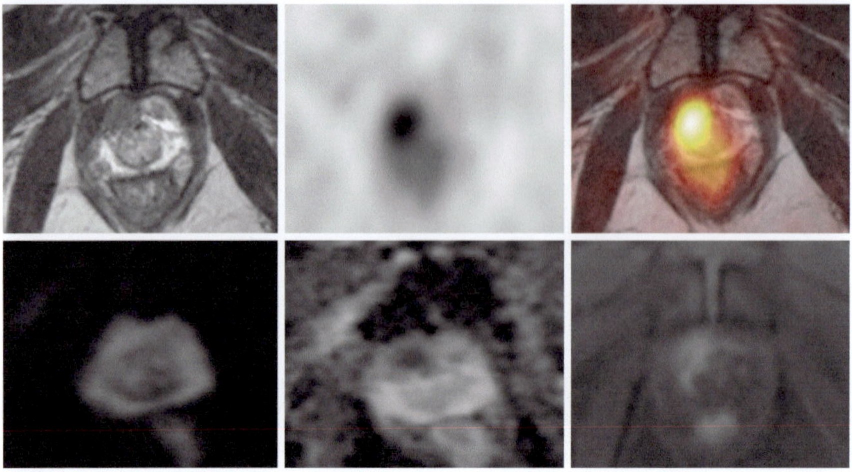

Fig. 25.2 Concordant detection of prostate cancer by MP-MRI and Ga-68-PSMA-11 PET/MR in a patient with elevated PSA (10.1 ng/mL) and a negative prostate biopsy. The MP-MRI study shows a T2 hypo-intense, contrast enhancing lesion with restricted diffusion on the ADC map (PIRADS 5). There intense tracer uptake on the corresponding PET images. Prostate cancer was confirmed on targeted biopsy (Gleason 4 + 3)

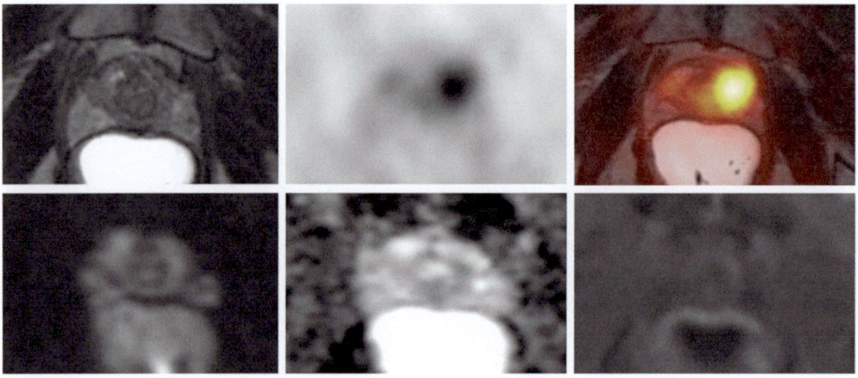

Fig. 25.3 Detection of MP-MRI occult prostate cancer by Ga-68-PSMA-11 PET/MR in a patient with elevated PSA (9.2) and a negative prostate biopsy. MP-MR images of the prostate (T2 weighted, diffusion weighted, ADC map and T1 contrast enhanced) shows no evidence of prostate cancer (PIRADS score 1). In contrast, there is intense tracer uptake in the left prostate, consistent with malignancy. Prostate cancer (Gleason 4 + 3) was confirmed by targeted biopsy

25.2.8 PET/MR in Children

The radiation exposure of the CT part of a PET/CT contributes to up to two-thirds of the total effective dose of a PET/CT scan with FDG if the CT is performed as a "diagnostic" CT [4, 53]. Using a so-called low-dose CT approach, the radiation exposure from CT can be markedly reduced, but at the cost of a significant loss of anatomical information and spatial resolution. Many institutions, therefore, acquire low-dose CTs that still result in about the same effective dose as an FDG PET/CT scan.

There is a long-standing controversy if reducing radiation exposure from CT is meaningful in adult patients [54, 55]. However, for pediatric patients, there is more or less consensus that radiation exposure from imaging studies should be as low as reasonably achievable. Acquiring high-quality anatomic images with MR instead of CT is therefore of significant interest. Furthermore, bone and soft tissue sarcomas are common tumor types in children, and MR is the imaging method of choice for staging because of its high soft-tissue contrast [56]. However, a limitation of PET/MR in younger children is the long acquisition times, which require anesthesia. Monitoring anesthesized children inside the PET/MR can be logistically challenging, because the PET/MR scans need to be coordinated with the anesthesiology department, and all equipment needs to be compatible with the magnetic field of the MR. Repeated anesthesia in early childhood, e.g., for follow-up imaging studies, may have long-term adverse effects on cognitive development [57]. Therefore, the development of optimized imaging protocols that limit scan duration will be important for the broader use of PET/MR in pediatric patients [53].

25.3 Conclusions

Whole-body FDG PET/MR is feasible in oncologic patients, but overall does not provide a substantially higher accuracy for staging than FDG PET/CT. With the substantially higher costs of PET/MR systems and the longer acquisition times, it is unlikely that FDG PET/MR will replace FDG PET/CT, except perhaps in pediatric patients. However, as PET/CT has replaced standalone CT for certain indications (e.g., treatment monitoring in lymphoma), PET/MR may replace standalone MR for some specific applications where the anatomic information from MR is fundamental for tumor detection and staging, but diagnostic accuracy can be improved by additional functional or molecular information from a PET scan. Currently developing applications in this area include imaging of head and neck cancers, gynecologic malignancies, and prostate cancer (with PSMA ligands). In these areas, truly multimodal and multiparametric imaging, i.e., imaging that fully utilizes the diagnostic capabilities of PET and MR may become feasible in the near future.

References

1. Bailey DL, Barthel H, Beyer T, Boellaard R, Guckel B, Hellwig D et al (2013) Summary report of the first international workshop on PET/MR imaging, March 19–23, 2012, Tubingen, Germany. Mol Imaging Biol 15:361–371
2. Bailey DL, Antoch G, Bartenstein P, Barthel H, Beer AJ, Bisdas S et al (2015) Combined PET/MR: the real work has just started. Summary report of the third international workshop on PET/MR imaging; February 17–21, 2014, Tubingen, Germany. Mol Imaging Biol 17:297–312

3. Grueneisen J, Schaarschmidt BM, Heubner M, Suntharalingam S, Milk I, Kinner S et al (2015) Implementation of FAST-PET/MRI for whole-body staging of female patients with recurrent pelvic malignancies: a comparison to PET/CT. Eur J Radiol 84:2097–2102
4. Grueneisen J, Sawicki LM, Schaarschmidt BM, Suntharalingam S, von der Ropp S, Wetter A et al (2016) Evaluation of a fast protocol for staging lymphoma patients with integrated PET/MRI. PLoS One 11:e0157880
5. Grueneisen J, Sawicki LM, Wetter A, Kirchner J, Kinner S, Aktas B et al (2017) Evaluation of PET and MR datasets in integrated 18F-FDG PET/MRI: a comparison of different MR sequences for whole-body restaging of breast cancer patients. Eur J Radiol 89:14–19
6. Kirchner J, Sawicki LM, Suntharalingam S, Grueneisen J, Ruhlmann V, Aktas B et al (2017) Whole-body staging of female patients with recurrent pelvic malignancies: ultra-fast 18F-FDG PET/MRI compared to 18F-FDG PET/CT and CT. PLoS One 12:e0172553
7. Spick C, Herrmann K, Czernin J (2016) 18F-FDG PET/CT and PET/MRI perform equally well in cancer: evidence from studies on more than 2,300 patients. J Nucl Med 57:420–430
8. Kuhn FP, Hullner M, Mader CE, Kastrinidis N, Huber GF, von Schulthess GK et al (2014) Contrast-enhanced PET/MR imaging versus contrast-enhanced PET/CT in head and neck cancer: how much MR information is needed? J Nucl Med 55:551–558
9. Platzek I, Beuthien-Baumann B, Schneider M, Gudziol V, Kitzler HH, Maus J et al (2014) FDG PET/MR for lymph node staging in head and neck cancer. Eur J Radiol 83:1163–1168
10. Schaarschmidt BM, Heusch P, Buchbender C, Ruhlmann M, Bergmann C, Ruhlmann V et al (2016) Locoregional tumour evaluation of squamous cell carcinoma in the head and neck area: a comparison between MRI, PET/CT and integrated PET/MRI. Eur J Nucl Med Mol Imaging 43:92–102
11. Chan SC, Yeh CH, Yen TC, Ng SH, Chang JT, Lin CY et al (2018) Clinical utility of simultaneous whole-body (18)F-FDG PET/MRI as a single-step imaging modality in the staging of primary nasopharyngeal carcinoma. Eur J Nucl Med Mol Imaging 45:1297–1308
12. Hayashi K, Kikuchi M, Imai Y, Yamashita D, Hino M, Ito K et al (2019) Clinical value of fused PET/MRI for surgical planning in patients with Oral/oropharyngeal carcinoma. Laryngoscope 130:367
13. Kubiessa K, Purz S, Gawlitza M, Kuhn A, Fuchs J, Steinhoff KG et al (2014) Initial clinical results of simultaneous 18F-FDG PET/MRI in comparison to 18F-FDG PET/CT in patients with head and neck cancer. Eur J Nucl Med Mol Imaging 41:639–648
14. Platzek I (2016) (18)F-Fluorodeoxyglucose PET/MR imaging in head and neck cancer. PET Clin 11:375–386
15. Sekine T, de Galiza Barbosa F, Kuhn FP, Burger IA, Stolzmann P, Huber GF et al (2017) PET+MR versus PET/CT in the initial staging of head and neck cancer, using a trimodality PET/CT+MR system. Clin Imaging 42:232–239
16. Szyszko TA, Cook GJR (2018) PET/CT and PET/MRI in head and neck malignancy. Clin Radiol 73:60–69
17. Hope TA, Pampaloni MH, Nakakura E, VanBrocklin H, Slater J, Jivan S et al (2015) Simultaneous (68)Ga-DOTA-TOC PET/MRI with gadoxetate disodium in patients with neuroendocrine tumor. Abdom Imaging 40:1432–1440
18. Kirchner J, Sawicki LM, Deuschl C, Gruneisen J, Beiderwellen K, Lauenstein TC et al (2017) 18 F-FDG PET/MR imaging in patients with suspected liver lesions: value of liver-specific contrast agent Gadobenate dimeglumine. PLoS One 12:e0180349
19. Mayerhoefer ME, Ba-Ssalamah A, Weber M, Mitterhauser M, Eidherr H, Wadsak W et al (2013) Gadoxetate-enhanced versus diffusion-weighted MRI for fused Ga-68-DOTANOC PET/MRI in patients with neuroendocrine tumours of the upper abdomen. Eur Radiol 23:1978–1985
20. Lee DH, Lee JM, Hur BY, Joo I, Yi NJ, Suh KS et al (2016) Colorectal cancer liver metastases: diagnostic performance and prognostic value of PET/MR imaging. Radiology 280:782–792

21. Reiner CS, Stolzmann P, Husmann L, Burger IA, Hullner MW, Schaefer NG et al (2014) Protocol requirements and diagnostic value of PET/MR imaging for liver metastasis detection. Eur J Nucl Med Mol Imaging 41:649–658
22. Beiderwellen K, Geraldo L, Ruhlmann V, Heusch P, Gomez B, Nensa F et al (2015) Accuracy of [18F]FDG PET/MRI for the detection of liver metastases. PLoS One 10:e0137285
23. Beiderwellen K, Grueneisen J, Ruhlmann V, Buderath P, Aktas B, Heusch P et al (2015) [(18) F]FDG PET/MRI vs. PET/CT for whole-body staging in patients with recurrent malignancies of the female pelvis: initial results. Eur J Nucl Med Mol Imaging 42:56–65
24. Sawicki LM, Kirchner J, Grueneisen J, Ruhlmann V, Aktas B, Schaarschmidt BM et al (2018) Comparison of (18)F-FDG PET/MRI and MRI alone for whole-body staging and potential impact on therapeutic management of women with suspected recurrent pelvic cancer: a follow-up study. Eur J Nucl Med Mol Imaging 45:622–629
25. Steiner A, Narva S, Rinta-Kiikka I, Hietanen S, Hynninen J, Virtanen J (2021) Diagnostic efficiency of whole-body (18)F-FDG PET/MRI, MRI alone, and SUV and ADC values in staging of primary uterine cervical cancer. Cancer Imaging 21:16
26. Tsuyoshi H, Tsujikawa T, Yamada S, Okazawa H, Yoshida Y (2020) Diagnostic value of (18)F-FDG PET/MRI for staging in patients with endometrial cancer. Cancer Imaging 20:75
27. Tsuyoshi H, Tsujikawa T, Yamada S, Okazawa H, Yoshida Y (2020) Diagnostic value of [(18) F]FDG PET/MRI for staging in patients with ovarian cancer. EJNMMI Res 10:117
28. Melsaether AN, Raad RA, Pujara AC, Ponzo FD, Pysarenko KM, Jhaveri K et al (2016) Comparison of whole-body (18)F FDG PET/MR imaging and whole-body (18)F FDG PET/CT in terms of lesion detection and radiation dose in patients with breast cancer. Radiology 281:193–202
29. Botsikas D, Bagetakos I, Picarra M, Da Cunha Afonso Barisits AC, Boudabbous S, Montet X et al (2019) What is the diagnostic performance of 18-FDG-PET/MR compared to PET/CT for the N- and M- staging of breast cancer? Eur Radiol 29:1787–1798
30. Bruckmann NM, Kirchner J, Umutlu L, Fendler WP, Seifert R, Herrmann K et al (2021) Prospective comparison of the diagnostic accuracy of 18F-FDG PET/MRI, MRI, CT, and bone scintigraphy for the detection of bone metastases in the initial staging of primary breast cancer patients. Eur Radiol 31:8714–8724
31. Morawitz J, Bruckmann NM, Dietzel F, Ullrich T, Bittner AK, Hoffmann O et al (2022) Comparison of nodal staging between CT, MRI, and [(18)F]-FDG PET/MRI in patients with newly diagnosed breast cancer. Eur J Nucl Med Mol Imaging 49:992–1001
32. Grueneisen J, Nagarajah J, Buchbender C, Hoffmann O, Schaarschmidt BM, Poeppel T et al (2015) Positron emission tomography/magnetic resonance imaging for local tumor staging in patients with primary breast cancer: a comparison with positron emission tomography/computed tomography and magnetic resonance imaging. Investig Radiol 50:505–513
33. Pace L, Nicolai E, Luongo A, Aiello M, Catalano OA, Soricelli A et al (2014) Comparison of whole-body PET/CT and PET/MRI in breast cancer patients: lesion detection and quantitation of 18F-deoxyglucose uptake in lesions and in normal organ tissues. Eur J Radiol 83:289–296
34. Botsikas D, Kalovidouri A, Becker M, Copercini M, Djema DA, Bodmer A et al (2016) Clinical utility of 18F-FDG-PET/MR for preoperative breast cancer staging. Eur Radiol 26:2297–2307
35. Wang J, Shih TT, Yen RF (2017) Multiparametric evaluation of treatment response to neoadjuvant chemotherapy in breast cancer using integrated PET/MR. Clin Nucl Med 42:506–513
36. Kasivisvanathan V, Rannikko AS, Borghi M, Panebianco V, Mynderse LA, Vaarala MH et al (2018) MRI-targeted or standard biopsy for prostate-cancer diagnosis. N Engl J Med 378:1767–1777
37. Ahmed HU, El-Shater Bosaily A, Brown LC, Gabe R, Kaplan R, Parmar MK et al (2017) Diagnostic accuracy of multi-parametric MRI and TRUS biopsy in prostate cancer (PROMIS): a paired validating confirmatory study. Lancet 389:815–822

38. Lindenberg ML, Turkbey B, Mena E, Choyke PL (2017) Imaging locally advanced, recurrent, and metastatic prostate cancer: a review. JAMA Oncol 3:1415–1422
39. Rosenkrantz AB, Ginocchio LA, Cornfeld D, Froemming AT, Gupta RT, Turkbey B et al (2016) Interobserver reproducibility of the PI-RADS version 2 lexicon: a multicenter study of six experienced prostate radiologists. Radiology 280:793–804
40. Li M, Huang Z, Yu H, Wang Y, Zhang Y, Song B (2019) Comparison of PET/MRI with multiparametric MRI in diagnosis of primary prostate cancer: a meta-analysis. Eur J Radiol 113:225–231
41. Eiber M, Weirich G, Holzapfel K, Souvatzoglou M, Haller B, Rauscher I et al (2016) Simultaneous (68)Ga-PSMA HBED-CC PET/MRI improves the localization of primary prostate cancer. Eur Urol 70:829–836
42. Al-Bayati M, Grueneisen J, Lutje S, Sawicki LM, Suntharalingam S, Tschirdewahn S et al (2018) Integrated 68Gallium labelled prostate-specific membrane Antigen-11 positron emission tomography/magnetic resonance imaging enhances discriminatory power of multi-parametric prostate magnetic resonance imaging. Urol Int 100:164–171
43. Taneja S, Jena A, Taneja R, Singh A, Ahuja A (2018) Effect of combined (68) Ga-PSMAHBED-CC uptake pattern and multiparametric MRI derived with simultaneous PET/MRI in the diagnosis of primary prostate cancer: initial experience. AJR Am J Roentgenol 210:1338–1345
44. Hicks RM, Simko JP, Westphalen AC, Nguyen HG, Greene KL, Zhang L et al (2018) Diagnostic accuracy of (68)Ga-PSMA-11 PET/MRI compared with multiparametric MRI in the detection of prostate cancer. Radiology 289:730–737
45. Jambor I, Kuisma A, Kahkonen E, Kemppainen J, Merisaari H, Eskola O et al (2018) Prospective evaluation of (18)F-FACBC PET/CT and PET/MRI versus multiparametric MRI in intermediate- to high-risk prostate cancer patients (FLUCIPRO trial). Eur J Nucl Med Mol Imaging 45:355–364
46. Jena A, Taneja R, Taneja S, Singh A, Kumar V, Agarwal A et al (2018) Improving diagnosis of primary prostate cancer with combined (68)Ga-prostate-specific membrane antigen-HBED-CC simultaneous PET and multiparametric MRI and clinical parameters. AJR Am J Roentgenol 211:1246–1253
47. Lee MS, Cho JY, Kim SY, Cheon GJ, Moon MH, Oh S et al (2017) Diagnostic value of integrated PET/MRI for detection and localization of prostate cancer: comparative study of multiparametric MRI and PET/CT. J Magn Reson Imaging 45:597–609
48. Park SY, Zacharias C, Harrison C, Fan RE, Kunder C, Hatami N et al (2018) Gallium 68 PSMA-11 PET/MR imaging in patients with intermediate- or high-risk prostate cancer. Radiology 288:495–505
49. de Perrot T, Rager O, Scheffler M, Lord M, Pusztaszeri M, Iselin C et al (2014) Potential of hybrid (1)(8)F-fluorocholine PET/MRI for prostate cancer imaging. Eur J Nucl Med Mol Imaging 41:1744–1755
50. Emmett L, Buteau J, Papa N, Moon D, Thompson J, Roberts MJ et al (2021) The additive diagnostic value of prostate-specific membrane antigen positron emission tomography computed tomography to multiparametric magnetic resonance imaging triage in the diagnosis of prostate cancer (PRIMARY): a prospective multicentre study. Eur Urol 80:682–689
51. Buteau JP, Moon D, Fahey MT, Roberts MJ, Thompson J, Murphy DG et al (2024) Clinical trial protocol for PRIMARY2: a multicentre, phase 3, randomised controlled trial investigating the additive diagnostic value of [(68)Ga]Ga-PSMA-11 positron emission tomography/computed tomography in men with negative or equivocal multiparametric magnetic resonance imaging for the diagnosis of clinically significant prostate cancer. Eur Urol Oncol 7:544–552
52. Meissner VH, Rauscher I, Schwamborn K, Neumann J, Miller G, Weber W et al (2022) Radical prostatectomy without prior biopsy following multiparametric magnetic resonance imaging and prostate-specific membrane antigen positron emission tomography. Eur Urol 82:156–160

53. Muehe AM, Theruvath AJ, Lai L, Aghighi M, Quon A, Holdsworth SJ et al (2018) How to provide gadolinium-free PET/MR cancer staging of children and young adults in less than 1 h: the Stanford approach. Mol Imaging Biol 20:324–335
54. Siegel JA, Pennington CW, Sacks B (2017) Subjecting radiologic imaging to the linear no-threshold hypothesis: a non sequitur of non-trivial proportion. J Nucl Med 58:1–6
55. Weber W, Zanzonico P (2017) The controversial linear no-threshold model. J Nucl Med 58:7–8
56. Kwatra NS, Lim R, Gee MS, States LJ, Vossough A, Lee EY (2019) PET/MR Imaging:: current updates on pediatric applications. Magn Reson Imaging Clin N Am 27:387–407
57. Schneuer FJ, Bentley JP, Davidson AJ, Holland AJ, Badawi N, Martin AJ et al (2018) The impact of general anesthesia on child development and school performance: a population-based study. Paediatr Anaesth 28:528–536

Clinical Applications of Advanced Ultrasound Imaging

26

Martin Krix and Anne Rix

Abbreviations

CEUS	Contrast-enhanced ultrasound
FNH	Focal nodular hyperplasia
HCC	Hepatocellular carcinoma
KDR	Kinase insert domain receptor
MTM	Macrotrabecular-massive subtype
mULM	Motion model ultrasound localization microscopy
MVI	Microvascular invasion
RCC	Renal cell carcinoma
VEGFR2	Vascular endothelial growth factor receptor-2
VETC	Vessels encapsulating tumor clusters
WFUMB	World Federation for Ultrasound in Medicine and Biology

M. Krix (✉)
University of Heidelberg, Heidelberg, Germany
e-mail: martin.krix@bracco.com

A. Rix
Institute of Experimental Molecular Imaging, RWTH Aachen University Hospital, Aachen, Germany
e-mail: arix@ukaachen.de

O. Schober et al. (eds.), *Molecular Imaging in Oncology - Volume 2*, Recent Results in Cancer Research 225, https://doi.org/10.1007/978-3-032-21415-7_8

26.1 Introduction

Ultrasound is a noninvasive imaging modality that provides anatomical and functional information of various human body areas. It is one of the most widely used imaging modalities worldwide, with frequent use in oncology [1, 2]. Novel ultrasound techniques, such as elastography and contrast-enhanced ultrasound, have evolved and have led to new clinical applications beyond conventional anatomical imaging with conventional ultrasound or blood flow assessment using Doppler ultrasound. Contrast-enhanced ultrasound (CEUS) uses microbubbles as a contrast medium. Such microbubbles can also be applied in different alternative ways, e.g., as a molecular tracer when microbubbles are targeted, as a carrier for targeted therapy, to enhance focused ultrasound therapy, or as a blood–brain barrier opener. Specific contrast-enhanced ultrasound techniques have been developed, making CEUS an extremely sensitive imaging modality. Classic microbubbles remain strictly intravascular due to their size and can be detected down to the capillary level. Together with the most recent techniques (super-resolution imaging), bubbles even allow for an extremely high spatial resolution ultrasound imaging beyond the wavelength barrier.

The ultrasound technologies related to molecular imaging and its probes are described in Part I (Chaps. 5 and 10, in Vol. I). In Part II (Chap. 17, in Vol. I) the results of preclinical studies with molecular ultrasound imaging are presented. This chapter provides an overview of current applications in humans. Since specific microbubbles are not yet available as commercial products and their wide clinical use is still limited. Results of first experiences with molecular ultrasound imaging in humans are presented. Furthermore, to give an overview in a broader sense—not only of molecular ultrasound imaging but also of contrast-enhanced ultrasound for molecular or specific diagnosis—also related studies with nonspecific, commercial ultrasound contrast agents are briefly described within the field of molecular diagnosis and the monitoring of targeted therapies in oncology. Furthermore, first experiences in humans with super-resolution ultrasound imaging as a potential breakthrough technique are presented.

26.2 CEUS in Molecular Diagnosis

Ultrasound contrast agents such as SonoVue® (Lumason® in the US) (Bracco Imaging Spa, Milan, Italy), Definity® (Luminity® in Europe) (Lantheus Medical Imaging, Billerica, USA), Optison® (GE Healthcare, Marlborough, USA), and Sonazoid® (GE Healthcare) are approved in several countries. Its range of approved indications, however, is relatively narrow. SonoVue® has the broadest indications, covering also the use of CEUS in oncology for the characterization of liver or breast lesions. Several off-label applications of ultrasound contrast agents have also been reported. These approved microbubbles based ultrasound contrast agents are nonspecific blood pool agents consisting of a shell based on phospholipids or albumin (Optison®) with an encapsulated inert gas (halogenated hydrocarbons). Sonazoid®

has a liver-specific late imaging phase since its microbubbles are strongly taken up by macrophages, including Kupffer cells [3].

26.2.1 Liver

CEUS in oncology is most commonly used for the diagnosis of liver lesions, in particular for the characterization or detection of metastases or hepatocellular carcinoma (HCC). A specific diagnosis of liver lesions relies on the identification of specific vascular features of liver lesions (e.g., a cottonwool-like peripheral globular enhancement of hemangioma, or a wheel-spoke arterial enhancement of focal nodular hyperplasias (FNHs)). Furthermore, malignant liver lesions typically show a fast washout phenomenon compared to the surrounding liver tissue at the late phase (starting at about 1 min after contrast injection) [4]. CEUS uses an intravasal contrast agent (blood pool agent) and can sensitively detect the microbubbles within the microvasculature. Therefore, it is highly suitable for the characterization of liver lesions with a diagnostic performance similar to MRI and similar or even better than CT [5, 6].

Attempts have been made to further characterize liver lesions down to their histopathological subtype using CEUS, in particular for HCCs. For this purpose, quantitative CEUS (see Chap. 5, in Vol. I) provides several parameters of tumor vascularity that are complementary to morphologic features. Microvascular invasion (MVI) of HCC is a relevant risk factor of HCC, and noninvasive imaging modalities are needed to predict this aggressive feature. CEUS, together with clinical parameters, can provide potential biomarkers for this risk assessment [7]. As for other imaging applications, the implementation of artificial intelligence may further improve models in predicting MVI of HCCs [8].

A more detailed HCC subtype analysis has been tried as well; CEUS patterns together with clinical parameters may characterize vessels encapsulating tumor clusters (VETC) HCCs or macrotrabecular-massive subtype (MTM) HCCs. MTM and VETC patterns may be associated with a poor prognosis, and CEUS may predict the prognosis preoperatively [9, 10].

26.2.2 Others

CEUS can be applied everywhere where conventional ultrasound is used, and several guidelines support applications of CEUS outside the liver for oncologic imaging, although currently not necessarily in common use [11]. Nonliver tumors do not always present lesion-specific vascular or other features, thus not always allowing for an imaging-based specific lesion type diagnosis as feasible for liver lesions. However, the principles of CEUS and quantitative CEUS remain applicable also outside the liver, and vascular features or quantitative parameters identified by CEUS have been used to further characterize molecular tumor subtypes.

Another potential, relevant application of CEUS in oncology, and in the label for SonoVue®, is the characterization of breast lesions. Conventional ultrasound radiomics together with clinical parameters have been investigated to noninvasively predict subtypes such as HER-2 low expression breast cancer or to differentiate the luminal from the nonluminal type [12]. Adding CEUS features [13] or using a multimodality approach (plus elastography) may further improve the ultrasound-based noninvasive molecular diagnosis of breast cancer [14].

For example, CEUS is an accurate approach for the characterization of cystic renal lesions [11] and has been used to further sub-characterize solid renal lesions as well, for instance to differentiate clear cell renal cell carcinoma (RCC), papillary renal cell carcinoma, and chromophobe renal cell carcinoma [15], or to differentiate Xp11.2 translocation renal cell carcinoma (RCC) from other RCC subtypes [16].

Thus, CEUS using nonselective microbubbles is established for the characterization of tumorous lesions, in particular of the liver. Several studies in humans have investigated whether CEUS (semi)-quantitative parameters or qualitative vascular patterns, together with other biomarkers, are able to further characterize and noninvasively diagnose molecular cancer subtypes, with promising results for HCC, breast cancer, or RCC. However, confirmatory or larger multicenter studies are lacking. In particular, it is not clear which concrete CEUS parameters or patterns are best suited for molecular diagnosis, and whether these may vary depending on the specific tumor entity and patient condition. Thus, as for other imaging modalities, the potential accuracy and benefit of CEUS for noninvasive lesion subtype diagnosis, its prognostic value, and the impact on individual patient management need to be further investigated.

26.2.3 CEUS in Monitoring of Targeted Therapy

Assessing tumor response to anticancer therapies is one of the main applications of imaging modalities. Traditional chemotherapy eliminates cancer cells and reduces the size of a tumor. Tumor size is a classic parameter used, e.g., by the World Health Organization (WHO) response criteria and the Response Evaluation Criteria in Solid Tumours (RECIST) to assess treatment response in solid tumors [17]. However, conventional assessment may not be sufficient for novel systemic targeted oncological therapies, such as anti-angiogenic therapies and immunotherapies, or even future molecular-specific treatment, as they may affect tumor viability and vascularity without immediately reducing the size. Contrast-enhanced imaging modalities such as CEUS are particularly suitable for monitoring such therapies, as they evaluate the viability of a tumor by measuring tumor perfusion and vascular environment.

The role of CEUS in monitoring early responses and in predicting responses to modern systemic targeted oncological therapy is supported by several studies in patients with liver metastasis of colorectal cancer [18–20] and other solid tumors [21] treated with targeted anti-angiogenic therapy. In these studies, CEUS enhancement parameters, either before treatment or during treatment, correlated with tumor response and other clinical outcomes. The guidelines of the World Federation for Ultrasound in Medicine and Biology (WFUMB) note that dynamic CEUS can be used in the quantitative assessment of response to targeted therapies in patients with malignant tumors of the liver [22]. As for CEUS in molecular diagnosis, however, confirmatory studies are lacking, and it is unclear which CEUS parameters may be best suited for an accurate monitoring of targeted therapy. Also, the robustness of a chosen CEUS parameter in clinical use may need to be considered. An example of a relatively robust parameter is the integral area under the curve (AUC) of the time-intensity curve delivered by dynamic CEUS [22]. Further studies are needed to investigate if CEUS allows accurate therapy monitoring of targeted therapies and for guiding clinical decision-making, e.g., for the early identification of patients who are unlikely to respond and may benefit from alternative treatments, thereby avoiding unnecessary costly therapy.

26.3 Molecular Imaging with Ultrasound

The actual molecular imaging in ultrasound uses modified ultrasound contrast agents to actively target disease-associated molecular markers. Such microbubbles are equipped with site-specific ligands. In the preclinical part (Chap. 17, in Vol. I) specific microbubbles are described which have been developed and studied in non-humans so far. None of them are yet clinically approved; however, some first experiences in humans and early clinical trials exist, which are presented in the following.

Microbubbles, which target the vascular endothelial growth factor receptor-2 (VEGFR2) (BR55, Bracco Research SA, Geneva, Switzerland), are in the most advanced development stage. Molecular markers related to neo-angiogenesis are considered particularly relevant for Molecular Imaging Diagnostics, as angiogenesis is involved in several major diseases (cardiovascular, inflammatory diseases), including tumor angiogenesis in oncology. Furthermore, in oncology, there is a concrete medical need for better patient management to early monitor the response of tumors to novel targeted systemic chemotherapies. As some of them are directly targeting neo-angiogenesis (e.g., Bevacizumab), specific ultrasound contrast agents related to angiogenesis would be particularly useful and may early identify changes in tumors or their environment caused by these therapies, beyond the assessment of tumor viability or just of tumor size.

A first report on the use in humans of the specific VEGFR2 (or kinase insert domain receptor, KDR) ultrasound molecular contrast agent BR55 was published already in 2014 [23]. BR55 was tested in prostate cancer patients, and these preliminary results demonstrated the capacity of this targeted agent to reach detectable level of binding to VEGFR2 in patients. First smaller clinical studies with BR55 in oncological patients have then been published in 2017 [24, 25]. In both studies the injection of the molecular contrast agent was considered safe.

Willmann performed a first-in-human clinical trial on ultrasound molecular imaging in patients with breast and ovarian lesions using BR55. Twenty-four women (age 48–79 years) with focal ovarian lesions and 21 women (age 34–66 years) with focal breast lesions were examined and underwent surgical resection of the tumors afterwards. KDR expression on immunohistochemistry matched well with imaging signal on molecular ultrasound imaging in 93% of breast and 85% of ovarian malignant lesions (Fig. 26.1). Strong KDR-targeted signal with BR55 was present in 77% of malignant ovarian lesions, with no targeted signal seen in 78% of benign ovarian lesions. Similarly, strong targeted signal was seen in 93% of malignant breast lesions with no targeted signal present in 67% of benign breast lesions.

Smeenge et al. described the feasibility and safety of BR55 for the detection of prostate cancer. In 24 patients with biopsy-proven prostate cancer scheduled for radical prostatectomy, BR55-CEUS was performed using clinical standard technology. In patients who were scanned with an improved dosing protocol, a total of 28 malignant lesions were determined. Nineteen (68%) of them were seen during BR55 ultrasound molecular imaging, whereas 9 (32%) were not identified.

Since then, the clinical development is ongoing, although no further peer-reviewed publications of major clinical studies with molecular ultrasound contrast agents have been published so far. In the National Library of Medicine (clinicaltrials.gov), four further clinical development studies have been reported. The first one was another pilot trial using the BR55 ultrasound contrast agent in the assessment of prostate cancer. Primary objectives were to obtain safety data and to assess the ability of BR55 at a dose of 0.03 mL/kg to identify prostate cancer lesions with a Gleason score ≥7 using histopathology as the truth standard. Eighteen patients were dosed, and 13 of them could be analyzed. Of 17 lesions with a Gleason score > = 7,

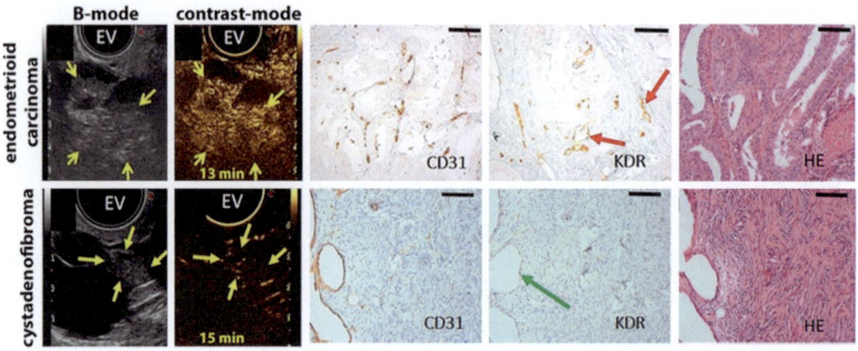

Fig. 26.1 Assessment of KDR expression in focal ovarian lesions of patients. Upper panel: Endometrioid carcinoma in a 50-year-old woman: the transverse endovaginal (EV) B-mode ultrasound image of the right ovary shows a 5.2 cm large mixed cystic and solid lesion (yellow arrows = solid lesion) that shows a strong imaging signal 13 min after intravenous injection of BR55. Kinase insert domain receptor (KDR)-expression on the tumor-associated neovasculature (CD31-positive, red arrows) was confirmed by immunohistology. Lower panel: Benign serous cystadenofibroma in a 65-year-old woman: the transverse endovaginal B-mode ultrasound image of the right ovary presents a 4.8 cm large, mixed cystic and solid ovarian mass (yellow arrows = solid lesion) with only minimal background signal after injection of BR55. Immunohistochemistry shows minimal KDR-expression (green arrow) on CD31-positive vasculature. Scalebar immunohistochemistry images: 100 mm. (Reproduced with permission from Willmann et al. [24] ©Wolters Kluwer Health, Inc.)

8 showed binding with the VEGFR2-specific microbubbles. In two other studies, BR55 was used in the diagnosis of ovarian cancer. One was an exploratory phase II, single-center, open-label, prospective study of BR55 CEUS for the characterization of ovarian lesions in subjects with suspected ovarian cancer. The second was an exploratory, single-center, open-label, prospective study of BR55 to determine the optimal phase of the menstrual cycle for performing BR55 CEUS of the target ovary in premenopausal women scheduled to undergo preventative surgery because of high familial/hereditary or genetic risk for ovarian cancer. Both studies were terminated due to recruitment issues caused by a tragic event of the principal investigator. In the first studies, 14 patients were examined, and only three training cases were performed in the second study. The fourth study was an exploratory, single-center, open-label, parallel-dose, and prospective study of BR55 CEUS for the characterization of solid pancreatic lesions in subjects with suspected pancreatic ductal adenocarcinoma using transabdominal US. Also, this study needed to be terminated for the same reason, and only four participants could be enrolled.

A most recent study of the development program for BR55 has been published on the Chinese clinical trials web-platform (chictr.org.cn). It was a multicenter, randomized, double-blind, dose-finding phase II study using BR55 for ultrasound molecular imaging of VEGFR2 (KDR) in patients with cancer and chronic inflammatory diseases. The primary objective was to determine the dose of BR55 for ultrasound imaging assessment of angiogenic areas in patients with a known or suspected diagnosis of cancer (breast, thyroid, and ovarian cancer) or chronic inflammatory diseases (inflammatory bowel disease and rheumatoid arthritis) by comparing the enhancing effects of 3 doses of the investigational product, using immunohistochemistry as the gold standard. In the oncology arm breast cancer, ovarian cancer and thyroid cancer patients were enrolled with confirmed or suspected cancer based on diagnostic imaging and plan to undergo pathologic confirmation. The trial was completed in 2024 with 240 patients enrolled; however, the results are not yet published.

BR55 is currently the only specific microbubble with advanced experience in humans. Besides BR55, polymeric microbubbles targeted to integrins have been GMP produced and are currently prepared for first-in-human use [26]. However, currently, no scientific reports exist for other potential molecular ultrasound contrast agents.

26.4 Super-Resolution Ultrasound

As described in the technical part (Chap. 5, in Vol. I), with super-resolution ultrasound, an ultrasound contrast agent-based technique has evolved that can image micron-scale vessels at a clinically relevant imaging depth without tissue destruction [27]. This can open the door for new clinical applications. Although it is not (yet) a specific molecular imaging modality and rather an improved, potentially breakthrough CEUS examination technique using conventional unspecific ultrasound contrast agents, its first experiences in humans are briefly described here.

First experiences applying super-resolution technique to CEUS datasets obtained from humans for tumor characterization were reported in 2018 by Opacic et al. A super-resolution CEUS approach called motion model ultrasound localization microscopy (mULM) was introduced as an advanced tracking technique adapted to clinical settings [28]. With mULM, within less than a minute and using a conventional US device operating at standard frame rates, super-resolution images and novel parameters can be extracted, as shown in Fig. 26.2. The feasibility was further assessed by additional studies in different tumors, such as those of the breast, the pancreas [29], or of lymph nodes [30]. Currently, larger clinical studies using super-resolution ultrasound imaging are lacking and are needed to demonstrate that this technique is robust and fast enough for clinical use and that relevant clinical information can be obtained beyond what is retrievable by conventional CEUS examinations.

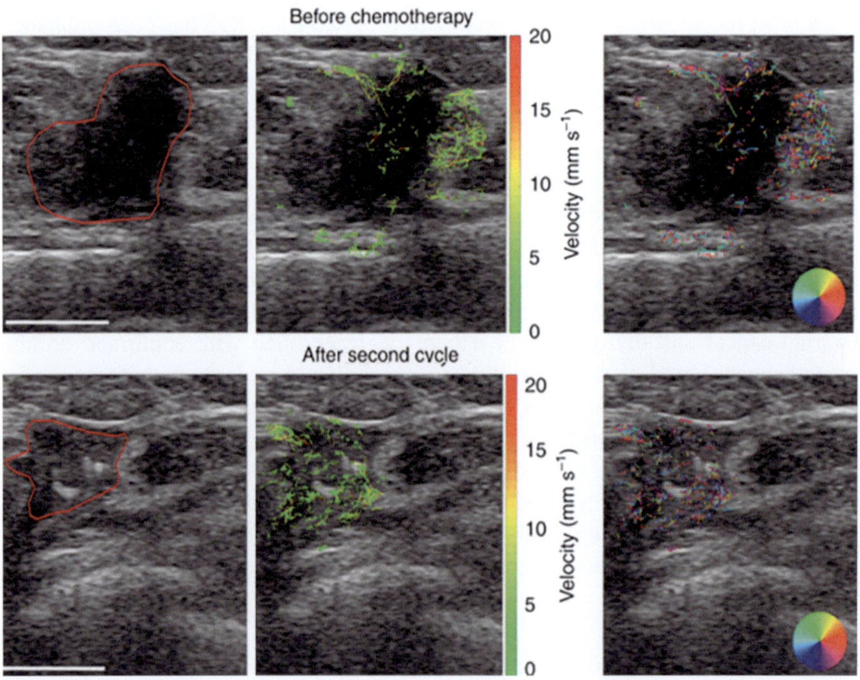

Fig. 26.2 First super-resolution ultrasound data in humans. In a triple negative breast cancer patient treated with neoadjuvant chemotherapy, CEUS measurements were performed with a conventional US device and phospholipid microbubbles. Measurements are shown before and after the second cycle of chemotherapy. The first column shows B-mode images with the tumor borders highlighted in red, the second and third columns display the mULM velocity and direction maps. At the baseline measurement, the tumor vascularization was present mainly in the peripheral areas. After the second cycle of treatment, the tumor volume decreased, while the level of vascularization remained stable. (This is an open-access article distributed under the terms of the Creative Commons CC BY 4.0 license, which permits unrestricted use, distribution, and reproduction in any medium, provided the original work is properly cited [28])

26.5 Conclusion

Modern ultrasound technologies are attractive for molecular imaging using specific ultrasound contrast agents based on targeted microbubbles, with a very high spatial resolution and detection sensitivity. Its potential has been widely investigated in vitro and in animal studies. Although in comparison to other drugs, its translation into clinical use is more difficult, first clinical experiences in humans have been obtained. Especially, BR55, microbubbles targeting VEGF receptor-2, are undergoing the clinical development program. Ultrasound is not (yet) considered a classical molecular imaging modality, like nuclear medicine is. On the other hand, ultrasound is one of the most widely used and inexpensive imaging modalities, and CEUS with unspecific contrast agents has established clinical applications with promising additional options. Thus, a broader implementation of molecular imaging information in clinical oncology may be easier to realize with the use of ultrasound. Angiogenesis-related targets, such as VEGRF2, with its specific but nevertheless broad potential clinical application options and benefits, may be particularly promising to take the step toward clinical molecular ultrasound imaging.

Disclosure Martin Krix is an employee of Bracco, Global Medical and Regulatory Affairs, Konstanz, Germany.

References

1. Wang S, Hossack JA, Klibanov AL (2020) From anatomy to functional and molecular biomarker imaging and therapy: ultrasound is safe, ultrafast, portable, and inexpensive. Investig Radiol 55(9):559–572
2. National Health Service (NHS) England. Facilities for diagnostic imaging and interventional radiology. 31 January 2024. Available at: https://www.england.nhs.uk/wp-content/uploads/2021/05/HBN_6_V1_DSSA.pdf
3. Yanagisawa K, Moriyasu F, Miyahara T et al (2007) Phagocytosis of ultrasound contrast agent microbubbles by Kupffer cells. Ultrasound Med Biol 33(2):318–325
4. Dietrich CF, Nolsoe CP, Barr RG et al (2020) Guidelines and good clinical practice recommendations for contrast-enhanced ultrasound (CEUS) in the liver-update 2020 WFUMB in cooperation with EFSUMB, AFSUMB, AIUM, and FLAUS. Ultrasound Med Biol 46(10):2579–2604
5. Barr RG (2018) Contrast-enhanced ultrasound for focal liver lesions: how accurate is it? Abdom Radiol 43(5):1128–1133
6. Westwood M, Joore M, Grutters J et al (2013) Contrast-enhanced ultrasound using SonoVue(R) (Sulphur hexafluoride microbubbles) compared with contrast-enhanced computed tomography and contrast-enhanced magnetic resonance imaging for the characterisation of focal liver lesions and detection of liver metastases: a systematic review and cost-effectiveness analysis. Health Technol Assess 17(16):1–243
7. Hu HT, Wang Z, Huang XW et al (2019) Ultrasound-based radiomics score: a potential biomarker for the prediction of microvascular invasion in hepatocellular carcinoma. Eur Radiol 29(6):2890–2901
8. Zhang W, Guo Q, Zhu Y et al (2024a) Cross-institutional evaluation of deep learning and radiomics models in predicting microvascular invasion in hepatocellular carcinoma: validity, robustness, and ultrasound modality efficacy comparison. Cancer Imaging 24(1):142

9. Xu W, Huang B, Zhang R et al (2024) Diagnostic and prognostic ability of contrast-enhanced ultrasound and biomarkers in hepatocellular carcinoma subtypes. Ultrasound Med Biol 50(4):617–626
10. Luo M, Liu X, Yong J et al (2023) Preoperative prediction of macrotrabecular-massive hepatocellular carcinoma based on B-mode US and CEUS. Eur Radiol 33(6):4024–4033
11. Sidhu PS, Cantisani V, Dietrich CF et al (2018) The EFSUMB guidelines and recommendations for the clinical practice of contrast-enhanced ultrasound (CEUS) in non-hepatic applications: update 2017 (long version). Ultraschall Med 39(2):e2–e44
12. Zhang X, Wu S, Zu X et al (2024b) Ultrasound-based radiomics nomogram for predicting HER2-low expression breast cancer. Front Oncol 14:1438923
13. Li X, Zhang J, Zhang G et al (2024) Contrast-enhanced ultrasound and conventional ultrasound characteristics of breast cancer with different molecular subtypes. Clin Breast Cancer 24(3):204–214
14. Zhu JY, He HL, Jiang XC et al (2023) Multimodal ultrasound features of breast cancers: correlation with molecular subtypes. BMC Med Imaging 23(1):57
15. Liang RX, Wang H, Zhang HP et al (2021) The value of real-time contrast-enhanced ultrasound combined with CT enhancement in the differentiation of subtypes of renal cell carcinoma. Urol Oncol 39(12):837.e19–837.e28
16. Ma W, Zhang F, Huang H et al (2022) Contrast-enhanced ultrasound features of adult Xp11.2 translocation renal cell carcinoma: differential diagnosis with three main renal cell carcinoma subtypes. J Ultrasound Med 41(11):2673–2685
17. Eisenhauer EA, Therasse P, Bogaerts J et al (2009) New response evaluation criteria in solid tumours: revised RECIST guideline (version 1.1). Eur J Cancer 45(2):228–247
18. Tranquart F, Dujardin P-A, Bouché O et al (2018) Value of contrast-enhanced ultrasound quantification criteria for identifying patients not responding to bevacizumab-based therapy for colorectal liver metastases. Ultraschall Med 39(05):544–558
19. Zhou B-Y, Liu H, Pu Y-Y et al (2024) Quantitative analysis of pre-treatment dynamic contrast-enhanced ultrasound for assessing the response of colorectal liver metastases to chemotherapy plus targeted therapy: a dual-institutional study. Abdom Radiol 49(2):414–424
20. Zhang X-L, Wang H-T, Tang Y et al (2024c) Colorectal liver metastases: correlations of contrast-enhanced ultrasound features with tumor clinicopathological factors and clinical outcomes following conversion therapy. Clin Hemorheol Microcirc 86(3):339–356
21. Lassau N, Coiffier B, Kind M et al (2016) Selection of an early biomarker for vascular normalization using dynamic contrast-enhanced ultrasonography to predict outcomes of metastatic patients treated with bevacizumab. Ann Oncol 27:1922–1928
22. Dietrich CF, Correas JM, Cui XW et al (2024) EFSUMB technical review – update 2023: dynamic contrast-enhanced ultrasound (DCE-CEUS) for the quantification of tumor perfusion. Ultraschall Med 45(1):36–46
23. Tranquart F, Arditi M, Bettinger T et al (2014) Ultrasound contrast agents for ultrasound molecular imaging. Gastroenterol 52(11):1268–1276
24. Willmann JK, Bonomo L, Testa AC et al (2017) Ultrasound molecular imaging with BR55 in patients with breast and ovarian lesions: first-in-human results. J Clin Oncol 35(19):2133–2140
25. Smeenge M, Tranquart F, Mannaerts CK et al (2017) First-in-human ultrasound molecular imaging with a VEGFR2-specific ultrasound molecular contrast agent (BR55) in prostate cancer: a safety and feasibility pilot study. Investig Radiol 52(7):419–427
26. Qi J, Chen J, von Stillfried S et al (2025) Molecular ultrasound imaging with clinically translatable cRGD-coated microbubbles to assess integrin-αvβ3 expression in inflammatory bowel disease. Invest Radiol. https://doi.org/10.1097/RLI.0000000000001143. Online ahead of print
27. Song P, Rubin JM, Lowerison MR (2023) Super-resolution ultrasound microvascular imaging: is it ready for clinical use? Z Med Phys 33(3):309–323
28. Opacic T, Dencks S, Theek B et al (2018) Motion model ultrasound localization microscopy for preclinical and clinical multiparametric tumor characterization. Nat Commun 9(1):1527

29. Huang C, Zhang W, Gong P et al (2021) Super-resolution ultrasound localization microscopy based on a high framerate clinical ultrasound scanner: an in-human feasibility study. Phys Med Biol 66(8):08NT01
30. Zhu J, Zhang C, Christensen-Jeffries K et al (2022) Super-resolution ultrasound localization microscopy of microvascular structure and flow for distinguishing metastatic lymph nodes – an initial human study. Ultraschall Med 43(6):592–598

Image-Guided Radiooncology: The Potential of Artificial Intelligence in Clinical Application

27

Samuel M. Vorbach, Stephanie E. Combs, Benedikt Wiestler, and Jan C. Peeken

Abbreviations

AI	Artificial intelligence
ANN	Artificial neural network
ART	Adaptive radiotherapy

Benedikt Wiestler and Jan C. Peeken contributed equally as senior authors.

S. M. Vorbach
Department of Radiation Oncology, TUM University Hospital Rechts der Isar, Technical University of Munich, Munich, Germany

Department of Radiation Oncology, Medical University of Innsbruck, Innsbruck, Austria
e-mail: samuel.vorbach@i-med.ac.at

S. E. Combs · J. C. Peeken (✉)
Department of Radiation Oncology, TUM University Hospital Rechts der Isar, Technical University of Munich, Munich, Germany

Department of Radiation Sciences (DRS), Institute of Radiation Medicine (IRM), Helmholtz Zentrum München, Neuherberg, Germany

Deutsches Konsortium Für Translationale Krebsforschung (DKTK), Partner Site Munich, Munich, Germany
e-mail: stephanie.combs@tum.de; jan.peeken@tum.de

B. Wiestler
AI for Image-Guided Diagnosis and Therapy, TUM School of Medicine and Health, Technical University of Munich, Munich, Germany
e-mail: b.wiestler@tum.de

O. Schober et al. (eds.), *Molecular Imaging in Oncology - Volume 2*, Recent Results in Cancer Research 225, https://doi.org/10.1007/978-3-032-21415-7_9

BMs	Brain metastases
BraTs	Brain Tumor Segmentation Challenge
CBCT	Cone beam computed tomography
CE	Contrast-enhancing
CI	Concordance index
CNNs	Convolutional neural networks
CT	computed tomography
CTV	Clinical target volume
DL	Deep learning
DLAS	Deep-learning-based autosegmentation
DSC	Dice Similarity Coefficient
EGFR	Epidermal growth factor receptor
ENR	Elastic net regularization
FET	18F-fluoroethyl-l-tyrosine
FLAIR	Fluid-attenuated inversion recovery
GAN	Generative adversarial network
GLCM	Gray level co-occurrence matrix
GLRLM	Gray level run length matrix
GLSZM	Gray level size zone matrix
GTV	Gross tumor volume
HER2	Human epidermal growth factor 2
HNC	Head and neck cancer
IBSI	Imaging Biomarker Standardization Initiative
IDH	Isocitrate dehydrogenase
LBP	Local binary pattern
LF	Local failure
LINAC	Linear accelerator
LLMs	Large language models
ML	Machine learning
MRI	Magnetic resonance imaging
NE	Non-enhancing
OARs	Organs at risk
OS	Overall survival
pCR	Pathologic complete response
PET	Positron emission tomography
PTV	Planning target volume
RANO	Response Assessment in Neuro-Oncology
RECIST	Response Evaluation Criteria in Solid Tumors
SRT	Stereotactic radiotherapy
STS	Soft tissue sarcomas
SSL	Self-supervised learning
VOI	Volume of interest
VLMs	Vision-language models

27.1 Current Artificial Intelligence Models: The State of the Art

27.1.1 Radiomics

The term "radiomics" was introduced in the early 2010s [1]. It describes the systematic extraction of large amounts of quantitative features from medical images, with the aim of uncovering subtle patterns that may not be visually apparent. These features capture various aspects of the image, such as intensity distribution, textural patterns, and the shape of the region or volume of interest (VOI). By converting medical images into high-dimensional data, radiomics provides a foundation for developing imaging biomarkers that can aid in diagnosis, prognosis, and treatment response assessment across a range of clinical applications. Depending on the exact implementation of such a predefined feature, however, results from the same image may differ significantly, impairing reproducibility and hence clinical usefulness. The Imaging Biomarker Standardization Initiative (IBSI) has defined guidelines on the extraction of radiomic parameters, image preprocessing, recommendations on the reporting of radiomics studies, and tools to verify radiomics software implementations [2]. The main focus of IBSI was the exact mathematical description to allow for better comparability of radiomics features used in scientific studies. This aims to improve reproducibility and facilitate clinical applications. The authors provide a detailed mathematical description of all radiomic features and preprocessing steps.

The most commonly used feature types are described in the following (see Fig. 27.1):

27.1.1.1 First-Order: Intensity Features

First-order intensity features describe the distribution of voxel intensity values within the VOI. They summarize the original image by simple statistical measures such as "mean," "range," or "kurtosis."

27.1.1.2 Second-Order: Texture Features

Texture features include multiple distinct feature types that derive information from the spatial distribution of intensity values. Intensity values must be discretized before textural analysis.

The *Gray Level Co-occurrence Matrix (GLCM)* quantifies the frequency of gray level pairs that are neighbored in a predefined direction and distance. Features are generated by quantifying the *GLCM* (such as "Cluster Tendency" as a measure for the grouping of similar intensity voxels) (see Fig. 27.1 for an exemplary GLCM).

The *Gray Level Run Length Matrix (GLRLM)* assesses the length of a sequence of equal gray values in neighboring voxels in a predefined direction. An exemplary feature, the "Long Run Emphasis," is a measure of the distribution of long-run length, indicating the coarseness of a texture.

If the *GLCM* or *GLRLM* features are averaged for every possible directional angle, the mean of these values represents a rotationally invariant measure, which is frequently used in radiomic studies.

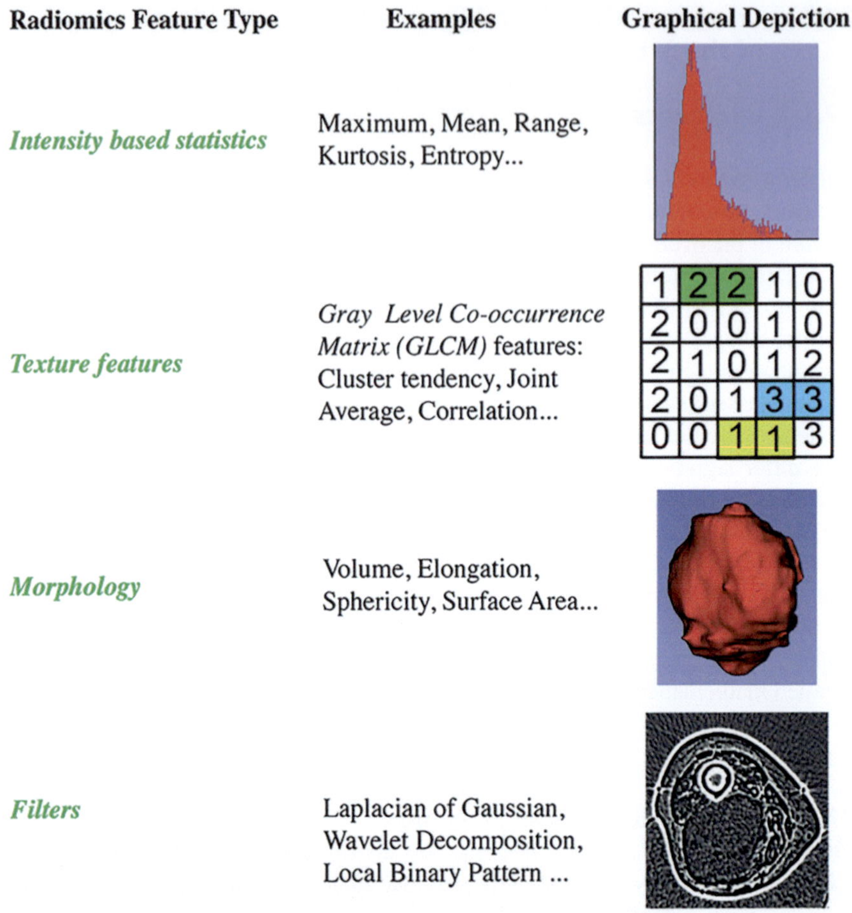

Fig. 27.1 Exemplary illustration of the radiomics features types. (Subfigures were adapted from Peeken et al. [3])

The *Gray Level Size Zone Matrix (GLSZM)* quantifies the occurrence of voxel zones with an equal gray value connected in all directions, yielding a rotational invariant matrix. An exemplary feature, the "Zone Entropy" quantifies the randomness in the distribution of gray level zone sizes, indicating a measure of heterogeneity.

In the *Gray Level Dependence Matrix,* the number of dependent voxels, which are defined as neighboring voxels in a predefined distance with a predefined maximal gray value difference, is quantified, yielding a rotationally invariant matrix. The exemplary feature "Dependence Non-Uniformity" assesses the similarity between all dependencies within the VOI as an indicator of the homogeneity of a texture.

The *Neighboring Gray Tone Difference Matrix* determines the mean difference in gray values between the voxel of interest and its connected voxels, yielding a rotational invariant matrix. An exemplary feature represents the "Busyness," which assesses the number of rapid intensity changes between voxels and their surroundings.

Finally, the less common *Gray Level Distance Zone matrix* combines the gray value zone matrix obtained as for the *GLSZM* features and a distance map assessing the distance of each voxel to the VOI edge. The combined matrix assesses the number of voxel groups with equal gray value and equal distance to the VOI edge. The feature derivation is similar to the *GLRLM*. In this case, the "Large distance emphasis" assesses gray zones with a large distance to the VOI edge.

27.1.1.3 Morphology Features

Morphology or "shape" features quantify the geometrical shape of a VOI. Thus, the features are independent of image gray values and only depend on the specific VOI mask. Important variables include the number of voxels, the surface area, or the axis length. Features range from the VOI "volume," over the quantification of the "elongation" (the relationship between the two principal axis lengths) to "sphericity" (a measure to quantify the roundness of a shape).

27.1.1.4 Image Filtering

First-order and second-order features can be calculated from the original image or from a transformed image, which has been modified by the application of a *filter*. As for the above-mentioned features, filters find frequent application in image processing. Depending on the filter type, certain properties of the image are altered, leading to different feature values. Thus, a radiomic feature is always defined by the applied filter and the actual feature algorithm. By multiplying the available feature algorithm and a series of different filters, a large number of radiomic features can be extracted from single images.

The "Laplacian of Gaussian" filter computes the second spatial derivative of the input image, which highlights areas of rapid intensity change such as edges. To reduce the effect of noise, a Gaussian smoothing filter is applied beforehand. The "wavelet decomposition" filter yields eight distinct decompositions. Each decomposition consists of a unique combination of applying a low-pass or high-pass filter in all three dimensions.

The "Local Binary Pattern" (LBP) filter assigns a new value to each voxel defined by the relative intensity of the neighboring voxels. LBP-based features introduce directionality in addition to rotational invariance. Each surrounding voxel is labeled with 1 or 0 depending on whether the intensity value is larger or smaller than the voxel of interest. Each combination of all surrounding voxels is assigned as a novel intensity value. As a consequence, semantic structures such as edges or corners can be quantified.

27.1.2 Machine Learning: The Toolbox for the Generation of Radiomic Models

In order to make a prediction on clinically relevant questions, radiomic features need to be used as input features for predictive models. Since a large proportion of radiomic features are intercorrelated, feature reduction methods are often used to reduce radiomic features to the most important ones. Common techniques include "least absolute shrinkage and selection operator," "minimum redundancy maximum relevance," or "principal component analysis." The remaining features can be used for model building.

If a sufficient feature reduction is possible, *statistical methods* such as logistic regression or Cox proportional hazard models can be trained. These methods bear the advantage of simple interpretability with the disadvantage of small input feature numbers and the incapability of modeling non-linear relationships. Other statistical methods, such as ridge regression, can fit prediction models based on a large number of input features by reducing the regression coefficients of unimportant features without setting them to zero.

Alternatively, a diverse set of *Machine Learning (ML) methods* can be applied for predictive modeling, allowing larger input feature numbers, potential handling of missing data points, and modeling of interaction or non-linear relationships at the expense of interpretability. Commonly used models include decision tree methods such as random forest, bagging, or boosting techniques, support vector machines, or neural networks.

Scientific studies have compared the performance of different ML methods. Depending on the specific dataset, predictive performances differed significantly between arbitrarily chosen models. Ensemble learning strategies in which several distinct ML models are combined into one model may compensate for this disadvantage.

27.1.3 Deep Learning

DL has emerged as a transformative force in AI, particularly within the field of medical imaging and radiomics [4]. By advancing beyond traditional ML and "classic" radiomics approaches, DL introduces a paradigm shift: it automates the extraction of features directly from raw imaging data, eliminating the need for manually engineered radiomic features. This end-to-end learning capability enables models to identify complex, hierarchical patterns in data—patterns that are often imperceptible to human experts or conventional algorithms. As a result, DL not only reduces human intervention but also enhances reproducibility and scalability in clinical applications. Its impact has been profound, achieving state-of-the-art performance across a wide array of computational image analysis tasks, including image classification, segmentation, and synthesis.

At its foundation, DL leverages *artificial neural networks (ANNs)*, computational models loosely inspired by the structure and functionality of the human brain.

While the analogy to biological neural systems is limited, ANNs consist of interconnected layers of nodes (neurons), each performing mathematical operations to process input data. The term "deep" in DL refers to the concatenation of multiple stacked layers, which allow the model to progressively learn increasingly abstract and complex representations of the input data. This hierarchical feature extraction is achieved through a training process that iteratively adjusts the network's internal parameters (weights) using backpropagation—a technique that minimizes prediction errors by optimizing a cost function. The choice of this cost function, along with the network architecture itself, is critical to achieving high model performance for specific tasks and datasets.

A pivotal breakthrough in DL for medical image analysis was the development of *convolutional neural networks (CNNs)*. These architectures introduced convolutional filters, which are particularly effective for analyzing spatial hierarchies in images. CNNs have excelled in tasks such as detecting abnormalities, segmenting organs or tissues, and classifying diseases in medical images like X-rays, magnetic resonance imaging (MRI), and computed tomography (CT) scans. Their layered structure enables them to learn features at varying levels of abstraction: early layers capture basic elements like edges or textures, while deeper layers identify more intricate structures such as tumors or specific anatomical features (Fig. 27.2). This hierarchical approach allows CNNs to achieve remarkable accuracy in medical image analysis, often matching or surpassing human experts in certain diagnostic tasks.

Building on the success of CNNs, transformers have emerged as a powerful alternative for medical image analysis, offering unique advantages through their self-attention mechanisms [5]. Unlike CNNs, which focus primarily on local features within an image, transformers excel at capturing global relationships across an entire image. This capability is especially valuable in medical imaging, where understanding contextual relationships—such as interactions between a lesion and surrounding tissues—is critical for accurate diagnosis. By processing all parts of an image simultaneously and modeling long-range dependencies, transformers enable a more holistic analysis. Positional encoding further ensures that spatial relationships within images are preserved—an essential feature for tasks such as organ

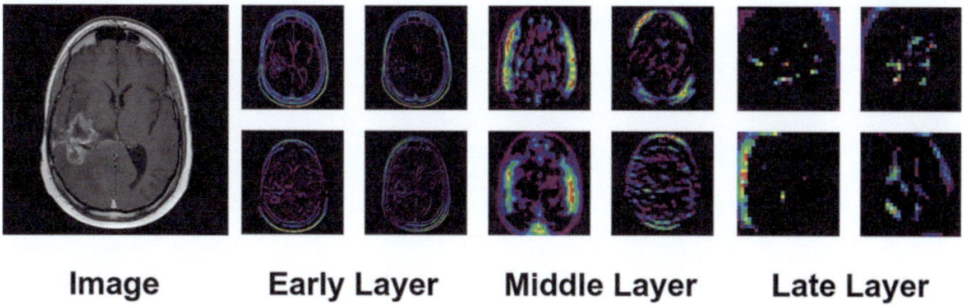

Fig. 27.2 In a typical CNN, early layers learn coarse shapes (such as edges), while in later layers, more detailed object parts and semantic concepts are learned

segmentation or tumor detection. While transformers often require large datasets and significant computational resources for training, they have demonstrated exceptional performance across various applications, including classification, segmentation, and anomaly detection. Their ability to enhance diagnostic accuracy makes them an invaluable tool for supporting clinical decision-making.

In parallel with advancements in network architectures like CNNs and transformers, self-supervised learning (SSL) has emerged as a transformative training paradigm addressing one of the most persistent challenges in medical image analysis: limited labeled data. Traditional supervised learning relies heavily on expert-annotated datasets, which are time-consuming and costly to produce at scale. SSL circumvents this bottleneck by leveraging vast amounts of unlabeled medical data routinely generated during clinical practice. Through pretext tasks—such as predicting missing parts of an image, restoring shuffled patches, or distinguishing between augmented views of the same image—SSL enables models to learn meaningful representations directly from the underlying structure of the data itself. These pretrained models can then be fine-tuned with minimal labeled samples for specific applications like disease detection, segmentation, or classification. This approach not only reduces annotation costs but also improves model generalization across diverse clinical settings. As SSL continues to evolve, it holds immense potential to unlock the value of unannotated medical data and pave the way for scalable AI-driven healthcare solutions. Using multiple foundation models for different imaging modalities also enables new multimodal classifiers, where the information from both image inputs is embedded using a specialized transformer-based encoder, allowing the integration of this information via subsequent adapters. Based on a simple neural network classifier, such as a multi-layer perceptron or transformer architecture, the embeddings are then processed to generate output classification (see Fig. 27.3).

Together, these innovations—spanning network architectures like CNNs and transformers as well as training paradigms like SSL—are revolutionizing how medical images are analyzed and interpreted. DL continues to push the boundaries of diagnostic accuracy and efficiency while offering promising avenues for addressing longstanding challenges in healthcare delivery.

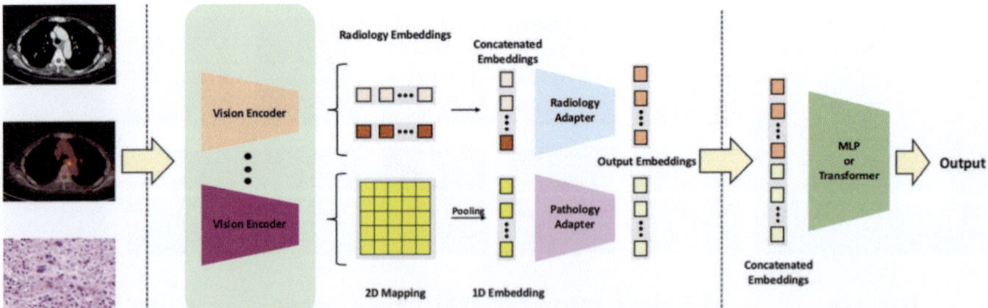

Fig. 27.3 Visualization of a multimodal foundation model-based approach combining information from different modalities in the embedding space

27.2 Clinical Applications of AI in (Radiation) Oncology

27.2.1 Image-Based Classification

The integration of advanced image analysis strategies based on ML and DL has opened new possibilities for automated, preoperative classification, and diagnosis of tumors, particularly in brain tumors. DL models, in particular, have demonstrated remarkable potential in automating tasks such as tumor detection and segmentation, classification, and even detailed prediction of genetic mutations, thereby enhancing diagnostic accuracy and informing clinical decision-making already preoperatively. This section will explore potential clinical applications of DL in image-based tumor classification, with a special focus on brain tumors.

AI-driven tools for radiological analysis offer several potential use cases across various tumor types. These include lesion detection, segmentation, and classification. For instance, in breast cancer imaging, AI has been employed for risk stratification, tumor subtype identification, and prognosis prediction. Similarly, in soft tissue tumors, ML models have successfully distinguished between benign and malignant lesions using MRI-derived radiomics features. These applications underscore the versatility of AI in addressing complex diagnostic challenges across oncological imaging. In the domain of brain tumors, DL has been particularly transformative. Brain tumors such as gliomas are notoriously heterogeneous and challenging to both segment and classify using conventional methods. DL models trained on MRI data have shown promise in distinguishing between different tumor types and grades, as well as predicting molecular markers critical for personalized treatment strategies.

The basis for automated tumor analysis is the reliable detection and segmentation of tumors on MRI. Automating this process holds significant clinical relevance as it addresses the challenges of manual tumor delineation, which is both time-consuming and prone to interobserver variability. Accurate segmentation is crucial for quantifying tumor volume, guiding treatment planning, and monitoring disease progression or response to therapy. By enabling precise and reproducible measurements, automated methods can improve diagnostic workflows and support personalized treatment strategies, particularly in complex and morphologically heterogeneous gliomas. The Brain Tumor Segmentation (BraTS) Challenge has played a pivotal role in advancing this field by providing standardized datasets and benchmarking platforms for evaluating state-of-the-art segmentation algorithms [6]. Since its inception in 2012, BraTS has fostered innovation by encouraging the development of robust ML models capable of segmenting distinct tumor subregions, such as enhancing tumor, nonenhancing (NE) core, and edema. These efforts have not only improved algorithmic performance to levels comparable with expert radiologists but have also facilitated the integration of automated segmentation tools into clinical practice, setting a benchmark for future advancements in neuro-oncology imaging.

Building upon segmented tumor outlines, DL models have demonstrated remarkable capabilities in distinguishing between distinct brain tumor types and predicting clinically significant genomic alterations, such as isocitrate dehydrogenase (IDH) mutations in gliomas [7]. Segmentation provides precise delineation of tumor subregions, enabling DL algorithms to extract detailed spatial and textural features critical for classification tasks. For instance, by analyzing the unique imaging characteristics of segmented regions, DL models can differentiate between glioblastomas, lower-grade gliomas, and other tumor types with high accuracy. Beyond classification, DL has also advanced the field of radiogenomics by linking imaging phenotypes to molecular markers. IDH mutation status, a key prognostic and therapeutic biomarker in gliomas, can now be predicted noninvasively using DL models trained on multiparametric MRI data. These models leverage radiomic features from segmented tumor regions to identify subtle imaging patterns associated with IDH mutations, obviating the need for invasive biopsies and guiding treatment and surgical decisions, as detailed in recent Response Assessment in Neuro-Oncology (RANO) reviews. Such applications not only enhance diagnostic precision but also support personalized treatment planning by providing valuable molecular insights directly from imaging data.

These advancements highlight the potential of DL to augment traditional diagnostic workflows by providing noninvasive, rapid, and highly accurate assessments of tumors. Moreover, DL models can outperform expert radiologists in specific tasks by identifying subtle imaging patterns that may elude human interpretation.

Despite these successes, several challenges remain before widespread clinical adoption can be realized. Developing robust DL models requires large annotated datasets, which are often scarce due to privacy concerns and the labor-intensive nature of manual labeling. Additionally, model interpretability and generalizability issues must be addressed to ensure that AI tools can be reliably applied across diverse patient populations and imaging settings. As the field evolves, collaboration between clinicians, data scientists, and regulatory bodies will be essential to harness the full potential of AI in oncological imaging.

27.2.2 Therapy Planning

27.2.2.1 Segmentation

The integration of AI, particularly DL, has not only revolutionized tumor segmentation in radiological analysis but also holds transformative potential for radiotherapy planning through automated delineation of organs at risk (normal tissue, OARs), gross tumor volume (GTV), clinical target volume (CTV), and planning target volume (PTV). Their manual segmentation, traditionally performed by radiation oncologists, is a labor-intensive, time-consuming process and is subject to variability both within and between radiotherapy centers. Differences in individual expertise and institutional protocols contribute to inter- and intra-observer discrepancies, potentially affecting treatment planning and, ultimately, treatment outcomes.

Early attempts to automate segmentation relied on conventional methods such as intensity analysis, shape modeling, and atlas-based approaches. Intensity-based methods differentiate tissue types by analyzing pixel or voxel intensity variations in imaging modalities, while shape modeling introduced statistical shape and appearance models to create anatomical references. Atlas-based models use a library of presegmented images (an atlas) or a synthetic body model as a reference to guide segmentation in new cases. While these techniques represented a step forward, they were constrained by limited adaptability, accuracy, and availability, especially for complex anatomical variations. Moreover, they were restricted to recurring anatomy and impossible to segment individual structures such as GTVs. Thus, despite their potential, these methods still required substantial manual correction, which limited their practical efficiency in routine clinical workflows. Nevertheless, many commercially available software solutions used in clinical routine still rely on atlas-based segmentation techniques.

The advent of DL, particularly CNNs, has further improved segmentation accuracy. Architectures such as the U-Net have proven particularly effective, using an encoder-decoder structure to transfer spatial and contextual information from the input image while preserving important macro-scale details in the final segmentation map.

Each patient requires an individualized contouring process to ensure accurate treatment planning. Inadequate contouring of OARs can result in excessive radiation exposure to healthy tissue, increasing the risk of toxicity and impairing the patient's quality of life. There are already several commercially available software solutions for automated segmentation with certified medical products. Most of them are based on the U-Net-based architecture. Recent research has shown the potential of AI-based segmentation. For example, Lustberg et al. demonstrated that deep learning contouring of OARs in patients with non-small cell lung cancer saved a median of 10 min compared to manual contouring [8]. In addition, the DL approach outperformed an atlas-based segmentation method. However, while deep learning achieves high accuracy in segmenting well-defined anatomical structures, the performance is sometimes inconsistent for small, irregular, or mobile organs (e.g., the optic chiasm and stomach), where variability in position and shape poses a challenge to reliable delineation.

Delineation of the GTV, which is the basis for defining the CTV and PTV, is particularly challenging due to the wide variability in case-specific tumor burden, requiring expert assessment of imaging modalities and clinical data. Semi- or fully automated algorithms provide a faster GTV delineation, which may be more standardized. Recent studies have shown that these segmentations achieve performance levels comparable to expert manual segmentation and have resulted in significant time savings, reducing segmentation time from several minutes per patient to just a few seconds. Despite these benefits, refinement of AI-generated contours is still often required prior to clinical implementation, particularly for challenging tumor regions such as the head and neck and, especially in cases where multimodal imaging is warranted for precise segmentation [9].

The CTV encompasses the GTV and surrounding tissues to account for potential microscopic tumor infiltration. Thus, CTV delineation requires anatomical and pathological considerations, making its segmentation inherently complex. DL methods can assist in automatically generating CTVs while integrating anatomical constraints to prevent excessive expansion into adjacent structures. Advanced methods now incorporate anatomical barrier-aware expansion techniques, which refine CTV contours by excluding regions unlikely to harbor microscopic disease. DL models have been developed for CTV delineation in a variety of different tumor sites, such as head and neck, lung, rectal, and cervical cancers. For example, deep-learning-based autosegmentation (DLAS) of individual lymph node target volumes in patients with head and neck cancer (HNC) was found to be clinically acceptable, with no or only minor adjustments required in 99% of cases. However, many DLAS models are developed and validated within single institutions, using the guidelines followed by the developing institutions. This limits their generalizability to different clinical settings.

A recent joint guideline from the European Society for Radiotherapy and Oncology and the American Association of Physicists in Medicine highlights the complexity of validating AI-driven segmentation, and emphasizes that defining a true "gold standard" remains a challenge [10]. The guideline recommends that once a reference segmentation has been established, both qualitative (e.g., Likert scale) and quantitative (e.g., Hausdorff distance) metrics should be used. In addition, a time trial assessment is recommended to determine the practical utility of AI-based segmentation models in clinical workflows.

In conclusion, AI-based segmentation is transforming radiation oncology by improving efficiency, accuracy, and consistency in delineating OARs, GTV, and CTV. DL models have already outperformed traditional approaches in many clinical applications, significantly reducing interobserver variability, increasing precision, and accelerating treatment workflows. However, further external validation, regulatory guidelines, and continued research are essential to ensure the full integration into daily clinical practice. In addition, as advances continue, AI-based real-time segmentation and adaptive radiotherapy (ART) could enable faster, more personalized treatments, ultimately improving patient care.

27.2.2.2 Growth Models

Biophysical tumor growth models are emerging as a powerful and innovative tool to address the inherent complexity of CTV delineation, enabling individualized target volume definition and radiotherapy planning. Particular progress has been made in glioblastoma, the most aggressive primary brain tumor. A hallmark of these tumors is their highly infiltrative nature, which cannot fully be revealed in conventional imaging. However, re-tracing the infiltrative growth is key to a personalized target volume definition. Biophysical tumor growth models, therefore, aim to predict the spatial distribution of tumor cells, including infiltrative regions beyond what is visible in standard imaging modalities such as MRI. By addressing the limitations of conventional radiotherapy planning, which relies on uniform margins around visible tumors, these models offer the potential for more precise and patient-specific treatment strategies. Biophysical tumor growth models typically rely on partial differential equations to describe tumor dynamics, incorporating processes like cell proliferation and diffusion. In this context, the "inverse problem" involves calibrating these models to patient-specific data, such as MRI scans, to estimate parameters that define tumor behavior. Solving this problem is crucial for uncovering otherwise invisible tumor cell infiltration into surrounding healthy tissue, which is often a source of recurrence. However, the inverse problem is computationally challenging due to its ill-posed nature and the high dimensionality of the parameter space.

A "traditional" way to solve these problems is by iterating over possible parameter combinations in many forward simulations. Lipkova et al., for example, proposed a Bayesian framework that integrates mathematical tumor models with multimodal imaging data, including MRI and 18F-fluoroethyl-l-tyrosine (FET) positron emission tomography (PET) scans [11]. Their approach uses the Fisher–Kolmogorov equation to model tumor growth and employs Bayesian inference to estimate patient-specific parameters while quantifying uncertainties in both imaging and modeling. This framework enables robust tumor cell density distribution predictions, even from single time-point data, making it suitable for standard clinical workflows. However, the Bayesian approach is computationally expensive, often requiring days of computation on specialized hardware.

To address this limitation, more recent approaches leverage DL to solve the inverse problem. Ezhov et al. introduced the "Learn-Morph-Infer" pipeline [12]. Their approach uses a CNN trained on synthetic data to predict tumor model parameters directly from MRI scans. The method achieves real-time inference while maintaining accuracy across different tumor models by leveraging the spatial alignment between patient-specific anatomy and a brain atlas. Unlike traditional optimization or sampling-based methods, this approach eliminates the need for iterative simulations during inference, reducing computation time from hours or days to minutes. However, its reliance on synthetic training data may limit its robustness when applied to real-world clinical scenarios, and, crucially, such approaches lack the inherent safety and convergence guarantees of traditional optimization-based approaches such as the one introduced by Lipkova et al.

To unite the "best of both worlds," Weidner et al. recently proposed a hybrid framework that combines DL with optimization techniques to overcome the limitations of both approaches [13]. In their method, a DL ensemble provides an initial estimate of tumor model parameters, which serves as a prior for subsequent optimization using the Covariance Matrix Adaptation Evolution Strategy. This combination leverages the speed of DL for parameter initialization and the precision of sampling-based methods for fine-tuning. The hybrid approach achieves a fivefold acceleration in convergence time compared to traditional sampling while maintaining high accuracy. This synergy allows for rapid yet reliable personalization of biophysical tumor models, making it feasible for clinical integration.

The synthesis of data-driven and physics-based approaches for glioblastoma modeling opens new avenues for personalized radiotherapy and a deeper understanding of tumor biology. Future research will focus on developing more complex models and further personalizing the modeling approach, for example, by incorporating genetic information from biopsies, paving the way for clinical translation.

27.2.2.3 Online Adaptive Radiotherapy

Advances in highly conformal techniques, such as volumetric-modulated arc therapy and treatment planning improvements, have enabled dose delivery with tight margins and steep gradients. However, these techniques are inherently more sensitive to anatomical and physiological changes, which can reduce treatment efficacy or increase toxicity. ART is an advanced approach to improving treatment quality, "by systematically monitoring treatment variations and incorporating them to re-optimize the treatment plan early on during the course of treatment" [14].

ART can be performed in three different timeframes: offline, between fractions; online, immediately before a fraction; and real-time, where modifications are made during a fraction. Despite the known benefits, the widespread implementation of ART in clinical routine remains limited due to its labor-intensive nature. The process requires procedures throughout the entire workflow, placing a significant workload on radiation oncology staff.

Given the challenges in implementing ART, AI has emerged as a transformative tool to streamline workflows, automate key processes, and enhance efficiency. By reducing manual labor and enhancing adaptive strategies, AI can make ART more accessible and clinically feasible, especially for anatomically complex regions such as HNC. Head and neck radiation therapy is particularly complex due to the high prescription doses required, the complicated anatomy with critical structures in close proximity to the target volumes, and the risk of malnutrition and weight loss during treatment. It therefore requires careful contouring and individualized planning. A recent systematic review examined the impact of AI on CT-based ART for HNC, focusing on its role in synthetic CT generation, autosegmentation, and predictive modeling [14]. The results presented below highlight the ability of AI to optimize treatment planning and improve patient-specific adaptation.

One of the fundamental challenges in ART is acquiring high-quality images suitable for accurate dose calculations. Cone beam computed tomography (CBCT) is widely used for target position verification and setup corrections; however, it exhibits increased image artifacts, including shading, cupping, and streaking, as well as reduced contrast. In addition, CBCT does not provide accurate Hounsfield unit values, making it unsuitable for direct dose calculations.

To overcome these limitations, AI-based synthetic CT generation has been developed. A CNN using a U-Net architecture provided improvements in mean absolute error, signal-to-noise ratio, and structural similarity. Deep residual U-Net and conditional generative adversarial networks (GAN) demonstrated superior performance to nondeep learning atlas-based approaches, ensuring dosimetric accuracy and fast image generation. One specific GAN model also proved effective for generalization across different accelerators. Building on these advancements, a novel model, the "self-attention-residual U-Net," enhanced imaging quality by an additional 11% over the standard U-Net, particularly excelling in limited-data scenarios. These innovations in synthetic CT generation enable more accurate dose calculations without repeated diagnostic CT scans and open the door for online ART.

As discussed in a previous chapter, AI-driven autosegmentation has significantly improved contouring accuracy and efficiency in radiation oncology, reducing interobserver variability and streamlining treatment workflows. These advances are particularly beneficial in the context of ART, where frequent anatomical changes necessitate repeated segmentation throughout the course of treatment. This capability is indispensable to allow for online ART, where resegmentation is performed while the patient is on the treatment table. Algorithm speed and quality are therefore decisive for an efficient workflow where manual input has to be minimized.

Beyond automation, AI could play a role in predictive modeling, allowing clinicians to anticipate the need for treatment adaptation before significant anatomical changes occur. Radiomic feature analysis can help identify patients needing ART by detecting volumetric changes. For example, a deep neural network was trained to predict anatomical changes in the parotid glands during radiation therapy by analyzing longitudinal deformation patterns between planning CT and weekly CBCTs. The model demonstrated high accuracy, achieving a Dice Similarity Coefficient (DSC) of approximately 0.8. In addition, ML algorithms incorporating the features of mean oral cavity dose, body mass index, number of fractions, DSC of CTV, and rate of changes in DSC over time could achieve over 90% accuracy in predicting which patients required ART in a retrospective study [14].

All major manufacturers of clinical linear accelerators (LINACs) have developed or are currently developing advanced treatment systems that enable online ART. One prominent solution leverages state-of-the-art CBCT-based LINACs, offering improved image quality and incorporating novel software workflows powered by AI at multiple stages. Another innovative approach combines a LINAC with MRI, providing superior soft-tissue contrast and enabling real-time monitoring through cine-MRI sequences during treatment. This MRI-guided method is particularly advantageous in abdominal treatments, significantly enhancing the effectiveness of online ART.

The primary aim of these emerging workflows is to maximize clinical efficiency, thereby promoting widespread implementation in routine practice. The capability for daily online ART facilitates reduced PTV safety margins, which consequently improves sparing of OARs. Initial clinical results have demonstrated reduced toxicity associated with these methods; however, larger clinical trials are necessary to confirm these findings comprehensively.

27.2.3 Response Assessment

The integration of AI into medical imaging can not only enhance diagnostic accuracy but also transform the way treatment response is assessed across multiple oncology disciplines. Traditional response assessment methods rely on subjective interpretation of imaging criteria, which can be inconsistent and time-consuming. As previously discussed, AI-driven approaches have demonstrated remarkable potential in automating image analysis. This capability is now being leveraged for response assessment, enabling automated, reproducible, and quantitative analysis of tumor changes over time. These methods could support personalized treatment adjustments by providing a more detailed characterization of tumor behavior in response to therapy.

In neuro-oncology, particularly in high-grade gliomas, a major challenge is to distinguish treatment-related effects such as pseudoprogression and radiation necrosis from true tumor recurrence following radiochemotherapy or immunotherapy. The lack of reliable imaging biomarkers and the risks associated with brain biopsy, as well as the co-existence of progressive disease and treatment effects in tissue samples, make follow-up imaging the standard approach for differentiation. However, this approach can delay clinical decision-making, potentially leading to unaddressed tumor progression. To address these challenges, the Artificial Intelligence for Response Assessment in Neuro-Oncology working group seeks to incorporate AI-based approaches into the established RANO criteria to improve standardized response criteria for brain tumors. In their recently published policy review, they summarized and provided a critical assessment of the work in this field [7, 15].

They emphasized that, despite not being routinely used in many centers, advanced MRI sequences improve the performance of AI-based approaches in differentiating pseudoprogression from tumor recurrence. For example, the integration of multiparametric MRI with advanced imaging sequences, such as diffusion-weighted imaging and T2-weighted fluid-attenuated inversion recovery (FLAIR), significantly improved differentiation performance compared to any single modality using a DL approach. The potential of combining imaging features from multiple modalities was also demonstrated by the development of an FET-PET AI model, which was able to identify all patients with pseudoprogression in a test cohort. Such AI-based approaches hold promise as noninvasive tools for distinguishing tumor from treatment-related effects. However, current studies are limited by their restricted generalizability across diverse datasets and potential confounding factors inherent to retrospective study designs.

As previously discussed, another crucial area in AI-driven tumor analysis and response assessment is automated tumor segmentation, which serves as the foundation for generating reliable quantitative response metrics. A notable example of fully automated quantitative tumor response assessment is the work by Kickingereder and colleagues, who developed a so-called U-Net neural network trained on a single-institution dataset to automatically segment contrast-enhancing (CE) tumors and NE T2-signal abnormalities on MRI scans [16]. Independent testing was performed on both a longitudinal dataset from the same institution and a multi-institutional dataset from a prospective phase 2/3 study at 34 institutions across Europe. The AI model demonstrated high accuracy, with median DSCs of 0.89 in the single institution dataset and 0.91 in the multicenter dataset for CE tumors and 0.93 for NEs in both datasets. More importantly, time-to-progression based on AI quantitative assessment of tumor response proved to be a significantly better surrogate endpoint for overall survival (OS) than the centrally performed conventional RANO assessment. The AI achieved a 36% improvement in reliability compared to RANO within the clinical trial. In addition, in a simulated clinical setting, the U-Net successfully processed MRI scans and performed quantitative tumor response assessments on demand fully automatically. These results demonstrate the potential for seamless integration into clinical workflows, objective, accurate, and high-throughput analysis in real-world neuro-oncology settings.

Despite these advances, AI response assessment, as discussed here with neuro-oncology as an example, still faces several limitations. The lack of reliable reference standards for differentiating tumor progression and treatment effects complicates model validation, as ground truth itself is unreliable and inconsistent. In addition, the low incidence of many cancer entities, such as gliomas, limits the availability of sufficiently large, diverse datasets required for robust model training and generalization. Another challenge is the continuous evolution of tumor classification systems, which requires frequent re-training of AI models with revised reference labels.

27.2.4 Outcome Prediction

Biomarkers in oncology play a critical role in disease monitoring, treatment selection, and outcome prediction. A biomarker is a measurable characteristic that indicates normal biological processes, pathogenic processes, or responses to therapeutic interventions. Depending on their clinical application, biomarkers can be classified into several categories, with prognostic and predictive biomarkers being the most clinically relevant in oncology.

A prognostic biomarker provides information about a disease-related endpoint. These biomarkers help clinicians identify patients at higher risk of poor outcomes who may benefit from more aggressive treatment strategies. Conversely, patients with favorable prognostic markers may be candidates for treatment de-escalation, reducing exposure to unnecessary side effects. While most established prognostic biomarkers are based on genomic and molecular assays—such as Decipher in prostate cancer—these methods are often costly and require invasive tissue sampling, limiting their applicability for continuous monitoring throughout the course of the disease.

A predictive biomarker, on the other hand, helps determine a patient's likelihood of responding to a particular treatment. In oncology, a biomarker is considered predictive if treatment effects differ significantly based on biomarker status. For example, human epidermal growth factor 2 (HER2) status in breast or gastric cancer guides the use of HER2-targeted therapies, while epidermal growth factor receptor (EGFR) mutations in non-small cell lung cancer determine eligibility for treatment with EGFR tyrosine kinase inhibitors. These biomarkers play a critical role in tailoring treatment strategies to individual patients, ensuring personalized oncology care [17].

Recent advances in AI have enabled the development of AI-enabled imaging biomarkers, which rely on extracting quantitative features from radiological images to provide valuable insights into tumor biology, prognosis, and treatment response. Advantages of AI-enabled imaging biomarkers include their ability to capture phenotypic tumor characteristics noninvasively, unlike molecular assays that require tissue biopsies. Since they use routine clinical images—such as MRI, CT, and PET scans—these biomarkers are relatively inexpensive and compatible with existing clinical workflows. They also enable comprehensive tumor characterization across its entire three-dimensional structure, minimizing the risk of sampling errors associated with biopsies from heterogeneous tumors. In the following section, radiomics-based prediction for soft tissue sarcomas (STS) and brain metastases (BMs) will be discussed.

The standard of care for high-grade STS is a multimodality approach, including surgery, radiation therapy, and/or chemotherapy. Neoadjuvant treatment approaches provide an opportunity to assess treatment response, which could guide therapy escalation for individual patients. Pathologic complete response (pCR) is a biomarker in STS that has been correlated with improved OS. However, conventional imaging methods, including assessments such as Response Evaluation Criteria in Solid Tumors (RECIST) and tumor volume changes, have shown limited accuracy in predicting pCR. In this context, delta-radiomics has emerged as a promising approach for predicting treatment response and outcomes. Unlike static radiomics models, delta-radiomics captures temporal changes in radiomic features extracted from sequential imaging, thereby quantifying treatment-related changes in tumor characteristics and potentially providing improved insight into tumor characteristics.

In a previous study, Peeken et al. investigated the potential of MRI-based delta-radiomics in predicting pCR in patients with high-grade STS undergoing neoadjuvant therapy [18]. Their retrospective analysis included two independent patient cohorts: a training cohort of 103 patients and a test cohort of 53 patients. They extracted 105 radiomic features from T1-weighted contrast-enhanced fat-saturated and T2-weighted fat-saturated MRI sequences obtained before and after neoadjuvant therapy. Delta-radiomic features were calculated by absolute subtraction of post-therapeutic feature values from pretherapeutic values. Three techniques were compared for pCR prediction: random forest, elastic net regression, and LogitBoost. In nested cross-validation, the random forest models achieved the best mean performance and were selected to train the final models. The combined delta-radiomic models demonstrated superior predictive performance, achieving the best area under the receiver operating characteristic curve of 0.75 in the test cohort, surpassing single time point models, RECIST criteria, and tumor volume changes. Delta-radiomic models also demonstrated better reproducibility than single time point models, RECIST, or the peri-therapeutic volume changes. Interestingly, although association with pCR was the primary hypothesis, delta-radiomic models were significantly associated with OS in multivariate Cox regression. Taken together, this study highlights the potential of delta-radiomics as a predictive imaging biomarker for assessing treatment response in STS. As a noninvasive tool, it offers a promising avenue for optimizing treatment strategies, allowing for tailored treatment escalation or de-escalation based on individual response profiles.

BMs are the most common malignant brain tumors. Surgical resection followed by stereotactic radiotherapy (SRT) is recommended for patients with symptomatic or large BMs. A significant proportion of patients experience local failure (LF), which negatively impacts prognosis and quality of life. Identifying patients at high risk for local recurrence could allow for risk-adapted strategies, such as intensified follow-up, dose escalation of SRT, or systemic therapy.

Buchner et al. conducted a multicenter study to develop and externally validate a radiomics-based model to predict freedom from LF in patients with resected BMs undergoing postoperative SRT [19]. They analyzed MRI data from 352 patients, with a training cohort of 253 patients from two centers and an external validation cohort of 99 patients from five additional centers. CE metastases and the surrounding edema were segmented on T1-contrast-enhanced MRI and T2-FLAIR sequences, respectively. Feature selection was performed in several steps to improve model robustness. A minimum redundancy–maximum relevance ensemble feature selection framework was used to select relevant features. Three different ML models were tested: random forest, extreme gradient boosting, and generalized linear models with elastic net regularization learner (ENR). Among them, ENR achieved the best performance in the internal validation. Different combinations of radiomic and clinical features, such as patient age, tumor histology, and location of the primary tumor, were compared. The best performing model incorporated both radiomic and clinical features. It achieved a concordance index (CI) of 0.77 in the external test cohort, significantly outperforming clinical models (best CI: 0.70). The model stratified patients into a low- and a high-risk group for LF, with Kaplan–Meier analysis demonstrating a significant LF difference between these groups. At 24 months post-treatment, LF was observed in only 9% of low-risk patients compared to 74% in the high-risk group, highlighting the ability of the model to meaningfully differentiate outcomes. Furthermore, the model retained its predictive capability when applied to tumor segmentations generated by a previously trained neural network, demonstrating its feasibility for automated workflows.

This study highlights the potential of radiomics as a predictive imaging biomarker for assessing local control in patients with BMs. By incorporating MRI-derived quantitative features into an ML framework, the proposed model outperformed clinical models, providing an opportunity for personalized treatment adaptation.

Both studies discussed exemplify the potential of AI-based outcome prediction as a powerful predictive tool in oncology. Such approaches have the potential to enhance risk stratification, guide personalized treatment decisions, and ultimately improve patient outcomes. However, further validation through prospective, multicenter studies, and standardized implementation is essential to fully translate these findings into routine clinical practice.

27.3 Future Perspectives of AI Application

27.3.1 Foundation Models

Foundation AI models represent a transformative advancement in AI, marking a significant departure from traditional narrow DL systems. Unlike conventional DL models designed specifically for singular, supervised tasks, foundation models are trained on extensive and heterogeneous datasets using SSL techniques. This approach eliminates the necessity of task-specific human annotations, instead leveraging large-scale unlabeled data, which is abundantly available in various domains, including research and clinical practice.

Large language models (LLMs) exemplify this paradigm shift, demonstrating remarkable flexibility in generating context-appropriate responses from text prompts. These models' capabilities extend far beyond static, task-specific applications; by simply altering the input prompt, LLMs can perform a multitude of different tasks utilizing a single pretrained model. Moreover, the concept of multimodal foundation models builds upon this capability, integrating multiple data modalities, such as text, images, and potentially other sensory inputs, into a unified framework.

From the architectural side, multimodal foundation models typically use so-called "encoders," specific foundation models that transform the original input into a meaningful latent space embedding. These embeddings are then fed into architecture components that enable direct cross-attention between the multimodal input, often based on the transformer architecture. Depending on the amount of training data, frozen LLM transformers can be used with trainable adapters in between or can be directly fine-tuned. For output generation, a set of decoders can be employed to generate novel outputs, such as language or images.

In clinical contexts, multimodal foundation models hold substantial promise. They can autonomously interpret medical images, extract and synthesize pertinent clinical information from associated documentation, and perform sophisticated analyses that transcend basic imaging tasks. For instance, vision-language models (VLMs) integrate visual data, such as pathology images, with textual reports, enabling simultaneous verbal description and quantitative analysis. This holistic integration of diverse data sources allows for enhanced patient-specific analyses, aiding clinicians in making more informed and precise diagnostic and therapeutic decisions.

For radiation oncology specifically, multimodal VLMs with segmentation capabilities are of special interest. In recent months, a series of models have been introduced that allow text-to-segmentation capabilities. Based on a text prompt, specific structures such as OARs can be directly segmented. While current solutions suffer from only a few target variables, future models may contain a rich set of target volumes. If such models become clinically available, manual segmentation could transition to a novel type of interactive segmentation using written or spoken language with specific adaptations using point or box prompts.

Despite their considerable potential and expanding applicability, foundation AI models currently face several limitations. Primarily, these systems continue to depend significantly on human supervision and intervention. Issues such as data biases, ethical considerations, interpretability of model outputs, and the need for rigorous validation in clinical settings remain critical challenges. Addressing these limitations through ongoing research and interdisciplinary collaboration will be essential for fully realizing the transformative impact of foundation AI models in healthcare and beyond.

27.3.2 Explainability

A key challenge in implementing AI is ensuring that models not only make accurate predictions but also provide transparent and interpretable decision-making processes. Clinicians need to understand how an AI system arrives at its conclusions, especially when its recommendations influence treatment strategies. Explainability, therefore, plays a critical role in fostering trust, regulatory acceptance, and clinical adoption of AI tools. To enhance transparency and clinical usability, multimodal VLMs have emerged as a promising approach, bridging the gap between medical imaging interpretation and clinical decision-making. These models, which simultaneously process and integrate visual and textual information, can potentially transform automated reporting systems in radiation oncology through several mechanisms. First, VLMs can interpret medical images (CT, MRI, and PET) alongside relevant clinical notes, previous treatment plans, and dose distribution maps to generate comprehensive, context-aware reports that mimic the cognitive process of expert radiation oncologists. This capability extends beyond simple annotation to include reasoned assessments of tumor response, critical structure constraints, and potential treatment adaptations. Second, these models offer enhanced explainability through their ability to localize specific regions of interest while providing natural language explanations for their assessments, creating an interpretable decision trail that supports clinical validation. For example, when identifying potential areas of treatment failure or radiation-induced toxicity, VLMs can highlight relevant imaging features while generating explanatory text that references established radiological criteria and dosimetric thresholds. This explanation capability addresses one of the most significant barriers to clinical AI adoption: the "black box" problem that has limited physician trust in algorithmic recommendations. Third, multimodal approaches show promise in standardizing radiation oncology reporting across institutions, potentially reducing interobserver variability while maintaining the nuanced interpretation necessary for personalized treatment planning. Looking forward, the implementation of foundation model architectures with domain-specific fine-tuning presents an opportunity to develop systems that continuously learn from institutional feedback while maintaining alignment with expert clinical judgment. Early research suggests that multimodal VLMs may achieve superior performance in tasks requiring complex reasoning, such as adaptive planning decisions and treatment response assessment, compared to unimodal approaches. However, significant challenges remain, including the need for carefully curated multimodal datasets that maintain patient privacy, methods to evaluate hallucination risk in generated reports, and regulatory frameworks to govern the implementation of these systems in clinical practice.

Despite these challenges, the trajectory of technological advancement suggests that within the next decade, multimodal VLMs could become essential tools in radiation oncology departments, serving not as replacements for human expertise but as augmentative systems that enhance clinical decision-making through improved information synthesis and communication. As the field progresses, interdisciplinary collaboration between radiation oncologists, medical physicists, and AI researchers will be crucial to ensure these systems are developed with appropriate clinical validation metrics and integrated into workflows in ways that enhance rather than complicate the radiation oncology treatment process.

27.3.3 AI Agents

So far, the integration of AI in radiation oncology has focused primarily on specialized tasks, including tumor segmentation, radiotherapy planning, or response assessment, as discussed in the previous sections. However, routine clinical workflows involve a wide range of interrelated tasks. Identifying, selecting, and optimizing appropriate AI tools for each of these steps is challenging and resource-intensive, significantly limiting the practicality and widespread adoption of single-purpose AI models in clinical routine. The novel concept of "AI agents" may fill these gaps, generating a new class of AI tools that can operate autonomously and thereby fulfill a whole series of independent tasks.

AI agents are autonomous AI systems designed to operate independently by understanding specific tasks and the broader context and goals of their environment [20]. Unlike conventional AI models that execute narrowly defined tasks, AI agents evaluate multiple factors within a given scenario to make informed decisions. They typically achieve this by having an internal representation of available resources, including various specialized AI tools, each with distinct characteristics and capabilities.

Structurally, AI agents are usually composed of several interconnected components: perception modules for gathering and interpreting data; decision-making modules that evaluate contexts and determine optimal actions; and execution modules that select and utilize the appropriate AI tools or resources to carry out these actions. These subcomponents often require iterative looping, either between different modules or after the completion of subtasks, to refine outcomes, adapt to new information, or adjust strategies dynamically. By integrating these modules with iterative feedback loops, AI agents autonomously select relevant data, choose the most suitable tools, and determine the timing of their application, thus effectively addressing complex problems that require contextual awareness and adaptive reasoning.

This holistic capability can be illustrated by imagining an advanced AI agent supporting the management of patients with HNC in radiation oncology. During multidisciplinary tumor board discussions, the AI agent leverages various analytical tools, including specialized DL models and comprehensive multimodal foundation models, to thoroughly analyze multimodal patient data such as PET, CT, and MRI, histopathological images and reports, genomic profiles, and patient comorbidities. Utilizing an LLM backbone, the AI agent summarizes all patient information and integrates it with relevant medical guidelines, which are retrieved via augmented generation systems tailored specifically to the patient's clinical context. Based on this comprehensive analysis, the agent formulates detailed treatment recommendations, extending beyond basic treatment modality selection to include specific suggestions such as proton therapy. Importantly, rather than acting autonomously, the agent fosters interactive discussions within the tumor board, encouraging clinicians to deliberate carefully on treatment implications, potential toxicities, and the balance between therapeutic efficacy and patient quality of life.

In addition, multiple AI agents can work together to manage a patient's treatment. For instance, an additional agent specialized in radiation treatment planning may take responsibility for generating and subsequently re-optimizing treatment plans throughout the course of therapy. During this procedure, target volume definition would be conducted by combining patient-specific information, imaging findings, and target delineation guidelines, and executing the target volume definition via a multimodal vision language segmentation model. The resulting target volumes, after acceptance by a radiation oncologist, could be further processed by dosimetrist AI agents. Potential plan adaptations could further be conducted by a quality assurance AI agent.

Currently, this advanced AI agent framework is primarily being explored outside of medicine in sectors such as autonomous driving, logistics, and robotics; its potential applicability to healthcare is increasingly recognized. With ongoing developments, such integrated AI agent systems may soon transition from theoretical and experimental stages into practical clinical reality in the coming years. However, current medical device regulations are not yet prepared for these advanced AI agent techniques and will require significant adaptation to accommodate their integration.

In conclusion, the emerging concept of "AI agents," autonomous systems with interconnected modules for perception, decision-making, and execution, aims to manage complex, interrelated clinical workflows dynamically and contextually. By evaluating multimodal patient data and integrating medical guidelines, these agents could significantly enhance personalized treatment planning and interdisciplinary clinical decision-making.

References

1. Peeken JC, Nüsslin F, Combs SE (2017) Radio-oncomics. Strahlenther Onkol 193(10):767–779. https://doi.org/10.1007/s00066-017-1175-0
2. Whybra P, Zwanenburg A, Andrearczyk V, Schaer R, Apte AP, Ayotte A et al (2024) The image biomarker standardization initiative: standardized convolutional filters for reproducible Radiomics and enhanced clinical insights. Radiology 310(2):e231319. https://doi.org/10.1148/radiol.231319
3. Peeken JC, Bernhofer M, Spraker MB, Pfeiffer D, Devecka M, Thamer A et al (2019) CT-based radiomic features predict tumor grading and have prognostic value in patients with soft tissue sarcomas treated with neoadjuvant radiation therapy. Radiother Oncol 135:187–196. https://doi.org/10.1016/j.radonc.2019.01.004
4. LeCun Y, Bengio Y, Hinton G (2015) Deep learning. Nature 521(7553):436–444. https://doi.org/10.1038/nature14539
5. Dosovitskiy A, Lucas B, Kolesnikov A, Weissenborn D, Zhai X, Thomas U, Dehghani M, Minderer M, Heigold G, Sylvain G, Uszkoreit J, Houlsby N (2021) An image is worth 16×16 words: transformers for image recognition at scale. International conference on learning representations 2021

6. Bakas S, Reyes M, Jakab A, Bauer S, Rempfler M, Crimi A, et al (2018) Identifying the best machine learning algorithms for brain tumor segmentation, progression assessment, and overall survival prediction in the BRATS challenge. arXiv preprint arXiv:181102629
7. Villanueva-Meyer JE, Bakas S, Tiwari P, Lupo JM, Calabrese E, Davatzikos C et al (2024) Artificial intelligence for response assessment in neuro oncology (AI-RANO), part 1: review of current advancements. Lancet Oncol 25(11):e581-e8. https://doi.org/10.1016/s1470-2045(24)00316-4
8. Lustberg T, van Soest J, Gooding M, Peressutti D, Aljabar P, van der Stoep J et al (2018) Clinical evaluation of atlas and deep learning based automatic contouring for lung cancer. Radiother Oncol 126(2):312–317. https://doi.org/10.1016/j.radonc.2017.11.012
9. Erdur AC, Rusche D, Scholz D, Kiechle J, Fischer S, Llorian-Salvador O et al (2025) Deep learning for autosegmentation for radiotherapy treatment planning: state-of-the-art and novel perspectives. Strahlenther Onkol 201(3):236–254
10. Hurkmans C, Bibault JE, Brock KK, van Elmpt W, Feng M, David Fuller C et al (2024) A joint ESTRO and AAPM guideline for development, clinical validation and reporting of artificial intelligence models in radiation therapy. Radiother Oncol 197:110345. https://doi.org/10.1016/j.radonc.2024.110345
11. Lipkova J, Angelikopoulos P, Wu S, Alberts E, Wiestler B, Diehl C et al (2019) Personalized radiotherapy design for glioblastoma: integrating mathematical tumor models, multimodal scans, and Bayesian inference. IEEE Trans Med Imaging 38(8):1875–1884. https://doi.org/10.1109/tmi.2019.2902044
12. Ezhov I, Scibilia K, Franitza K, Steinbauer F, Shit S, Zimmer L et al (2023) Learn-morph-infer: a new way of solving the inverse problem for brain tumor modeling. Med Image Anal 83:102672. https://doi.org/10.1016/j.media.2022.102672
13. Weidner J, Ezhov I, Balcerak M, Metz MC, Litvinov S, Kaltenbach S et al (2025) A learnable prior improves inverse tumor growth modeling. IEEE Trans Med Imaging 44(3):1297–1307. https://doi.org/10.1109/tmi.2024.3494022
14. Mastella E, Calderoni F, Manco L, Ferioli M, Medoro S, Turra A et al (2025) A systematic review of the role of artificial intelligence in automating computed tomography-based adaptive radiotherapy for head and neck cancer. Phys Imaging Radiat Oncol:100731
15. Bakas S, Vollmuth P, Galldiks N, Booth TC, Aerts H, Bi WL et al (2024) Artificial intelligence for response assessment in neuro oncology (AI-RANO), part 2: recommendations for standardisation, validation, and good clinical practice. Lancet Oncol 25(11):e589–e601. https://doi.org/10.1016/s1470-2045(24)00315-2
16. Kickingereder P, Isensee F, Tursunova I, Petersen J, Neuberger U, Bonekamp D et al (2019) Automated quantitative tumour response assessment of MRI in neuro-oncology with artificial neural networks: a multicentre, retrospective study. Lancet Oncol 20(5):728–740. https://doi.org/10.1016/s1470-2045(19)30098-1
17. Bera K, Braman N, Gupta A, Velcheti V, Madabhushi A (2022) Predicting cancer outcomes with radiomics and artificial intelligence in radiology. Nat Rev Clin Oncol 19(2):132–146. https://doi.org/10.1038/s41571-021-00560-7
18. Peeken JC, Asadpour R, Specht K, Chen EY, Klymenko O, Akinkuoroye V et al (2021) MRI-based delta-radiomics predicts pathologic complete response in high-grade soft-tissue sarcoma patients treated with neoadjuvant therapy. Radiother Oncol 164:73–82. https://doi.org/10.1016/j.radonc.2021.08.023
19. Buchner JA, Kofler F, Mayinger M, Christ SM, Brunner TB, Wittig A et al (2024) Radiomics-based prediction of local control in patients with brain metastases following postoperative stereotactic radiotherapy. Neuro-Oncology 26(9):1638–1650. https://doi.org/10.1093/neuonc/noae098
20. Lee Y, Ferber D, Rood JE, Regev A, Kather JN (2024) How AI agents will change cancer research and oncology. Nat Cancer 5(12):1765–1767. https://doi.org/10.1038/s43018-024-00861-7

Non-invasive Imaging Techniques: From Histology to *In-vivo* Imaging

28

Elena Corbetta, Anja Silge, Hyeonsoo Bae, Marko Rodewald, Fisseha Bekele Legesse, Tobias Meyer, Jürgen Popp, and Thomas Bocklitz

28.1 Introduction

All imaging techniques are based on the interactions of particles or waves with the molecules or atoms of the sample.[1] Examples of particles used for imaging are photons of different energies or electrons, while ultrasound waves are examples of waves used for similar applications. After the interaction with the sample takes place, either newly generated particles/waves or missing particles/waves are measured [1]. The particles and waves used for imaging can be diverse and must be selected according to the samples to be imaged. For example, ultrasound waves

[1] Due to the wave-particle duality, the separation between particles and waves is not strict and an object can be described as wave or particle.

E. Corbetta · T. Bocklitz (✉)
Research Department of Photonic Data Science, Leibniz Institute of Photonic Technology, Jena, Germany

Institute of Physical Chemistry (IPC) and Abbe Center of Photonics (ACP), Friedrich Schiller University Jena, Jena, Germany
e-mail: elena.corbetta@uni-jena.de; thomas.bocklitz@uni-jena.de

A. Silge · H. Bae · M. Rodewald · F. B. Legesse · T. Meyer
Institute of Physical Chemistry (IPC), Friedrich Schiller University Jena, Jena, Germany
e-mail: anja.silge@leibniz-ipht.de; hyeonsoo.bae@uni-jena.de; marko.rodewald@polimi.it; tobias.meyer@leibniz-ipht.de

J. Popp
Institute of Physical Chemistry (IPC) and Abbe Center of Photonics (ACP), Friedrich Schiller University Jena, Jena, Germany

Research Department of Spectroscopy and Imaging, Leibniz Institute of Photonic Technology, Jena, Germany
e-mail: juergen.popp@leibniz-ipht.de

O. Schober et al. (eds.), *Molecular Imaging in Oncology - Volume 2*, Recent Results in Cancer Research 225, https://doi.org/10.1007/978-3-032-21415-7_10

are used in ultrasound imaging, where the detected signal represents the fraction of waves that are not absorbed. It is beyond the scope of this chapter to review all the interactions and the corresponding imaging techniques. Therefore, we will focus on photon–matter interactions and emphasize interactions that do not destroy the molecules of the sample [2]. The imaging methods that are derived from these interactions can be used for non-destructive tissue imaging and *in-vivo* applications. As photon–matter interaction is composition dependent, all these imaging methods can be used to highlight the general chemical composition of the sample or the spatial distribution of specific molecules or molecular groups within the sample. An overview of the techniques described in this chapter is visualized in Fig. 28.1.

Photon–matter interactions can be classified into three broad categories: absorption-based, emission-based and scattering-based interactions. In the first type of interaction, a photon is absorbed and its energy is transferred to an electron of the molecule, transferring this electron to an excited state.[2] After a certain time, the system exits the excited state by re-emitting part of the energy, often as a photon. In contrast, scattering interactions are working instantaneously, i.e. without time delay. The scattering processes generate a time-dependent dipole in the molecule, which subsequently radiates. All types of photon–matter interactions and the corresponding imaging techniques can be further categorized into linear or nonlinear processes according to their dependence on the excitation intensity, which is called the order of the process.

In addition to the intensity dependence of the physical processes discussed above, two additional aspects are important for bioimaging techniques. The first

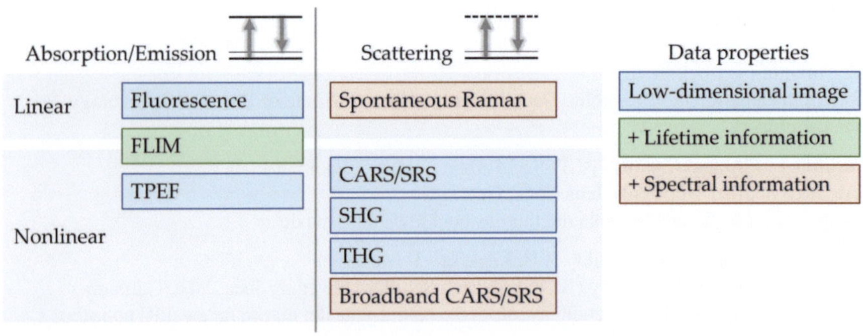

Fig. 28.1 Overview of non-invasive imaging techniques described in this chapter. The schematic represents various imaging techniques that are located in the chart according to the photon–matter interaction type (absorption/emission or scattering), and the physical process involved (linear or nonlinear, according to the dependence on the excitation intensity). In addition, the colours indicate whether the basic implementations of the methods provide single-channel images, additional lifetime information or additional spectral information that generates multi–/hyper-spectral images. (See text for more details)

[2] It should be noted here that an absorption can also occur in vibrational states. The corresponding imaging technique based on IR absorption is not described in this section.

aspect is whether the measurement results in (hyper)spectral scans or in low-dimensional images: the former approach is called spectral imaging, while the latter is called band integration or imaging mode. This property has an impact on the information depth and on the measurement time, which are higher for spectral imaging. The second aspect is the need for specific labels for imaging. We have decided to review methods that do not necessarily require a label for measurement. Therefore, all the techniques presented can be applied under *in-vivo* conditions, because they are also label-free and non-destructive [2].

In this chapter, we give a brief introduction and review the applications of the following scattering-based techniques: spontaneous Raman spectral imaging, coherent anti-Stokes Raman scattering (CARS), stimulated Raman scattering (SRS), second harmonic generation (SHG) and third harmonic generation (THG). Additionally, we present absorption-based techniques: two-photon excited fluorescence (TPEF) and fluorescence lifetime imaging (FLIM). In both fluorescence-based imaging techniques, we focus on the label-free version of the technique, where intrinsic fluorophores of the samples are visualized. We do not review IR-absorption-based imaging in this chapter, because an *in-vivo* application seems challenging at the current state of the art. At the end of the chapter, we briefly review chemometric and machine learning methods that are essential for the use of the presented imaging methods in diagnostic applications.

28.2 Raman Spectral Imaging/Spectroscopy

The first imaging technique to be reviewed is Raman spectral imaging, which is a scattering technique based on inelastic light scattering from the vibrational states of the molecules in the sample. Raman spectroscopy is suitable for measuring biological specimens because it is non-destructive and label-free. In addition, it can be combined with a microscope to generate an imaging modality that allows a non-invasive and label-free measurement of the composition of samples of biomedical interest.

The initial step of Raman spectral imaging is the irradiation of a sample with laser light. The backscattered radiation from the illuminated area of the sample is detected spectroscopically and the elastic (Rayleigh) scattered photons, which have the same frequency as the incoming photons, are filtered out. In addition to this elastic scattered light, only a small percentage of the scattered light is frequency shifted due to inelastic scattering. The frequency shifts are specific for the molecular vibrations within the excited sample area and indirectly represent the molecular composition. The result of the spectroscopic measurement of the inelastic scattered light is called the Raman spectrum. The scattering process can cause frequency shifts to lower energies ω_{L-vib} compared to the incoming radiation ω_L, which is called Stokes–Raman scattering. The scattering process also causes frequency shifts to higher energies ω_{L+vib}, which is called anti-Stokes Raman scattering. The Raman imaging techniques described below make use of Stokes–Raman scattering, as this is the dominant effect at room temperature.

Raman scattering can be observed through a microscope, applying the instrumental set-up presented in Fig. 28.2a. The laser light ω_L enters the microscope through a small pinhole and is focused by an objective to a spot size corresponding to the diffraction limit. Typically, the scattered light from the illuminated spot is collected by the same objective in back-scattering geometry and the Raman-scattered light ω_{L-vib} is selectively guided to the spectrometer coupled to the microscope. This implementation allows to collect spectra from spatially resolved image points. To build a Raman spectral scan, the focused laser can be moved over the sample by galvanometer mirror systems, or the sample can be moved relative to the laser focus using high-precision piezo stages. Due to the confocal pinhole, i.e. an aperture, only the light from the respective focal volume is detected, leading to a depth resolution (Fig. 28.2a). Raman imaging produces datasets of several thousand individual spectra. The subsequent computer-based image generation can be best described by a hyper-spectral data cube, visualized in Fig. 28.2b. The x and y directions represent the spatial dimension of the image for a single focal plane. The spectral dimension is plotted in the third direction and is indicated by λ. Within the data cube, each pixel at position x, y is containing a Raman spectrum. Therefore, each pixel contains the molecular fingerprint within the respective sampling volume on a given point x, y [3, 4].

The data analysis pipeline for such a Raman spectral data cube is described in Sect. 28.6 in detail, but it is roughly sketched here. To generate an image based on a Raman spectral scan, the hyperspectral data cube is reoriented into a 2D data

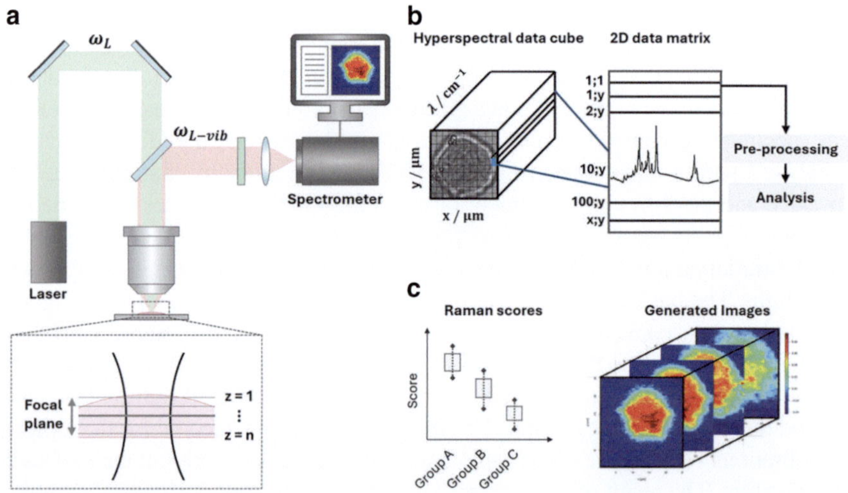

Fig. 28.2 Principles of the Raman spectral image generation. (**a**) Schematic of a confocal Raman microscope, designed to probe spatially resolved image points. The sample is probed by a laser ω_L focused through a microscope objective. The Stokes–Raman scattered light ω_{L-vib} is guided to a spectrometer and detected. (**b**) Hyperspectral data cube, each pixel at position x, y represents a unique spectrum. On the right, data pipeline for feature extraction and generation of molecular images. (See text for more details) (**c**) Example results obtained upon application of the data pipeline, showing extracted features and false-colour Raman images

matrix. In this matrix, every spectrum is pre-processed for a robust data analysis of the entire Raman scan. The pre-processing procedure includes calibration routines and corrections for artefacts and noise contributions. From every wavenumber slice of the data cube, a Raman false colour image can be generated (Fig. 28.2c). In this manner, the spatial distribution of defined marker signals, e.g. Raman bands, can be visualized. For a deeper understanding, clustering algorithms, as well as classification and regression methods, are applied. The output of these multivariate methods can be utilized to translate the measured Raman spectra into biomedical information that can be further used by biologists or physicians [5]. An example of such information would be the appearance of biomarkers, biochemical alterations or the detection of the concentration of substances described by the generated Raman score or images. This translation is explained in more detail in Sect. 28.6.

In the field of cancer research, in vitro Raman spectral imaging is often employed for diagnostic and therapy assessment: by identifying changes in the biochemical composition of proteins, biofluids, cells and tissues, it is possible to reveal *spectral biomarkers* to monitor disease progression [8]. For example, cell models are analysed to detect subcellular structures and spectral changes induced by a treatment with chemotherapeutic agents or due to a changed metabolism (Fig. 28.3A) [9–11]. Other studies explored intracellular lipid accumulations using Raman spectral imaging, which provided new insights into inflammation processes and cancer progression [6, 12]. In the field of cytopathology, Raman spectral signatures have been utilized to differentiate between cell types like normal and tumour cells circulating in body fluids, for example, for oral cancer diagnosis [13, 14].

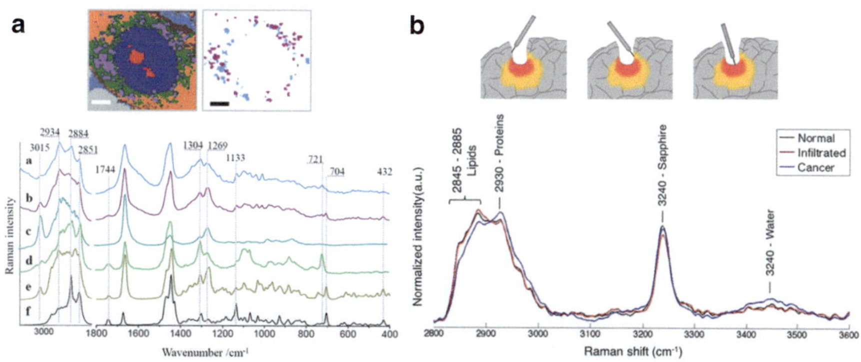

Fig. 28.3 Example Raman measurements of human cells and tissue. (**A**) Top figures: k-means cluster analysis on Raman measurements of human endothelial cells exposed to tumour necrosis (left) and lipid bodies (right). Bottom plot: Raman spectra of subclasses of lipid bodies (a, b) are compared to analytical standards of lipids, namely arachidonic acid (c), phosphatidylcholine (d), cholesteryl arachidonate (e) and cholesteryl stearate (f). Scale bar: 6 μm. Image taken and adapted from [6], under Creative Commons Attribution 4.0 International License (**B**) Top figure: Schematic of *in-vivo* Raman measurements of normal brain (left), infiltrated brain (centre) and dense cancer (right) taken in the surgical cavity during glioma resection. (Image taken and adapted from [7], under Creative Commons Attribution 4.0 International License (https://creativecommons.org/licenses/by/4.0/))

For detecting alterations in tissues, Raman imaging can be an alternative method for in situ, low-invasive and real-time clinical investigation and can offer some advantages compared to golden standards like bioassays and staining procedures. Thanks to these properties, Raman microspectroscopy has been investigated for intraoperative applications [15]. In this context, *spectral histopathology* is a term that refers to the use of optical and spectroscopic techniques for the investigation of the morphochemistry of tissues. This investigation involves a wide variety of optical techniques described in this chapter, including Raman imaging. By using this spectral histopathology, chemical and molecular changes can be directly obtained from the examined samples and correlated with the histopathological gold standard Hematoxylin and Eosin staining (H&E) [16]. Then, the Raman spectral signatures of a specimen are linked to the pathologist's diagnosis to construct a classification model that can be applied for the differential diagnosis of new samples, e.g. the discrimination between normal and tumour regions and the visualization of tumour margins [17]. In [18], the adenoma-carcinoma-sequence was studied using a Raman-based spectral histopathology. The introduced Raman-based workflow featured 100% mean sensitivity for the prediction of normal and tumour tissue compared to the gold standard diagnosis of an experienced pathologist. This spectral histopathology workflow was also tested for the Raman spectral imaging of brain metastases and a prediction of the primary tumour could be achieved with high sensitivity [19]. A further development of the Raman spectral imaging concept is its use within a core needle biopsy system. The system allows an in situ tumour analysis by applying molecular Raman imaging and a differentiation between healthy and tumour tissue before tissue harvesting. This approach has been successfully tested in brain surgery, as shown in Fig. 28.3B, with the development of intraoperative, label-free devices that can improve cancer targeting and reduce the risk of patients undergoing multiple biopsies [7].

28.3 Coherent Raman Spectroscopy and Spectromicroscopy: CARS and SRS

Linear Raman spectroscopy-based imaging has several advantages, as described above. Nevertheless, it has one major drawback, which is the low efficiency of the process, leading to long measurement times. This drawback can be circumvented by nonlinear Raman-spectroscopic techniques, which are applied to biomedical imaging. The most commonly applied imaging methods are coherent anti-Stokes Raman scattering (CARS) and stimulated Raman scattering (SRS) [20–23], which are third-order processes. Opposite to second-order processes, which can be generated only under specific symmetry conditions of materials, third-order processes can be induced in all materials, resulting in a wide range of potential applications. Both techniques, CARS and SRS, address one of the major limitations of linear Raman spectroscopy-based methods, which is the small scattering cross section of spontaneous Raman scattering and the resulting low signal. This drawback leads to severe limitations in the field of imaging and results in the need for long acquisition times, constantly requiring a trade-off between image size and image resolution.

Spontaneous in this context means that in linear Raman spectroscopy all individual molecular vibrations are excited independently of one another by a single laser frequency and do not exhibit any phase relationship. In coherent Raman spectroscopy, instead of the single laser frequency used in spontaneous Raman, two frequencies ω_p (p = pump) and ω_S (S = Stokes) are used. As depicted in Fig. 28.4, by matching the difference frequency (i.e. the beat-frequency) $\omega_p - \omega_S$ to a specific Raman-active molecular vibration ω_R, those vibrations can be driven coherently. From simple energy conservation, $\omega_{aS} = 2\omega_p - \omega_S$ arises. Therefore, in CARS spectroscopy, a third photon ω_{aS} can then be inelastically scattered from this ensemble of coherently vibrating molecules. Because of the shift of the anti-Stokes scattered photon to higher energies (blue shift), the CARS signal does not interfere with fluorescence, which is a major drawback of Raman spectral imaging. Additionally, the CARS signal is significantly enhanced compared to spontaneous Raman spectroscopy, opening the possibilities for fast imaging of large areas with high resolution and even video rate. These benefits come at the expense of lower spectral information, since the choice of ω_p and ω_S targets only a specific resonance. To overcome this limitation, broadband laser sources for the excitation beams have been developed [24–26] leading to CARS and SRS spectra. Other drawbacks, such as the need to meet specific phase matching criteria, are not an issue under the tight focusing conditions of microscope lenses and therefore do not cause inconveniences in the context of imaging [20]. The CARS signal is always accompanied by a non-resonant background caused by a four-wave mixing process that can be induced by the same laser pulses ($2\omega_p = \omega_S + \omega_a S$, in Fig. 28.4), leading to a relatively poor contrast in CARS imaging. The non-resonant background is largely independent from the resonant signal, and its effect is therefore more severe for modes with low Raman intensities.

In SRS spectroscopy, a photon of frequency ω_S stimulates the emission of a second photon at the same frequency upon interaction with the virtual state reached by ω_p if $\omega_p - \omega_S$ matches the vibrational resonance ω_R. This leads to an energy transfer from the pump beam to the Stokes beam. Depending on whether the intensity loss

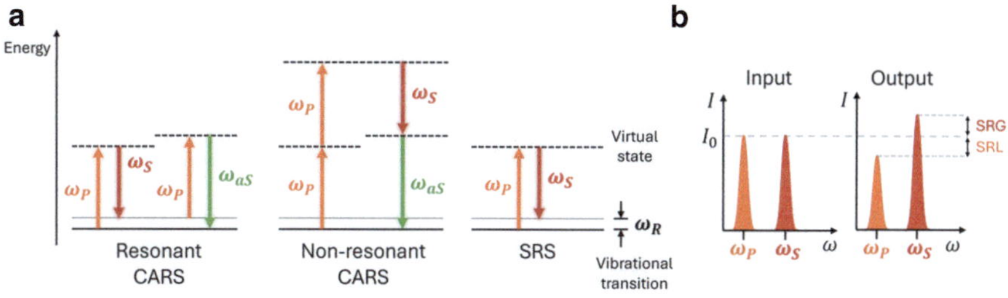

Fig. 28.4 Energy level diagram of different CARS and SRS processes. (**a**) The panel shows, from left to right, the resonant CARS, the non-resonant CARS and the SRS process. (**b**) Representation of stimulated Raman gain (SRG) and stimulated Raman loss (SRL) induced during SRS processes

of the pump beam or the intensity gain of the Stokes beam is detected, the technique is called stimulated Raman loss spectroscopy (SRLS), or stimulated Raman gain spectroscopy (SRGS). Since these losses or gains are usually small compared to the initial laser power, SRLS and SRGS rely on very sophisticated detection methods. In contrast to CARS, the generated signal is linearly dependent on the analyte concentration and has no intrinsic background, leading to easier quantification and better contrast in imaging applications, especially when dealing with low analyte concentrations. It does, however, interfere with fluorescence caused by ω_p. Nevertheless, this drawback can be suppressed by lock-in detection.

Both CARS and SRS microscopy provide molecular information that can be linked with pathological conditions [22, 27]. This molecular information is intrinsic to the respective sample, eliminating the need for labels or staining techniques. Figure 28.5 shows an example CARS image of a human tissue. In this figure, three vibrational resonances (2845 cm^{-1}, 2930 cm^{-1} and 3030 cm^{-1}) were measured, and the corresponding images are shown on the left. The combination of the individual images, shown on the right, leads to a non-invasive tissue characterization. In this combination, image nuclei are shown in green, the cytoplasm is represented in red and water is shown in cyan. Thus, also CARS and SRS might be used as spectral histopathology techniques, as they might not only add to the repertoire of pathologists, but potentially even replace common staining techniques. The combination with computer-aided data analysis, such as machine learning or deep learning, promises high diagnostic performance. The ultimate goal in this regard is fast and reliable on-site diagnostics, including *in-vivo* imaging during surgery [28–30].

Typical samples for CARS and SRS microscopy are tissue sections and cell assays, but bulk samples can also be studied. The 3D imaging capabilities of the techniques vary depending on the sample type and the laser frequencies but usually penetration

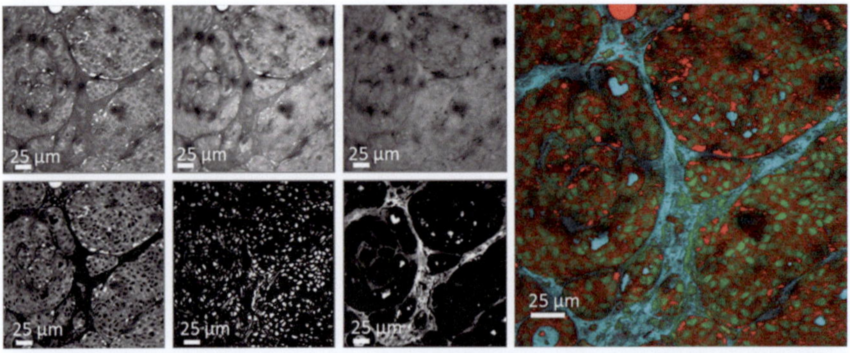

Fig. 28.5 Example CARS image of a human tissue. The small images on the top row correspond to different mapped vibrations, namely, from left to right, 2845 cm^{-1}, 2930 cm^{-1} and 3030 cm^{-1}. The images in the lower row show difference images generated by subtracting the images in the top row from one another to highlight the tissue features corresponding to different chemical stretches. The combined false colour image on the right highlights nuclei in green, cytoplasm in red and water in cyan. (Reprinted and adapted with permission from Ref. [27], Taylor & Francis Group, LLC)

depths of 100–200 μm are achievable, with some studies reporting even larger penetration depths by using adaptive optics [31]. The maximum resolution for a given set of wavelengths is slightly better than in diffraction-limited-white light microscopy due to the nonlinear nature of the processes. In fact, thanks to the nonlinear intensity dependence of the processes, the CARS/SRS signal is generated only in confined regions with high excitation intensity. Nevertheless, a compromise must be found between image size, acquisition speed and resolution. To meet clinical needs, considerable effort is put into miniaturizing the devices, as well as making them more reliable and user-friendly. In view of the on-site diagnostic potential, many groups worldwide are currently working on integrating the technique into endoscopic devices [32–34].

Other imaging modalities like second harmonic generation (SHG) and two-photon excited fluorescence (TPEF) are often seamlessly integrated into the same set-up since the corresponding signals are generated by the same strong laser fields as a side effect, thus providing additional valuable information. These techniques are described in the next section.

As mentioned above, single-frequency CARS/SRS techniques give signal levels that are orders of magnitude higher than linear Raman spectroscopy under appropriate conditions. However, the lower spectral information is not feasible to investigate complex systems, such as cells and tissues, where chemical species overlap in heterogeneous structures. Broadband implementations of CARS and SRS can be applied to overcome this limitation while keeping the high acquisition speed and signal level of coherent Raman processes. The two main experimental implementations of broadband microspectroscopy are based on hyperspectral or multiplex approaches. In hyperspectral techniques, narrow pump and Stokes pulses are tuned to scan the full spectral range of interest. In multiplex approaches, at least one among the pump and Stokes beam is broad in the frequency range, and the detected signal is acquired by a multichannel detector or by a Fourier transform approach. The mentioned techniques are still under development and are not yet established in clinical settings [35]. Recent studies have demonstrated the successful differentiation of tumorous and healthy cells with pixel dwell times down to 1 ms with a multiplex broadband CARS set-up [36]. However, this acquisition speed is not suitable for imaging large tissue sections and performing spectral histopathology studies. Alternative time-domain approaches have achieved much higher acquisition speeds, but these have mostly been applied to non-biological materials and require complex implementations [37]. Nevertheless, recent studies have demonstrated the diagnostic values of broadband methods for the study of body fluids, comparing these techniques to other experimental approaches [38].

28.4 Nonlinear Processes (SHG, THG, TPEF)

As described in the previous chapter, nonlinear phenomena such as CARS or SRS occur when high-intensity light interacts with molecules in biological samples. In addition to these Raman-related processes, other nonlinear processes are triggered by high intensities, such as two photon excited fluorescence (TPEF), second harmonic generation (SHG) and third harmonic generation (THG). These processes can be used in microscopic imaging techniques to achieve rapid and non-invasive investigation of cells and tissues with high resolution and depth of penetration, thanks to the generation of the nonlinear processes only in confined regions of the samples with high excitation intensity. These techniques also offer intrinsic optical sectioning and thus enable imaging inside thick tissue samples. The energy level diagrams for these nonlinear processes are depicted in Fig. 28.6a–c.

TPEF is a nonlinear fluorescence technique in which two photons of frequency ω are simultaneously absorbed to excite a fluorophore, which subsequently emits a fluorescence photon of frequency ω_{TPEF}. SHG is a second-order coherent scattering optical process wherein two incident photons of frequency ω are converted into a photon of twice their frequency ($\omega_{SHG} = 2\omega$). Analogous to SHG, THG converts three photons of frequency ω into a photon of three times their frequency ($\omega_{THG} = 3\omega$).

These nonlinear techniques have been employed as a contrast mechanism for optical imaging purposes and have readily been incorporated into laser scanning microscopy (LSM) set-ups, as the different nonlinear processes can be induced by the same excitation beam and collected by proper detection units [39, 40]. In LSMs, a laser beam is focused into a diffraction-limited spot and is raster-scanned across the sample. The tight focusing and small temporal width of pulsed laser sources lead to high peak intensities that are strong enough to induce nonlinear effects. A typical LSM used for nonlinear imaging is shown in Fig. 28.6d. The output of a tuneable pulsed near-infrared laser source is coupled to the galvanometer mirrors of the LSM. The scanning module of the LSM, consisting of a scan and tube lens, directs the beam onto the rear aperture of the objective, thereby translating the angular deflections of the galvanometer mirrors into lateral scanning of the focal spot in the focal plane. The generated signal is then collected either in the forward direction or in the epi-direction. Beam splitters are then needed to separate the generated signal from the excitation beam. The signal is eventually detected using a photo-multiplier tube (PMT) after passing through a series of detection filters, which are selected

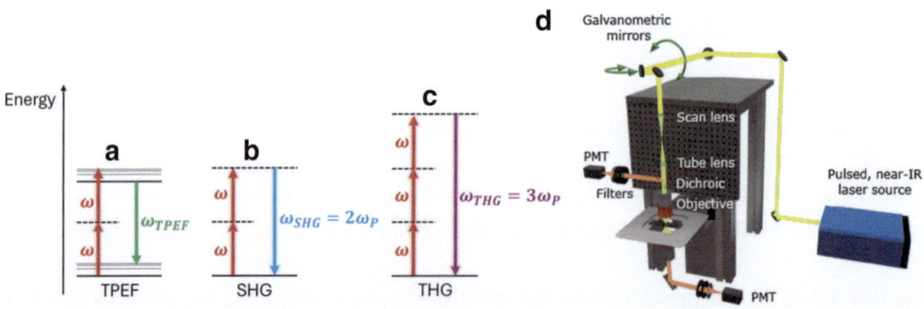

Fig. 28.6 Energy diagrams for nonlinear processes. Jablonski diagram of (**a**) two photon excited fluorescence (TPEF), (**b**) second harmonic generation (SHG) and (**c**) third harmonic generation (THG). (**d**) A laser scanning microscope (LSM) for nonlinear imaging

according to the specific nonlinear modality in order to extract the frequency generated by the process.

TPEF microscopy has been used to image several endogenous fluorophores in mammalian tissue. Among these fluorophores are porphyrins, amino acids, macromolecular proteins like collagen and elastin, as well as cofactors such as FAD and NAD(P)H [42]. Autofluorescence information, particularly from NAD(P)H, has been shown to be useful in differentiating between healthy and cancerous tissue [43]. In this regard, TPEF microscopy has been used for tumour tissue imaging and cancer diagnostics [42, 44].

SHG is a consequence of second-order nonlinear susceptibility; therefore, the incoming photons must interact simultaneously in a non-centrosymmetric medium to generate the signal of double frequency. Consequently, SHG maps the distribution of anisotropic biological structures with large hyperpolarizability [45, 46]. Most of the SHG signal in mammalian tissue arises from collagen, a highly ordered non-centrosymmetric structure [47]. The imaging of collagen with SHG has been demonstrated to provide information regarding the ageing, healing and tumour progression [44, 48].

Unlike the SHG process, THG is the result of third-order nonlinear susceptibility, which exists for all materials [40]. The THG signal is dependent on optical heterogeneities of objects in the probed medium, which allows the imaging of otherwise transparent samples [49]. For instance, THG has been used to image lipid droplets in the aqueous environment of the cell cytoplasm using the significant differences in the optical properties of lipid and water [50]. THG also has found versatile applications in cell and tissue research within the context of cancer diagnostics [51].

As mentioned before, these techniques are applied for spectral histopathology studies because they allow the label-free characterization of morphological changes associated with malignant transformation, such as increases in nuclear size and nuclei to cytoplasm ratio and loss of epithelial architecture [52, 53]. An example image of human tissue section measured by an endomicroscopic system combining CARS (red), SHG (blue) and TPEF (green) is shown in Fig. 28.7 together with a H&E stain of the same section [41]. In this figure, different tissue structures can be differentiated either using the stained section or the multimodal image. In this image, connective tissue is highlighted by SHG in blue (collagen fibres) and by TPEF in green (elastin fibres), while lipids from adipocytes are highlighted by CARS (red bubbles).

In recent studies, multimodal nonlinear imaging has been applied for the detection of different kinds of cancer [54, 55], and it has been integrated into endomicroscopic devices [56, 57].

The direct use of multimodal images in clinical settings remains a challenge because pathologists are trained to interpret stained images of tissues. To overcome this limitation and to exploit the information extracted from multimodal nonlinear imaging, new strategies are being investigated that involve the generation of virtual stained images from multimodal microscopy measurements using deep neural

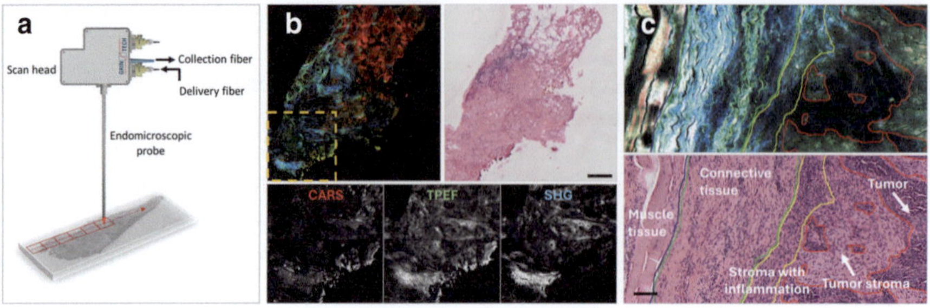

Fig. 28.7 Multimodal image of head and neck tissue section. (**a**) Schematics of the *ex-vivo* multimodal nonlinear measurement acquired by an endomicroscopic system. (**b**) Multimodal image of head and neck tissue section (top-left) and the same section after a H&E stain (top-right). In the bottom panels, single channels are displayed in greyscale for the image crop highlighted by the yellow dashed frame: red, green and blue represent CARS, TPEF and SHG measurements. Scale bar: 500 μm. (**c**) Multimodal and stained region of another tissue slice from the same study, with lines and annotations showing different kinds of tissue. Scale bar: 100 μm. (The images were taken and adapted from [41], distributed under a Creative Commons Attribution License 4.0 (CC BY, https://creativecommons.org/licenses/by/4.0/). See text for more details)

networks. These approaches combine the advantages of multimodal measurements with the interpretability of stained images [58, 59].

28.5 Fluorescence Lifetime Imaging (FLIM)

In addition to the above described TPEF, other fluorescence-based imaging methods exist. The most prominent fluorescence-based imaging technique is one-photon fluorescence imaging, which is usually applied in combination with exogenous labelling. After labelling, the spatial distribution of the labels and hence the spatial distribution of the labelled structures can be visualized. Important information about the fluorophore of interest is encoded not only in the fluorescence intensity, but also in the fluorescence lifetime, which is the average time a fluorophore remains in the excited state before decaying back to the ground state by emitting a fluorescence photon. Fluorophores can be often differentiated by their lifetime even though a differentiation based on their intensities is not possible, leading to an increased multiplexing capability of fluorescence lifetime imaging (FLIM). The fluorescence lifetime of endogenous fluorophores in biological samples typically varies in the range from hundreds to thousands of picoseconds [60, 61]. Because the fluorescence lifetime is sensitive to the local micro-environment of the fluorophore, FLIM can be used to monitor subtle changes in the chemical composition of tissues induced by disease progression, e.g. by cancer growth [62, 63].

In general, two dominant implementations are used for FLIM: the time-domain technique and the frequency-domain technique. In the time domain technique, the fluorescence signal is acquired as a function of time delay, while the frequency domain method measures the phase difference between excitation and fluorescence signals. According to the target application, variations for each approach can be selected by changing the sampling technique, the detection technique and the type of microscope [20]. The most applied (time-domain) FLIM detection techniques are Time-Correlated Single Photon Counting (TCSPC) or time-gated CCD acquisitions. In addition, fibre-based FLIM measurement concepts also exist [65].

FLIM is also combined with multiphoton techniques, such as TPEF. For example, two-photon FLIM (2p-FLIM) set-ups are based on laser scanning microscopes equipped with ultrafast pulsed lasers in the near-infrared as the excitation light source. This technique enables single-point fluorescence lifetime measurements with significantly reduced photobleaching and provides deeper penetration into tissue samples. An example of the 2p-FLIM system and fluorescence decay curves of different dyes are described in Fig. 28.8 [64]. The beam is scanned by scanning mirrors (one is a resonant scanning mirror (RM) for the fast axis, and another is a galvo-mirror (GM) for the slow axis) and focused on the sample. The synchronization of the data sampling clock of the detected signal from PMT and the laser pulse clock is precisely tuned to secure time-locked sampling of each data set.

FLIM has demonstrated extensive medical applicability. For example, it enables the imaging of the metabolic activity within cells and tissues by differentiating quantitative shifts in the fluorescence lifetime of NAD(P)H. Thus, FLIM has the potential to study possible metabolic rearrangements in various pathologies, particularly in cancer [63, 66]. Recent studies have demonstrated the huge potential of FLIM, thanks to its applicability *in-vivo* and in intraoperative settings [68–70].

Figure 28.9A [66] presents 2p-FLIM images of live cells and an example of the fitting procedure applied to retrieve the fluorescence lifetime. In addition to this, FLIM can track the metabolic changes in NADH fluorescence due to the applied treatment. Figure 28.9B shows an example differentiation of normal and pre-cancerous tissue by FLIM: the panel shows a 3d image stack of fluorescence lifetime components and their fractional distribution for normal and pre-cancerous sample, where the distribution of each fluorophore is visualized in color-coded images [67].

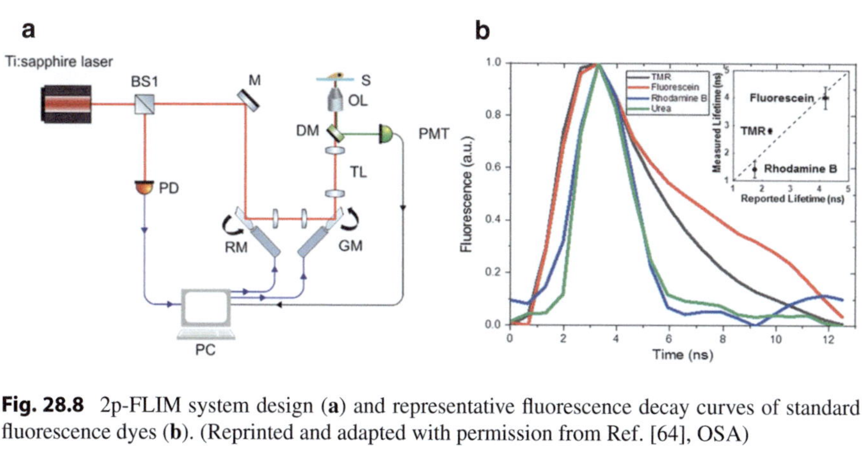

Fig. 28.8 2p-FLIM system design (**a**) and representative fluorescence decay curves of standard fluorescence dyes (**b**). (Reprinted and adapted with permission from Ref. [64], OSA)

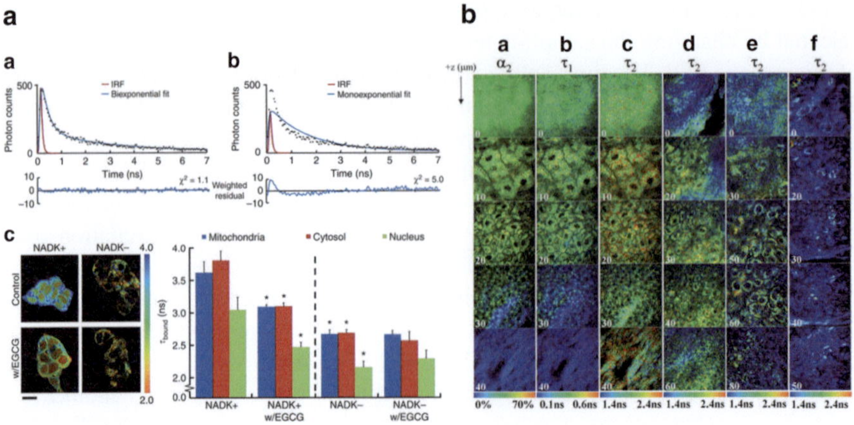

Fig. 28.9 FLIM images. (**A**) FLIM measurements to separate NADH and NADPH fluorescence in live cells. Panels (a) and (b) show that a biexponential decay model can describe the NAD(P)H fluorescence decay with a better fit than the monoexponential model. (c) Color-coded images of the mean lifetime τ_{bound} in NADK+ and NADK− HEK293 cells before and after a treatment to inhibit NADPH binding. Reprinted and adapted from [66]. (**B**) Multiphoton FLIM images of normal and pre-cancerous hamster cheek pouch. Panel (a–c) represents normal tissue and (d–f) shows altered tissue. The column (a) represents α_2, e.g. the contribution of the long lifetime component, while column (b) shows the short lifetime component τ_1 and columns (c–f) show the long lifetime component. The image size is 100 μm × 100 μm. (Reprinted and adapted with permission from Ref. [67], SPIE)

28.6 Machine Learning for Spectral and Image Data

The imaging modalities presented in the previous sections result in either images or spectral scans. In order to use these measurements for diagnostic purposes, the data must be translated into medically relevant information. For images this translation can—in principle—be done by manual inspection, whereas for higher-dimensional spectral scans, this approach is not possible. Although manual inspection is feasible for image data, an automated approach is preferable for both types of data, as it can convert spectral features and image structures into medical information more quickly and reliably. In addition, the measurement process is always constrained by a trade-off between imaging speed, spatial resolution, signal-to-noise ratio and sample health. In fact, only one of these aspects can usually be optimized, and biomedical applications always require the avoidance of sample degradation caused by light exposure. For this reason, it is not possible to rely only on optimizing the measurement process, but it is necessary to implement data processing and analysis methods to retrieve the information encoded in the measured data. This requires the implementation of standardized data pipelines to translate the measurement of the sample into medical knowledge (Fig. 28.10). These data pipelines are composed of processing and analysis steps, and include either machine learning and/or chemometric algorithms [71]. The two techniques are not very different, but 'machine learning' is a general term that is often used for images [72], as it can be applied to a variety

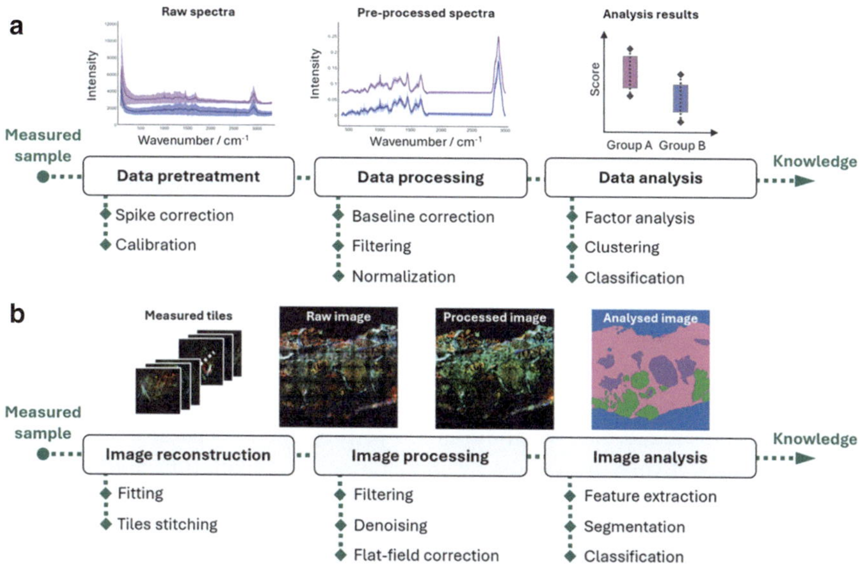

Fig. 28.10 Schematic of data pipelines for spectral and image data. Example data pipelines for spectral data (Raman spectra) (**a**) and image data (in this figure, multimodal nonlinear images composed of CARS, TPEF and SHG channels) (**b**) are implemented to extract quantitative knowledge from the measured samples. They include spectra pretreatment, image generation or reconstruction, processing and analysis algorithms. The figure shows possible algorithms implemented for each step, depending on the measurement technique. Multimodal nonlinear images in panel **b** are taken and adapted from [41], distributed under a Creative Commons Attribution License 4.0 (CC BY, https://creativecommons.org/licenses/by/4.0/). (See text for more details)

of data types, while 'chemometrics' [73] is a more specific term utilized for spectral data analysis models and it is related to the extraction of information from chemical systems. We will stick to this terminology throughout this section.

If chemometrics is utilized to analyse spectral data, such as the described Raman (Sect. 28.2), CARS and SRS spectra (Sect. 28.3), automatic spectral data pipelines are constructed (Fig. 28.10a). The pipelines combine data pre-treatment, data pre-processing and analysis methods. For Raman spectra, the pretreatment consists of spike correction, wavenumber and intensity calibration, baseline correction and smoothing [74]. In the case of CARS spectra, additional processing must be applied to deal with the non-resonant background, such as phase retrieval methods or deep learning based approaches [75, 76]. Thereafter, baseline correction, filtering and normalization have to be combined to pre-process and standardize the data. Analysis methods can be applied afterwards to the pretreated and pre-processed spectra. The analysis methods can be either factor analysis methods, clustering or classification methods. While factor methods can be utilized for dimension reduction, clustering methods can be used to highlight different groups in the data without prior knowledge. Instead, if prior knowledge is available, classification methods can be utilized to model group differences in a supervised manner. After training, the classification model can be used as a diagnostic model [72, 73].

When the experimental technique provides image data, image data pipelines are constructed (Fig. 28.10b) and machine learning can be included for data processing and analysis [71]. Image data can be derived in the case of TPEF, SHG, THG, FLIM, CARS and SRS microscopy. Some techniques require the prior generation of the image from the raw data. For example, an image reconstruction step must be added to fuse different views of the sample to generate three-dimensional datasets, or to align and stitch multiple tiles acquired from a large tissue section, as shown in Fig. 28.10b. In the case of FLIM, the image must be generated by fitting the experimental signal with exponential functions to retrieve the lifetime of the imaged fluorophores and their distribution [77]. Once the raw image is available, the data pipeline should address the various experimental artefacts that prevent a correct interpretation of the image content. The most common image artefacts include, but are not limited to, noise, loss of spatial resolution and uneven illumination of the sample. The artefacts can be removed, respectively, by denoising algorithms, deconvolution and/or super-resolution image reconstruction, and flat-field correction [78, 79]. Depending on prior information available and problem complexity, the processing methods can be implemented with different strategies. Calibration measurements estimate the degradation introduced by the optical system by measuring a reference sample prior to the actual measurement. Inverse modelling methods enhance the image quality by modelling the artefacts using the physical knowledge of the measurement process. As an alternative, deep learning methods can achieve powerful image restoration capabilities and have been explored for various types of imaging applications. Once the quality of the data has been enhanced, the images are analysed using standard methods or machine learning. The aim of image analysis is to extract quantitative knowledge from the image by identifying clearly the image content. Classification methods allocate the measured samples in a set of defined categories, including, for example, different kinds of tissue. Object detection methods aim at identifying the location of specific structures in the image, and can be paired with object tracking methods to follow the objects in a time-lapse move. Segmentation is applied to partition the image in regions of interest (i.e. a set of pixels) according to the different structures present in the measurement; if a classification label is assigned to each region, this is referred to as semantic segmentation. In case of classical machine learning, these image analysis tasks are performed by extracting prior image features, and then applying the chemometric techniques described above [71]. Alternatively, deep learning methods perform an intrinsic feature extraction and modelling [80, 81]. Deep learning constructs a highly parameterized model, which can be used as feature extraction method in combination with a classification model [72, 73].

Figure 28.11 shows the pipeline implemented for deep learning-based spectral histopathology to obtain an automatic semantic segmentation of human head and neck tissue slices.

Optical nonlinear measurements of CARS, TPEF and SHG signals were acquired by an endomicroscopic system and utilized to differentiate different tissue types, in

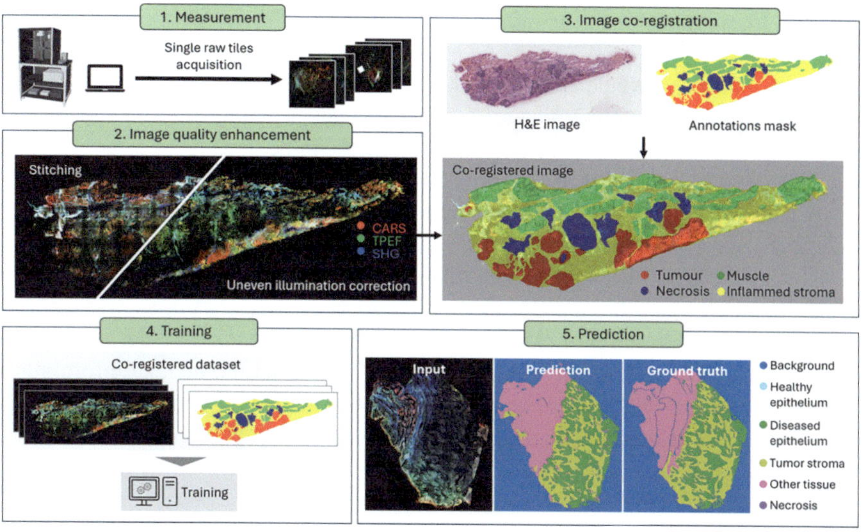

Fig. 28.11 Data pipeline from sample measurement to spectral histopathology analysis for head and neck human tissue. The experimental pipeline to perform deep learning based spectral histopathology starts with the measurement of the sample with multimodal nonlinear techniques (1), the application of image reconstruction and processing steps for image quality enhancement (2), and the co-registration of the multimodal measurements with annotation masks generated by an expert pathologist after staining the measured tissue slices (3). Then, a supervised deep learning model is trained on the pairs of multimodal images and annotation masks to generate semantic segmentation of the multimodal measurements (4). Finally, the trained model is utilized to obtain predictions directly from multimodal images (5). (The images were taken and adapted from [41], distributed under a Creative Commons Attribution License 4.0 (CC BY, https://creativecommons.org/licenses/by/4.0/))

particular to identify healthy and diseased areas. These processing and analysis methods enable the enhancement of image quality by removing the experimental artefacts introduced by the endomicroscopic system, such as uneven illumination, and the prediction of semantic segmentation masks for the identification of healthy and diseased areas [41].

Deep learning models have proven to be able to identify, in a fast and label-free manner, tumour infiltration in brain tissue measured just after resection during surgical operation [82]. In addition, as mentioned above, deep learning has been used to digitally generate alternative measurement modalities. Examples include the generation of virtual stained images from fluorescence and nonlinear microscopy measurements, and the generation of alternative microscopy modalities with resolution enhancement. These approaches reduce the experimental time required to obtain the target images and demonstrate that relevant information is encoded in multiple microscopy modalities. In this way, it is possible to measure relevant samples using minimally invasive techniques and then digitally translate the images into alternative modalities that may be more suitable for human interpretation [58, 59, 83].

28.7 Summary

In this chapter, we have described label-free and non-destructive bioimaging methods that enable the quantification of bio-chemical composition of samples. Therefore, the imaging techniques presented here can be used to measure samples of biomedical interest, and the information can be used for diagnostic applications or to gain a deeper insight into the ongoing processes in the sample. We have described several measurement techniques, namely Raman spectral imaging, CARS, SRS, TPEF, FLIM, 2p-FLIM, SHG and THG, and we shortly reviewed the application of these techniques for measurements of biological samples with a focus on cancer diagnostics and oncological applications. At the end, we described how chemometrics and machine learning are utilized to extract biomedical information from the generated data, an essential step to utilize the imaging modalities for diagnostic applications or to gain a deeper insight into the biological samples.

References

1. Popp J, Tuchin VV, Chiou A, Heinemann S (eds) (2011) Handbook of biophotonics: vol. 1: basics and techniques. Wiley-VCH
2. Vogler N, Heuke S, Bocklitz TW, Schmitt M, Popp J (2015) Multimodal imaging spectroscopy of tissue. Annu Rev Anal Chem 8:359–387
3. Abramczyk H, Brozek-Pluska B (2013) Raman imaging in biochemical and biomedical applications. Diagnosis and treatment of breast cancer. Chem Rev 113(8):5766–5781
4. Stewart S, Priore RJ, Nelson MP, Treado PJ (2012) Raman imaging. Annu Rev Anal Chem 5:337–360
5. Bocklitz TW, Guo S, Ryabchykov O, Vogler N, Popp J (2016) Raman based molecular imaging and analytics: a magic bullet for biomedical applications!? Anal Chem 88:133–151
6. Czamara K, Majzner K, Selmi A, Baranska M, Ozaki Y, Kaczor A (2017) Unsaturated lipid bodies as a hallmark of inflammation studied by Raman 2D and 3D microscopy. Sci Rep 7:40889
7. Desroches J, Jermyn M, Pinto M, Picot F, Tremblay M-A, Obaid S, Marple E, Urmey K, Trudel D, Soulez G et al (2018) A new method using Raman spectroscopy for in vivo targeted brain cancer tissue biopsy. Sci Rep 8(1):1792
8. El-Mashtoly SF, Gerwert K (2022) Diagnostics and therapy assessment using label-free Raman imaging. Anal Chem 94(1):120–142
9. Bräutigam K, Bocklitz T, Schmitt M, Rösch P, Popp J (2013) Raman spectroscopic imaging for the real-time detection of chemical changes associated with docetaxel exposure. ChemPhysChem 14:550–553
10. Mignolet A, Wood BR, Goormaghtigh E (2018) Intracellular investigation on the differential effects of 4 polyphenols on MCF-7 breast cancer cells by Raman imaging. Analyst 143(1):258–269
11. Cutshaw G, Uthaman S, Hassan N, Kothadiya S, Wen X, Bardhan R (2023) The emerging role of Raman spectroscopy as an omics approach for metabolic profiling and biomarker detection toward precision medicine. Chem Rev 123(13):8297–8346
12. Tirinato L, Liberale C, Di Franco S, Candeloro P, Benfante A, La Rocca R, Potze L, Marotta R, Ruffilli R, Rajamanickam VP et al (2015) Lipid droplets: a new player in colorectal cancer stem cells unveiled by spectroscopic imaging. Stem Cells 33(1):35–44
13. Traynor D, Behl I, O'Dea D, Bonnier F, Nicholson S, O'Connell F, Maguire A, Flint S, Galvin S, Healy CM, Martin CM, O'Leary JJ, Malkin A, Byrne HJ, Lyng FM (2021) Raman spectral cytopathology for cancer diagnostic applications. Nat Protoc 16(7):3716–3735

14. Behl I, Calado G, Vishwakarma A, Traynor D, Flint S, Galvin S, Healy CM, Pimentel ML, Malkin A, Byrne HJ, Lyng FM (2022) Classification of cytological samples from oral potentially malignant lesions through Raman spectroscopy: a pilot study. Spectrochim Acta A Mol Biomol Spectrosc 266:120437
15. Jermyn M, Desroches J, Aubertin K, St-Arnaud K, Madore W-J, De Montigny E, Guiot M-C, Trudel D, Wilson BC, Petrecca K, Leblond F (2016) A review of Raman spectroscopy advances with an emphasis on clinical translation challenges in oncology. Phys Med Biol 61(23):R370
16. Krafft C, Schmitt M, Schie IW, Cialla-May D, Matthäus C, Bocklitz T, Popp J (2017) Label-free molecular imaging of biological cells and tissues by linear and nonlinear Raman spectroscopic approaches. Angew Chem Int Ed 56(16):4392–4430
17. Chenzhou Wu, Gleysteen J, Teraphongphom NT, Li Y, Rosenthal E (2018) In-vivo optical imaging in head and neck oncology: basic principles, clinical applications and future directions. Int J Oral Sci 10(2):10
18. Vogler N, Bocklitz T, Salah FS, Schmidt C, Bräuer R, Cui T, Mireskandari M, Greten F, Schmitt M, Stallmach A, Petersen I, Popp J (2015) Systematic evaluation of colorectal tissue diagnostics based on the statistical analysis of Raman spectra. J Biophotonics 9:533–541
19. Bergner N, Bocklitz T, Romeike BFM, Reichart R, Kalff R, Krafft C, Popp J (2012) Identification of primary tumors of brain metastases by Raman imaging and support vector machines. Chemom Intell Lab Syst 117:224–232
20. Popp J, Tuchin VV, Chiou A, Heinemann SH (2013) Handbook of biophotonics. Wiley-VCH Verlag GmbH & Co. KGaA, Weinheim
21. Müller M, Zumbusch A (2007) Coherent anti-stokes Raman scattering microscopy. Chemphyschem 8(15):2156–2170
22. Krafft C, Dietzek B, Popp J (2009) Raman and CARS microspectroscopy of cells and tissues. Analyst 134(6):1046–1057
23. Rodriguez LG, Lockett SJ, Holtom GR (2006) Coherent anti-stokes Raman scattering microscopy: a biological review. Cytometry Part A 69(8):779–791
24. Pohling C, Bocklitz T, Duarte AS, Emmanuello C, Ishikawa MS, Dietzeck B, Buckup T, Uckermann O, Schackert G, Kirsch M, Schmitt M, Popp J, Motzkus M (2017) Multiplex coherent anti-stokes Raman scattering microspectroscopy of brain tissue with higher ranking data classification for biomedical imaging. J Biomed Opt 22:22–25
25. Bocklitz T, Meyer T, Schmitt M, Rimke I, Hoffmann F, von Eggeling F, Ernst G, Guntinas-Lichius O, Popp J (2018) Comparison of hyperspectral coherent Raman scattering microscopies for biomedical applications. APL Photonics 3:092404
26. Charles H Jr, Camp YJ, Lee JM, Heddleston CM, Hartshorn AR, Walker H, Rich JN, Lathia JD, Cicerone MT (2014) High-speed coherent Raman fingerprint imaging of biological tissues. Nat Photonics 8:627–634
27. Lee M, Downes A, Chau Y-Y, Serrels B, Hastie N, Elfick A, Brunton V, Frame M, Serrels A (2015) In vivo imaging of the tumor and its associated microenvironment using combined CARS/2-photon microscopy. Intravital 4(1):e1055430
28. Weng S, Xiaoyun X, Li J, Wong STC (2017) Combining deep learning and coherent anti-stokes Raman scattering imaging for automated differential diagnosis of lung cancer. J Biomed Opt 22(10):1–10
29. Chernavskaia O, Heuke S, Vieth M, Friedrich O, Schürmann S, Atreya R, Stallmach A, Neurath MF, Waldner M, Petersen I, Schmitt M, Bocklitz T, Popp J (2016) Beyond endoscopic assessment in inflammatory bowel disease: real-time histology of disease activity by non-linear multimodal imaging. Sci Rep 6:29239
30. Rodner E, Bocklitz T, von Eggeling F, Ernst G, Chernavskaia O, Popp J, Denzler J, Guntinas-Lichius O (2018) Fully convolutional networks in multimodal nonlinear microscopy images for automated detection of head and neck carcinoma: a pilot study. Head Neck, online:1–6
31. Wright AJ, Poland SP, Girkin JM, Freudiger CW, Evans CL, Xie XS (2007) Adaptive optics for enhanced signal in CARS microscopy. Opt Express 15(26):18209–18219

32. Lombardini A, Mytskaniuk V, Sivankutty S, Andresen ER, Chen X, Wenger J, Fabert M, Joly N, Louradour F, Kudlinski A, Rigneault H (2018) High-resolution multimodal flexible coherent Raman endoscope. Light Sci Appl 7(1):aaa8870
33. Haohua T, Boppart SA (2014) Coherent anti-stokes Raman scattering microscopy: overcoming technical barriers for clinical translation. J Biophotonics 7(1–2):9–22
34. Zirak P, Matz G, Messerschmidt B, Meyer T, Schmitt M, Popp J, Uckermann O, Galli R, Kirsch M, Winterhalder MJ, Zumbusch A (2018) Invited article: a rigid coherent anti-stokes Raman scattering endoscope with high resolution and a large field of view. APL Photonics 3(9):092409
35. Polli D, Kumar V, Valensise CM, Marangoni M, Cerullo G (2018) Broadband coherent Raman scattering microscopy. Laser Photonics Rev 12(9):1800020
36. Vernuccio F, Vanna R, Ceconello C, Bresci A, Manetti F, Sorrentino S, Ghislanzoni S, Lambertucci F, Motiño O, Martins I, Kroemer G, Bongarzone I, Cerullo G, Polli D (2023) Full-spectrum cars microscopy of cells and tissues with ultrashort whitelight continuum pulses. J Phys Chem B 127(21):4733–4745
37. Nakamura T, Hashimoto K, Ideguchi T (2024) Broadband coherent Raman scattering spectroscopy at 50,000,000 spectra per second. Ultrafast Sci 4:0076
38. Farnesi E, Calvarese M, Liu C, Messerschmidt C, Vafaeinezhad MS, Meyer-Zedler T, Cialla-May D, Krafft C, Ballmaier J, Guntinas-Lichius O, Schmitt M, Popp J (2024) Advancing cerumen analysis: exploring innovative vibrational spectroscopy techniques with respect to their potential as new point-of-care diagnostic tools. Analyst 149:5381–5393
39. Denk W, Strickler JH, Webb WW (1990) Two-photon laser scanning fluorescence microscopy. Science 248(4951):73–76
40. Barad Y, Eisenberg H, Horowitz M, Silberberg Y (1997) Nonlinear scanning laser microscopy by third harmonic generation. Appl Phys Lett 70(8):922–924
41. Calvarese M, Corbetta E, Contreras J, Bae H, Lai C, Reichwald K, Meyer-Zedler T, Pertzborn D, Mühlig A, Hoffmann F, Messerschmidt B, Guntinas-Lichius O, Schmitt M, Bocklitz T, Popp J (2024) Endomicroscopic AI-driven morphochemical imaging and fs-laser ablation for selective tumor identification and selective tissue removal. Sci Adv 10(50):eado9721
42. Zipfel WR, Williams RM, Christie R, Nikitin AY, Hyman BT, Webb WW (2003) Live tissue intrinsic emission microscopy using multiphoton-excited native fluorescence and second harmonic generation. Proc Natl Acad Sci 100(12):7075–7080
43. Richards-Kortum R, Sevick-Muraca E (1996) Quantitative optical spectroscopy for tissue diagnosis. Annu Rev Phys Chem 47(1):555–606
44. Meyer T, Guntinas-Lichius O, von Eggeling F, Ernst G, Akimov D, Schmitt M, Dietzek B, Popp J (2013) Multimodal nonlinear microscopic investigations on head and neck squamous cell carcinoma: toward intraoperative imaging. Head Neck 35(9):E280–E287
45. Fine S, Hansen WP (1971) Optical second harmonic generation in biological systems. Appl Opt 10(10):2350–2353
46. Pavone FS, Campagnola PJ (2013) Second harmonic generation imaging. CRC Press
47. Mohler W, Millard AC, Campagnola PJ (2003) Second harmonic generation imaging of endogenous structural proteins. Methods 29(1):97–109
48. Cicchi R, Vogler N, Kapsokalyvas D, Dietzek B, Popp J, Pavone FS (2013) From molecular structure to tissue architecture: collagen organization probed by SHG microscopy. J Biophotonics 6:129–142
49. Müller M, Squier J, Wilson KR, Brakenhoff GJ (1998) 3D microscopy of transparent objects using third-harmonic generation. J Microsc 191(3):266–274
50. Débarre D, Supatto W, Pena A-M, Fabre A, Tordjmann T, Combettes L, Schanne-Klein M-C, Beaurepaire E (2006) Imaging lipid bodies in cells and tissues using third-harmonic generation microscopy. Nat Methods 3(1):47
51. Weigelin B, Bakker G-J, Friedl P (2016) Third harmonic generation microscopy of cells and tissue organization. J Cell Sci:jcs–152272
52. Heuke S, Vogler N, Meyer T, Akimov D, Kluschke F, Röwert-Huber H-J, Lademann J, Dietzek B, Popp J (2013) Multimodal mapping of human skin. Br J Dermatol 169(4):794–803

53. Adur J, Carvalho HF, Cesar CL, Casco VH (2014) Nonlinear optical microscopy signal processing strategies in cancer. Cancer Informat 13:CIN–S12419
54. Ali N, Quansah E, Köhler K, Meyer T, Schmitt M, Popp J, Niendorf A, Bocklitz T (2019) Automatic label-free detection of breast cancer using nonlinear multimodal imaging and the convolutional neural network ResNet50. Transl Biophotonics 1(1–2):e201900003
55. Heuke S, Vogler N, Meyer T, Akimov D, Kluschke F, Röwert-Huber H-J, Lademann J, Dietzek B, Popp J (2013) Detection and discrimination of non-melanoma skin cancer by multimodal imaging. Healthcare (Basel, Switzerland) 1:64–83
56. Bae H, Rodewald M, Meyer-Zedler T, Bocklitz TW, Matz G, Messerschmidt B, Press AT, Bauer M, Guntinas-Lichius O, Stallmach A, Schmitt M, Popp J (2023) Feasibility studies of multimodal nonlinear endoscopy using multicore fiber bundles for remote scanning from tissue sections to bulk organs. Sci Rep 13(1):13779
57. Pshenay-Severin E, Bae H, Reichwald K, Matz G, Bierlich J, Kobelke J, Lorenz A, Schwuchow A, Meyer-Zedler T, Schmitt M, Messerschmidt B, Popp J (2021) Multimodal nonlinear endomicroscopic imaging probe using a double-core double-clad fiber and focus-combining micro-optical concept. Light Sci Appl 10(1):207
58. Borhani N, Bower AJ, Boppart SA, Psaltis D (2019) Digital staining through the application of deep neural networks to multi-modal multiphoton microscopy. Biomed Opt Express 10(3):1339–1350
59. Pradhan P, Meyer T, Vieth M, Stallmach A, Waldner M, Schmitt M, Popp J, Bocklitz T (2021) Computational tissue staining of non-linear multimodal imaging using supervised and unsupervised deep learning. Biomed Opt Express 12(4):2280–2298
60. Richards-Kortum R, Sevick-Muraca E (1996) Quantitative optical spectroscopy for tissue diagnosis. Annu Rev Phys Chem 47:555–606
61. Elson D, Requejo-Isidro J, Munro I, Reavell F, Siegel J, Suhling K, Tadrous P, Benninger R, Lanigan P, McGinty J, Talbot C, Treanor B, Webb S, Sandison A, Wallace A, Davis D, Lever J, Neil M, Phillips D, Stamp G, French P (2004) Time-domain fluorescence lifetime imaging applied to biological tissue. Photochem Photobiol Sci 3(8):795–801
62. Dowling K, Dayel MJ, Lever MJ, French PMW, Hares JD, Dymoke-Bradshaw AKL (1998) Fluorescence lifetime imaging with picosecond resolution for biomedical applications. Opt Lett 23(10):810–812
63. Becker L, Janssen N, Layland SL, Mürdter TE, Nies AT, Schenke-Layland K, Marzi J (2021) Raman imaging and fluorescence lifetime imaging microscopy for diagnosis of cancer state and metabolic monitoring. Cancer 13(22)
64. Bower AJ, Li J, Chaney EJ, Marjanovic M, Spillman DR, Boppart SA (2018) High-speed imaging of transient metabolic dynamics using two-photon fluorescence lifetime imaging microscopy. Optica 5(10):1290–1296
65. Liu J, Sun Y, Qi J, Marcu L (2012) A novel method for fast and robust estimation of fluorescence decay dynamics using constrained least-squares deconvolution with Laguerre expansion. Phys Med Biol 57(4):843
66. Blacker TS, Mann ZF, Gale JE, Ziegler M, Bain AJ, Szabadkai G, Duchen MR (2014) Separating NADH and NADPH fluorescence in live cells and tissues using FLIM. Nat Commun 5:3936
67. Skala MC, Riching KM, Bird DK, GendronFitzpatrick A, Eickhoff J, Eliceiri KW, Keely PJ, Ramanujam N (2007) In vivo multiphoton fluorescence lifetime imaging of protein-bound and free nicotinamide adenine dinucleotide in normal and precancerous epithelia. J Biomed Opt 12(2):024014
68. Alfonso-Garcia A, Anbunesan SN, Bec J, Lee HS, Jin L-W, Bloch O, Marcu L (2023) In vivo characterization of the human glioblastoma infiltrative edge with label-free intraoperative fluorescence lifetime imaging. Biomed Opt Express 14:2196–2208
69. Mark Marsden, Weyers BW, Bec J, Sun T, Gandour- Edwards RF, Birkeland AC, Abouyared M, Bewley AF, Farwell DG, Marcu L (2021) Intraoperative margin assessment in oral and oropharyngeal cancer using label-free fluorescence lifetime imaging and machine learning. IEEE Trans Biomed Eng 68(3):857–868

70. König K (2020) Review: clinical in vivo multiphoton FLIM tomography. Methods Appl Fluoresc 8(3):034002
71. Thomas Bocklitz, Schmitt M, Popp J (2014) Image processing – chemometric approaches to analyze optical molecular images. In: Ex-vivo and in-vivo optical molecular pathology. Wiley-VCH Verlag GmbH & Co. KGaA, pp 215–248
72. Bishop CM (2011) Pattern recognition and machine learning, Information Science and Statistics. Springer
73. Tauler R, Walczak B, Brown SD (eds) (2009) Comprehensive chemometrics: chemical and biochemical data analysis. Elsevier
74. Guo S, Popp J, Bocklitz T (2021) Chemometric analysis in Raman spectroscopy from experimental design to machine learning-based modeling. Nat Protoc 16(12):5426–5459
75. Houhou R, Barman P, Schmitt M, Meyer T, Popp J, Bocklitz T (2020) Deep learning as phase retrieval tool for CARS spectra. Opt Express 28:21002–21024
76. Valensise CM, Giuseppi A, Vernuccio F, De la Cadena A, Cerullo G, Polli D (2020) Removing non-resonant background from CARS spectra via deep learning. APL Photonics 5(6):061305
77. Mannam V, Zhang Y, Yuan X, Ravasio C, Howard SS (2020) Machine learning for faster and smarter fluorescence lifetime imaging microscopy. J Phys Photonics 2(4):042005
78. Chernavskaia O, Bocklitz T, Meyer T, Vogler N, Akimov D, Heuke S, Guo S, Heintzmann R, Popp J (2017) Correction of mosaicking artefacts in multimodal images caused by uneven illumination. J Chemom 31(6):e2901
79. Joris Roels, Jan Aelterman, Jonas De Vylder, Saskia Lippens, Hiêp Q. Luong, Christopher J. Guérin, and Wilfried Philips. Image degradation in microscopic images: avoidance, artifacts, and solutions, pages 41–67. Springer International Publishing, Cham, 2016
80. Liu Z, Jin L, Chen J, Fang Q, Ablameyko S, Yin Z, Xu Y (2021) A survey on applications of deep learning in microscopy image analysis. Comput Biol Med 134:104523
81. Pradhan P, Guo S, Ryabchykov O, Popp J, Bocklitz TW (2020) Deep learning a boon for biophotonics? J Biophotonics 13(6):e201960186
82. Kondepudi A, Pekmezci M, Hou X, Scotford K, Jiang C, Rao A, Harake ES, Chowdury A, Al-Holou W, Wang L, Pandey A, Lowenstein PR, Castro MG, Koerner LI, Roetzer-Pejrimovsky T, Widhalm G, Camelo-Piragua S, MovahedEzazi M, Orringer DA, Lee H, Freudiger C, Berger M, Hervey-Jumper S, Hollon T (2024) Foundation models for fast, label-free detection of glioma infiltration. Nature 637:439
83. Wang H, Rivenson Y, Jin Y, Wei Z, Gao R, Günaydın H, Bentolila LA, Kural C, Ozcan A (2019) Deep learning enables cross-modality super-resolution in fluorescence microscopy. Nat Methods 16(1):103–110

Image-Guided Brain Tumor Surgery 29

Stephanie Schipmann, Michael Schwake,
and Walter Stummer

29.1 Introduction

Over the past few decades, brain tumor surgery has undergone significant changes as medical technology and surgical expertise have advanced. A pivotal moment was the introduction of the microscope and microsurgical techniques by Yasargil [1]. The paradigm of brain tumor surgery has shifted from removing tumors visible to the naked eye to resecting malignant cells beyond the scope of the microscope and visual inspection, aided by technological innovations. In the treatment of gliomas, an independent factor for better outcome regarding overall survival (OS) and progression-free-survival (PFS) that can be directly influenced by the neurosurgeon is the extent of resection (EOR) [2–6].

It is well known that gliomas infiltrate surrounding brain parenchyma in a manner that is imperceptible to the human eye, even with the aid of a surgical microscope. Moreover, an infiltrated brain often cannot be distinguished from normal brain tissue based on tactile features alone.

Consequently, numerous efforts have been made over recent decades to develop techniques for improved tumor visualization and identification, aiming to achieve a greater EOR. These include neuronavigation, intraoperative ultrasound, intraoperative magnetic resonance imaging (iMRI), and, more recently, fluorescence-guided surgery (FGS). FGS, in particular, has elevated intraoperative tissue visualization to a new level, offering the potential for real-time tumor imaging without interrupting surgery.

S. Schipmann (✉)
Department of Neurosurgery, University Hospital Bergen, Bergen, Norway

M. Schwake · W. Stummer
Department of Neurosurgery, University Hospital Münster, Münster, Germany
e-mail: michael.schwake@ukmuenster.de; walter.stummer@ukmuenster.de

O. Schober et al. (eds.), *Molecular Imaging in Oncology - Volume 2*, Recent Results in Cancer Research 225, https://doi.org/10.1007/978-3-032-21415-7_11

Recently, other highly precise techniques have been introduced and are being translated into clinical practice, promising even more accurate delineation of tumor tissue. These include confocal microscopy, Raman spectroscopy, and targeted fluorescence, which are opening new frontiers in real-time intraoperative molecular and cellular imaging.

A promising technology is hyperspectral imaging (HSI), which can provide detailed spectral information of different tissues. The combination of HSI with deep-learning algorithms has further enhanced its capabilities for automated tissue classification and improved visualization.

All these tools aim to enhance the surgeon's ability to identify tumor tissue and distinguish it from normal brain parenchyma. This chapter will discuss the various techniques, their applicability in brain tumor surgery, and their benefits and limitations.

29.2 Conventional Intraoperative Imaging

Conventional intraoperative imaging techniques like neuronavigation and ultrasound are the basis for most cases in brain tumor surgery and have been well integrated into the operative setting in neurosurgery.

29.2.1 Ultrasound

Intraoperative ultrasound provides a safe, cost-effective, and rapidly available imaging technique that integrates easily into surgical workflows, allowing real-time imaging during surgery. It can be used to locate lesions prior to durotomy and to identify residual tumor during tumor resection [7]. This dynamic method enables visualization of tumor borders and adjacent normal brain structures [8]. Studies have shown that ultrasound can increase the EOR and thus improve outcomes [9, 10]. Ultrasound is particularly effective with cystic and heterogeneous lesions with echogenicity different from the cortex.

Modern navigation systems can integrate ultrasound data and co-register it with preoperative acquired imaging, enabling better interpretation of ultrasound data and navigation of complex brain anatomy. Recent advancements include the creation of 3D volume models based on 2D intraoperative ultrasound data [11].

Importantly, intraoperative acquired ultrasound data can be used to update navigation systems, helping to mitigate the effects of brain shift during surgery [11, 12] (Fig. 29.1a).

29.2.2 Neuronavigation

Neuronavigation has become an essential and widely available tool for the surgical treatment of brain tumors. It relies on three-dimensional preoperative radiological

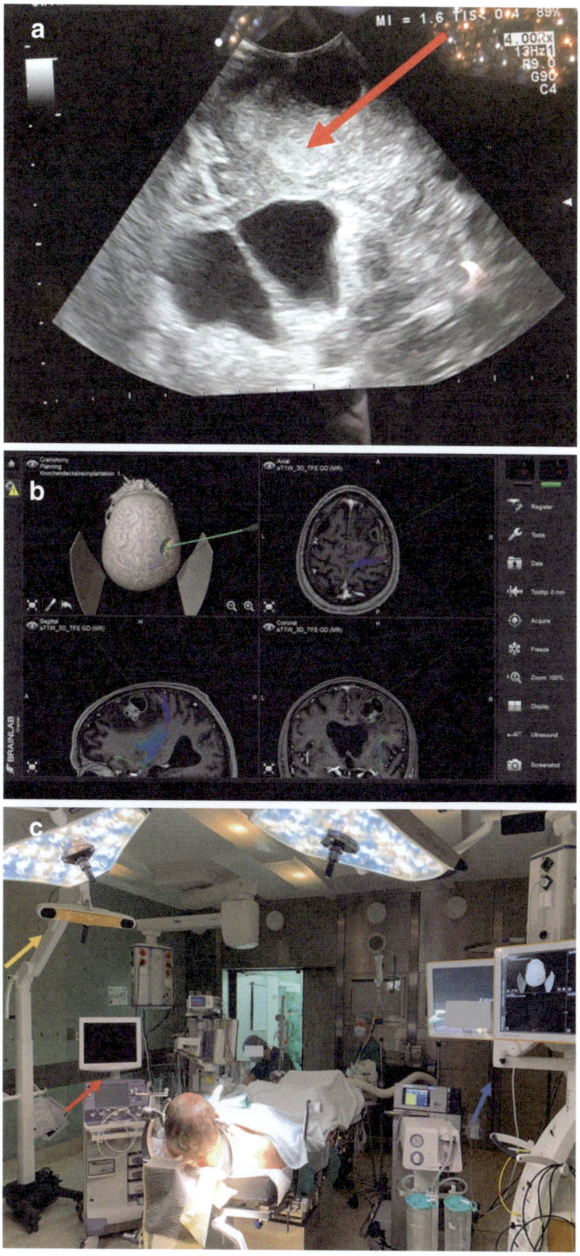

Fig. 29.1 Techniques for intraoperative imaging. (**a**) Ultrasound. The lesion can be seen transdurally and can be clearly distinguished from normal brain structures (red arrow). (**b**) MRI: Patient with fiber tracking (pyramid tract) for intraoperative orientation and planning of surgical approach. (**c**) Setting in the operating room with simultaneous use of ultrasound (red arrow), neuronavigation with display (blue arrow), and camera (yellow arrow)

imaging data that is aligned with the patient's anatomy through a registration process [13]. The navigation system consists of a reference arm attached to the head clamp, which is fixed to the surgical table. Infrared cameras track the position of the probe relative to the fixed reference arm, and preoperative imaging is shown on the screen with the real-time intraoperative position of the probe [8]. Various types of preoperative imaging, such as CT, MRI, and PET scans, can be incorporated into the neuronavigation software. This provides the neurosurgeon with near real-time localization and orientation. Modern systems allow for 3D reconstruction of imaging. Anatomical information and data on the extent of the tumor and its relation to adjacent structures can be gained from the system, leading to higher surgical accuracy and precision for the resection of brain tumors [13].

Furthermore, functional data can be integrated into the neuronavigation system. Functional MRI (fMRI) can help identifying localization of functional brain regions, such as those for language and motor functions [14]. Data from transcranial magnetic stimulation can also aid in motor mapping [15].

Diffusion tensor imaging (DTI) is based on the preferential diffusion of water in the direction of white matter tracts within the central nervous system [8, 16]. These data can be added to the navigation system to provide detailed information on subcortical fiber tracts, such as the corticospinal tract, which may be at risk during tumor resection [17]. In addition, neuronavigation is highly useful for planning the surgical approach and craniotomy [18].

However, neuronavigation has some limitations. A major issue is loss of accuracy due to intraoperative brain shift caused by positioning, administration of mannitol, drainage of cerebrospinal fluid (CSF), and tumor resection, as navigational systems rely on preoperative imaging. The use of navigated ultrasound can help account for brain shift by updating navigational data [11, 12]. Another limitation is that most navigational systems display the information used during surgery on a screen outside the surgical field, forcing surgeons to divert their attention from the surgical site. However, modern neuronavigational systems are beginning to address this by projecting navigational information into the surgical microscope (Fig. 29.1b, c).

29.2.3 Intraoperative MRI (iMRI)

Intraoperative magnetic resonance imaging (iMRI) was first introduced in the 1990s [19] and has since undergone several improvements. This technology allows surgeons to obtain images during surgery and update navigation systems to account for anatomical changes due to brain shift [20]. Intraoperative MRI is also valuable for identifying residual tumor and improving the extent of tumor resection. Additionally, it can help detect early intraoperative complications like ischemia or hemorrhage, allowing prompt intervention.

A randomized controlled trial by Senft et al. evaluating the benefit of iMRI in glioma surgery showed a gross total resection (GTR) rate of 96% in the iMRI group versus 68% in the control group using conventional microsurgery [21]. Roder et al. found a complete resection rate of 81% for iMRI in their prospective multicenter trial comparing iMRI and 5-aminolevulinic acid (5-ALA) resection of glioblastoma, showing no superiority of iMRI over 5-ALA [22].

Intraoperative MRI has shown promise in the treatment of low-grade gliomas (LGG), with several studies reporting that 30–60% of patients returned to surgery after initial resection to address residual tumor identified by iMRI [23–25].

Despite its increasing use, iMRI has some disadvantages. It is expensive, time-consuming, and prolongs the duration of surgery and anesthesia, and cannot be used for patients with ferromagnetic implants.

29.3 Fluorescence-Guided Brain Surgery

For neurosurgeons, the ability to differentiate abnormal from normal tissues is crucial for safe and effective procedures. Fluorescence-guided surgery (FGS) has proven to be a valuable tool for visualizing and delineating pathological tissues. The principle behind FGS involves administering optical imaging agents to patients before or during surgery, which selectively accumulate in tumor tissues. George E. Moore first described FGS for neurosurgery in 1947, demonstrating that glioma and meningioma cells could be better visualized through fluorescence after intravenous application of fluorescein [26]. This technique for real-time intraoperative detection of tumor tissue has significantly advanced in recent years, offering the major advantage of visualizing tumor tissue independently of neuronavigation, which can be affected by brain shift [27]. In addition to fluorescein, two other agents have been introduced into the field of neuro-oncological surgery: 5-aminolevulinic acid (5-ALA) [28] and indocyanine green (ICG) [29].

29.3.1 5-Aminolevulinic Acid (5-ALA)

5-aminolevulinic acid (5-ALA) is a natural metabolite in the hemoglobin pathway. It is metabolized into Protoporphyrin IX (PpIX), a strongly fluorescent precursor of heme. Glioma cells selectively take up 5-ALA and convert this to PpIX, resulting in tumor cell fluorescence [30, 31]. Fluorescence can be visualized by coupling the surgical microscope to a xenon light source that is capable of switching between white and violet-blue light (wavelength: 370–440 nm). An emission filter is added to visualize the red tumor fluorescence at a peak of 635 and 704 nm [31]. These filters also enable sufficient background discrimination, allowing surgeons to perform significant portions of the procedure under conditions suitable for visualizing fluorescence. Currently, all modern surgical microscopes offer attachments capable of visualizing PpIX fluorescence. 5-ALA (brand name Gliolan® in the European Union or Gleolan® in the United States) is administered as an oral solution at a dose of 20 mg/kg body weight 3 h before anesthesia induction. Plasma clearance occurs within 2 h after administration [32]. Peak fluorescence is typically observed after 6–8 h, with fluorescence beginning to become visible after about 3 h [31, 33, 34]. High-grade gliomas typically display solid red fluorescence with slightly pink fluorescence at the tumor margins, representing the infiltrating zone [35]. Multiple studies have demonstrated the toxicological safety of 5-ALA. The most common side effects are transient skin phototoxicity or temporarily elevated liver enzymes [36, 37].

5-ALA is the most extensively studied fluorescent agent worldwide and has been approved by both the US Food and Drug Administration (FDA) and the European Medicines Agency (EMA) as the only optical agent for real-time visualization of malignant tissue during glioma surgery. Beyond its clinical application in malignant gliomas, several studies have confirmed its benefit for resection in other primary and metastatic brain tumors, including meningiomas, brain metastases, and pediatric brain tumors [38–40].

29.3.1.1 5-Aminolevulinic Acid in High-Grade Gliomas

High-grade gliomas (HGGs) are the most frequent primary malignant brain tumors in adults, known for their highly infiltrative nature [41]. Glioblastoma, a particularly aggressive form of HGG, has a poor prognosis with a median survival of just 15 months and a 5-year survival rate of 6.9% [42, 43]. These tumors typically consist of a solid core surrounded by normal brain tissue infiltrated with cancer cells, lacking a clear, histologically defined border. Although surgery can never completely cure HGGs due to their infiltrative nature, numerous studies have shown that complete removal of the contrast-enhancing tumor significantly improves overall survival. This evidence supports the approach of maximal safe resection [2–6, 22]. However, identifying and fully removing the contrast-enhancing tumor solely based on visual appearance or tactile information is virtually impossible to achieve [44].

5-ALA has emerged as a valuable tool for visualizing glioma tissue during surgery. Its first clinical use, reported in 1998 in a small study of nine HGG patients, showed impressive results with 85% sensitivity and 100% specificity in detecting malignant tissue [28]. A subsequent phase III randomized controlled multicenter trial demonstrated that 5-ALA significantly improved complete resection rates of contrast-enhancing tumors (65% of patients assigned to the 5-ALA group compared with 36% of those assigned to the conventional surgery white light group, $p < 0.001$). This led to better 6-month progression-free-survival rates (41.0% in the 5-ALA group vs. 21.1% in the white light group) [36]. Since this landmark study, 5-ALA has become widely adopted in surgery for high-grade gliomas.

Resection rates have further improved, now ranging from 80% to 100%, thanks to increased experience and the integration of advanced intraoperative monitoring and brain mapping techniques. These advancements allow for safe resections even in eloquent regions [45, 46].

Strong 5-ALA fluorescence correlates closely with contrast enhancement on MRI scans. Interestingly, weaker, pink fluorescence often extends beyond the contrast-enhancing margins, representing the tumor's infiltration zone [47] (Fig. 29.2). Strong correlations between histological grading, features of malignancy, a higher Ki-67/MIB-1 index, and the intensity of 5-ALA fluorescence were observed [48, 49].

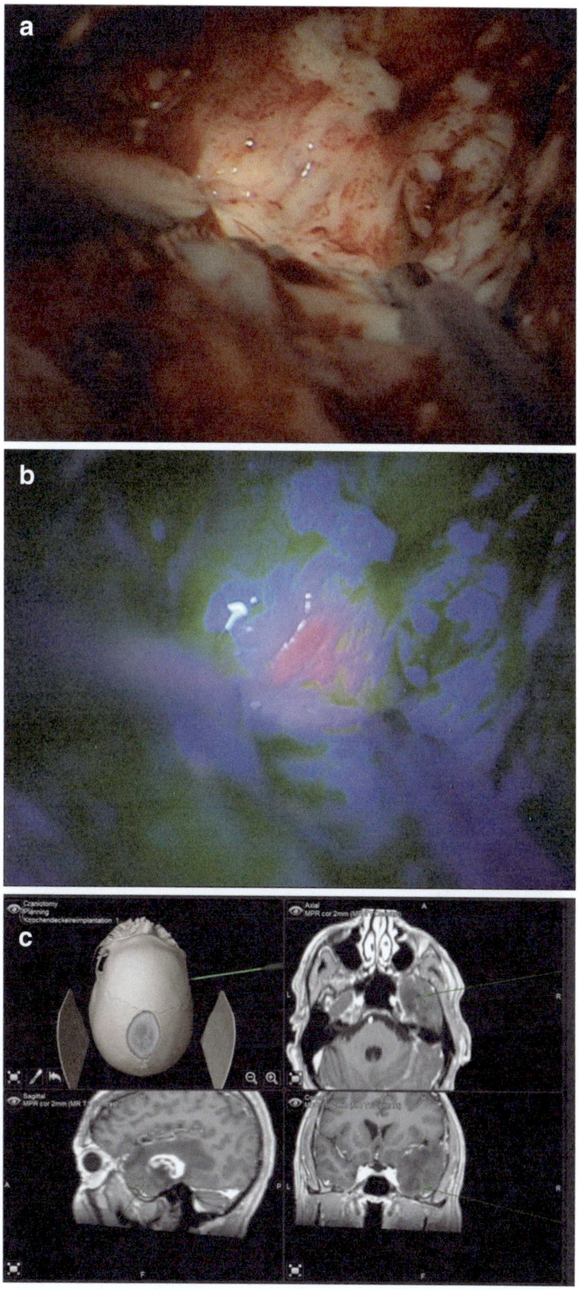

Fig. 29.2 5-ALA-guided resection of glioblastoma. (**a**) Tumor under white light, delineation between tumor and normal tissue is almost impossible. (**b**) Tumor under violet light, showing a clear and solid fluorescence in tumor tissue and a vague fluorescence at the border and infiltrating zone. (**c**) Screenshot from neuronavigation, demonstrating the area of the above images. 5-ALA fluorescence goes beyond the borders of the contrast-enhancement on MRI, enabling a higher extent of resection

29.3.1.2 5-Aminolevulinic Acid in Recurrent High-Grade Gliomas

Several small, nonrandomized studies of patients with recurrent HGG suggest that more complete resection of contrast-enhancing tumor leads to improved survival rates [50–52]. Given these findings, 5-ALA-guided resection appears to be a promising approach for recurrent glioma cases, as supported by multiple studies. Using 5-ALA, researchers have reported average rates of complete tumor resection as high as 98% [53, 54]. In addition, patients with recurrent gliomas who underwent 5-ALA fluorescence-guided surgery (FGS) showed longer overall survival compared to those who had repeat surgery without 5-ALA [54]. However, the utility of 5-ALA might be impacted by post-therapeutic tissue changes such as gliosis, necrosis, and vascular hyalinization [55–57], affecting specificity and sensitivity. Positive fluorescence was reported in the vast majority of recurrent high-grade gliomas and was considered a good predictor for the presence of tumor [54, 58–60]. However, unlike in primary gliomas, the absence of fluorescence in recurrent tumors is not essentially a reliable marker for the absence of tumor [61]. In some cases, no active tumor tissue could be diagnosed despite visible fluorescence linked to reactive tissue changes or inflammation [58, 60]. In summary, the use of 5-ALA appears to be feasible in recurrent gliomas, keeping in mind possible false positive or negative fluorescence and the not yet fully understood impact of adjuvant tumor treatment on the degree of fluorescence.

29.3.1.3 5-Aminolevulinic Acid in Low-Grade Gliomas

There is clear evidence that more extensive resection of low-grade gliomas (LGG) results in improved outcomes [62–64]. Consequently, the aim of surgery is maximal safe tumor resection. A challenge in the surgery of LGG is the fact that these tumors often show only slight differences in texture and consistency compared to the normal brain. LGG frequently exhibits histological heterogeneity with circumscribed areas showing malignant transformation (anaplastic foci) [65]. Most LGGs do not display visible 5-ALA fluorescence; however, several studies demonstrated correlations between 5-ALA fluorescence and patchy/faint contrast-enhancement on preoperative MRI, areas with higher metabolic activity in PET, and higher proliferation rate [66–69]. Consequently, the use of 5-ALA enables intraoperative identification of anaplastic foci, more precise histopathological diagnoses, reduces the risk of histopathological undergrading, and enables allocation of patients to appropriate adjuvant treatment. At present, the use of 5-ALA in suspected LGG is recommended in case of patchy or faint contrast-enhancement on MRI and in case of ^{18}F-FET-PET hot spots with a standardized uptake value (SUV) greater than 1.9 [67] (Fig. 29.3).

It is known that even in those LGG without visible fluorescence under a standard surgical microscope, lower levels of PPIX fluorescence can be detected using spectroscopy [70].

The reasons for poor PpIX accumulation in low-grade gliomas may include: lower tumor cell density, proliferation, and metabolic characteristics, and varying degrees of blood-brain barrier (BBB) permeability [70]. The application of double-dose 5-ALA in low-grade gliomas can aid in increasing the PpIX concentration in tumor regions where PpIX concentration is below the visibility threshold with

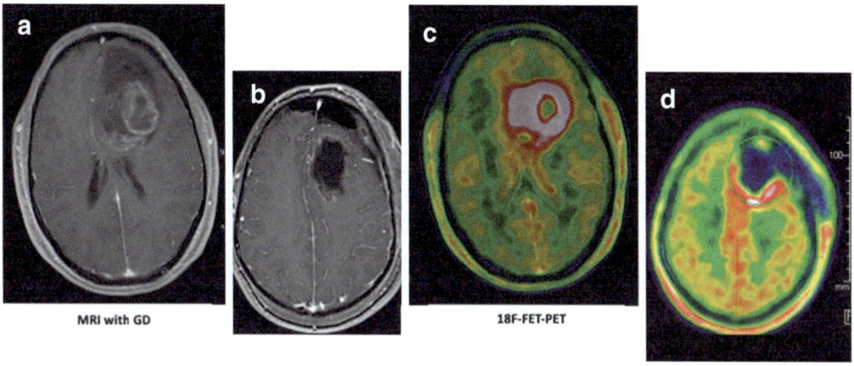

Fig. 29.3 (**a**) MRI T1 + Gd before and after surgery (**a** and **b**) with corresponding F18-FET-PET imaging pre- and postoperatively (**c** and **d**). The enhanced metabolism of the tumor can be visualized using PET imaging

single doses. However, this does not increase the incidence of strongly fluorescent tumor areas [70]. Ongoing advancements in visualization technology and standardized fluorescence quantification methods may further enhance the utility of 5-ALA fluorescence in low-grade glioma resection [71].

29.3.1.4 5-Aminolevulinic Acid in Other Brain Tumors

5-ALA has shown promising results in surgery for various brain tumors beyond its well-established use in glioma resection. In meningioma surgery, 5-ALA fluorescence helps surgeons identify residual tumor, infiltration into surrounding structures like the dura, brain, and bone, as well as satellite lesions. This allows for a more complete tumor removal [40, 72–75] (Fig. 29.4).

For cerebral metastases, which often recur locally even after seemingly complete resection, 5-ALA has been studied as a potential aid [76]. However, only about half of the metastases studied showed 5-ALA fluorescence [39, 77, 78]. Current evidence suggests that 5-ALA does neither allow reliable visualization of residual tumor after resection, nor does it improve the EOR or patient survival. There are no known predictors for positive 5-ALA fluorescence in metastasis [39, 76, 79].

In spinal tumor surgery, 5-ALA has shown encouraging results, particularly for ependymomas, astrocytomas, and meningiomas, enabling more extensive tumor removal [80].

Promising results have also been found in pediatric brain tumors with the use of 5-ALA for resection of astrocytomas, glioblastomas, ependymomas, and medulloblastoma [38, 81–83].

In cases of cerebral lymphoma, application of 5-ALA can assist in obtaining representative biopsy samples as most lymphomas exhibit positive 5-ALA fluorescence [84, 85]. In addition, 5-ALA fluorescence-guided surgery has been described in single cases for resection of hemangioblastoma [86], subependymomas [87], and germ cell tumors [88].

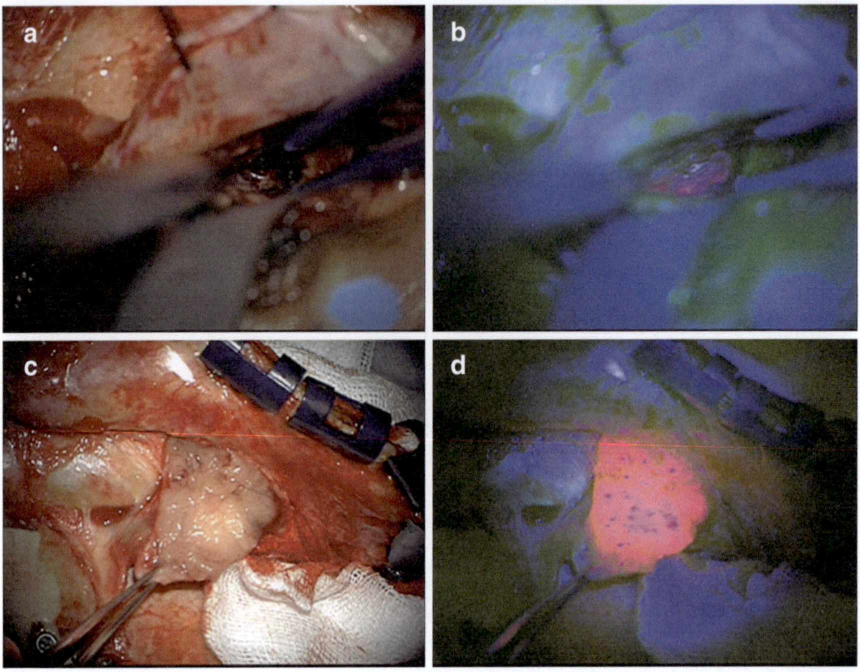

Fig. 29.4 Usage of 5-ALA in meningioma. After dural opening, 5-ALA-induced fluorescence of tumor tissue is visible (**a**, **c**: white light; **b**, **d**: violet light)

While 5-ALA shows potential for various non-glial brain tumors, the current evidence is largely limited to case reports. Further, prospective studies are needed to fully evaluate the benefits and value of 5-ALA guided surgery in these tumor types.

29.3.2 Fluorescein

Fluorescein sodium, discovered 150 years ago, has become a cornerstone in ophthalmology, primarily used for detecting corneal abrasions and performing retinal angiography [89, 90]. Its potential application in neurosurgery was first proposed by George E. Moore in 1947, who demonstrated that glioma and meningioma cells could be differentially visualized through fluorescence following intravenous administration of fluorescein [26]. Fluorescein is regarded as a robust, cost-effective, and safe fluorescent biomarker, characterized by its distinctive yellow-green fluorescence. Its peak absorption spectrum occurs at 465–490 nm with emission peaks from 500 to 530 nm. Notably, fluorescein fluorescence can also be discriminated under white light [91, 92]. After intravenous administration fluorescein is systemically distributed via the bloodstream and extravasates into regions with increased vascular permeability, abnormal vasculature, and neovascularization [26]. Under normal circumstances, the BBB prevents circulating fluorescein from entering normal brain tissue [93]. However, in cases BBB disruption, such as in tumors, fluorescein accumulates in the extracellular space of tumor tissue and can be visualized under yellow-filtered (560 nm) light [91].

A surgical microscope enabling visualization of fluorescein was introduced for the resection of high-grade gliomas [91]. Nowadays, a variety of fluorescent filters are available, including the YELLOW 560 system (Carl Zeiss) or the FL560 System (Leica Microscopes).

Fluorescein can also be visualized as a yellow dye under the white light of surgical microscopes at high concentrations. However, lower concentrations of fluorescein can be used when using specialized microscopes equipped with appropriate emission filters. A dose of 3–5 mg/kg body weight is administered intravenously after induction of anesthesia [94, 95]. Fluorescein is eliminated renally and mostly free of side effects apart from leading to transient discoloration of skin and urine after administration. Single cases of anaphylactic shock have been reported [96].

29.3.2.1 Critical Points and Problems with the Usage of Fluorescein

Recent studies have confirmed fluorescein staining not to be tumor-cell specific [94]. Additionally, fluorescein primarily marks areas with BBB breakdown, which are related to but not strictly confined to tumor tissue. Thus, fluorescein serves as an excellent marker of edema propagation [97, 98]. There is no real consensus on timing of administration of fluorescein before surgery and dosage in the current literature, although this is critical due to the fact that extravasation and distribution of this agent follow a certain time course regarding plasma fluorescein contents, perfusion of brain, and finally extravasation. After a half-life of 4 and ½ h, intravascular fluorescein will slowly subside, resulting in prolonged staining of normal perfused brain, while being extravasated and traveling with edema through peritumoral tissue, raising the danger of staining nontumorous tissue [97]. Consequently, the timing of surgery is critical and duration of craniotomy and preparation before reaching the lesion have to be considered. A further aspect confounding applicability of fluorescein is the problem with surgical injury of normal brain tissue, which will lead to unselective extravasation of fluorescein from the blood stream along the cut margins.

Consequently, further studies are required to evaluate fluorescein in the context of tumor histology, timing of administration, illumination, tissue perfusion, and edema. In summary, from the current point of view, the abovementioned confounders have to be considered using a fluorophore that does not have a specific tumor–fluorophore interaction and is rather a marker of BBB integrity.

29.3.2.2 Fluorescein-Guided Surgery for High-Grade Gliomas

Following the success of 5-ALA-guided glioma resection in improving the EOR, researchers have explored the potential of fluorescein, a more cost-effective alternative, for enhancing EOR in malignant gliomas [90, 99–102]. The groups of Schebesch and Acerbi reported gross total resection rates of 80% in their series of $n = 35$ and $n = 20$, respectively, high-grade glioma patients using YELLOW 560 filter [93, 99]. Other studies reported GTR in up to 100% of cases using fluorescein, while also demonstrating a strong correlation between intraoperative fluorescence and contrast enhancement on MRI scans [94, 103]. Sensitivity and specificity analyses following low-dose fluorescein administration yielded a sensitivity of 94% and a specificity of 90% [99]. Results of a phase II trial (FLUOGLIO) showed that the use of fluorescein is safe, feasible, and associated with a high percentage of complete resections in high-grade gliomas [103]. An ongoing prospective study (FLUOCERTUM) is evaluating fluorescein's efficacy in the resection of various CNS pathologies, with a preliminary subgroup analysis of glioblastoma patients showing an 82% GTR rate using fluorescein [104, 105].

Despite these promising findings, the current evidence supporting fluorescein use in high-grade gliomas remains limited due to a lack of randomized controlled trials investigating its potential benefits in terms of survival and EOR.

Interestingly, the simultaneous usage of fluorescein with 5-ALA has been investigated for the resection of high-grade glioma. This approach results in better background discrimination from circulating fluorescein, while retaining the selectivity of 5-ALA-induced porphyrins for discriminating tumor [106, 107].

29.3.2.3 Fluorescein-Guided Surgery for Cerebral Metastases

Gross total resection (GTR) of cerebral metastases is recognized as an independent predictor of patient survival. As a result, there is a growing focus on intraoperative imaging techniques that can help increase the EOR to improve patient outcomes. While 5-aminolevulinic acid (5-ALA) shows positive fluorescence in approximately 50% of metastases, fluorescein appears to be more effective, with up to 94% of lesions exhibiting bright fluorescence (Fig. 29.5) [108, 109].

Studies have demonstrated a significantly higher rate of GTR when using fluorescein compared to traditional white light surgery for metastasis resection, suggesting that fluorescein-guided surgery for brain metastasis may offer improved patient outcome [95, 109–111]. However, it is important to note that further randomized controlled trials are necessary to conclusively prove the efficacy of fluorescein in metastasis surgery.

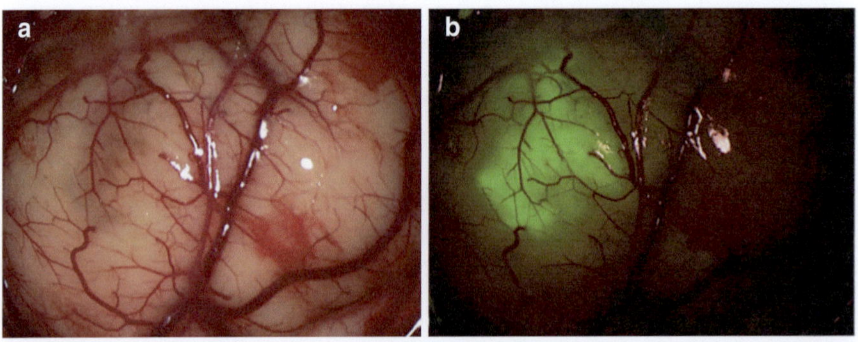

Fig. 29.5 Fluorescein-guided resection of brain metastasis. Intraoperative view of a metastasis under white light (**a**) and after application of fluorescein under YELLOW 560 filter (**b**) before corticotomy. (Reprinted with permission [110])

29.3.2.4 Fluorescein-Guided Surgery for Other CNS Tumors

Similar to the growing use of 5-ALA-guided surgery, an increasing number of studies are now reporting on fluorescein-guided resection of various CNS tumors. However, these studies are currently limited by small sample sizes and a lack of standardized protocols for fluorescein administration. Fluorescein has been described as helpful for resection of convexity meningioma, enabling visualization and differentiation of meningioma and its dural tail from normal brain and dura [112]. Furthermore, fluorescein might help enhance contrast between normal brain structures and cranial nerves and meningiomas in skull base surgery [113]. While primary central nervous system (CNS) lymphomas are typically managed with radio- and chemotherapy, a surgical biopsy is often necessary for diagnosis. Fluorescein has demonstrated utility in this context by helping to visualize lymphomas by delineating malignant tissue from normal brain [95, 104, 114].

29.3.3 Indocyanine Green (ICG)

Indocyanine green (ICG) is a tricarbocyanine with fluorescence in the near-infrared range with a peak emission at 780 nm and excitation at 810 nm. The US Food and Drug Administration (FDA) approved ICG in 1959 for assessing liver and cardiovascular functions. It later gained widespread use in ophthalmology [115, 116]. Raabe and colleagues pioneered the use of ICG for visualizing blood flow in cerebral vessels during surgery, a technique now known as ICG videoangiography [29]. ICG videoangiography was originally used to provide augmented information on cerebrovascular pathologies, and especially used for vascular cases (aneurysms and arterio-venous malformations) [117, 118]. ICG has also proven useful in understanding the angioarchitecture of hypervascular tumors, like hemangioblastomas, or in identifying surrounding vessels, enhancing surgical safety. Following the intravenous administration of 0.2–0.5 mg ICG/kg, NIR light (range 700–850 nm) is used to excite the dye, and an NIR camera—integrated in the latest generations of surgical microscopes—captures the emission at 780–950 nm of the molecules flowing through the vessels.

ICG is generally safe, with severe adverse reactions (such as hypotension, arrhythmia, or anaphylactic shock) occurring in only 0.05% of cases. Mild to moderate side effects (like nausea, skin eruption, and pruritus) are reported in 0.2% of cases [29].

A growing body of research has led to the utilization of ICG in neuro-oncological surgery as well. One technique has been referred to as second window ICG (SWIG), a procedure in which higher doses up to 5 mg/kg are administered to the patient up to 24 h in advance of surgery, with intraoperative imaging [119]. Within 24 h, ICG accumulates in the tumor tissue due to enhanced permeability within the tumor and selective retention effects [120]. It is assumed that ICG binds to serum albumin and can pass through the disrupted BBB. ICG is retained, possibly due to a lack of drainage [119, 120]. However, the exact mechanisms of retention are not fully understood.

Unlike 5-ALA-PpIX and fluorescein, which emit fluorescence within the visible spectrum, ICG's excitation and emission are in the near-infrared (NIR) region of the spectrum [121]. These properties enable visualization of the ICG fluorophore situated deeper in the tissue since longer wavelength excitation and emission light undergo less absorption than shorter wavelength [121]. Therefore, ICG permits visualization of tumors up to a depth of 2 cm and through the dura, facilitating planning of dural opening and corticotomy.

Studies revealed ICG fluorescence to be detectable in contrast-enhancing gliomas and have discussed ICG's value for the detection of tumor margins. Strong tumor-to-background fluorescence ratios were observed, and fluorescence appeared to correlate with the degree of contrast-enhancement on preoperative MRI [119]. So far, there are no studies demonstrating a benefit for EOR in glioma surgery. Furthermore, ICG is not tumor-specific, incorporating the risk of resection of normal false-positive tissue.

In addition, some authors suggest the usage of second-window-ICG in order to visualize residual tumor and the margins in surgery for metastases and meningioma [122, 123]. A recently published study underlines the capability of residual ICG fluorescence after resection of brain metastases as a promising variable for predicting the EOR [124]. However, the benefit of this intraoperative tool warrants further investigation.

29.4 Novel Techniques

Despite several advantages and the broad use of wide-field fluorescence imaging techniques, there are some limitations regarding sensitivity for the detection of malignant cells. Researchers are actively working on enhancing FGS and developing new methods to improve brain tumor resection. Many of these cutting-edge technologies are still in their early stages and are currently the focus of extensive research efforts.

29.4.1 Next-Generation Agents for Fluorescence-Guided Brain Tumor Surgery

Targeted fluorescence imaging, using fluorescent-labeled probes with tumor-specific molecular targets, is the next obvious step toward a higher accuracy for discriminating tumor-infiltrated tissue from normal brain.

Next-generation fluorescent agents should ideally have a high binding affinity for tumor cells, easily pass the BBB, allow for excellent optical visualization, and at the same time simplify the surgical workflow [125].

Tumor-targeting peptides that possess a specific affinity for receptors or molecules overexpressed on the tumor surface are under growing investigation [125]. One example is peptides targeting anti-epidermal growth-factor receptor (EGFR).

Studies on EGFR antibody-conjugated infrared dye have shown promising results in terms of safety and glioblastoma visualization [126].

Current preclinical research focuses on activable imaging probes. These are triggered by disease-relevant enzymes or molecules overexpressed in cancer cells, considering the tumor microenvironment [125]. The use of nanosystems, engineered to specifically target brain tumor cells, is also under present research [125]. These advancements aim to enhance the precision and effectiveness of fluorescence-guided surgery for brain tumors.

29.4.1.1 BLZ-100 Fluorescence-Guided Brain Tumor Surgery

The combination of a fluorophore with a tumor-specific peptide can enhance the specificity for the detection of malignant cells. One such advanced molecule is BLZ-100, also known as tozuleristide. This compound consists of two key components: chlorotoxin, a tumor-targeting peptide derived from scorpion venom, and ICG (indocyanine green), a near-infrared fluorophore [127].

Chlorotoxin has been shown to bind specifically to gliomas and tumors of neuroectodermal origin, making it an ideal targeting agent [128]. BLZ-100 is administered intravenously 24 h prior to surgery. During the procedure, surgeons can visualize the ICG fluorescence using a near-infrared camera. Studies have demonstrated that BLZ-100 has a high affinity for human gliomas, providing clear intraoperative imaging and potentially increasing the extent of tumor resection [129, 130]. However, further trials are needed to determine the utility of BLZ-100 in glioma surgery.

29.4.1.2 Tumor-Targeted Alkylphosphocholine Analogs for Intraoperative Visualization

Another promising approach targeting cancer cells involves the use of alkylphosphocholine (APC) analogs. Researchers are currently exploring the potential of APCs linked to fluorescent molecules for real-time visualization of tumor cells during surgery. APC analogs are small synthetic phospholipid ether molecules that are absorbed by tumor cells through overexpressed lipid rafts and undergo prolonged retention due to decreased catabolism [131, 132]. Initially developed for PET imaging and targeted radiotherapy, APC analogs have shown broad potential in targeting various types of tumors [132]. Two fluorescent APCs (CLR1501-green fluorescence and CLR1502-near infrared fluorescence) have demonstrated high selectivity in labeling cancer cells in a glioblastoma xenograft model [120]. As this technology progresses toward clinical application, researchers are working on developing a dual-labeled APC. This advanced version would combine near-infrared fluorescence, which allows for deep tissue imaging, with PET imaging capabilities in a single agent. Such a development could revolutionize cancer management by enabling synergistic diagnostic detection of tumor cells and proving useful across multiple stages of treatment, including tumor removal, cancer staging, and localized radiotherapy. However, to date, these are preclinical data, and the benefit in the management of brain tumor patients has yet to be determined and will require further research and clinical trials [133, 134].

29.4.2 Advanced Imaging Technologies

29.4.2.1 Confocal Laser Endomicroscopy

A significant challenge in wide-field fluorescence-guided surgery is the lack of high-resolution imaging and the subjective interpretation of fluorescence intensities. This makes it difficult to accurately distinguish between normal brain tissue and tumor tissue, especially in glioma surgery and at tumor margins. Preoperative imaging often fails to provide reliable predictions of tumor grade in glioma surgery [135]. As a result, surgeons frequently rely on time-consuming intraoperative frozen-section analyses. However, frozen-section pathology has its limitations and can sometimes be inconclusive or misleading [136]. To address these issues, confocal laser endomicroscopy has recently been introduced in neurosurgery. This technique allows for real-time intraoperative standard neuropathological diagnostics with high accuracy [137–139].

The system consists of a handheld probe that uses a single optical fiber both for illumination and detection, displaying high-resolution images with up to 1000-fold magnification on a mobile LCD workstation [140]. Tissue contrast is achieved by administration of fluorescent dyes, e.g., fluorescein [138].

This "optical biopsy" enables surgeons to detect tumor remnants at resection margins more accurately. In critical and eloquent brain regions, where an aggressive maximal EOR is not possible, confocal laser endomicroscopy can be used to measure tumor cell densities before resection.

In cases of LGG, which often do not show visible PPIX fluorescence, intraoperative confocal endomicroscopy is able to visualize the presence of even small amounts of fluorescence in tumor cells [141]. The combination of confocal laser endomicroscopy with Fluorescein has shown promising results, demonstrating high accuracy in histological assessments and detecting regions with infiltrating tumor [142, 143].

Confocal laser endomicroscopy has been successfully used to visualize tumor cells in various brain tumors, including meningiomas, pituitary adenomas, hemangioblastomas, gliomas, and neurocytomas [137, 144].

It is important to note that confocal laser endomicroscopy has a limited field of view, approximately 0.5 mm in diameter. Therefore, it cannot be used to scan the entire tumor area but is particularly useful at the end of surgery to detect remaining malignant tissue. Interpreting the images requires knowledge of histopathology or the presence of a neuropathologist [145].

29.4.2.2 Raman Spectroscopy

All previously mentioned visualization techniques rely on labeling agents that have limitations in terms of sensitivity or specificity for tumor detection. Recently, label-free techniques have emerged in the field of intraoperative tumor visualization. These new methods depend on the intrinsic biochemical properties of normal versus pathological tissue to provide image contrast [146–148].

Raman spectroscopy is one such technique based on the findings of C.V. Raman in 1928 [149]. The Raman effect refers to the scattering of monochromatic light.

While most photons in the visible spectrum are scattered elastically when interacting with tissue or media, a small portion of photons either absorb energy or transfer energy to or from the object being imaged. The transfer of energy results in inelastic scattering, known as the Raman effect. The Raman effect can be captured using a sensitive spectrometer. Raman spectroscopy provides information on the chemical composition of different tissues, such as their lipid and protein ratios, providing a structural fingerprint.

Studies have shown that Raman spectroscopy is helpful in distinguishing normal brain parenchyma from various types of brain tumors, including meningiomas, gliomas, and metastasis [150]. It can also help define tumor margins, detect residual tumor [146], and rapidly classify gliomas into common genetic subtypes [151].

Handheld probes for Raman spectroscopy are available for in vivo intraoperative use [152] (Fig. 29.6). These devices allow for immediate and precise tissue characterization, eliminating the delay associated with traditional histopathological examinations. This real-time information enables informed decision-making during critical procedures, potentially reducing operative time and improving surgical outcomes. The integration of machine learning algorithms for data analysis expands the possibilities of Raman spectroscopy in brain tumor surgery [153, 154].

While showing great promise, the clinical translation of Raman spectroscopy still faces challenges. Technological advancements are necessary to streamline its integration into the surgical workflow. There is also a need for standardization of

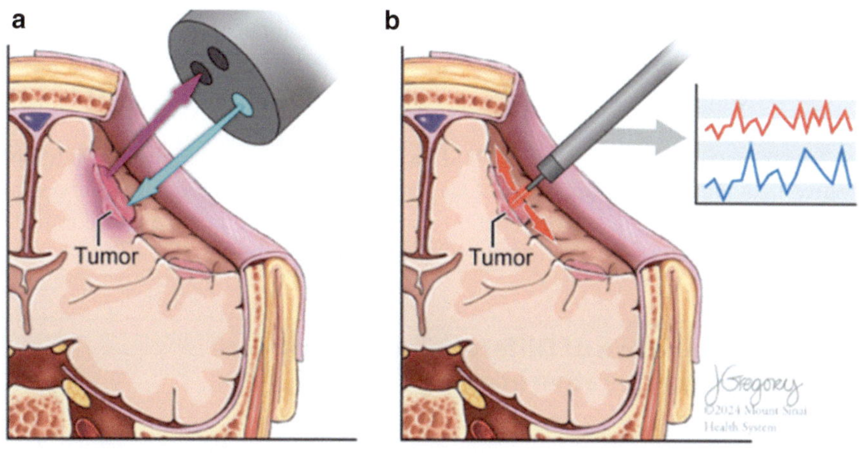

Fig. 29.6 Raman spectroscopy. (**a**) An intraoperative Raman spectroscopy probe emits a laser onto brain tissue during surgery, differentiating between tumor and healthy tissue in real time. The laser light interacts with molecular structures, generating a Raman signal that reveals biochemical differences. (**b**) The Raman spectrum displays distinct frequency peaks that differentiate tumor tissue from the surrounding normal brain parenchyma. The clear separation of spectral signatures highlights the effectiveness of Raman spectroscopy in identifying pathological tissues during surgery. (Reproduced under the terms and conditions of the Creative Commons Attribution license from [154])

data acquisition and analysis, as well as further studies to validate the data generated by Raman spectroscopy [154].

29.4.2.3 Hyperspectral Imaging

Hyperspectral imaging (HSI) is a noninvasive, emerging optical imaging technique offering surgeons enhanced visualization and tissue characterization in real time [155]. HSI captures and processes information from across the electromagnetic spectrum, typically focusing on the visible and near-infrared ranges. It collects detailed spectral information for each pixel, forming a large dataset that can be analyzed to identify specific tissue types based on their unique spectral signatures. This capability allows surgeons to detect tumors that might be invisible to the human eye or standard imaging technologies, potentially aiding in more extensive resections.

HSI in the field of neurosurgery is still under research; algorithms and protocols for data analysis are being developed and validated. As HSI technology progresses, there is potential for it to be combined with other imaging modalities, such as fluorescence-guided surgery (FGS).

A current limitation in the use of 5-ALA is its use in low-grade glioma surgery, as lower concentrations of PpIX fluorescence cannot be visualized with the currently applied surgical microscopes and filters. Obtaining quantitative maps of protoporphyrin IX (PpIX) concentration in tissue with the use of HIS could address this limitation and potentially extend the benefits of FGS to patients with low-grade gliomas, possibly allowing for higher EOR. Additionally, HSI can differentiate true PpIX fluorescence from autofluorescence and other photoproducts' fluorescence, allowing for more precise tumor identification.

Application of machine learning models not only facilitates automatic evaluation of acquired imaging data but also has the potential to use the generated information to classify tumor type, margin, WHO grade, and molecular status, e.g., IDH mutation status [156].

Together with machine learning, HSI has the potential to revolutionize intraoperative imaging in neuro-oncological surgery by providing surgeons with unprecedented insights into tissue composition and enabling more precise and complete tumor resections.

29.5 Combination of Different Techniques for Intraoperative Imaging

The combination of different imaging modalities, such as neuronavigation with MRI and PET with specific biomarkers and FGS, provides comprehensive information on tumor location, extent, anatomy, metabolism, and function [157, 158].

Emerging techniques may offer additional insights into the chemical or molecular composition of tissue. By combining different modalities, surgeons can overcome limitations of individual techniques, such as brain shift, while leveraging synergistic effects and maximizing the benefits of each approach [159–161].

29.6 Future Directions

Current developments in intraoperative visualization aim to enhance accuracy and EOR. However, established clinical methods face individual limitations, necessitating further research. For methods utilizing induced tissue fluorescence, there is a need to move from qualitative to quantitative assessments. Currently, the determination of "fluorescent" tissue relies on the surgeon's subjective impression. Efforts to measure and quantify fluorescence objectively are underway. One promising technology enabling quantitative information is fluorescence spectroscopy. Small handheld devices for intraoperative spectroscopy can determine actual protoporphyrin IX (PpIX) concentrations in tumor tissue during 5-ALA FGS, even when fluorescence is not visible under the microscope [47, 162, 163]. This method enables objective measurements of tissue fluorescence and can detect invisible PpIX accumulation in LGGs, which might otherwise go unnoticed. Studies have shown a 100-fold increase in fluorescence detection sensitivity in LGGs using handheld spectroscopy [164].

Research is ongoing into more specific labeling of tumor cells, such as targeted fluorescence imaging.

Innovations in neurosurgical microscopes and other optical technologies will enhance the view of the surgical field using various visualization tools, detecting additional optical features in tumor tissue [121]. Newer technologies like hyperspectral imaging can provide detailed spectral information of different tissues. When combined with deep learning algorithms, this approach can enable automated tissue classification [156]. The future of intraoperative imaging lies in multimodality and the development of new techniques. This approach will provide comprehensive information from different sources regarding biological, metabolic, anatomical, and functional properties of tissue. Neurosurgeons are increasingly integrating these imaging concepts into their daily routine for brain tumor surgery, aiming to improve the EOR while minimizing the risk of removing functional nontumor tissue.

References

1. Tew JM Jr, Gazi Yasargil M (1999) neurosurgery's man of the century. Neurosurgery 45(5):1010–1014
2. Brown TJ, Brennan MC, Li M, Church EW, Brandmeir NJ, Rakszawski KL et al (2016) Association of the extent of resection with survival in glioblastoma: a systematic review and meta-analysis. JAMA Oncol 2(11):1460–1469. https://doi.org/10.1001/jamaoncol.2016.1373
3. Lacroix M, Abi-Said D, Fourney DR, Gokaslan ZL, Shi W, DeMonte F et al (2001) A multivariate analysis of 416 patients with glioblastoma multiforme: prognosis, extent of resection, and survival. J Neurosurg 95(2):190–198. https://doi.org/10.3171/jns.2001.95.2.0190
4. Marko NF, Weil RJ, Schroeder JL, Lang FF, Suki D, Sawaya RE (2014) Extent of resection of glioblastoma revisited: personalized survival modeling facilitates more accurate survival prediction and supports a maximum-safe-resection approach to surgery. J Clin Oncol 32(8):774–782. https://doi.org/10.1200/JCO.2013.51.8886

5. Sanai N, Polley MY, McDermott MW, Parsa AT, Berger MS (2011) An extent of resection threshold for newly diagnosed glioblastomas. J Neurosurg 115(1):3–8. https://doi.org/10.3171/2011.2.JNS10998; https:doi.org/10.3171/2011.7.JNS10238
6. Stummer W, Reulen HJ, Meinel T, Pichlmeier U, Schumacher W, Tonn JC et al (2008) Extent of resection and survival in glioblastoma multiforme: identification of and adjustment for bias. Neurosurgery 62(3):564–576; discussion -76. https://doi.org/10.1227/01.neu.0000317304.31579.17
7. Klein Gunnewiek K, van Baarsen KM, Graus EHM, Brink WM, Lequin MH, Hoving EW (2024) Navigated intraoperative ultrasound in pediatric brain tumors. Childs Nerv Syst 40(9):2697–2705. https://doi.org/10.1007/s00381-024-06492-8
8. Orringer DA, Golby A, Jolesz F (2012) Neuronavigation in the surgical management of brain tumors: current and future trends. Expert Rev Med Devices 9(5):491–500. https://doi.org/10.1586/erd.12.42
9. Mahboob S, McPhillips R, Qiu Z, Jiang Y, Meggs C, Schiavone G et al (2016) Intraoperative ultrasound-guided resection of gliomas: a meta-analysis and review of the literature. World Neurosurg 92:255–263. https://doi.org/10.1016/j.wneu.2016.05.007
10. Saether CA, Torsteinsen M, Torp SH, Sundstrom S, Unsgard G, Solheim O (2012) Did survival improve after the implementation of intraoperative neuronavigation and 3D ultrasound in glioblastoma surgery? A retrospective analysis of 192 primary operations. J Neurol Surg A Cent Eur Neurosurg 73(2):73–78. https://doi.org/10.1055/s-0031-1297247
11. Aleo D, Elshaer Z, Pfnur A, Schuler PJ, Fontanella MM, Wirtz CR et al (2022) Evaluation of a navigated 3D ultrasound integration for brain tumor surgery: first results of an ongoing prospective study. Curr Oncol 29(9):6594–6609. https://doi.org/10.3390/curroncol29090518
12. Dixon L, Lim A, Grech-Sollars M, Nandi D, Camp S (2022) Intraoperative ultrasound in brain tumor surgery: a review and implementation guide. Neurosurg Rev 45(4):2503–2515. https://doi.org/10.1007/s10143-022-01778-4
13. Schulz C, Waldeck S, Mauer UM (2012) Intraoperative image guidance in neurosurgery: development, current indications, and future trends. Radiol Res Pract 2012:197364. https://doi.org/10.1155/2012/197364
14. Villanueva-Meyer JE, Mabray MC, Cha S (2017) Current clinical brain tumor imaging. Neurosurgery 81(3):397–415. https://doi.org/10.1093/neuros/nyx103
15. Picht T (2014) Current and potential utility of transcranial magnetic stimulation in the diagnostics before brain tumor surgery. CNS Oncol 3(4):299–310. https://doi.org/10.2217/cns.14.25
16. Basser PJ, Mattiello J, LeBihan D (1994) Estimation of the effective self-diffusion tensor from the NMR spin echo. J Magn Reson B 103(3):247–254
17. Elhawary H, Liu H, Patel P, Norton I, Rigolo L, Papademetris X et al (2011) Intraoperative real-time querying of white matter tracts during frameless stereotactic neuronavigation. Neurosurgery 68(2):506–516; discussion 16. https://doi.org/10.1227/NEU.0b013e3182036282
18. Jung TY, Jung S, Kim IY, Park SJ, Kang SS, Kim SH et al (2006) Application of neuronavigation system to brain tumor surgery with clinical experience of 420 cases. Minim Invasive Neurosurg 49(4):210–215. https://doi.org/10.1055/s-2006-948305
19. Sutherland GR, Kaibara T, Louw D, Hoult DI, Tomanek B, Saunders J (1999) A mobile high-field magnetic resonance system for neurosurgery. J Neurosurg 91(5):804–813. https://doi.org/10.3171/jns.1999.91.5.0804
20. Jolesz FA (2011) Intraoperative imaging in neurosurgery: where will the future take us? Acta Neurochir Suppl 109:21–25. https://doi.org/10.1007/978-3-211-99651-5_4
21. Senft C, Bink A, Franz K, Vatter H, Gasser T, Seifert V (2011) Intraoperative MRI guidance and extent of resection in glioma surgery: a randomised, controlled trial. Lancet Oncol 12(11):997–1003. https://doi.org/10.1016/S1470-2045(11)70196-6
22. Roder C, Stummer W, Coburger J, Scherer M, Haas P, von der Brelie C et al (2023) Intraoperative MRI-guided resection is not superior to 5-Aminolevulinic acid guidance in

newly diagnosed glioblastoma: a prospective controlled multicenter clinical trial. J Clin Oncol 41(36):5512–5523. https://doi.org/10.1200/JCO.22.01862
23. Kremer P, Tronnier V, Steiner HH, Metzner R, Ebinger F, Rating D et al (2006) Intraoperative MRI for interventional neurosurgical procedures and tumor resection control in children. Childs Nerv Syst 22(7):674–678. https://doi.org/10.1007/s00381-005-0030-2
24. Senft C, Franz K, Ulrich CT, Bink A, Szelenyi A, Gasser T et al (2010) Low field intraoperative MRI-guided surgery of gliomas: a single center experience. Clin Neurol Neurosurg 112(3):237–243. https://doi.org/10.1016/j.clineuro.2009.12.003
25. Senft C, Seifert V, Hermann E, Franz K, Gasser T (2008) Usefulness of intraoperative ultra low-field magnetic resonance imaging in glioma surgery. Neurosurgery 63(4 Suppl 2):257–266; discussion 66–7. https://doi.org/10.1227/01.NEU.0000313624.77452.3C
26. Moore GE (1947) Fluorescein as an agent in the differentiation of normal and malignant tissues. Science 106(2745):130–131. https://doi.org/10.1126/science.106.2745.130-a
27. Hadjipanayis CG, Widhalm G, Stummer W (2015) What is the surgical benefit of utilizing 5-Aminolevulinic acid for fluorescence-guided surgery of malignant gliomas? Neurosurgery 77(5):663–673. https://doi.org/10.1227/NEU.0000000000000929
28. Stummer W, Stocker S, Wagner S, Stepp H, Fritsch C, Goetz C et al (1998) Intraoperative detection of malignant gliomas by 5-aminolevulinic acid-induced porphyrin fluorescence. Neurosurgery 42(3):518–525; discussion 25–6
29. Raabe A, Beck J, Gerlach R, Zimmermann M, Seifert V (2003) Near-infrared indocyanine green video angiography: a new method for intraoperative assessment of vascular flow. Neurosurgery 52(1):132–139; discussion 9
30. Colditz MJ, Leyen K, Jeffree RL (2012) Aminolevulinic acid (ALA)-protoporphyrin IX fluorescence guided tumour resection. Part 2: theoretical, biochemical and practical aspects. J Clin Neurosci 19(12):1611–1616. https://doi.org/10.1016/j.jocn.2012.03.013
31. Stummer W, Stepp H, Moller G, Ehrhardt A, Leonhard M, Reulen HJ (1998) Technical principles for protoporphyrin-IX-fluorescence guided microsurgical resection of malignant glioma tissue. Acta Neurochir 140(10):995–1000
32. Stummer W, Stepp H, Wiestler OD, Pichlmeier U (2017) Randomized, prospective double-blinded study comparing 3 different doses of 5-Aminolevulinic acid for fluorescence-guided resections of malignant gliomas. Neurosurgery 81(2):230–239. https://doi.org/10.1093/neuros/nyx074
33. Kaneko S, Suero Molina E, Ewelt C, Warneke N, Stummer W (2019) Fluorescence-based measurement of real-time kinetics of Protoporphyrin IX after 5-Aminolevulinic acid administration in human in situ malignant gliomas. Neurosurgery 85:E739
34. Stummer W, Suero ME (2017) Fluorescence imaging/agents in tumor resection. Neurosurg Clin N Am 28(4):569–583. https://doi.org/10.1016/j.nec.2017.05.009
35. Stummer W, Novotny A, Stepp H, Goetz C, Bise K, Reulen HJ (2000) Fluorescence-guided resection of glioblastoma multiforme by using 5-aminolevulinic acid-induced porphyrins: a prospective study in 52 consecutive patients. J Neurosurg 93(6):1003–1013. https://doi.org/10.3171/jns.2000.93.6.1003
36. Stummer W, Pichlmeier U, Meinel T, Wiestler OD, Zanella F, Reulen HJ et al (2006) Fluorescence-guided surgery with 5-aminolevulinic acid for resection of malignant glioma: a randomised controlled multicentre phase III trial. Lancet Oncol 7(5):392–401. https://doi.org/10.1016/S1470-2045(06)70665-9
37. Teixidor P, Arraez MA, Villalba G, Garcia R, Tardaguila M, Gonzalez JJ et al (2016) Safety and efficacy of 5-Aminolevulinic acid for high grade glioma in usual clinical practice: a prospective cohort study. PLoS One 11(2):e0149244. https://doi.org/10.1371/journal.pone.0149244
38. Schwake M, Schipmann S, Muther M, Kochling M, Brentrup A, Stummer W (2019) 5-ALA fluorescence-guided surgery in pediatric brain tumors-a systematic review. Acta Neurochir 161(6):1099–1108. https://doi.org/10.1007/s00701-019-03898-1
39. Utsuki S, Miyoshi N, Oka H, Miyajima Y, Shimizu S, Suzuki S et al (2007) Fluorescence-guided resection of metastatic brain tumors using a 5-aminolevulinic acid-induced proto-

porphyrin IX: pathological study. Brain Tumor Pathol 24(2):53–55. https://doi.org/10.1007/s10014-007-0223-3
40. Valdes PA, Millesi M, Widhalm G, Roberts DW (2019) 5-aminolevulinic acid induced protoporphyrin IX (ALA-PpIX) fluorescence guidance in meningioma surgery. J Neuro-Oncol 141(3):555–565. https://doi.org/10.1007/s11060-018-03079-7
41. Carlsson SK, Brothers SP, Wahlestedt C (2014) Emerging treatment strategies for glioblastoma multiforme. EMBO Mol Med 6(11):1359–1370. https://doi.org/10.15252/emmm.201302627
42. Koshy M, Villano JL, Dolecek TA, Howard A, Mahmood U, Chmura SJ et al (2012) Improved survival time trends for glioblastoma using the SEER 17 population-based registries. J Neuro-Oncol 107(1):207–212. https://doi.org/10.1007/s11060-011-0738-7
43. Ostrom QT, Price M, Neff C, Cioffi G, Waite KA, Kruchko C et al (2023) CBTRUS statistical report: primary brain and other central nervous system tumors diagnosed in the United States in 2016–2020. Neuro-Oncology 25(12 Suppl 2):iv1–iv99. https://doi.org/10.1093/neuonc/noad149
44. Orringer D, Lau D, Khatri S, Zamora-Berridi GJ, Zhang K, Wu C et al (2012) Extent of resection in patients with glioblastoma: limiting factors, perception of resectability, and effect on survival. J Neurosurg 117(5):851–859. https://doi.org/10.3171/2012.8.JNS12234
45. Coburger J, Hagel V, Wirtz CR, Konig R (2015) Surgery for glioblastoma: impact of the combined use of 5-Aminolevulinic acid and intraoperative MRI on extent of resection and survival. PLoS One 10(6):e0131872. https://doi.org/10.1371/journal.pone.0131872
46. Della Puppa A, De Pellegrin S, d'Avella E, Gioffre G, Rossetto M, Gerardi A et al (2013) 5-aminolevulinic acid (5-ALA) fluorescence guided surgery of high-grade gliomas in eloquent areas assisted by functional mapping. Our experience and review of the literature. Acta Neurochir 155(6):965–972; discussion 72. https://doi.org/10.1007/s00701-013-1660-x
47. Stummer W, Tonn JC, Goetz C, Ullrich W, Stepp H, Bink A et al (2014) 5-Aminolevulinic acid-derived tumor fluorescence: the diagnostic accuracy of visible fluorescence qualities as corroborated by spectrometry and histology and postoperative imaging. Neurosurgery 74(3):310–319; discussion 9–20. https://doi.org/10.1227/NEU.0000000000000267
48. Idoate MA, Diez Valle R, Echeveste J, Tejada S (2011) Pathological characterization of the glioblastoma border as shown during surgery using 5-aminolevulinic acid-induced fluorescence. Neuropathology 31(6):575–582. https://doi.org/10.1111/j.1440-1789.2011.01202.x
49. Roberts DW, Valdes PA, Harris BT, Fontaine KM, Hartov A, Fan X et al (2011) Coregistered fluorescence-enhanced tumor resection of malignant glioma: relationships between delta-aminolevulinic acid-induced protoporphyrin IX fluorescence, magnetic resonance imaging enhancement, and neuropathological parameters. Clinical article. J Neurosurg 114(3):595–603. https://doi.org/10.3171/2010.2.JNS091322
50. Perrini P, Gambacciani C, Weiss A, Pasqualetti F, Delishaj D, Paiar F et al (2017) Survival outcomes following repeat surgery for recurrent glioblastoma: a single-center retrospective analysis. J Neuro-Oncol 131(3):585–591. https://doi.org/10.1007/s11060-016-2330-7
51. Ringel F, Pape H, Sabel M, Krex D, Bock HC, Misch M et al (2016) Clinical benefit from resection of recurrent glioblastomas: results of a multicenter study including 503 patients with recurrent glioblastomas undergoing surgical resection. Neuro-Oncology 18(1):96–104. https://doi.org/10.1093/neuonc/nov145
52. Suchorska B, Weller M, Tabatabai G, Senft C, Hau P, Sabel MC et al (2016) Complete resection of contrast-enhancing tumor volume is associated with improved survival in recurrent glioblastoma-results from the DIRECTOR trial. Neuro-Oncology 18(4):549–556. https://doi.org/10.1093/neuonc/nov326
53. Della Puppa A, Ciccarino P, Lombardi G, Rolma G, Cecchin D, Rossetto M (2014) 5-Aminolevulinic acid fluorescence in high grade glioma surgery: surgical outcome, intraoperative findings, and fluorescence patterns. Biomed Res Int 2014:232561. https://doi.org/10.1155/2014/232561
54. Hickmann AK, Nadji-Ohl M, Hopf NJ (2015) Feasibility of fluorescence-guided resection of recurrent gliomas using five-aminolevulinic acid: retrospective analysis of surgical and neu-

rological outcome in 58 patients. J Neuro-Oncol 122(1):151–160. https://doi.org/10.1007/s11060-014-1694-9
55. Brandes AA, Tosoni A, Spagnolli F, Frezza G, Leonardi M, Calbucci F et al (2008) Disease progression or pseudoprogression after concomitant radiochemotherapy treatment: pitfalls in neurooncology. Neuro-Oncology 10(3):361–367. https://doi.org/10.1215/15228517-2008-008
56. de Wit MC, de Bruin HG, Eijkenboom W, Sillevis Smitt PA, van den Bent MJ (2004) Immediate post-radiotherapy changes in malignant glioma can mimic tumor progression. Neurology 63(3):535–537
57. Taal W, Brandsma D, de Bruin HG, Bromberg JE, Swaak-Kragten AT, Smitt PA et al (2008) Incidence of early pseudo-progression in a cohort of malignant glioma patients treated with chemoirradiation with temozolomide. Cancer 113(2):405–410. https://doi.org/10.1002/cncr.23562
58. Kamp MA, Felsberg J, Sadat H, Kuzibaev J, Steiger HJ, Rapp M, et al. 5-ALA-induced fluorescence behavior of reactive tissue changes following glioblastoma treatment with radiation and chemotherapy. Acta Neurochir 2015;157(2):207–213; discussion 13–4. doi:https://doi.org/10.1007/s00701-014-2313-4
59. Nabavi A, Thurm H, Zountsas B, Pietsch T, Lanfermann H, Pichlmeier U et al (2009) Five-aminolevulinic acid for fluorescence-guided resection of recurrent malignant gliomas: a phase ii study. Neurosurgery 65(6):1070–1076; discussion 6–7. https://doi.org/10.1227/01.NEU.0000360128.03597.C7
60. Utsuki S, Oka H, Sato S, Shimizu S, Suzuki S, Tanizaki Y, et al. Histological examination of false positive tissue resection using 5-aminolevulinic acid-induced fluorescence guidance. Neurol Med Chir (Tokyo) 2007;47(5):210–213; discussion 3–4
61. Lau D, Hervey-Jumper SL, Chang S, Molinaro AM, McDermott MW, Phillips JJ et al (2016) A prospective phase II clinical trial of 5-aminolevulinic acid to assess the correlation of intraoperative fluorescence intensity and degree of histologic cellularity during resection of high-grade gliomas. J Neurosurg 124(5):1300–1309. https://doi.org/10.3171/2015.5.JNS1577
62. Smith JS, Chang EF, Lamborn KR, Chang SM, Prados MD, Cha S et al (2008) Role of extent of resection in the long-term outcome of low-grade hemispheric gliomas. J Clin Oncol 26(8):1338–1345. https://doi.org/10.1200/JCO.2007.13.9337
63. Sanai N, Berger MS (2008) Glioma extent of resection and its impact on patient outcome. Neurosurgery 62(4):753–764; discussion 264–6. https://doi.org/10.1227/01.neu.0000318159.21731.cf
64. Hervey-Jumper SL, Berger MS (2014) Role of surgical resection in low- and high-grade gliomas. Curr Treat Options Neurol 16(4):284. https://doi.org/10.1007/s11940-014-0284-7
65. Paulus W, Peiffer J (1989) Intratumoral histologic heterogeneity of gliomas. A quantitative study. Cancer 64(2):442–447
66. Ewelt C, Floeth FW, Felsberg J, Steiger HJ, Sabel M, Langen KJ et al (2011) Finding the anaplastic focus in diffuse gliomas: the value of Gd-DTPA enhanced MRI, FET-PET, and intraoperative, ALA-derived tissue fluorescence. Clin Neurol Neurosurg 113(7):541–547. https://doi.org/10.1016/j.clineuro.2011.03.008
67. Jaber M, Wolfer J, Ewelt C, Holling M, Hasselblatt M, Niederstadt T et al (2016) The value of 5-Aminolevulinic acid in low-grade gliomas and high-grade gliomas lacking glioblastoma imaging features: an analysis based on fluorescence, magnetic resonance imaging, 18F-Fluoroethyl tyrosine positron emission tomography, and tumor molecular factors. Neurosurgery 78(3):401–411; discussion 11. https://doi.org/10.1227/NEU.0000000000001020
68. Kaneko S, Suero Molina E, Sporns P, Schipmann S, Black D, Stummer W (2022) Fluorescence real-time kinetics of protoporphyrin IX after 5-ALA administration in low-grade glioma. J Neurosurg 136(1):9–15. https://doi.org/10.3171/2020.10.JNS202881
69. Widhalm G, Kiesel B, Woehrer A, Traub-Weidinger T, Preusser M, Marosi C et al (2013) 5-Aminolevulinic acid induced fluorescence is a powerful intraoperative marker for precise

histopathological grading of gliomas with non-significant contrast-enhancement. PLoS One 8(10):e76988. https://doi.org/10.1371/journal.pone.0076988
70. Suero Molina E, Black D, Kaneko S, Muther M, Stummer W (2022) Double dose of 5-aminolevulinic acid and its effect on protoporphyrin IX accumulation in low-grade glioma. J Neurosurg 137(4):943–952. https://doi.org/10.3171/2021.12.JNS211724
71. Almekkawi AK, El Ahmadieh TY, Wu EM, Abunimer AM, Abi-Aad KR, Aoun SG et al (2020) The use of 5-Aminolevulinic acid in low-grade glioma resection: a systematic review. Oper Neurosurg (Hagerstown) 19(1):1–8. https://doi.org/10.1093/ons/opz336
72. Della Puppa A, Rustemi O, Gioffre G, Troncon I, Lombardi G, Rolma G et al (2014) Predictive value of intraoperative 5-aminolevulinic acid-induced fluorescence for detecting bone invasion in meningioma surgery. J Neurosurg 120(4):840–845. https://doi.org/10.3171/2013.12.JNS131642
73. Millesi M, Kiesel B, Mischkulnig M, Martinez-Moreno M, Wohrer A, Wolfsberger S et al (2016) Analysis of the surgical benefits of 5-ALA-induced fluorescence in intracranial meningiomas: experience in 204 meningiomas. J Neurosurg 125(6):1408–1419. https://doi.org/10.3171/2015.12.JNS151513
74. Wadiura LI, Millesi M, Makolli J, Wais J, Kiesel B, Mischkulnig M et al (2021) High diagnostic accuracy of visible 5-ALA fluorescence in meningioma surgery according to histopathological analysis of tumor bulk and peritumoral tissue. Lasers Surg Med 53(3):300–308. https://doi.org/10.1002/lsm.23294
75. Wilbers E, Hargus G, Wolfer J, Stummer W (2014) Usefulness of 5-ALA (Gliolan(R))-derived PPX fluorescence for demonstrating the extent of infiltration in atypical meningiomas. Acta Neurochir 156(10):1853–1854. https://doi.org/10.1007/s00701-014-2148-z
76. Kamp MA, Fischer I, Buhner J, Turowski B, Cornelius JF, Steiger HJ et al (2016) 5-ALA fluorescence of cerebral metastases and its impact for the local-in-brain progression. Oncotarget 7(41):66776–66789. https://doi.org/10.18632/oncotarget.11488
77. Kamp MA, Grosser P, Felsberg J, Slotty PJ, Steiger HJ, Reifenberger G et al (2012) 5-aminolevulinic acid (5-ALA)-induced fluorescence in intracerebral metastases: a retrospective study. Acta Neurochir 154(2):223–228; discussion 8. https://doi.org/10.1007/s00701-011-1200-5
78. Sarkis HM, Zawy Alsofy S, Stroop R, Lewitz M, Schipmann S, Unnewehr M et al (2024) Does 5-ALA fluorescence microscopy improve complete Resectability in cerebral/cerebellar metastatic surgery? A retrospective data analysis from a cranial center. Cancers (Basel) 16(12). https://doi.org/10.3390/cancers16122242
79. Shah HA, Leskinen S, Khilji H, Narayan V, Ben-Shalom N, D'Amico RS (2022) Utility of 5-ALA for fluorescence-guided resection of brain metastases: a systematic review. J Neuro-Oncol 160(3):669–675. https://doi.org/10.1007/s11060-022-04188-0
80. Albalkhi I, Shafqat A, Bin-Alamer O, Abou Al-Shaar AR, Mallela AN, Fernandez-de Thomas RJ et al (2023) Fluorescence-guided resection of intradural spinal tumors: a systematic review and meta-analysis. Neurosurg Rev 47(1):10. https://doi.org/10.1007/s10143-023-02230-x
81. Eicker S, Sarikaya-Seiwert S, Borkhardt A, Gierga K, Turowski B, Heiroth HJ et al (2011) ALA-induced porphyrin accumulation in medulloblastoma and its use for fluorescence-guided surgery. Cent Eur Neurosurg 72(2):101–103. https://doi.org/10.1055/s-0030-1252010
82. Ruge JR, Liu J (2009) Use of 5-aminolevulinic acid for visualization and resection of a benign pediatric brain tumor. J Neurosurg Pediatr 4(5):484–486. https://doi.org/10.3171/2009.6.PEDS08428
83. Stummer W, Rodrigues F, Schucht P, Preuss M, Wiewrodt D, Nestler U et al (2014) Predicting the "usefulness" of 5-ALA-derived tumor fluorescence for fluorescence-guided resections in pediatric brain tumors: a European survey. Acta Neurochir 156(12):2315–2324. https://doi.org/10.1007/s00701-014-2234-2
84. Evers G, Kamp M, Warneke N, Berdel W, Sabel M, Stummer W et al (2017) 5-Aminolaevulinic acid-induced fluorescence in primary central nervous system lymphoma. World Neurosurg 98:375–380. https://doi.org/10.1016/j.wneu.2016.11.011

85. Yamamoto T, Ishikawa E, Miki S, Sakamoto N, Zaboronok A, Matsuda M et al (2015) Photodynamic diagnosis using 5-Aminolevulinic acid in 41 biopsies for primary central nervous system lymphoma. Photochem Photobiol 91(6):1452–1457. https://doi.org/10.1111/php.12510
86. Utsuki S, Oka H, Kijima C, Miyajima Y, Hagiwara H, Fujii K (2011) Utility of intraoperative fluorescent diagnosis of residual hemangioblastoma using 5-aminolevulinic acid. Neurol India 59(4):612–615. https://doi.org/10.4103/0028-3886.84349
87. Bernal Garcia LM, Cabezudo Artero JM, Marcelo Zamorano MB, Gilete Tejero I (2015) Fluorescence-guided resection with 5-aminolevulinic Acid of subependymomas of the fourth ventricle: report of 2 cases: technical case report. Neurosurgery 11(Suppl 2):E364–E371; discussion E71. https://doi.org/10.1227/NEU.0000000000000682
88. Takeda J, Nonaka M, Li Y, Komori Y, Kamei T, Iwata R et al (2017) 5-ALA fluorescence-guided endoscopic surgery for mixed germ cell tumors. J Neuro-Oncol 134(1):119–124. https://doi.org/10.1007/s11060-017-2494-9
89. Rabb MF, Burton TC, Schatz H, Yannuzzi LA (1978) Fluorescein angiography of the fundus: a schematic approach to interpretation. Surv Ophthalmol 22(6):387–403
90. Schebesch KM, Brawanski A, Hohenberger C, Hohne J (2016) Fluorescein sodium-guided surgery of malignant brain tumors: history, current concepts, and future project. Turk Neurosurg 26(2):185–194. https://doi.org/10.5137/1019-5149.JTN.16952-16.0
91. Kuroiwa T, Kajimoto Y, Ohta T (1998) Development of a fluorescein operative microscope for use during malignant glioma surgery: a technical note and preliminary report. Surg Neurol 50(1):41–48; discussion 8–9
92. Shinoda J, Yano H, Yoshimura S, Okumura A, Kaku Y, Iwama T et al (2003) Fluorescence-guided resection of glioblastoma multiforme by using high-dose fluorescein sodium. Technical note. J Neurosurg 99(3):597–603. https://doi.org/10.3171/jns.2003.99.3.0597
93. Schebesch KM, Proescholdt M, Hohne J, Hohenberger C, Hansen E, Riemenschneider MJ et al (2013) Sodium fluorescein-guided resection under the YELLOW 560 nm surgical microscope filter in malignant brain tumor surgery–a feasibility study. Acta Neurochir 155(4):693–699. https://doi.org/10.1007/s00701-013-1643-y
94. Diaz RJ, Dios RR, Hattab EM, Burrell K, Rakopoulos P, Sabha N et al (2015) Study of the biodistribution of fluorescein in glioma-infiltrated mouse brain and histopathological correlation of intraoperative findings in high-grade gliomas resected under fluorescein fluorescence guidance. J Neurosurg 122(6):1360–1369. https://doi.org/10.3171/2015.2.JNS132507
95. Hamamcioglu MK, Akcakaya MO, Goker B, Kasimcan MO, Kiris T (2016) The use of the YELLOW 560 nm surgical microscope filter for sodium fluorescein-guided resection of brain tumors: our preliminary results in a series of 28 patients. Clin Neurol Neurosurg 143:39–45. https://doi.org/10.1016/j.clineuro.2016.02.006
96. Dilek O, Ihsan A, Tulay H (2011) Anaphylactic reaction after fluorescein sodium administration during intracranial surgery. J Clin Neurosci 18(3):430–431. https://doi.org/10.1016/j.jocn.2010.06.012
97. Stummer W (2015) Poor man's fluorescence? Acta Neurochir 157(8):1379–1381. https://doi.org/10.1007/s00701-015-2471-z
98. Stummer W, Gotz C, Hassan A, Heimann A, Kempski O (1993) Kinetics of Photofrin II in perifocal brain edema. Neurosurgery 33(6):1075–1081; discussion 81-2
99. Acerbi F, Broggi M, Eoli M, Anghileri E, Cavallo C, Boffano C et al (2014) Is fluorescein-guided technique able to help in resection of high-grade gliomas? Neurosurg Focus 36(2):E5. https://doi.org/10.3171/2013.11.FOCUS13487
100. Chen B, Wang H, Ge P, Zhao J, Li W, Gu H et al (2012) Gross total resection of glioma with the intraoperative fluorescence-guidance of fluorescein sodium. Int J Med Sci 9(8):708–714. https://doi.org/10.7150/ijms.4843
101. Neira JA, Ung TH, Sims JS, Malone HR, Chow DS, Samanamud JL et al (2017) Aggressive resection at the infiltrative margins of glioblastoma facilitated by intraoperative fluorescein guidance. J Neurosurg 127(1):111–122. https://doi.org/10.3171/2016.7.JNS16232

102. Rey-Dios R, Hattab EM, Cohen-Gadol AA (2014) Use of intraoperative fluorescein sodium fluorescence to improve the accuracy of tissue diagnosis during stereotactic needle biopsy of high-grade gliomas. Acta Neurochir 156(6):1071–1075; discussion 5. https://doi.org/10.1007/s00701-014-2097-6
103. Acerbi F, Broggi M, Schebesch KM, Hohne J, Cavallo C, De Laurentis C et al (2018) Fluorescein-guided surgery for resection of high-grade gliomas: a multicentric prospective phase II study (FLUOGLIO). Clin Cancer Res 24(1):52–61. https://doi.org/10.1158/1078-0432.CCR-17-1184
104. Falco J, Cavallo C, Vetrano IG, de Laurentis C, Siozos L, Schiariti M et al (2019) Fluorescein application in cranial and spinal tumors enhancing at preoperative MRI and operated with a dedicated filter on the surgical microscope: preliminary results in 279 patients enrolled in the FLUOCERTUM prospective study. Front Surg 6:49. https://doi.org/10.3389/fsurg.2019.00049
105. Falco J, Rubiu E, Broggi M, Farinotti M, Vetrano IG, Schiariti M et al (2022) Towards an established intraoperative oncological favorable tool: results of fluorescein-guided resection from a monocentric, prospective series of 93 primary glioblastoma patients. J Clin Med 12(1). https://doi.org/10.3390/jcm12010178
106. Pesaresi A, La Cava P, Bonada M, Zeppa P, Melcarne A, Cofano F et al (2024) Combined fluorescence-guided surgery with 5-Aminolevulinic acid and fluorescein in glioblastoma: technical description and report of 100 cases. Cancers (Basel) 16(16). https://doi.org/10.3390/cancers16162771
107. Suero Molina E, Wolfer J, Ewelt C, Ehrhardt A, Brokinkel B, Stummer W (2018) Dual-labeling with 5-aminolevulinic acid and fluorescein for fluorescence-guided resection of high-grade gliomas: technical note. J Neurosurg 128(2):399–405. https://doi.org/10.3171/2016.11.JNS161072
108. Ohadi MAD, Dashtkoohi M, Babaei MR, Zamani R, Dashtkoohi M, Hadjipanayis CG (2024) Sodium fluorescein-guided resection of brain metastases: a needed approach or an option? A systematic review and meta-analysis. Acta Neurochir 166(1):334. https://doi.org/10.1007/s00701-024-06223-7
109. Schebesch KM, Hohne J, Noeva E, Pukrop T, Araceli T, Schmidt NO et al (2023) Brain metastasis resection: the impact of fluorescence guidance (MetResect study). Neurosurg Focus 55(2):E10. https://doi.org/10.3171/2023.5.FOCUS23197
110. Hohne J, Hohenberger C, Proescholdt M, Riemenschneider MJ, Wendl C, Brawanski A et al (2017) Fluorescein sodium-guided resection of cerebral metastases-an update. Acta Neurochir 159(2):363–367. https://doi.org/10.1007/s00701-016-3054-3
111. Patchell RA, Tibbs PA, Regine WF, Dempsey RJ, Mohiuddin M, Kryscio RJ et al (1998) Postoperative radiotherapy in the treatment of single metastases to the brain: a randomized trial. JAMA 280(17):1485–1489
112. da Silva CE, da Silva VD, da Silva JL (2014) Convexity meningiomas enhanced by sodium fluorescein. Surg Neurol Int 5:3. https://doi.org/10.4103/2152-7806.124978
113. da Silva CE, da Silva JL, da Silva VD (2010) Use of sodium fluorescein in skull base tumors. Surg Neurol Int 1:70. https://doi.org/10.4103/2152-7806.72247
114. Schebesch KM, Hoehne J, Hohenberger C, Acerbi F, Broggi M, Proescholdt M et al (2015) Fluorescein sodium-guided surgery in cerebral lymphoma. Clin Neurol Neurosurg 139:125–128. https://doi.org/10.1016/j.clineuro.2015.09.015
115. Cherrick GR, Stein SW, Leevy CM, Davidson CS (1960) Indocyanine green: observations on its physical properties, plasma decay, and hepatic extraction. J Clin Invest 39:592–600. https://doi.org/10.1172/JCI104072
116. Reinhart MB, Huntington CR, Blair LJ, Heniford BT, Augenstein VA (2016) Indocyanine green: historical context, current applications, and future considerations. Surg Innov 23(2):166–175. https://doi.org/10.1177/1553350615604053
117. Hanggi D, Etminan N, Steiger HJ (2010) The impact of microscope-integrated intraoperative near-infrared indocyanine green videoangiography on surgery of arteriovenous malforma-

tions and dural arteriovenous fistulae. Neurosurgery 67(4):1094–1103; discussion 103–4. https://doi.org/10.1227/NEU.0b013e3181eb5049
118. Raabe A, Nakaji P, Beck J, Kim LJ, Hsu FP, Kamerman JD et al (2005) Prospective evaluation of surgical microscope-integrated intraoperative near-infrared indocyanine green videoangiography during aneurysm surgery. J Neurosurg 103(6):982–989. https://doi.org/10.3171/jns.2005.103.6.0982
119. Lee JY, Thawani JP, Pierce J, Zeh R, Martinez-Lage M, Chanin M et al (2016) Intraoperative near-infrared optical imaging can localize gadolinium-enhancing gliomas during surgery. Neurosurgery 79(6):856–871. https://doi.org/10.1227/NEU.0000000000001450
120. Swanson KI, Clark PA, Zhang RR, Kandela IK, Farhoud M, Weichert JP et al (2015) Fluorescent cancer-selective alkylphosphocholine analogs for intraoperative glioma detection. Neurosurgery 76(2):115–123; discussion 23–4. https://doi.org/10.1227/NEU.0000000000000622
121. Valdes PA, Roberts DW, Lu FK, Golby A (2016) Optical technologies for intraoperative neurosurgical guidance. Neurosurg Focus 40(3):E8. https://doi.org/10.3171/2015.12.FOCUS15550
122. Lee JYK, Pierce JT, Thawani JP, Zeh R, Nie S, Martinez-Lage M et al (2018) Near-infrared fluorescent image-guided surgery for intracranial meningioma. J Neurosurg 128(2):380–390. https://doi.org/10.3171/2016.10.JNS161636
123. Lee JYK, Pierce JT, Zeh R, Cho SS, Salinas R, Nie S et al (2017) Intraoperative near-infrared optical contrast can localize brain metastases. World Neurosurg 106:120–130. https://doi.org/10.1016/j.wneu.2017.06.128
124. Teng CW, Cho SS, Singh Y, De Ravin E, Somers K, Buch L et al (2021) Second window ICG predicts gross-total resection and progression-free survival during brain metastasis surgery. J Neurosurg 135(4):1026–1035. https://doi.org/10.3171/2020.8.JNS201810
125. Chirizzi C, Pellegatta S, Gori A, Falco J, Rubiu E, Acerbi F et al (2024) Next-generation agents for fluorescence-guided glioblastoma surgery. Bioeng Transl Med 9(3):e10608. https://doi.org/10.1002/btm2.10608
126. Miller SE, Tummers WS, Teraphongphom N, van den Berg NS, Hasan A, Ertsey RD et al (2018) First-in-human intraoperative near-infrared fluorescence imaging of glioblastoma using cetuximab-IRDye800. J Neuro-Oncol 139(1):135–143. https://doi.org/10.1007/s11060-018-2854-0
127. Parrish-Novak J, Byrnes-Blake K, Lalayeva N, Burleson S, Fidel J, Gilmore R et al (2017) Nonclinical profile of BLZ-100, a tumor-targeting fluorescent imaging agent. Int J Toxicol 36(2):104–112. https://doi.org/10.1177/1091581817697685
128. Lyons SA, O'Neal J, Sontheimer H (2002) Chlorotoxin, a scorpion-derived peptide, specifically binds to gliomas and tumors of neuroectodermal origin. Glia 39(2):162–173. https://doi.org/10.1002/glia.10083
129. Butte PV, Mamelak A, Parrish-Novak J, Drazin D, Shweikeh F, Gangalum PR et al (2014) Near-infrared imaging of brain tumors using the tumor paint BLZ-100 to achieve near-complete resection of brain tumors. Neurosurg Focus 36(2):E1. https://doi.org/10.3171/2013.11.FOCUS13497
130. Patil CG, Walker DG, Miller DM, Butte P, Morrison B, Kittle DS et al (2019) Phase 1 safety, pharmacokinetics, and fluorescence imaging study of Tozuleristide (BLZ-100) in adults with newly diagnosed or recurrent gliomas. Neurosurgery 85(4):E641–E6E9. https://doi.org/10.1093/neuros/nyz125
131. Hilgard P, Klenner T, Stekar J, Unger C (1993) Alkylphosphocholines: a new class of membrane-active anticancer agents. Cancer Chemother Pharmacol 32(2):90–95
132. Weichert JP, Clark PA, Kandela IK, Vaccaro AM, Clarke W, Longino MA et al (2014) Alkylphosphocholine analogs for broad-spectrum cancer imaging and therapy. Sci Transl Med 6(240):240ra75. https://doi.org/10.1126/scitranslmed.3007646
133. Kuo JS, Zhang RR, Pinchuk AN, Clark PA, Weichert JP (2016) Creation of a dual-labeled cancer-targeting Alkylphosphocholine analog for dual modality quantitative positron emission tomography and intraoperative tumor visualization. Neurosurgery 63(CN_suppl_1):208

134. Zhang RR, Swanson KI, Hall LT, Weichert JP, Kuo JS (2016) Diapeutic cancer-targeting alkylphosphocholine analogs may advance management of brain malignancies. CNS Oncol 5(4):223–231. https://doi.org/10.2217/cns-2016-0017
135. Muragaki Y, Chernov M, Maruyama T, Ochiai T, Taira T, Kubo O et al (2008) Low-grade glioma on stereotactic biopsy: how often is the diagnosis accurate? Minim Invasive Neurosurg 51(5):275–279. https://doi.org/10.1055/s-0028-1082322
136. Uematsu Y, Owai Y, Okita R, Tanaka Y, Itakura T (2007) The usefulness and problem of intraoperative rapid diagnosis in surgical neuropathology. Brain Tumor Pathol 24(2):47–52. https://doi.org/10.1007/s10014-007-0219-z
137. Byun YH, Won JK, Hong DH, Kang H, Kim JH, Yu MO et al (2024) A prospective multicenter assessor blinded pilot study using confocal laser endomicroscopy for intraoperative brain tumor diagnosis. Sci Rep 14(1):6784. https://doi.org/10.1038/s41598-024-52494-6
138. Foersch S, Heimann A, Ayyad A, Spoden GA, Florin L, Mpoukouvalas K et al (2012) Confocal laser endomicroscopy for diagnosis and histomorphologic imaging of brain tumors in vivo. PLoS One 7(7):e41760. https://doi.org/10.1371/journal.pone.0041760
139. Radtke K, Schulz-Schaeffer WJ, Oertel J (2024) Confocal laser endomicroscopy in glial tumors-a histomorphological analysis. Neurosurg Rev 47(1):65. https://doi.org/10.1007/s10143-024-02286-3
140. Hoffman A, Goetz M, Vieth M, Galle PR, Neurath MF, Kiesslich R (2006) Confocal laser endomicroscopy: technical status and current indications. Endoscopy 38(12):1275–1283. https://doi.org/10.1055/s-2006-944813
141. Sanai N, Snyder LA, Honea NJ, Coons SW, Eschbacher JM, Smith KA et al (2011) Intraoperative confocal microscopy in the visualization of 5-aminolevulinic acid fluorescence in low-grade gliomas. J Neurosurg 115(4):740–748. https://doi.org/10.3171/2011.6.JNS11252
142. Abramov I, Mathis AM, Xu Y, On TJ, Belykh E, Mignucci-Jimenez G et al (2024) Intraoperative confocal laser endomicroscopy during 5-aminolevulinic acid-guided glioma surgery: significant considerations for resection at the tumor margin. J Neurosurg:1–14. https://doi.org/10.3171/2024.5.JNS24140
143. Wagner A, Brielmaier MC, Kampf C, Baumgart L, Aftahy AK, Meyer HS et al (2024) Fluorescein-stained confocal laser endomicroscopy versus conventional frozen section for intraoperative histopathological assessment of intracranial tumors. Neuro-Oncology 26(5):922–932. https://doi.org/10.1093/neuonc/noae006
144. Sanai N, Eschbacher J, Hattendorf G, Coons SW, Preul MC, Smith KA et al (2011) Intraoperative confocal microscopy for brain tumors: a feasibility analysis in humans. Neurosurgery 68(2 Suppl Operative):282–290; discussion 90. https://doi.org/10.1227/NEU.0b013e318212464e
145. Belykh E, Martirosyan NL, Yagmurlu K, Miller EJ, Eschbacher JM, Izadyyazdanabadi M et al (2016) Intraoperative fluorescence imaging for personalized brain tumor resection: current state and future directions. Front Surg 3:55. https://doi.org/10.3389/fsurg.2016.00055
146. Hollon T, Lewis S, Freudiger CW, Sunney Xie X, Orringer DA (2016) Improving the accuracy of brain tumor surgery via Raman-based technology. Neurosurg Focus 40(3):E9. https://doi.org/10.3171/2015.12.FOCUS15557
147. Kalkanis SN, Kast RE, Rosenblum ML, Mikkelsen T, Yurgelevic SM, Nelson KM et al (2014) Raman spectroscopy to distinguish grey matter, necrosis, and glioblastoma multiforme in frozen tissue sections. J Neuro-Oncol 116(3):477–485. https://doi.org/10.1007/s11060-013-1326-9
148. Orringer DA, Pandian B, Niknafs YS, Hollon TC, Boyle J, Lewis S et al (2017) Rapid intraoperative histology of unprocessed surgical specimens via fibre-laser-based stimulated Raman scattering microscopy. Nat Biomed Eng 1. https://doi.org/10.1038/s41551-016-0027
149. Raman C, Krishnan K (1928) A new type of secondary radiation. Nature 121:501–502
150. Ember K, Dallaire F, Plante A, Sheehy G, Guiot MC, Agarwal R et al (2024) In situ brain tumor detection using a Raman spectroscopy system-results of a multicenter study. Sci Rep 14(1):13309. https://doi.org/10.1038/s41598-024-62543-9

151. Livermore LJ, Isabelle M, Bell IM, Scott C, Walsby-Tickle J, Gannon J et al (2019) Rapid intraoperative molecular genetic classification of gliomas using Raman spectroscopy. Neurooncol Adv 1(1):vdz008. https://doi.org/10.1093/noajnl/vdz008
152. Desroches J, Jermyn M, Mok K, Lemieux-Leduc C, Mercier J, St-Arnaud K et al (2015) Characterization of a Raman spectroscopy probe system for intraoperative brain tissue classification. Biomed Opt Express 6(7):2380–2397. https://doi.org/10.1364/BOE.6.002380
153. Bin-Alamer O, Abou-Al-Shaar H, Gersey ZC, Huq S, Kallos JA, McCarthy DJ et al (2023) Intraoperative imaging and optical visualization techniques for brain tumor resection: a narrative review. Cancers (Basel) 15(19). https://doi.org/10.3390/cancers15194890
154. Rivera D, Young T, Rao A, Zhang JY, Brown C, Huo L et al (2024) Current applications of Raman spectroscopy in intraoperative neurosurgery. Biomedicine 12(10). https://doi.org/10.3390/biomedicines12102363
155. Puustinen S, Vrzakova H, Hyttinen J, Rauramaa T, Falt P, Hauta-Kasari M et al (2023) Hyperspectral imaging in brain tumor surgery-evidence of machine learning-based performance. World Neurosurg 175:e614–ee35. https://doi.org/10.1016/j.wneu.2023.03.149
156. Black D, Byrne D, Walke A, Liu S, Di Ieva A, Kaneko S et al (2024) Towards machine learning-based quantitative hyperspectral image guidance for brain tumor resection. Commun Med (Lond) 4(1):131. https://doi.org/10.1038/s43856-024-00562-3
157. Laukamp KR, Lindemann F, Weckesser M, Hesselmann V, Ligges S, Wolfer J et al (2017) Multimodal imaging of patients with gliomas confirms (11)C-MET PET as a complementary marker to MRI for noninvasive tumor grading and intraindividual follow-up after therapy. Mol Imaging 16:1536012116687651. https://doi.org/10.1177/1536012116687651
158. Meyer GJ, Schober O, Hundeshagen H (1985) Uptake of 11C-L- and D-methionine in brain tumors. Eur J Nucl Med 10(7–8):373–376
159. Kracht LW, Miletic H, Busch S, Jacobs AH, Voges J, Hoevels M et al (2004) Delineation of brain tumor extent with [11C]L-methionine positron emission tomography: local comparison with stereotactic histopathology. Clin Cancer Res 10(21):7163–7170. https://doi.org/10.1158/1078-0432.CCR-04-0262
160. Schober O, Creutzig H, Meyer GJ, Becker H, Schwarzrock R, Dietz H et al (1985) 11C-methionine PET, IMP-SPECT, CT and MRI in brain tumors. Rofo 143(2):133–136. https://doi.org/10.1055/s-2008-1052777
161. Schober O, Meyer GJ, Stolke D, Hundeshagen H (1985) Brain tumor imaging using C-11-labeled L-methionine and D-methionine. J Nucl Med 26(1):98–99
162. Kim A, Khurana M, Moriyama Y, Wilson BC (2010) Quantification of in vivo fluorescence decoupled from the effects of tissue optical properties using fiber-optic spectroscopy measurements. J Biomed Opt 15(6):067006. https://doi.org/10.1117/1.3523616
163. Valdes PA, Leblond F, Kim A, Harris BT, Wilson BC, Fan X et al (2011) Quantitative fluorescence in intracranial tumor: implications for ALA-induced PpIX as an intraoperative biomarker. J Neurosurg 115(1):11–17. https://doi.org/10.3171/2011.2.JNS101451
164. Valdes PA, Jacobs V, Harris BT, Wilson BC, Leblond F, Paulsen KD et al (2015) Quantitative fluorescence using 5-aminolevulinic acid-induced protoporphyrin IX biomarker as a surgical adjunct in low-grade glioma surgery. J Neurosurg 123(3):771–780. https://doi.org/10.3171/2014.12.JNS14391

Imaging Immunotherapy

30

Egesta Lopci, Angelo Castello, Matteo Caracciolo,
Luigi Mansi, and Akram Al-Ibraheem

30.1 Introduction

Malignant cells develop immune evasion strategies through tumor-driven mechanisms that suppress host defenses. Cancer immunotherapy aims to enhance or reactivate immune system function by leveraging both adaptive and innate immunity mechanisms. Key approaches to stimulate tumor-specific immune responses include cytokine therapies, cancer vaccines, and immune checkpoint blockade [1, 2]. These processes enable cancers to establish an immunologically hostile microenvironment by impairing T cell cytotoxic activity, a phenomenon counteracted by checkpoint-blocking therapies [3]. In healthy biological systems, immune checkpoints (ICs) maintain self-tolerance and prevent autoimmune

E. Lopci (✉)
Nuclear Medicine Unit, IRCCS – Humanitas Research Hospital, Rozzano (MI), Italy
e-mail: egesta.lopci@humanitas.it; egesta.lopci@cancercenter.humanitas.it

A. Castello
Nuclear Medicine Unit, Fondazione IRCCS Ca' Granda, Ospedale Maggiore Policlinico, Milan, Italy
e-mail: angelo.castello@policlinico.mi.it

M. Caracciolo
Nuclear Medicine Unit, Oncological Medical and Specialists Department, University Hospital of Ferrara, Ferrara, Italy
e-mail: matteo.caracciolo@ospfe.it

L. Mansi
Interuniversity Research Center for Sustainable Development (CIRPS), Section Health and Development, Naples, Italy

A. Al-Ibraheem
Department of Nuclear Medicine and PET/CT, King Hussein Cancer Center (KHCC), Amman, Jordan

O. Schober et al. (eds.), *Molecular Imaging in Oncology - Volume 2*, Recent Results in Cancer Research 225, https://doi.org/10.1007/978-3-032-21415-7_12

reactions through response modulation. Key regulatory proteins in this context include Cytotoxic T Lymphocyte Associated protein 4 (CTLA-4) and Programmed Cell Death protein 1 (PD-1), along with its binding partner Programmed Death Ligand 1 (PD-L1) [4]. This foundational understanding has driven the development of monoclonal antibodies (mAbs) targeting CTLA-4, PD-1, and PD-L1, establishing immune checkpoint inhibitors (ICIs) as a cornerstone of modern immunotherapeutic cancer treatment [5]. These breakthroughs have catalyzed advancements in adoptive T cell therapies as well, particularly chimeric antigen receptor–engineered T cells or genetically modified CAR T cell, whose infusion in hematological malignancies and more recently in solid tumors has shown promising clinical efficacy, signaling a paradigm shift in oncology treatment approaches [6–9].

Parallely to the clinical implementation of various immunotherapeutic agents, response assessment has been facing new challenges. In fact, immunotherapy response patterns often contrast with conventional chemotherapy, particularly regarding phenomena like pseudoprogression (Fig. 30.1), delayed clinical effects, and extended disease stabilization. To address these unique dynamics, revised response assessment guidelines have been established to enhance therapeutic development and clinical decision-making [11–14]. Alongside anatomical response criteria with computed tomography (CT), huge efforts have been made to improve and implement metabolic imaging with positron emission tomography/computed tomography (PET/CT) with 2-[^{18}F]fluoro-2-deoxy-D-glucose ([^{18}F]FDG)[15–17] (Fig. 30.2). Notwithstanding, the development of new immune-based

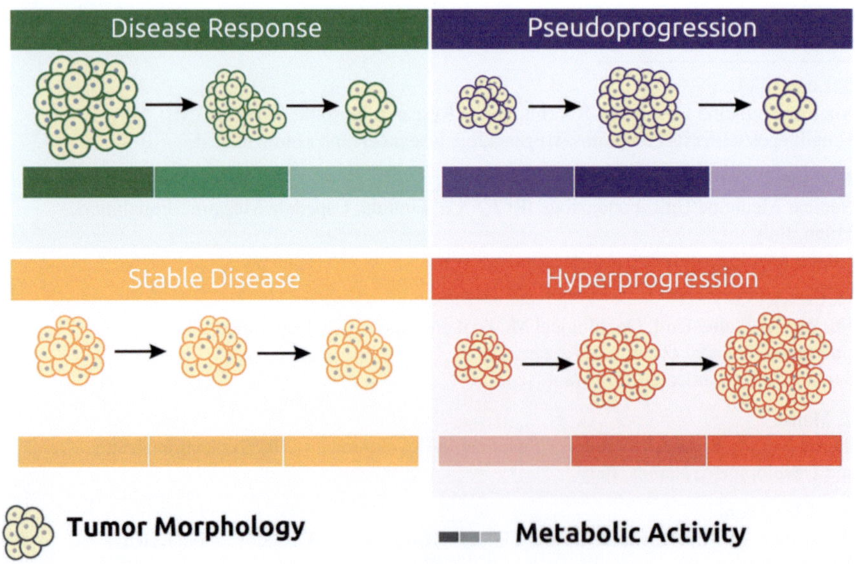

Fig. 30.1 Different response patterns achieved after immunotherapy administration. (Reproduced from Al-Ibraheem et al. [10] distributed under the terms and conditions of the Creative Commons Attribution (CC BY) license (https://creativecommons.org/licenses/by/4.0/))

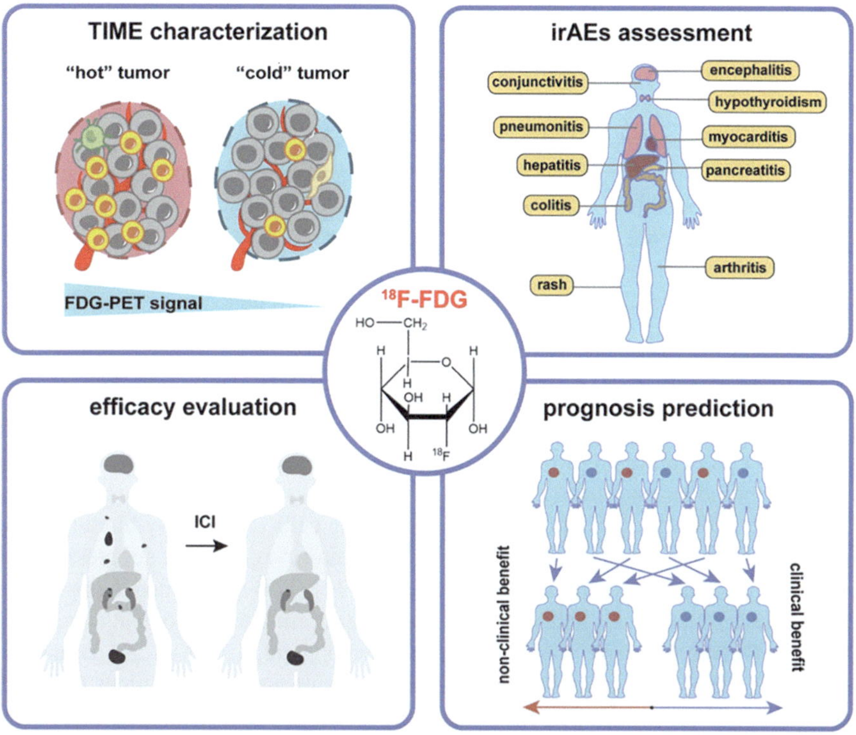

Fig. 30.2 The application of [^{18}F]FDG PET/CT imaging in cancer immunotherapy includes characterization of tumor immune microenvironment (TIME), assessment of immune-related adverse events (irAEs), evaluation of therapeutic efficacy, and prediction of prognosis. (Copyright © 2022 Gao, Wu, Chen, Ma, Zhang, Chen, Liao, and Liu. Distributed under the terms of the Creative Commons Attribution License (CC BY). [18])

radiopharmaceuticals for imaging ICI-expression and tumor microenvironment (TIME) [3, 19–22].

In this chapter, we aim to examine the most relevant aspects related to immunotherapy imaging, by illustrating the progression of immune-specific evaluation standards, their application in clinical practice, and their consequences, concluding with insights into future advancements in response classification systems.

30.2 Imaging Solid Tumors Treated with Checkpoint Inhibitors

Numerous ICIs have been approved by the US Food and Drug Administration (FDA) and the European Medicines Agency (EMA) for various cancer types, including PD-1 inhibitors such as Nivolumab, Pembrolizumab, and Cemiplimab; PD-L1 inhibitors like Atezolizumab, Durvalumab, and Avelumab; and the CTLA-4 inhibitor Ipilimumab [4, 23]. The number has expanded rapidly; as of January 2024, the FDA has approved 11 checkpoint inhibitors for a total of 43 indications across malignancies [24]. In Europe, the EMA has also played a significant role in the approval of ICIs, though the process typically takes longer. Despite this longer timeline, the EMA has approved a similar range of ICIs for various cancer types, reflecting the global impact of these therapies. Both agencies have continued to expand indications for existing ICIs, with line extensions and new approvals occurring regularly as additional clinical evidence emerges [25].

Ipilimumab (Yervoy) is the first immune checkpoint inhibitor antibody approved by the FDA in March 2011 for the treatment of advanced melanoma, demonstrating a notable increase in overall survival of patients [26, 27]. In addition to its use in melanoma, Yervoy has shown clinical benefit in combination with other immune checkpoint inhibitors for patients with advanced renal cell carcinoma, non-small cell lung cancer (NSCLC), malignant pleural mesothelioma, colorectal cancer, and squamous cell carcinoma of the esophagus [28, 29]. It targets CTLA-4, which is a transmembrane receptor found on activated T cells that interacts with the B7 ligands, CD80 and CD86, all present on antigen-presenting cells (APCs). By binding these ligands with great affinity, CTLA-4 delivers inhibitory signals that suppress T cell activation and reduce the immune response [30, 31]. This mechanism helps maintain immune homeostasis and self-tolerance under normal physiological conditions [30–32]. During the early stages of cancer development, CTLA-4 can dampen T cell activity, facilitating tumor growth. Therefore, using antibodies to block CTLA-4 can enhance T cell cytotoxic activity within the tumor microenvironment, promoting an anti-tumor immune response [30, 33].

Nivolumab (Opdivo), instead, was the first anti-PD-1 checkpoint inhibitor approved in 2014 for melanoma, and its use has since expanded to several other cancer types [34, 23]. PD-1 is a transmembrane receptor that is part of the CD28/CTLA-4 immunoglobulin superfamily. Its expression is induced upon activation of CD4+ and CD8+ T cells, as well as on B cells and monocytes [35, 36]. PD-1 has two ligands: PD-L1 (B7-H1) and PD-L2 (B7-DC). Of these, PD-L1 is more widely expressed across various cell types, including tumor cells, and plays a predominant role in immune evasion within the tumor microenvironment [37, 38]. When PD-1 binds to its ligands, it transmits inhibitory signals that suppress the activation of antigen-specific T cells both in the tumor microenvironment and in lymph nodes, a mechanism that cancer cells exploit by expressing PD-L1 to avoid immune detection and destruction [35, 37, 38]. Soon after the introduction of Nivolumab, other monoclonal antibodies targeting PD-1, such as pembrolizumab, and those directed against PD-L1, including avelumab and atezolizumab, were developed, marking significant progress in cancer immunotherapy [39–41].

30.2.1 Response Assessment to ICIs

While ICIs have led to significant improvements in outcomes for many cancer patients, only a minority achieve long-lasting responses [42]. Even in melanoma, which is among the cancers with the highest rates of response to ICIs, the majority of patients, about 60–70%, do not experience an objective response to anti-PD-1 therapy [43, 44]. Furthermore, of those who initially respond, 20–30% will eventually experience tumor relapse and disease progression [42, 45]. This pattern is not unique to melanoma; across various cancer types, the proportion of patients who benefit from durable responses to ICIs remains relatively low. For most cancers, objective response rates to ICIs generally range from 20% to 40%, and in some cases, are even lower [44, 46, 47]. As a result, ongoing research is focused on identifying predictive biomarkers and combination strategies to increase the proportion of patients who can achieve sustained benefit from ICIs.

Another peculiarity of immunotherapy with ICIs is represented by the patterns of response (Fig. 30.1). In fact, unlike the typical response patterns observed with chemotherapy, some patients receiving ICIs exhibit atypical responses characterized by a delayed therapeutic effect. This can manifest as a temporary increase in tumor size or the emergence of new lesions, a phenomenon known as "pseudoprogression," which is thought to result from the initial infiltration of immune cells into the tumor [12]. Traditional radiographic criteria [11], commonly used to assess responses to chemotherapy or targeted treatments, do not accommodate these unique response dynamics. Consequently, several adapted evaluation frameworks have been developed to better capture these patterns by allowing for the appearance of new lesions or transient tumor enlargement before confirming true disease progression. These include immune-related response criteria (irRC), which utilize bidimensional measurements, as well as unidimensional approaches such as immune-related RECIST (irRECIST), immune RECIST (iRECIST), and immune-modified RECIST (imRECIST) [12–14, 48]. Some of the principal characteristics of these new criteria can be listed as follows: irRC/irRECIST, implemented bidimensional (later unidimensional) measurements and integrated new lesions into total tumor burden calculations; Progressive disease (PD) criteria require confirmation ≥4 weeks post-initial progression, with thresholds (>25% tumor burden increase) or nontarget lesion progression; and iRECIST, introduced unconfirmed progressive disease (iUPD), requiring subsequent imaging to confirm iCPD (confirmed PD) or reclassify as iCR/iPR/iSD based on regression patterns. These immune-specific criteria prioritize temporal confirmation of progression and hybrid assessment models to account for delayed immune-mediated responses.

In parallel to the evolution of morphological response criteria for immunotherapy assessment, metabolic criteria have also adapted to fit the new scenario (Table 30.1). The evaluation of [^{18}F]FDG PET/CT scans in patients receiving immunotherapy must consider the various patterns of response, in particular the phenomenon of pseudoprogression, where apparent disease progression may not reflect true tumor growth [15]. To address this, several alternative metabolic response criteria have been developed to supplement or replace the traditional PERCIST criteria [50], but current evidence is insufficient to determine which approach is optimal [16, 55]. Firstly, the PET/CT Criteria for Early Prediction of Response to Immune Checkpoint Inhibitor Therapy (PECRIT) are considered [51]. In advanced melanoma treated with ICIs, PECRIT criteria integrate both morphological (RECIST) and metabolic parameters. In one study, this approach classified 20 patients according to clinical benefit, achieving 100% sensitivity and 93% specificity [56]. Once

Table 30.1 Immune-related response criteria: [^{18}F]FDG PET

Criteria	EORTC*1999	PERCIST 1.0*2009	PECRIT 2017	PERCIMT 2018	iPERCIST 2019	imPERCIST5 2019
Reference	Young et al. [49]	Wahl et al. [50]	Cho et al. [51]	Anwar et al. [52]	Goldfarb et al. [53]	Ito et al. [54]
Target lesions	Tumor lesion with the highest SUV uptake	Minimum tumor SUL 1.5× mean SUL liver, ≤5 target lesions/ patient	RECIST 1.1 PERCIST 1.0	Size (metabolically active lesion) >1.0 or 1.5 cm, ≤5 target lesions/ patient	Minimum tumor SUL 1.5× mean SUL liver, ≤5 target lesions/ patient	Minimum tumor SUL 1.5× mean SUL liver, ≤5 target lesions/ patient
New lesions	Progression	Progression	Progression	Metabolic progressive disease (PMD)	Immune unconfirmed metabolic progressive disease (iuPMD)	Need to be included in the sum of SULpeak, PMD if >30% increase in sum of SULpeak
Complete metabolic response (CMR)	Complete resolution of FDG uptake within the tumor volume so that it was indistinguishable from surrounding normal tissue.	Disappearance of all metabolically active lesions	Disappearance of all lesions	Disappearance of all metabolically active lesions	Disappearance of any uptake in target lesion	Disappearance of all metabolically active lesions
Partial metabolic response (PMR)	A reduction of a minimum of 15–25% in tumor SUV after one cycle of chemotherapy, and >25% after more than one treatment cycle	Reduction in sum of SULpeak in target lesions >30% *and* absolute drop in SUL >0.8 SUL units	≥30% decrease from baseline	Disappearance of some metabolically active lesions without any new lesions	Reduction in SULpeak in target lesions ≥30%	Reduction in sum of SULpeak in target lesions ≥30% and absolute drop in SUL by ≥0.8 SUL units

Criteria	EORTC*1999	PERCIST 1.0*2009	PECRIT 2017	PERCIMT 2018	iPERCIST 2019	imPERCIST5 2019
Stable metabolic disease (SMD)	An increase in SUV <25% or a decrease <15% and no visible increase in extent of FDG tumor uptake (>20% in the longest dimension).	Neither PMD, PMR, nor CMR	Neither PD, PR or CR, evaluation of change in SUL peak of the hottest lesion: >15.5% (clinical benefit), ≤15.5% (no clinical benefit)	Neither PMD, PMR, nor CMR	Neither PMD, PMR, nor CMR	Neither PMD, PMR, nor CMR
Progressive metabolic disease (PMD)	An increase in SUV >25% within the tumor region defined on the baseline scan, visible increase in the extent of FDG tumor uptake (>20% in the longest dimension), or the appearance of new FDG uptake in metastatic lesions.	Increase in sum of SULpeak of >30% or the appearance of a new lesion	≥20% increase in the nadir of the sum of target lesions (> 5 mm)	≥4 new lesions of <1 cm or ≥3 new lesions of >1 cm or ≥2 new lesions of >1.5 cm	≥30% increase in SULpeak or new metabolically active lesions: Immune unconfirmed PMD (iuPMD)	>30% increase in SULpeak, with >0.8 SUL unit increase in tumor SULpeak
Confirmed PMD (cPMD)	Na	Na	Na	Na	PET at 4–8 weeks: Confirmed PMD	Na
Delay for confirmation of PMD	Undetermined	Undetermined	3–4 weeks	3 months	2 months	3 months

Modified from Lopci et al. [15] licensed under a Creative Commons Attribution 4.0 http://creativecommons.org/licenses/by/4.0/

Notes:* Although originally developed for chemotherapy and targeted treatments, EORCT and PERCIST criteria can be used even in the case of immunotherapeutic regimens again, in patients with melanoma, the PET Response Evaluation Criteria for Immunotherapy (PERCIMT) criteria were proposed [52] to overcome the limitations of [^{18}F]FDG PET/CT with pseudoprogression. Unlike traditional criteria that rely on standardized uptake value (SUV) changes, PERCIMT emphasizes the number of new FDG-avid lesions as a more accurate predictor of clinical outcomes during ICI therapy [17, 57]. Specifically, disease progression is defined by the emergence of four or more new lesions smaller than 1 cm, three or more new lesions larger than 1 cm, or two or more new lesions larger than 1.5 cm (Fig. 30.3). Fewer new lesions suggest pseudoprogression rather than true progression [15, 58]. PERCIMT was originally validated in a cohort of 41 metastatic melanoma patients treated with ipilimumab, using clinical response as the reference standard. Further studies in different melanoma populations and treatment regimens have shown promising results for patient stratification, especially compared to EORTC criteria [59].

Derived from PERCIST, the immunotherapy-modified PERCIST (imPERCIST) criteria instead do not consider the appearance of new lesions alone as sufficient for classifying progressive disease [54]. Whereas, the sum of SULpeak (peak standardized uptake value normalized for lean body mass) of up to five lesions is calculated

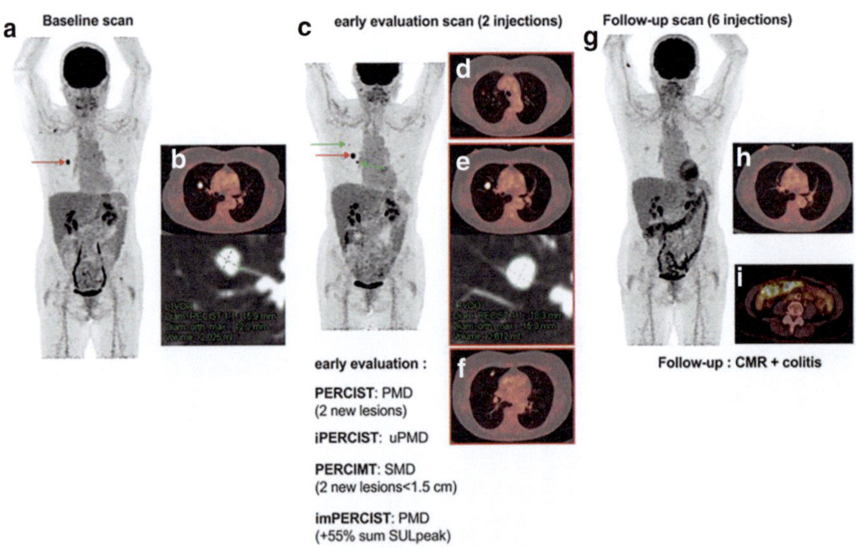

Fig. 30.3 Comparison of PERCIST, iPERCIST, imPERCIST, and PERCIMT criteria in a patient with metastatic cutaneous melanoma experiencing pseudoprogression at early evaluation. Serial maximal intensity projection (MIP) images at baseline before introduction of immunotherapy (**a**, **b**) and after two courses of nivolumab (**c**–**f**), showing two new lung lesions (**d**, **f**; green arrows) as well as a progression in tracer uptake and RECIST measurements of the main lung metastasis (**e**; red arrows). Follow-up scan (**g**–**i**) shows complete disappearance of lung lesions, classifying the patient as CMR and retrospectively the early evaluation as pseudoprogression. (Reproduced from Lopci et al. [15] licensed under a Creative Commons Attribution 4.0 http://creativecommons.org/licenses/by/4.0/)

at baseline and follow-up. Progressive metabolic disease (PMD) is defined as at least a 30% increase in this sum. New lesions are only included if they have higher uptake than existing target lesions or if fewer than five target lesions were present at baseline. Studies indicate that imPERCIST may offer slightly better prognostic accuracy than standard PERCIST [60]. Based on a similar concept as iRECIST guidelines, another recent adaptation of PERCIST incorporate a "wait-and-see" approach, resulting in the iPERCIST criteria [53]. Herein, patients with new lesions or a significant increase in SULpeak are initially classified as having unconfirmed progressive metabolic disease (uPMD). If clinically stable, these patients undergo a repeat PET/CT 4–8 weeks later to confirm or refute progression. This approach reduces the risk of prematurely discontinuing immunotherapy in patients who may ultimately benefit, as a substantial proportion of early uPMD cases are later reclassified as pseudoprogression or atypical responders [61].

While several PET/CT-based criteria have been proposed to better assess immunotherapy response and manage the challenge of pseudoprogression, robust validation in larger, prospective studies is still needed. Meanwhile, given the lack of validated methods to distinguish true progression from pseudoprogression based on a single scan, joint International guidelines recommend continuing immunotherapy in clinically stable patients and repeating [^{18}F]FDG PET/CT after 4–8 weeks before making definitive treatment decisions [15]. This strategy aims to prevent unnecessary discontinuation of potentially effective therapy in patients who may later show a favorable response. Moreover, a thorough checklist is proposed to systematically approach cancer patients undergoing immunotherapy, starting with baseline assessment, to interim response monitoring, and lastly proceeding with the follow-up or end-of-treatment evaluation (Table 30.2).

30.2.2 Immune Organs and Immune-Related Adverse Events

Immunotherapy can trigger a wide range of toxicities affecting various organs, caused by autoimmune reactions due to inappropriate activation of the immune system [17, 62]. Commonly observed adverse effects include pneumonitis, colitis, hepatitis, pancreatitis, thyroiditis, hypophysitis, synovitis, arthritis, as well as sarcoid-like granulomatosis and lymphadenopathy [63]. Imaging techniques are capable of detecting approximately 74% of these immune-related adverse events (irAEs) [64, 65]. IrAEs represent a novel and critical concept in cancer imaging, as they can be challenging to differentiate from tumor response or progression [66]. This difficulty arises because T cell-driven inflammation can cause swelling in the tumor microenvironment that mimics tumor growth, as well as apparent disease spread in healthy tissues [67]. Prompt and accurate identification of irAEs is vital for managing immunotherapy patients effectively. While mild irAEs can often be managed with corticosteroids, severe cases may be life-threatening and necessitate discontinuation of the causative immunotherapy. Despite their potential severity, irAEs have been associated with improved survival outcomes in several cancers, including melanoma and non–small cell lung cancer [68, 69]. This association may partly

Table 30.2 Checklist of requirements and recommendations to consider when approaching [18F]FDG PET/CT imaging during treatment with ICIs

	Checklist
History	Type of immunomodulatory treatment ICI: e.g., anti-CTLA-4, anti-PD-1/PD-L1, or combination. Intra-tumoral immunotherapies. Cell-based immunotherapies. Number of cycles received and date of the last injection If intra-tumoral administration is the site of injection Prior lines of treatment If combination treatment, the type of treatment or, in case of radiation, the site of irradiation Clinical symptoms suggesting immune-related adverse events For diabetic patients, check whether drugs likely to mimic colitis (biguanides) have been given Previous or ongoing use of corticosteroids and antibiotics should be noted
Therapy response	Response of target lesion(s) If the appearance of new lesions: The number of new anatomical sites and the number of new lesions. Could new lesions be explained by other processes, such as sarcoidosis or other irAES? If new nodal sites. Located in the drainage area of the main tumor? In a distribution suggestive of sarcoid-like lymphadenopathy. If possible, include MTV/TLG at baseline and subsequent studies If there is doubt whether there is progression or pseudoprogression, especially on the first posttreatment evaluation and a confirmatory follow-up [18F]FDG PET/CT study in >4 weeks later in the setting of clinical stability or biopsy should be recommended
ASSESSING IMMUNE ORGANS	Report spleen to liver ratio
Manifestations of immune-related adverse events	Different ICIs have differing side-effect profiles (e.g., colitis is more common in anti-CTLA-4 and pneumonitis is more common in anti-PD-1/PD-L1) Sarcoidosis can have variable presentations and can involve lymph nodes and other organs Increased bone marrow activity and inversion of spleen-to-liver [18F]FDG uptake ratio may support systemic immune response If available comparison with baseline study, it is critical to monitor the metabolic activity within the organs Preferably, the brain should be included, [18F]FDG uptake in the pituitary gland should be checked and compared it to the baseline study When immune-related adverse events are shown on [18F]FDG PET/CT check patient's recovery on subsequent studies

reflect that patients who respond well to immunotherapy tend to receive treatment for longer durations, increasing their risk of developing irAEs [17, 70]. Monitoring irAEs is another critical aspect of patient evaluation [71]. Although some studies suggest that the occurrence of irAEs is associated with improved survival, there is limited research specifically examining irAEs detected by PET imaging [72, 73]. For example, in melanoma patients treated with ipilimumab, PET findings of colitis correlated with clinically significant diarrhea, but neither PET-detected colitis nor diarrhea independently predicted treatment response [74]. More recently, evidence has shown that [^{18}F]FDG PET/CT can frequently identify significant irAEs before they become clinically apparent, particularly in patients receiving combination immune checkpoint inhibitors [75, 76].

In addition to identifying irAEs and using conventional or immunotherapy-adapted PET response criteria [77], baseline metabolic parameters and immune organ tracer uptake can provide valuable prognostic information (Fig. 30.2) [78]. The initial evidence of immune system activation on PET/CT is often seen as either splenic enlargement or increased splenic uptake, which can result in the spleen-to-liver uptake ratio (SLR) becoming equal to or surpassing that of the liver [16]. Some investigators have also proposed other markers, including the bone marrow-to-liver ratio (BLR) and uptake at the ileocecal valve [79, 80]. While much of the PET imaging community has concentrated on SLR as a predictor of immune activation, where heightened splenic uptake is thought to indicate robust T cell responses and a potentially favorable prognosis, several studies have found that an elevated SLR at baseline or during follow-up may actually signal a worse prognosis [71], possibly due to underlying inflammation or higher tumor burden [15, 16]. Meaning that, alongside response assessment, PET imaging also plays a potentially remarkable role in the early detection of immune activation, as well as identification and monitoring of irAEs in patients undergoing immunotherapy.

30.3 Immunotherapy Imaging in Lymphoma

Recent advancements in lymphoma treatment have increasingly prioritized immunotherapy, demonstrated by the expanding array of approved options tailored to specific disease stages and subtypes. Checkpoint inhibitors, particularly PD-1 blockers like pembrolizumab and nivolumab, have reshaped lymphoma treatment by countering immune evasion mechanisms. These agents are most effective in classic Hodgkin lymphoma (cHL) and primary mediastinal B cell lymphoma (PMBCL) [81], where Reed-Sternberg cells exploit PD-L1/PD-L2 overexpression to suppress T cell activity. By blocking PD-1/PD-L1 interactions, these drugs restore immune recognition, achieving high response rates in relapsed/refractory cases. This therapeutic approach has redefined lymphoma management by targeting tumor biology alongside localized disease control. Clinical trials have demonstrated durable remissions even in transplant-ineligible patients, leading to FDA approvals for third-line therapy and exploration in frontline combinations with chemotherapy or targeted agents [82–84]. However, challenges persist in non-Hodgkin lymphomas due to immunosuppressive tumor microenvironments and limited predictive biomarkers beyond PD-L1 expression [85]. Significant progress over the years has led, however, to the approval of other immunotherapeutic agents, particularly those focused on chimeric antigen receptor-engineered (CAR) T cells [8]. CAR-T cell therapy, such as axicabtagene ciloleucel and tisagenlecleucel, genetically engineers T cells to target CD19, a surface protein abundant in B cell lymphomas. This approach has shown remarkable efficacy in aggressive subtypes like diffuse large B cell lymphoma (DLBCL), particularly for relapsed/refractory cases post-chemotherapy. While CAR-T therapy achieves long-term remissions in some patients, challenges include cytokine release syndrome, neurotoxicity, and variable durability [86]. In the upcoming paragraphs, we will discuss the major aspects related to immunotherapeutic agents in malignant lymphomas, focusing on both response assessment and irAEs.

30.3.1 Checkpoint Inhibitors

Consolidated evidence reports PET/CT imaging essential for response assessment in FDG-avid lymphomas, offering both metabolic evaluation and prognostic insights [87]. Derived metabolic parameters serve as critical predictors in the absence of validated alternative biomarkers [10, 88]. The current paradigm of response to first-line therapy in Hodgkin's lymphoma is based on the type of response that is reached at interim evaluation, with patients showing a complete metabolic response (i.e., Deauville Score: DS 1, 2, 3) being more likely to have a complete response at the end of treatment and a better outcome compared to patients without a complete metabolic response at interim (DS 4, 5).[89, 90]. Initial clinical findings on PD-1 inhibitors for Hodgkin lymphoma emerged in late 2014, combining CT-based morphologic assessments with FDG-PET metabolic imaging to confirm complete responses [82]. Subsequent trials, including the KEYNOTE-013 study led by Armand et al., adopted the International Harmonization Project or Cheson 2007 guidelines for response evaluation [83, 91]. These frameworks, along with their later iterations, became widely utilized across immunotherapy trials in Hodgkin lymphoma [92, 93]. Early PET-based response assessments for checkpoint inhibitors relied predominantly on retrospective analyses, with studies consistently applying the Cheson 2014 (Lugano) criteria while cross-referencing outcomes against the Lymphoma response to immunomodulatory therapy criteria (LYRIC) framework [89]. LYRIC criteria, introduced in 2016, adapted the Lugano classification by incorporating immune-specific response patterns initially developed for solid tumors [89]. Designed primarily for assessing checkpoint inhibitors in Hodgkin lymphoma, LYRIC addressed challenges in distinguishing true progression from pseudoprogression by introducing an indeterminate response (IR) category with three subtypes: IR1: ≥50% tumor burden increase (measured by sum of product diameters [SPD] of up to six lesions) within the first 12 weeks, without clinical decline. IR2: New lesions or ≥50% growth of existing lesions without overall progression (<50% tumor burden increase). IR3: Elevated FDG uptake without size/

number changes in lesions. LYRIC explicitly excluded FDG avidity increases (without size progression) from constituting progressive disease (PD). Thereon, biopsies were recommended for IR1/IR2 cases, with reassessment after 12 weeks using specific thresholds (e.g., >10% size increase for IR1). The criteria retained Lugano's definitions for complete (CMR) and partial metabolic response (PMR) while accommodating clinical observations.

The Gustave Roussy team pioneered the characterization of immunotherapy response kinetics and imaging patterns in lymphoma [94, 95]. Their initial analysis of 16 patients revealed a median time to nadir of 12.7 months (range: 3–23 months), with four CMR observed within 6 months, three detected at the three-month evaluation, and one converting from PMR. Notably, 78% of patients showing metabolic responses at 3 months (CMR/PMR) maintained disease control at 1 year. Subsequent imaging analysis of this cohort demonstrated strong predictive performance, with 3- and 6-month assessments achieving 88%/97% positive predictive value (PPV) and 92%/97% negative predictive value (NPV) using lesion-based Deauville scores (DS). All early PET parameter changes correlated with ultimate treatment outcomes.

Further validation emerged from another study involving 43 Hodgkin lymphoma patients evaluated at eight and 17 weeks posttreatment initiation [88]. DS-based visual analysis effectively differentiated responders from nonresponders at both timepoints ($P = 0.003$ early; $P = 0.008$ interim), with interim responders exhibiting significantly reduced progression/death risk (HR 0.13; $P = 0.01$). Comparative analyses of Lugano and LYRIC criteria revealed discrepancies: while Gustave Roussy reported 71% (5/7) of indeterminate responses (IR) confirming as progression, multicenter data showed frequent LYRIC downgrading (e.g., DS 4–5 cases recategorized as PR/IR). However, consistent findings across retrospective studies remain limited, underscoring the need for prospective validation of LYRIC's clinical utility.

Other comparative analyses between Lugano and LYRIC criteria reveal significant reclassification patterns. In one study [95], 71% (5/7) of patients categorized as IR under LYRIC ultimately progressed, while only 29% (2/7) exhibited pseudoprogression. Another investigation demonstrated that Lugano-classified Deauville scores 4–5 (15/30 patients) were frequently reassigned under LYRIC as partial responses (27%) or IR subtypes: IR1 (13%), IR2 (53%), and IR3 (7%) [96]. A separate analysis found minimal discrepancy between the systems, though 75% (3/4) of Lugano-defined progressive disease cases were reclassified as IR1 using LYRIC [88]. While these findings suggest potential clinical value for LYRIC, prospective validation remains critical to confirm its utility.

30.3.2 CAR-T Cell Therapy

[^{18}F]FDG PET/CT imaging plays a pivotal role in lymphoma management by enhancing treatment response evaluation also in case of CAR-T cell therapy (Fig. 30.4) [7, 8, 10]. Its integration into therapeutic protocols has proven critical for optimizing patient outcomes. With the emergence of CAR-T cell therapies, timely metabolic imaging has become essential to distinguish responders from nonresponders, predict survival

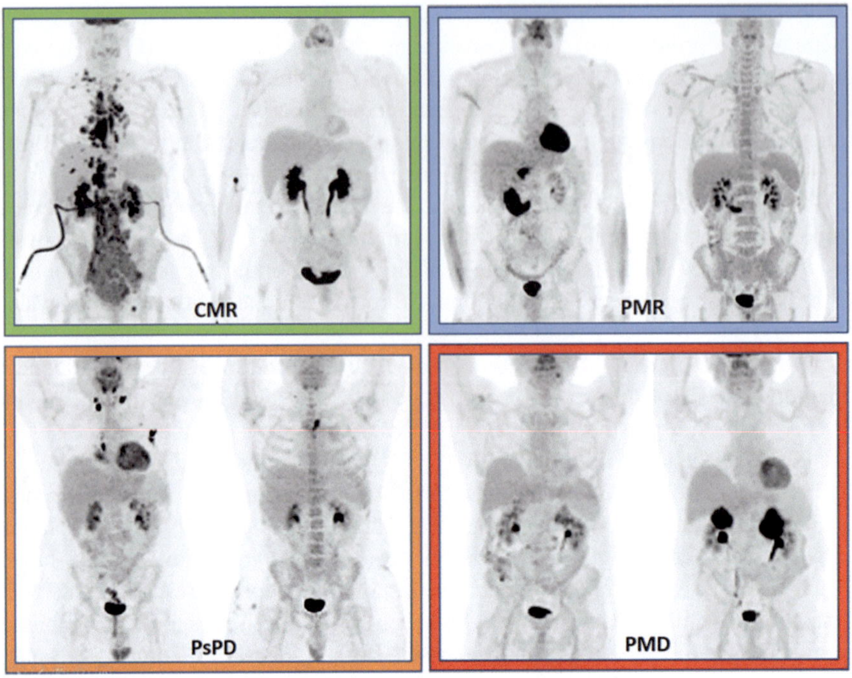

Fig. 30.4 Different patterns of response in patients with DLBCL undergoing CAR-T cell therapy and assessed with [^{18}F]FDG PET/CT before (**a**, **c**, **e**, **g**) and one month after CAR-T infusion (**b**, **d**, **f**, **h**). MIP (maximal intensity projection) images presented with complete metabolic response (**a**, **b**), partial metabolic response (**c**, **d**), pseudoprogressive (**e**, **f**), or progressive metabolic disease (**g**, **h**)

outcomes, and detect early treatment failure. In CAR-T protocols, patients typically undergo four key PET/CT assessments (Fig. 30.5): pre-infusion scans at the decision-making (TD) and transfusion (TT) phases, followed by posttreatment evaluations at 1 month (M1) and 3 months (M3). M1/M3 scans demonstrate high diagnostic accuracy (99% sensitivity, 100% specificity) for initial response assessment [97, 98]. While repeated imaging poses minimal patient burden mitigated by modern PET/CT systems and optimized protocols per EANM guidelines, clinical practices often omit TT scans [99], leaving uncertainty about whether early post-infusion responses reflect CAR-T efficacy or prior therapies (e.g., bridging regimens). This ambiguity underscores the need for standardized imaging timelines, particularly as bridging therapy strategies remain under investigation.

Several PET parameters are commonly employed in clinical practice to interpret imaging data in lymphoma cases undergoing CAR-T cells, including the Deauville 5-point scale (DS), SUVmax, and its change over time (ΔSUVmax), as well as volumetric analyses [7]. To distinguish between responders and nonresponders after CAR-T cell therapy, Cohen and colleagues recommended utilizing both the visual score and semi-quantitative parameters. Specifically, a DS greater than 3 on PET/CT

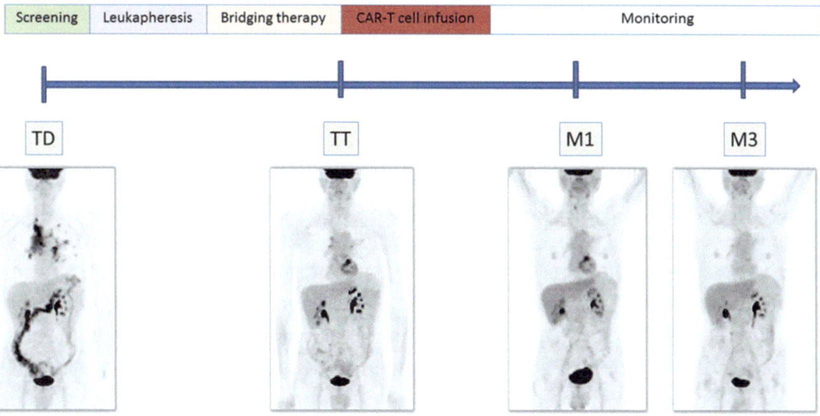

Fig. 30.5 Time line for CAR-T cell therapy and corresponding schedules for [^{18}F]FDG PET/CT imaging, respectively at TD (time of decision), TT (time of transfusion), M1 (1 month after CAR-T cell infusion), and M3 (3 months evaluation after CAR-T cell infusion). (Reproduced from Linguanti et al. [7] distributed under the terms and conditions of the Creative Commons Attribution (CC BY) license (https://creativecommons.org/licenses/by/4.0/))

scans performed one month post-infusion (M1-PET/CT), as well as ΔSUVmax comparing M1 to the time of decision (TD-SUVmax), were identified as strong predictors of poor overall survival [7, 100]. The prognostic value of the DS at M1-PET/CT was further validated by other studies, which confirmed that the quality of response determined by this scale significantly impacts patient outcomes, with patients exhibiting DS3–4 responses facing a notably higher risk of early relapse [101].

In contrast, Breen and colleagues evaluated the prognostic significance of SUVmax at M1-PET/CT and identified a threshold value of 10 as a meaningful predictor for patients with partial response or stable disease [102], a finding later supported by Al Zaki et al., who also advocated for SUVmax >10 as a relevant biomarker at this time point [103]. Additionally, Shah et al. assessed quantitative PET/CT parameters in a small cohort of CAR-T treated patients, finding that those without residual metabolically active tumor volume (MTV) at M1-PET/CT remained in complete remission during follow-up, while patients with persistent or increased MTV were less likely to sustain remission [104]. Despite the limited sample size, their data suggest that M1-PET/CT is effective for distinguishing responders, particularly those with durable responses. Overall, these findings indicate that PET/CT evaluation at one month post-CAR-T infusion is optimal for response assessment and could guide subsequent therapeutic decisions [7, 8, 10].

30.3.3 Immune-Related Adverse Events in Lymphoma

Immunotherapy has achieved significant success in treating lymphoma; however, it is often accompanied by a rise in immune-related toxicities [10, 16]. Fortunately, most of these adverse effects are not life threatening and can be effectively managed when accurately identified. The immune-related adverse events (irAEs) are triggered by inflammatory responses in various organs throughout the body [105]. For example, the most frequently observed adverse events during ICIs are inflammatory, with gastrointestinal inflammation (enterocolitis) being the most common, followed by lung and liver involvement [105, 106]. Other research has identified colitis, hepatitis, and myocarditis as the most prevalent adverse effects linked to ICI treatment [107].

Fortunately, irAEs are detectable through FDG PET/CT imaging (Fig. 30.6). For instance, increased FDG uptake in the thyroid may indicate autoimmune thyroiditis, which has been associated with better outcomes in some cases. Additionally, patients who show PET/CT evidence of at least one irAE (such as colitis or arthritis) tend to have improved progression-free survival compared to those without such findings [108]. Therefore, it is recommended to document all observed side effects in PET/CT reports, even if they are not clinically significant, to provide a comprehensive overview of the patient's response to immunotherapy [109]. However, care must be taken to interpret PET/CT results within the clinical context to avoid misdiagnosis or overestimation of disease activity.

Another metabolic imaging feature that may indicate immune activation is the reversal of the normal liver-to-spleen FDG uptake ratio (typically greater than 1) [16]. This inversion can suggest heightened immune activity before T cell expansion and may also be seen as reactive lymph nodes near the primary tumor site, which can complicate scan interpretation. Diffuse splenic enlargement and increased bone marrow activity are additional findings that may arise after immunotherapy or chemotherapy. While these changes are usually benign, they should be noted and monitored to ensure they resolve once therapy ends. Additionally, sarcoid-like

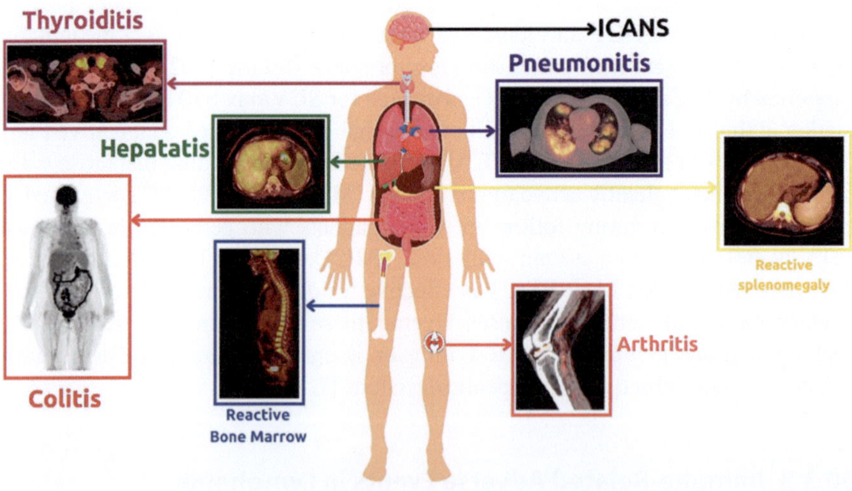

Fig. 30.6 Clinical examples of Immunotherapy-Related Adverse Effects observed during FDG PET/CT imaging in lymphoma patients receiving immunotherapy. (Reproduced from Al-Ibraheem et al. [10] distributed under the terms and conditions of the Creative Commons Attribution (CC BY) license (https://creativecommons.org/licenses/by/4.0/))

reactions, characterized by FDG-avid symmetrical lymphadenopathy in the chest, have been observed after ICI therapy [110]. Such findings often require follow-up to rule out metastatic disease, as they may occur with or without clinical symptoms.

Adverse effects are a common aspect of all cancer treatments, and CAR-T cell therapy is no exception. Unlike cytotoxic chemotherapy, which causes off-target effects due to permanent genetic alterations affecting cells throughout the body and can lead to long-lasting clinical consequences, the primary toxicities associated with CAR-T cell infusion are on-target. These toxicities arise from the specificity of the single-chain variable fragments of the antibody and the activation of T cells. Importantly, such adverse effects tend to be reversible once the targeted cells are eliminated or the CAR-T cell engraftment diminishes. The main challenges include cytokine release syndrome (CRS), immune effector cell-associated neurotoxicity syndrome (ICANS), and coagulation abnormalities (Fig. 30.6).

Cytokine release syndrome (CRS) is the most frequent adverse effect observed with CAR-T cell therapy [10, 111, 112]. CRS typically develops within the first few days following CAR-T cell infusion and may persist for up to 9 days [113]. While FDG PET/CT is not directly used to diagnose CRS, studies have demonstrated that PET-derived metrics can help predict its occurrence. In particular, research in relapsed or refractory non-Hodgkin lymphoma (R/R NHL) has established a strong association between tumor burden and CRS severity [112, 113]. Furthermore, elevated tumor burden reflected by parameters such as average standardized uptake value (SUVAvg), metabolic tumor volume (MTV), and total lesion glycolysis (TLG) has been identified as a significant risk factor for developing CRS of any grade [114].

The most common neurological symptoms of ICANS include encephalopathy, confusion, delirium, and changes in mental status, which can progress to coma, often without further specific characterization [114–116]. Brain [^{18}F]FDG PET/CT may have an important role in assessing this syndrome by analyzing metabolic patterns, similar to its use in evaluating metabolic stress and neuronal injury in other conditions. For example, Vernier et al. described a case where a patient developed CRS followed by neurotoxicity after CAR-T infusion, presenting with symptoms such as slowed cognition, comprehension difficulties, apraxia, cerebellar syndrome, and ataxia [117]. Despite normal findings on MRI and diffuse slow activity on EEG, [^{18}F]FDG PET/CT at day 14 post-infusion revealed widespread hypometabolism in the parietal and temporal cortices, sparing the limbic and cerebellar regions. Four months later, PET/CT showed persistent but more localized prefrontal and temporal hypometabolism. As highlighted by Vernier, the detection of hypometabolic areas on PET in the absence of MRI abnormalities is crucial for evaluating CAR-T cell-related neurotoxicity [117].

30.4 Immune-PET

ICIs have demonstrated remarkable efficacy across multiple clinical indications. However, not all patients respond favorably to ICIs, and some may experience treatment-related adverse effects. These challenges, along with difficulties in assessing treatment response, have prompted ongoing research to identify new predictive biomarkers that can help tailor ICI therapy to individual patients [3]. In this context, beyond the metabolic tracer [^{18}F]FDG [15], various other PET radiopharmaceuticals have been developed to target immune checkpoints or critical components of the immune system. Antibody-based imaging or Immune-PET has the potential to noninvasively detect the expression of the various checkpoints and the pattern of distribution and the features of the immune infiltrate (Fig. 30.7), providing a powerful approach for patient stratification [29, 118]. Early findings indicate that Immune-PET, using engineered antibodies, diabodies, or small molecules [119], can deliver a more holistic assessment of immune status compared to traditional immunohistochemistry, which is limited to sampling a single tissue site [17, 119–121]. This technology offers the potential for whole-body evaluation of immune responses, which could improve patient selection, guide therapy, and enhance monitoring of immunotherapy effectiveness [120, 121]. Key proteins targeted for this purpose include CTLA-4, PD-1, along with its ligand, PD-L1 (linked to lymphocyte exhaustion), CD8 (cytotoxic T cells), and markers of lymphocyte activation, such as Granzyme B, [^{18}F]F-AraG, [^{18}F]F-FLT, and so forth [3].

In recent years, several preclinical studies have investigated anti-CTLA-4 monoclonal antibodies labeled with [^{64}Cu] for imaging CTLA-4 expression in tumors. The first, conducted by Higashikawa et al. in 2014, developed a molecular imaging probe targeting CTLA-4 and demonstrated significant accumulation of [^{64}Cu]Cu-DOTA-anti-CTLA-4 mAb in CTLA-4-expressing CT26 tumors in mice, suggesting its utility as a noninvasive method to assess CTLA-4 levels [3, 122]. In 2017, researchers evaluated the biodistribution of [^{64}Cu]Cu-DOTA-ipilimumab in

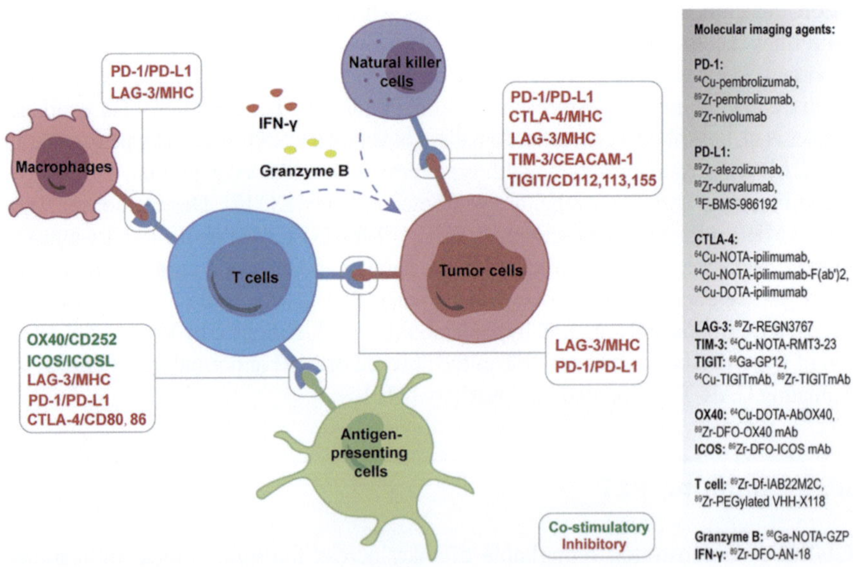

Fig. 30.7 New PET molecular probes targeting the compositions of tumor microenvironment (TIME). (Copyright © 2022 Gao, Wu, Chen, Ma, Zhang, Chen, Liao, and Liu. Distributed under the terms of the Creative Commons Attribution License (CC BY). [18])

mice with lung cancer xenografts expressing CTLA-4, showing that in vivo tracer uptake correlated with CTLA-4 expression in tumor cells; this was first confirmed in vitro across three NSCLC cell lines and then validated by PET imaging [122]. Further, in 2019, the same research group compared two [^{64}Cu]-labeled tracers, full-length ipilimumab and its F(ab')2 fragment, in humanized mouse models engrafted with peripheral blood lymphocytes. Full-length ipilimumab exhibited higher absolute uptake in target organs, while the F(ab')2 fragment provided better imaging contrast at earlier time points, albeit with lower total uptake. This study highlighted key differences between full antibodies and their fragments: full mAbs tend to clear from the bloodstream more slowly, resulting in less favorable target-to-background ratios and necessitating the use of long-lived radionuclides for repeated imaging. Despite these differences, both tracers were effective in localizing CTLA-4-positive tissues [122, 123]. When it comes to clinical studies [3], CTLA-4 PET/CT imaging using [^{89}Zr]Zr-ipilimumab has been investigated in melanoma patients. Imaging was conducted at 2, 72, and 144 h following tracer administration, which was injected within 2 h after the first therapeutic dose and again after 3 weeks at the second treatment cycle. The goal is to determine whether this imaging approach can serve as a predictive biomarker for therapy response. Preliminary results demonstrate that the tracer can successfully visualize and quantify ipilimumab uptake in tumors [124, 125].

The initial human study of PET imaging with [^{89}Zr]Zr-nivolumab was reported by Niemeijer and colleagues in 2018, involving 13 patients with advanced non-small cell lung cancer (NSCLC) prior to nivolumab therapy [126]. The research demonstrated that the procedure was safe and feasible in a clinical context, with the optimal imaging window identified at 5–7 days after tracer injection. Notably, the study found a correlation between [^{89}Zr]Zr-nivolumab uptake and the presence of PD-1-positive tumor-infiltrating immune cells, as determined by immunohistochemistry, indicating potential for noninvasive assessment of PD-1 status. Furthermore, tumors that responded to therapy exhibited higher SUVpeak values compared to nonresponding tumors, suggesting a relationship between tracer uptake and therapeutic response [127]. Pembrolizumab has also been labeled with [^{89}Zr] to evaluate tumor uptake and distribution before anti-PD-1 treatment, and to investigate associations with patient outcomes. In a study by Kok et al., [^{89}Zr]Zr-pembrolizumab PET imaging in 18 patients with advanced melanoma or NSCLC visualized major lymphoid tissues and revealed that lymph node metastases had the highest tracer uptake [21]. Higher [^{89}Zr]Zr-pembrolizumab uptake was linked to longer progression-free and overall survival [3]. A subsequent study by Niemeijer et al. in 12 patients with advanced NSCLC confirmed that responders to pembrolizumab generally had higher tracer uptake, though statistical significance was not reached [22, 127]. Other anti-PD-L1 agents, such as atezolizumab and durvalumab, have been radiolabeled and assessed in clinical imaging studies. Bensch et al. conducted the first [^{89}Zr]Zr-atezolizumab PET study in 25 patients with various cancers, documenting heterogeneous but high tumor uptake and a significant association between tracer uptake, treatment response, and survival outcomes [20]. Ongoing trials are further evaluating [^{89}Zr]Zr-atezolizumab in renal cell carcinoma and metastatic triple-negative breast cancer, with plans to correlate imaging findings with PD-L1 immunohistochemistry [3]. Durvalumab, too, has been studied with [^{89}Zr]Zr-durvalumab PET imaging [128, 129]. Initial results showed variable tumor uptake similar to previous studies, but no significant correlation between tracer uptake and treatment response. The specificity and stability of the tracer were confirmed, with imaging without a therapeutic predose of unlabeled durvalumab detecting more lesions [127]. Newer tracers, such as [^{89}Zr]Zr-DFO-KN035 targeting the anti-PD-L1 monodomain antibody KN035, as well as radiolabeled antibody fragments and small molecules, such as [^{18}F]F-BMS-986192 and [^{68}Ga]Ga-NOTA-WL12, are being developed to address limitations of full antibodies, including prolonged circulation times [130]. These smaller tracers enable imaging within hours of administration and have demonstrated correlations between PET uptake, PD-L1 expression, and treatment response in NSCLC patients [3].

Within the TIME components, the presence of tumor-infiltrating lymphocytes (TILs), particularly CD8+ cytotoxic T cells located within tumors or at their margins, critically impacts the success of checkpoint blockade therapies. Farwell et al. conducted a pioneering phase 1 study using [^{89}Zr]Zr-labeled anti-CD8 minibody PET imaging in 15 patients with metastatic solid tumors (melanoma, NSCLC, hepatocellular carcinoma) undergoing immunotherapy, demonstrating both safety and potential predictive value [131]. Earlier, Pandit-Taskar et al. reported preliminary data from a study of [^{89}Zr]Zr-IAB22M2C in six patients with solid tumors, confirming its ability to visualize CD8+ leukocyte distribution in tumors and CD8-rich tissues, with peak uptake at 24–48 hours post-injection [132]. Farwell's team observed elevated [^{89}Zr]Zr-Df-IAB22M2C uptake in tumors of three patients who later responded to therapy (Fig. 30.8), hinting at a correlation between CD8+ T cell presence and treatment success. Further insights are anticipated from an ongoing phase II trial (NCT03802123). Kist de Ruijter et al. explored a [^{89}Zr]Zr-labeled anti-CD8 antibody (89ZED88082A) in a phase 1/2 trial (NCT04029181) involving 38 patients with solid tumors [133]. Pre- and post-ICI PET scans revealed that baseline tracer uptake correlated with CD8+ T cell density on immunohistochemistry and autoradiography, while higher baseline uptake predicted improved overall survival, underscoring CD8 imaging's potential as a predictive biomarker. To address limitations of traditional antibodies, smaller tracers like [^{64}Cu]Cu-IAB22M2C and [68Ga]Ga-NODAGA-SNA006 have been developed [134]. Wang et al. preliminarily assessed [^{68}Ga]Ga-NODAGA-SNA006 in three cancer patients, noting strong correlations between tumor CD8 expression and tracer uptake [135]. Additional trials are evaluating [^{89}Zr]Zr-Df-Crefmirlimab in stage III melanoma (NCT05289193) and [^{18}F]F-GEH200521 in head/neck squamous cell carcinoma. ImmunoPET also enables early assessment of immunotherapy responses [136]. Zhou et al. investigated [^{68}Ga]Ga-grazytracer, targeting granzyme B-a protease released by cytotoxic T cells during tumor cell killing—in a clinical trial [137]. Patients with positive scans post-treatment exhibited better outcomes, suggesting granzyme B PET's predictive value. Similarly, [^{64}Cu]Cu-GRIP B (NCT05888532) is being tested in genitourinary cancers, while prior preclinical studies with [^{68}Ga]Ga-NOTA-GZP demonstrated its utility in predicting immunotherapy efficacy [138–140]. The fluorinated tracer

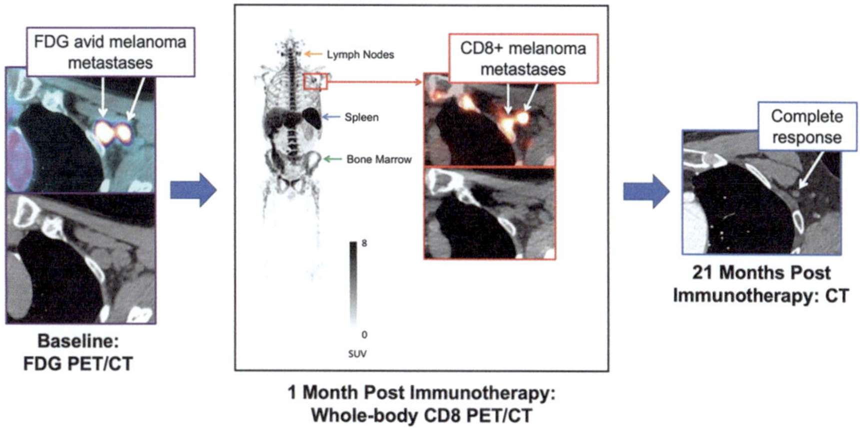

Fig. 30.8 Comparison of [^{18}F]FDG and [^{89}Zr]-df-IAB22M2C PET/CT in a patient with metastatic melanoma experiencing pseudoprogression in the left axilla, correctly identified with the CD8-targeted probe, also confirmed by the complete response after 21 months post-immunotherapy. © 2022 by the Society of Nuclear Medicine and Molecular Imaging. (Reproduced from [131] Creative Commons Attribution 4.0 International License (CC BY) allows users to share and adapt with attribution, excluding materials credited to previous publications. License: https://creativecommons.org/licenses/by/4.0/)

[^{18}F]F-AraG, which images activated T cells, has shown promise in evaluating immune response heterogeneity. A study in head/neck cancer patients revealed that stable or increasing [^{18}F]F-AraG signals post-anti-PD-1 therapy correlated with prolonged survival, while signal loss predicted poorer outcomes [141]. Ongoing phase 2 trials (e.g., NCT04401995) are assessing [^{18}F]F-AraG in melanoma and NSCLC patients [3]. Repurposed tracers like [^{18}F]F-FLT, typically used to measure cell proliferation, may also aid immunotherapy monitoring. Ribas et al. demonstrated its ability to track both tumor and immune cell proliferation in melanoma patients post-CTLA-4 blockade, highlighting dual utility in assessing responses [142].

30.5 Future Perspectives

Radiomics and artificial intelligence (AI) are advancing fields that transform digital medical images into large sets of quantitative features, enabling deeper analysis of tissue characteristics and disease biology [17, 143, 144]. Research increasingly demonstrates that AI-driven tools can extract imaging biomarkers that reveal tumor biology, supporting innovative approaches for prognosis, prediction, and therapy selection, especially in patients undergoing immunotherapy [144]. Although AI can process images from various modalities, computed tomography (CT) is most commonly used; its applications also extend to magnetic resonance imaging (MRI) and [^{18}F]FDG PET scans, particularly in studies of primary lung cancers and melanoma [143, 145]. Early or baseline imaging features identified by AI have shown potential in forecasting outcomes, treatment effectiveness, tumor characteristics (such as mutational burden), immune-related adverse events (irAEs), and indicators of the tumor immune environment, like CD8+ cell infiltration [143, 144, 146]. Despite promising results, widespread clinical adoption of radiomics and AI will require further translational research. Most studies are retrospective and single-center, underscoring the need for standardized protocols, harmonized radiomic feature definitions, external validation, and consistent use of quality control measures in imaging [17].

Patient anthropometric data, such as body composition measurements routinely collected during imaging and clinical assessments, represent an underutilized resource for guiding cancer treatment decisions [17]. Conditions like sarcopenia, characterized by reduced skeletal muscle mass, and cachexia have consistently been linked to poorer survival rates and increased complications across various tumor types and therapies [147–149]. Specifically, sarcopenia has been shown to negatively influence outcomes in patients receiving immunotherapy, with a notable impact in lung cancer [148–150]. Emerging evidence suggests that sarcopenia may also increase the risk of severe treatment-related toxicity and is associated with unfavorable responses to immune checkpoint inhibitors, such as anti-PD-1 therapies [147, 150, 151]. For example, patients with both sarcopenia and a high body mass index may experience worse outcomes when treated with immunotherapy [147]. Furthermore, cancer cachexia, a syndrome involving chronic inflammation and metabolic changes, can independently predict reduced survival and lower disease control rates in patients with advanced non-small cell lung cancer (NSCLC) undergoing immunotherapy [161]. Changes in anthropometric parameters during treatment, such as improvements in skeletal muscle mass, have been associated with better outcomes in patients treated with immune checkpoint inhibitors, suggesting these measures could serve as surrogate markers of treatment efficacy [151]. Additionally, advanced imaging techniques have identified that low subcutaneous fat mass before treatment may correlate with significantly worse outcomes in metastatic NSCLC, indicating a potential role for these measurements in personalizing immunotherapy dosing and management strategies [151]. Despite the growing body of evidence, further research is needed to standardize the assessment and integration of anthropometric characteristics into routine clinical practice.

Promising developments are expected in the field of immunotherapy assessment, and the impressive proliferation of theranostic applications should not be an exception [119]. Theranostic approaches hold indeed a great promise for immunotherapy, thanks to the possibility of coupling the diagnostic and therapeutic pairs targeting checkpoint inhibitors and elements of the TIME to boost response. By characterizing both baseline and treatment-induced changes in imaging phenotypes, new radiopharmaceuticals for radionuclide therapy could enable in vivo evaluation and targeting of the immune landscape across all tumor sites [17]. Immuno-theranostics, however, require proper investigations that are currently missing.

Lastly, the possibility to combine liquid biopsy and PET-based parameters across different cancer types and therapeutic settings represents another future development [152]. A variety of tests using body fluids to detect tumor-related molecular changes have been introduced, with many more under active development [153]. These methods, collectively known as liquid biopsies, cover a broad range of diagnostic tools, including the analysis of circulating tumor cells (CTCs), cell-free circulating tumor DNA (ctDNA), tumor-derived exosomes, and additional biomarkers, primarily found in the bloodstream [154]. Detecting these markers can provide valuable insights into tumor burden and the current status of the disease [155–157]. CTCs are cancerous cells that originate from primary or metastatic tumors and enter the bloodstream or lymphatic system, where they can potentially establish new metastatic sites [155]. Measuring CTCs offers promise as a biomarker for cancer diagnosis, prognosis, and monitoring treatment response, with evidence showing that higher CTC counts are linked to disease progression and poorer outcomes across various cancers [158]. ctDNA consists of DNA fragments released into circulation by dying cancer cells through apoptosis or necrosis. Analyzing ctDNA allows for the identification of tumor-specific mutations, gene amplifications, epigenetic changes, and microsatellite instability, thereby providing a molecular snapshot of tumor dynamics [159]. Also, exosomes, which are nano-sized vesicles secreted by tumor cells, carry diverse biomolecules and represent another promising class of biomarkers. Although they are more abundant and stable than CTCs or ctDNA in blood, their clinical utility is currently limited by challenges in standardizing isolation techniques [160]. In various cancer types, i.e., head and neck [161], lung [162], hematologic [163–165], gastro-intestinal [166–168], melanoma [169], sarcoma [170], bladder [171], brain [123], etc., the combination of metabolic parameters and liquid biopsy has proven usefull in detecting minimal residual disease, in predicting therapy response, survival, and time to progression. Consolidation of this evidences requires further investigations, possibly with large, prospective, multicenter trials.

Acknowledgments E.L. reports receiving grants from AIRC (Associazione Italiana per la Ricerca sul Cancro) and from the Italian Ministry of Health (Ministero della Salute), and faculty remuneration from MI&T congressi. No other potential conflict of interest.

References

1. Disis ML (2014) Mechanism of action of immunotherapy. Semin Oncol 41(S5):S3–S13
2. Mellman I, Coukos G, Dranoff G (2011) Cancer immunotherapy comes of age. Nature [Internet] 480(7378):480–489
3. Abenavoli EM, Linguanti F, Calabretta R, Delgado Bolton RC, Berti V, Lopci E (2023) Clinical application of ImmunoPET targeting checkpoint inhibitors. Cancers (Basel) 15(23):5675
4. Pardoll DM (2012) The blockade of immune checkpoints in cancer immunotherapy. Nat Rev Cancer 12:252–264
5. Borgeaud M, Sandoval J, Obeid M, Banna G, Michielin O, Addeo A, Friedlaender A (2023) Novel targets for immune-checkpoint inhibition in cancer. Cancer Treat Rev 120:102614
6. Jackson HJ, Rafiq S, Brentjens RJ (2016) Driving CAR T-cells forward. Nat Rev Clin Oncol [Internet] 13(6):370–383
7. Linguanti F, Abenavoli EM, Berti V, Lopci E (2022) Metabolic imaging in B-cell lymphomas during CAR-T cell therapy. Cancers (Basel) 14(19):4700

8. Abenavoli EM, Linguanti F, Dercle L, Berti V, Lopci E (2024) FDG-PET/CT imaging in chimeric antigen receptor-engineered T-cell treatment in patients with B-cell lymphoma: current evidence. PET Clin 19(4):505–513
9. Albelda SM (2024) CAR T cell therapy for patients with solid tumours: key lessons to learn and unlearn. Nat Rev Clin Oncol 21(1):47–66
10. Al-Ibraheem A, Abdlkadir AS, Juweid ME, Al-Rabi K, Ma'koseh M, Abdel-Razeq H, Mansour A (2023) FDG-PET/CT in the monitoring of lymphoma immunotherapy response: current status and future prospects. Cancers (Basel) 15(4):1063
11. Eisenhauer EA, Therasse P, Bogaerts J, Schwartz LH, Sargent D, Ford R et al (2009) New response evaluation criteria in solid tumours: revised RECIST guideline (version 1.1). Eur J Cancer 45:228–247
12. Wolchok JD, Hoos A, O'Day S, Weber JS, Hamid O, Lebbe C et al (2009) Guidelines for the evaluation of immune therapy activity in solid tumors: immune-related response criteria. Clin Cancer Res 15:7412–7420
13. Nishino M, Giobbie-Hurder A, Gargano M, Suda M, Ramaiya NH, Hodi FS (2013) Developing a common language for tumor response to immunotherapy: immune-related response criteria using unidimensional measurements. Clin Cancer Res 19:3936–3943
14. Seymour L, Bogaerts J, Perrone A et al (2017) iRECIST: guidelines for response criteria for use in trials testing immunotherapeutics. Lancet Oncol 18:e143–e152
15. Lopci E, Hicks RJ, Dimitrakopoulou-Strauss A, Dercle L, Iravani A, Seban RD, Sachpekidis C, Humbert O, Gheysens O, Glaudemans AWJM, Weber W, Wahl RL, Scott AM, Pandit-Taskar N, Aide N (2022) Joint EANM/SNMMI/ANZSNM practice guidelines/procedure standards on recommended use of [18F]FDG PET/CT imaging during immunomodulatory treatments in patients with solid tumors version 1.0. Eur J Nucl Med Mol Imaging 49(7):2323–2341
16. Aide N, Hicks RJ, Le Tourneau C, Lheureux S, Fanti S, Lopci E (2019) FDG PET/CT for assessing tumour response to immunotherapy: report on the EANM symposium on immune modulation and recent review of the literature. Eur J Nucl Med Mol Imaging 46(1):238–250
17. Dercle L, Sun S, Seban RD, Mekki A, Sun R, Tselikas L, Hans S, Bernard-Tessier A, Mihoubi Bouvier F, Aide N, Vercellino L, Rivas A, Girard A, Mokrane FZ, Manson G, Houot R, Lopci E, Yeh R, Ammari S, Schwartz LH (2023) Emerging and evolving concepts in cancer immunotherapy imaging. Radiology 306(1):32–46
18. Gao Y, Wu C, Chen X, Ma L, Zhang X, Chen J, Liao X, Liu M (2022) PET/CT molecular imaging in the era of immune-checkpoint inhibitors therapy. Front Immunol 13:1049043
19. Higashikawa K, Yagi K, Watanabe K, Kamino S, Ueda M, Hiromura M, Enomoto S (2014) 64Cu-DOTA-anti-CTLA-4 mAb enabled PET visualization of CTLA-4 on the T-cell infiltrating tumor tissues. PLoS One 9(11):e109866
20. Bensch F, van der Veen EL, Lub-de Hooge MN, Jorritsma-Smit A, Boellaard R, Kok IC, Oosting SF, Schröder CP, Hiltermann TJN, van der Wekken AJ et al (2018) 89Zr-atezolizumab imaging as a non-invasive approach to assess clinical response to PD-L1 blockade in cancer. Nat Med 24(12):1852–1858
21. Kok IC, Hooiveld JS, van de Donk PP, Giesen D, van der Veen EL, Lub-de Hooge MN, Brouwers AH, Hiltermann TJN, van der Wekken AJ, Hijmering-Kappelle LBM et al (2022) 89Zr-pembrolizumab imaging as a non-invasive approach to assess clinical response to PD-1 blockade in cancer. Ann Oncol 33(1):80–88
22. Niemeijer AN, Oprea-Lager DE, Huisman MC, Hoekstra OS, Boellaard R, de Wit-van der Veen BJ, Bahce I, Vugts DJ, van Dongen GAMS, Thunnissen E et al (2022) Study of 89Zr-Pembrolizumab PET/CT in patients with advanced-stage non-small cell lung cancer. J Nucl Med 63(3):362–367
23. Vaddepally RK, Kharel P, Pandey R, Garje R, Chandra AB (2020) Review of indications of FDA-approved immune check-point inhibitors per NCCN guidelines with the level of evidence. Cancers (Basel) 12(3):738
24. https://ascopubs.org/doi/10.1200/JCO.2024.42.16_suppl.11057
25. https://ascopubs.org/doi/10.1200/JCO.2019.37.15_suppl.e14062

26. Lipson EJ, Drake CG (2011) Ipilimumab: an anti-CTLA-4 antibody for metastatic melanoma. Clin Cancer Res 17(22):6958–6962
27. Hanaizi Z, van Zwieten-Boot B, Calvo G, Lopez AS, van Dartel M, Camarero J, Abadie E, Pignatti F (2012) The European medicines agency review of ipilimumab (Yervoy) for the treatment of advanced (unresectable or metastatic) melanoma in adults who have received prior therapy: summary of the scientific assessment of the Committee for Medicinal Products for human use. Eur J Cancer 48(2):237–242
28. Graziani G, Tentori L, Navarra P (2012) Ipilimumab: a novel immunostimulatory monoclonal antibody for the treatment of cancer. Pharmacol Res 65(1):9–22
29. Rossi S, Toschi L, Castello A, Grizzi F, Mansi L, Lopci E (2017) Clinical characteristics of patient selection and imaging predictors of outcome in solid tumors treated with checkpoint-inhibitors. Eur J Nucl Med Mol Imaging 44(13):2310–2325
30. Van Coillie S, Wiernicki B, Xu J (2020) Molecular and cellular functions of CTLA-4. Adv Exp Med Biol 1248:7–32. https://doi.org/10.1007/978-981-15-3266-5_2
31. Hossen MM, Ma Y, Yin Z, Xia Y, Du J, Huang JY, Huang JJ, Zou L, Ye Z, Huang Z (2023) Current understanding of CTLA-4: from mechanism to autoimmune diseases. Front Immunol 14:1198365
32. Buchbinder EI, Desai A (2016) CTLA-4 and PD-1 pathways: similarities, differences, and implications of their inhibition. Am J Clin Oncol 39(1):98–106
33. Rowshanravan B, Halliday N, Sansom DM (2018) CTLA-4: a moving target in immunotherapy. Blood 131(1):58–67
34. Shiravand Y, Khodadadi F, Kashani SMA, Hosseini-Fard SR, Hosseini S, Sadeghirad H, Ladwa R, O'Byrne K, Kulasinghe A (2022) Immune checkpoint inhibitors in cancer therapy. Curr Oncol 29(5):3044–3060
35. Han Y, Liu D, Li L (2020) PD-1/PD-L1 pathway: current researches in cancer. Am J Cancer Res 10(3):727–742
36. Folkl A, Bienzle D (2010) Structure and function of programmed death (PD) molecules. Vet Immunol Immunopathol 134(1-2):33–38
37. Yamane H, Isozaki H, Takeyama M, Ochi N, Kudo K, Honda Y, Yamagishi T, Kubo T, Kiura K, Takigawa N (2015) Programmed cell death protein 1 and programmed death-ligand 1 are expressed on the surface of some small-cell lung cancer lines. Am J Cancer Res 5(4):1553–1557
38. Hudson K, Cross N, Jordan-Mahy N, Leyland R (2020) The extrinsic and intrinsic roles of PD-L1 and its receptor PD-1: implications for immunotherapy treatment. Front Immunol 11:568931
39. Robert C, Schachter J, Long GV, Arance A, Grob JJ, Mortier L et al (2015) Pembrolizumab versus Ipilimumab in advanced Melanoma. N Engl J Med 372:2521–2532
40. Herbst RS, Giaccone G, de Marinis F, Reinmuth N, Vergnenegre A, Barrios CH et al (2020) Atezolizumab for first-line treatment of PD-L1–selected patients with NSCLC. N Engl J Med 383:1328–1339
41. Kaufman HL, Russell J, Hamid O, Bhatia S, Terheyden P, D'Angelo SP et al (2016) Avelumab in patients with chemotherapy-refractory metastatic Merkel cell carcinoma: a multicentre, single-group, open-label, phase 2 trial. Lancet Oncol 17:1374–1385
42. Bagchi S, Yuan R, Engleman EG (2021) Immune checkpoint inhibitors for the treatment of cancer: clinical impact and mechanisms of response and resistance. Annu Rev Pathol 16:223–249
43. Valero C, Lee M, Hoen D, Zehir A, Berger MF, Seshan VE, Chan TA, Morris LGT (2021) Response rates to anti-PD-1 immunotherapy in microsatellite-stable solid tumors with 10 or more mutations per Megabase. JAMA Oncol 7(5):739–743
44. Mao Y, Xie H, Lv M, Yang Q, Shuang Z, Gao F, Li S, Zhu L, Wang W (2023) The landscape of objective response rate of anti-PD-1/L1 monotherapy across 31 types of cancer: a system review and novel biomarker investigating. Cancer Immunol Immunother 72(7):2483–2498

45. Chen J, Rebibo D, Cao J, Mok SY, Patel N, Tseng PC, Zhang Z, Yip KY (2023) ICI efficacy information portal: a knowledgebase for responder prediction to immune checkpoint inhibitors. NAR. Cancer 5(1):zcad012
46. Garon EB, Rizvi NA, Hui R, Leighl N, Balmanoukian AS et al (2015) Pembrolizumab for the treatment of non-small-cell lung cancer. N Engl J Med 372(21):2018–2028
47. Ott PA, Bang Y-J, Piha-Paul SA, Razak ARA, Bennouna J et al (2019) T-cell-inflamed gene-expression profile, programmed death ligand 1 expression, and tumor mutational burden predict efficacy in patients treated with pembrolizumab across 20 cancers: KEYNOTE-028. J Clin Oncol 37(4):318–327
48. Hodi FS, Ballinger M, Lyons B, Soria JC, Nishino M, Tabernero J et al (2018) Immune-modified response evaluation criteria in solid tumors (imRECIST): refining guidelines to assess the clinical benefit of cancer immunotherapy. J Clin Oncol 36:850–858
49. Young H, Baum R, Cremerius U, Herholz K, Hoekstra O, Lammertsma AA, Pruim J, Price P (1999) Measurement of clinical and subclinical tumour response using [18F]-fluorodeoxyglucose and positron emission tomography: review and 1999 EORTC recommendations. European Organization for Research and Treatment of cancer (EORTC) PET study group. Eur J Cancer 35(13):1773–1782
50. Wahl RL, Jacene H, Kasamon Y, Lodge MA (2009) From RECIST to PERCIST: evolving considerations for PET response criteria in solid tumors. J Nucl Med 50(Suppl 1):122S–150S
51. Cho SY, Lipson EJ, Im HJ, Rowe SP, Gonzalez EM, Blackford A et al (2017) Prediction of response to immune checkpoint inhibitor therapy using early-time-point (18)F-FDG PET/CT imaging in patients with advanced melanoma. J Nucl Med 58:1421–1428
52. Anwar H, Sachpekidis C, Winkler J, Kopp-Schneider A, Haberkorn U, Hassel JC et al (2018) Absolute number of new lesions on (18)F-FDG PET/CT is more predictive of clinical response than SUV changes in metastatic melanoma patients receiving ipilimumab. Eur J Nucl Med Mol Imaging 45:376–383
53. Goldfarb L, Duchemann B, Chouahnia K, Zelek L, Soussan M (2019) Monitoring anti-PD-1-based immunotherapy in non-small cell lung cancer with FDG PET: introduction of iPERCIST. EJNMMI Res 9:8
54. Ito K, Teng R, Schoder H, Humm JL, Ni A, Michaud L et al (2019) (18)F-FDG PET/CT for monitoring of ipilimumab therapy in patients with metastatic melanoma. J Nucl Med 60:335–341
55. Aide N, De Pontdeville M, Lopci E (2020) Evaluating response to immunotherapy with 18F-FDG PET/CT: where do we stand? Eur J Nucl Med Mol Imaging 47(5):1019–1021
56. Unterrainer M, Ruzicka M, Fabritius MP, Mittlmeier LM, Winkelmann M, Rübenthaler J, Brendel M, Subklewe M, von Bergwelt-Baildon M, Ricke J, Kunz WG, Cyran CC (2020) PET/CT imaging for tumour response assessment to immunotherapy: current status and future directions. Eur Radiol Exp 4(1):63
57. Castello A, Lopci E (2020) Update on tumor metabolism and patterns of response to immunotherapy. Q J Nucl Med Mol Imaging 64(2):175–185
58. Lopci E (2021) Immunotherapy monitoring with immune checkpoint inhibitors based on [18F]FDG PET/CT in metastatic melanomas and lung cancer. J Clin Med 10(21):5160
59. Sachpekidis C, Anwar H, Winkler J, Kopp-Schneider A, Larribere L, Haberkorn U, Hassel JC, Dimitrakopoulou-Strauss A (2018) The role of interim 18F-FDG PET/CT in prediction of response to ipilimumab treatment in metastatic melanoma. Eur J Nucl Med Mol Imaging 45(8):1289–1296
60. Hughes DJ, Subesinghe M, Taylor B, Bille A, Spicer J, Papa S, Goh V, Cook GJR (2022) 18F FDG PET/CT and novel molecular imaging for directing immunotherapy in cancer. Radiology 304(2):246–264
61. Masse M, Chardin D, Tricarico P, Ferrari V, Martin N, Otto J, Darcourt J, Comte V, Humbert O (2024) [18F]FDG-PET/CT atypical response patterns to immunotherapy in non-small cell lung cancer patients: long term prognosis assessment and clinical management proposal. Eur J Nucl Med Mol Imaging 51(12):3696–3708

62. Gougis P, Jochum F, Abbar B, Dumas E, Bihan K, Lebrun-Vignes B, Moslehi J, Spano JP, Laas E, Hotton J, Reyal F, Hamy AS, Salem JE (2024) Clinical spectrum and evolution of immune-checkpoint inhibitors toxicities over a decade-a worldwide perspective. EClinicalMedicine 70:102536
63. Baxi S, Yang A, Gennarelli RL et al (2018) Immune-related adverse events for anti-PD-1 and anti-PD-L1 drugs: systematic review and meta-analysis. BMJ 360:k793
64. Mekki A, Dercle L, Lichtenstein P et al (2018) Detection of immune-related adverse events by medical imaging in patients treated with anti-programmed cell death 1. Eur J Cancer 96:91–104
65. Petrelli F, Grizzi G, Ghidini M et al (2020) Immune-related adverse events and survival in solid tumors treated with immune checkpoint inhibitors: a systematic review and meta-analysis. J Immunother 43(1):1–7
66. Postow MA, Sidlow R, Hellmann MD (2018) Immune-related adverse events associated with immune checkpoint blockade. N Engl J Med 378(2):158–168
67. Ramos-Casals M, Brahmer JR, Callahan MK et al (2020) Immune-related adverse events of checkpoint inhibitors. Nat Rev Dis Primers 6(1):38
68. Nakamura Y, Tanaka R, Asami Y et al (2017) Correlation between vitiligo occurrence and clinical benefit in advanced melanoma patients treated with nivolumab: a multi-institutional retrospective study. J Dermatol 44(2):117–122
69. Haratani K, Hayashi H, Chiba Y et al (2018) Association of immune-related adverse events with nivolumab efficacy in non-small-cell lung cancer. JAMA Oncol 4(3):374–378
70. Das S, Johnson DB (2019) Immune-related adverse events and anti-tumor efficacy of immune checkpoint inhibitors. J Immunother Cancer 7(1):306
71. Prigent K, Lasnon C, Ezine E, Janson M, Coudrais N, Joly E, Césaire L, Stefan A, Depontville M, Aide N (2021 Jul) Assessing immune organs on 18F-FDG PET/CT imaging for therapy monitoring of immune checkpoint inhibitors: inter-observer variability, prognostic value and evolution during the treatment course of melanoma patients. Eur J Nucl Med Mol Imaging 48(8):2573–2585
72. Mangas Losada M, Romero Robles L, Mendoza Melero A, García Megías I, Villanueva Torres A, Garrastachu Zumarán P, Boulvard Chollet X, Lopci E, Ramírez Lasanta R, Delgado Bolton RC (2023) [18F]FDG PET/CT in the evaluation of melanoma patients treated with immunotherapy. Diagnostics (Basel) 13(5):978
73. Kotwal A, Kottschade L, Ryder M (2020) PD-L1 inhibitor-induced thyroiditis is associated with better overall survival in cancer patients. Thyroid 30:177–184
74. Lang N, Dick J, Slynko A, Schulz C, Dimitrakopoulou-Strauss A, Sachpekidis C et al (2019) Clinical significance of signs of autoimmune colitis in (18)F-fluorodeoxyglucose positron emission tomography-computed tomography of 100 stage-IV melanoma patients. Immunotherapy 11:667–676
75. Wong A, Callahan J, Beresford J, Herschtal A, Fullerton S, Milne D (2016) Spleen to liver ratio (SLR): novel PET imaging biomarker for prediction of overall survival after ipilimumab and anti-PD1 in patients with metastatic melanoma. J Clin Oncol 34:9523–9533
76. Wong A, Callahan J, Keyaerts M, Neyns B, Mangana J, Aberle S et al (2020) (18)F-FDG PET/CT based spleen to liver ratio associates with clinical outcome to ipilimumab in patients with metastatic melanoma. Cancer Imaging 20:36
77. Costa LB, Queiroz MA, Barbosa FG, Nunes RF, Zaniboni EC, Ruiz MM, Jardim D, Gomes Marin JF, Cerri GG, Buchpiguel CA (2021) Reassessing patterns of response to immunotherapy with PET: from morphology to metabolism. Radiographics 41(1):120–143
78. Berz AM, Dromain C, Vietti-Violi N, Boughdad S, Duran R (2022) Tumor response assessment on imaging following immunotherapy. Front Oncol 12:982983. https://doi.org/10.3389/fonc.2022.982983. Erratum in: Front Oncol. 2023 Mar 07;13:1175321
79. Brezun J, Aide N, Peroux E, Lamboley J-L, Gutman F, Lussato D, Helissey C (2024) [18F]FDG PET/CT integration in evaluating immunotherapy for lung cancer: a clinician's practical approach. Diagnostics 14(18):2104

80. Seban RD, Nemer JS, Marabelle A, Yeh R, Deutsch E, Ammari S (2019) Prognostic and Theranostic 18F-FDG PET biomarkers for anti-PD1 immunotherapy in metastatic melanoma: association with outcome and transcriptomics. Eur J Nucl Med Mol Imaging 46:2298–2310
81. Hatic H, Sampat D, Goyal G (2021) Immune checkpoint inhibitors in lymphoma: challenges and opportunities. Ann Transl Med 9(12):1037
82. Ansell SM, Lesokhin AM, Borrello I, Halwani A, Scott EC, Gutierrez M, Schuster SJ, Millenson MM, Cattry D, Freeman GJ, Rodig SJ, Chapuy B, Ligon AH, Zhu L, Grosso JF, Kim SY, Timmerman JM, Shipp MA, Armand P (2015) PD-1 blockade with nivolumab in relapsed or refractory Hodgkin's lymphoma. N Engl J Med 372(4):311–319
83. Armand P, Shipp MA, Ribrag V, Michot JM, Zinzani PL, Kuruvilla J, Snyder ES, Ricart AD, Balakumaran A, Rose S, Moskowitz CH (2016) Programmed Death-1 blockade with Pembrolizumab in patients with classical Hodgkin lymphoma after Brentuximab Vedotin failure. J Clin Oncol 34(31):3733–3739
84. Lopci E, Meignan M (2020) Current evidence on PET response assessment to immunotherapy in lymphomas. PET Clin 15(1):23–34
85. Lin AY, Schnitter JM, Gordon LI (2022) Immune checkpoint blockade for the treatment of Hodgkin lymphoma. Immunotargets Ther 11:1–10
86. Lv Y, Luo X, Xie Z, Qiu J, Yang J, Deng Y, Long R, Tang G, Zhang C, Zuo J (2024) Prospects and challenges of CAR-T cell therapy combined with ICIs. Front Oncol 14:1368732
87. Manson G, Lemchukwu AC, Mokrane FZ, Lopci E, Aide N, Vercellino L, Houot R, Dercle L (2022) Interpretation of 2-[18F]FDG PET/CT in Hodgkin lymphoma patients treated with immune checkpoint inhibitors. Eur Radiol 32(9):6536–6544
88. Castello A, Grizzi F, Qehajaj D, Rahal D, Lutman F, Lopci E (2018) 18F-FDG PET/CT for response assessment in Hodgkin lymphoma undergoing immunotherapy with checkpoint inhibitors. Leuk Lymphoma 22:1–9
89. Cheson BD, Ansell S, Schwartz L et al (2016) Refinement of the Lugano classification lymphoma response criteria in the era of immunomodulatory therapy. Blood 128:2489–2496
90. Lopci E, Meignan M (2019) Deauville score: the Phoenix rising from ashes. Eur J Nucl Med Mol Imaging 46(5):1043–1045
91. Cheson BD, Pfistner B, Juweid ME, Gascoyne RD, Specht L, Horning SJ, Coiffier B, Fisher RI, Hagenbeek A, Zucca E, Rosen ST, Stroobants S, Lister TA, Hoppe RT, Dreyling M, Tobinai K, Vose JM, Connors JM, Federico M, Diehl V (2007) International harmonization project on lymphoma. Revised response criteria for malignant lymphoma. J Clin Oncol 25(5):579–586
92. Cheson BD, Fisher RI, Barrington SF, Cavalli F, Schwartz LH, Zucca E, Lister TA, Alliance, Australasian Leukaemia and Lymphoma Group, Eastern Cooperative Oncology Group, European Mantle Cell Lymphoma Consortium, Italian Lymphoma Foundation, European Organisation for Research, Treatment of Cancer/Dutch Hemato-Oncology Group, Grupo Español de Médula Ósea, German High-Grade Lymphoma Study Group; German Hodgkin's Study Group, Japanese Lymphorra Study Group; Lymphoma Study Association, NCIC Clinical Trials Group, Nordic Lymphoma Study Group, Southwest Oncology Group, United Kingdom National Cancer Research Institute (2014) Recommendations for initial evaluation, staging, and response assessment of Hodgkin and non-Hodgkin lymphoma: the Lugano classification. J Clin Oncol 32(27):3059–3068
93. Armand P, Zinzani PL, Lee HJ, Johnson NA, Brice P, Radford J, Ribrag V, Molin D, Vassilakopoulos TP, Tomita A, von Tresckow B, Shipp MA, Herrera AF, Lin J, Kim E, Chakraborty S, Marinello P, Moskowitz CH (2023) Five-year follow-up of KEYNOTE-087: pembrolizumab monotherapy for relapsed/refractory classical Hodgkin lymphoma. Blood 142(10):878–886
94. Dercle L, Ammari S, Seban RD, Schwartz LH, Houot R, Labaied N, Mokrane FZ, Lazarovici J, Danu A, Marabelle A, Ribrag V, Michot JM (2018) Kinetics and nadir of responses to immune checkpoint blockade by anti-PD1 in patients with classical Hodgkin lymphoma. Eur J Cancer 91:136–144

95. Dercle L, Seban RD, Lazarovici J, Schwartz LH, Houot R, Ammari S, Danu A, Edeline V, Marabelle A, Ribrag V, Michot JM (2018) 18F-FDG PET and CT scans detect new imaging patterns of response and progression in patients with Hodgkin lymphoma treated by anti-programmed death 1 immune checkpoint inhibitor. J Nucl Med 59(1):15–24
96. Rossi C, Gilhodes J, Maerevoet M, Herbaux C, Morschhauser F, Brice P, Garciaz S, Borel C, Ysebaert L, Obéric L, Lazarovici J, Deau B, Dupuis J, Chauchet A, Abraham J, Bijou F, Stamatoullas-Bastard A, Malfuson JV, Golfier C, Laurent C, Pericart S, Traverse-Glehen A, Kanoun S, Filleron T, Casasnovas RO, Ghesquières H (2018) Efficacy of chemotherapy or chemo-anti-PD-1 combination after failed anti-PD-1 therapy for relapsed and refractory Hodgkin lymphoma: a series from Lysa centers. Am J Hematol. https://doi.org/10.1002/ajh.25154
97. Jain T, Bar M, Kansagra A, Chong EA, Hashmi SK, Neelapu SS et al (2019) Use of chimeric antigen receptor T cell therapy in clinical practice for relapsed/refractory aggressive B cell non-Hodgkin lymphoma: an expert panel opinion from the American Society for Transplantation and Cellular Therapy. Biol Blood Marrow Transplant 25(12):2305–2321
98. Ruff A, Ballard HJ, Pantel AR, Namoglu EC, Hughes ME, Nasta SD et al (2021) 18F-Fluorodeoxyglucose positron emission tomography/computed tomography following chimeric antigen receptor T-cell therapy in large B-cell lymphoma. Mol Imaging Biol 23(6):818–826
99. Boellaard R, Delgado-Bolton R, Oyen WJ, Giammarile F, Tatsch K, Eschner W, Verzijlbergen FJ, Barrington SF, Pike LC, Weber WA, Stroobants S, Delbeke D, Donohoe KJ, Holbrook S, Graham MM, Testanera G, Hoekstra OS, Zijlstra J, Visser E, Hoekstra CJ, Pruim J, Willemsen A, Arends B, Kotzerke J, Bockisch A, Beyer T, Chiti A, Krause BJ, European Association of Nuclear Medicine (EANM) (2015) FDG PET/CT: EANM procedure guidelines for tumour imaging: version 2.0. Eur J Nucl Med Mol Imaging 42(2):328–354
100. Cohen D, Luttwak E, Beyar-Katz O, Hazut Krauthammer S, Bar-On Y, Amit O, Gold R, Perry C, Avivi I, Ram R, Even-Sapir E (2022) [18F]FDG PET-CT in patients with DLBCL treated with CAR-T cell therapy: a practical approach of reporting pre- and post-treatment studies. Eur J Nucl Med Mol Imaging 49(3):953–962
101. Kuhnl A, Roddie C, Kirkwood AA, Menne T, Cuadrado M, Marzolini MAV, Osborne W, Sanderson R, O'Reilly M, Townsend W, Benjamin R, Potter V, Patten PEM, Yallop D, Voo S, Petrides GS, Mulholland N, Kayani I (2022) Early FDG-PET response predicts CAR-T failure in large B-cell lymphoma. Blood Adv 6(1):321–326
102. Breen WG, Hathcock MA, Young JR, Kowalchuk RO, Bansal R, Khurana A et al (2022) Metabolic characteristics and prognostic differentiation of aggressive lymphoma using one-month post-CAR-T FDG PET/CT. J Hematol Oncol 15(1):36
103. Al Zaki A (2022) Day 30 SUVmax predicts progression in patients with lymphoma achieving PR/SD after CAR T-cell therapy. Blood Adv 6(9):2867–2871
104. Shah NN, Nagle SJ, Torigian EA, Farwell MD, Hwang WT, Frey N et al (2018) Early positron emission tomography/computed tomography as a predictor of response after CTL019 chimeric antigen receptor -T-cell therapy in B-cell non-Hodgkin lymphomas. Cytotherapy 20:1415–1418
105. Dougan M (2020) Understanding and overcoming the inflammatory toxicities of immunotherapy. Cancer Immunol Res 8(10):1230–1235
106. Shi Y, Su H, Song Y, Jiang W, Sun X, Qian W, Zhang W, Gao Y, Jin Z, Zhou J, Jin C, Zou L, Qiu L, Li W, Yang J, Hou M, Zeng S, Zhang Q, Hu J, Zhou H, Xiong Y, Liu P (2019) Safety and activity of sintilimab in patients with relapsed or refractory classical Hodgkin lymphoma (ORIENT-1): a multicentre, single-arm, phase 2 trial. Lancet Haematol 6(1):e12–e19
107. Conroy M, Naidoo J (2022) Immune-related adverse events and the balancing act of immunotherapy. Nat Commun 13(1):392
108. Bajwa R, Cheema A, Khan T, Amirpour A, Paul A, Chaughtai S, Patel S, Patel T, Bramson J, Gupta V, Levitt M, Asif A, Hossain MA (2019) Adverse effects of immune checkpoint inhibitors (programmed Death-1 inhibitors and cytotoxic T-lymphocyte-associated Protein-4 inhibitors): results of a retrospective study. J Clin Med Res 11(4):225–236

109. Ibis B, Aliazis K, Cao C, Yenyuwadee S, Boussiotis VA (2023) Immune-related adverse effects of checkpoint immunotherapy and implications for the treatment of patients with cancer and autoimmune diseases. Front Immunol 14:1197364
110. Gandy N, Arshad MA, Wallitt KL, Dubash S, Khan S, Barwick TD (2020) Immunotherapy-related adverse effects on 18F-FDG PET/CT imaging. Br J Radiol 93:20190832
111. Frey N, Porter D (2019) Cytokine release syndrome with chimeric antigen receptor T cell therapy. Biol Blood Marrow Transplant 25(4):e123–e127
112. Neelapu SS, Tummala S, Kebriaei P et al (2018) Chimeric antigen receptor T-cell therapy—assessment and management of toxicities. Nat Rev Clin Oncol 15:47–62
113. Giavridis T, van der Stegen SJC, Eyquem J, Hamieh M, Piersigilli A, Sadelain M (2018) CAR T cell-induced cytokine release syndrome is mediated by macrophages and abated by IL-1 blockade. Nat Med 24(6):731–738. https://doi.org/10.1038/s41591-018-0041-7
114. Buciuc AG, Tran S, Weber M, Padilla V, Rueda-Lara M, Espinel Z (2025) Immune effector cell-associated neurotoxicity syndrome after CAR T-cell therapy and other psychiatric manifestations: a review and case series. J Clin Med 14(5):1451
115. Sterner RC, Sterner RM (2022) Immune effector cell associated neurotoxicity syndrome in chimeric antigen receptor-T cell therapy. Front Immunol 13:879608
116. Nie EH, Su YJ, Baird JH, Agarwal N, Bharadwaj S, Weng WK, Smith M, Dahiya S, Han MH, Dunn JE, Kipp LB, Miklos DB, Scott BJ, Frank MJ (2024) Clinical features of neurotoxicity after CD19 CAR T-cell therapy in mantle cell lymphoma. Blood Adv 8(6):1474–1486
117. Vernier V, Ursu R, Belin C, Maillet D, Thieblemont C, Carpentier AF (2022) Hypometabolism on brain FDG-PET as a marker for neurotoxicity after CAR T-cell therapy: a case report. Rev Neurol (Paris) 178(3):282–284
118. Knowles SM, Wu A (2012) Advances in immuno–positron emission tomography: antibodies for molecular imaging in oncology. J Clin Oncol 30(31):3884–3892
119. Zhang T, Lei H, Chen X, Dou Z, Yu B, Su W, Wang W, Jin X, Katsube T, Wang B, Zhang H, Li Q, Di C (2024) Carrier systems of radiopharmaceuticals and the application in cancer therapy. Cell Death Discov 10(1):16
120. Menzies AM, Lastoria S (2022) PET imaging for cancer immunotherapy: the Immuno-PET. Ann Oncol 33(1):13–14
121. Hegi-Johnson F, Rudd S, Hicks RJ, De Ruysscher D, Trapani JA, John T, Donnelly P, Blyth B, Hanna G, Everitt S, Roselt P, MacManus MP (2022) Imaging immunity in patients with cancer using positron emission tomography. NPJ Precis Oncol 6(1):24
122. Ehlerding EB, England CG, Majewski RL, Valdovinos HF, Jiang D, Liu G, McNeel DG, Nickles RJ, Cai W (2017) ImmunoPET imaging of CTLA-4 expression in mouse models of non-small cell lung cancer. Mol Pharm 14(5):1782–1789
123. Gao F, Zhao W, Li M et al (2021) Role of circulating tumor cell detection in differentiating tumor recurrence from treatment necrosis of brain gliomas. Biosci Trends 15(2):107–117
124. Wei W, Rosenkrans ZT, Liu J, Huang G, Luo QY, Cai W (2020) ImmunoPET: concept, design, and applications. Chem Rev 120(8):3787–3851
125. Ehlerding EB, Lee HJ, Jiang D, Ferreira CA, Zahm CD, Huang P, Engle JW, McNeel DG, Cai W (2019) Antibody and fragment-based PET imaging of CTLA-4+ T-cells in humanized mouse models. Am J Cancer Res 9(1):53–63
126. Niemeijer AN, Leung D, Huisman MC, Bahce I, Hoekstra OS, van Dongen GAMS, Boellaard R, Du S, Hayes W, Smith R, Windhorst AD, Hendrikse NH, Poot A, Vugts DJ, Thunnissen E, Morin P, Lipovsek D, Donnelly DJ, Bonacorsi SJ, Velasquez LM, de Gruijl TD, Smit EF, de Langen AJ (2018) Whole body PD-1 and PD-L1 positron emission tomography in patients with non-small-cell lung cancer. Nat Commun 9(1):4664
127. Westdorp H, Verhoeff SR, Gotthardt M, van Herpen CML, van MM, Heuvel D, Heskamp S, Aarntzen EHJG. (2022) Toward a better understanding of immune checkpoint inhibitor radiolabeled PET imaging studies. J Nucl Med 63(3):359–361
128. Verhoeff SR, van de Donk PP, Aarntzen EHJG, Oosting SF, Brouwers AH, Miedema IHC, Voortman J, der Houven M-v, van Oordt WC, Boellaard R, Vriens D, Slingerland M, Hermsen R, Grunsven IVE, Heskamp S, van Herpen CML (2022) 89Zr-DFO-Durvalumab PET/CT

before Durvalumab treatment in patients with recurrent or metastatic head and neck cancer. J Nucl Med 63(10):1523–1530

129. Hegi-Johnson F, Rudd SE, Wichmann C, Akhurst T, Roselt P, Trinh J, John T, Devereux L, Donnelly PS, Hicks R, Scott AM, Steinfort D, Fox S, Blyth B, Parakh S, Hanna GG, Callahan J, Burbury K, MacManus M (2022) ImmunoPET: IMaging of cancer imMUNOtherapy targets with positron emission tomography: a phase 0/1 study characterising PD-L1 with 89Zr-durvalumab (MEDI4736) PET/CT in stage III NSCLC patients receiving chemoradiation study protocol. BMJ Open 12(11):e056708
130. Puyalto A, Rodríguez-Remírez M, López I, Iribarren F, Simón JA, Ecay M, Collantes M, Vilalta-Lacarra A, Francisco-Cruz A, Solórzano JL, Sandiego S, Peñuelas I, Calvo A, Ajona D, Gil-Bazo I (2023) A novel [89Zr]-anti-PD-1-PET-CT to assess response to PD-1/PD-L1 blockade in lung cancer. Front Immunol 14:1272570
131. Farwell MD, Gamache RF, Babazada H, Hellmann MD, Harding JJ, Korn R, Mascioni A, Le W, Wilson I, Gordon MS, Wu AM, Ulaner GA, Wolchok JD, Postow MA, Pandit-Taskar N (2022) CD8-targeted PET imaging of tumor-infiltrating T cells in patients with cancer: a phase I first-in-humans study of 89Zr-Df-IAB22M2C, a radiolabeled anti-CD8 minibody. J Nucl Med 63(5):720–726
132. Pandit-Taskar N, Postow MA, Hellmann MD, Harding JJ, Barker CA, O'Donoghue JA, Ziolkowska M, Ruan S, Lyashchenko SK, Tsai F, Farwell M, Mitchell TC, Korn R, Le W, Lewis JS, Weber WA, Behera D, Wilson I, Gordon M, Wu AM, Wolchok JD (2020) First-in-humans imaging with 89Zr-Df-IAB22M2C anti-CD8 Minibody in patients with solid malignancies: preliminary pharmacokinetics, biodistribution, and lesion targeting. J Nucl Med 61(4):512–519
133. Kist de Ruijter L, van de Donk PP, Hooiveld-Noeken JS, Giesen D, Elias SG, Lub-de Hooge MN, Oosting SF, Jalving M, Timens W, Brouwers AH et al (2022) Whole-body CD8+ T cell visualization before and during cancer immunotherapy: a phase 1/2 trial. Nat Med 28:2601–2610
134. Nagle VL, Henry KE, Hertz CAJ, Graham MS, Campos C, Parada LF, Pandit-Taskar N, Schietinger A, Mellinghoff IK, Lewis JS (2021) Imaging tumor-infiltrating lymphocytes in brain tumors with [64Cu]cu-NOTA-anti-CD8 PET. Clin Cancer Res 27(7):1958–1966
135. Wang Y, Wang C, Huang M, Qin S, Zhao J, Sang S, Zheng M, Bian Y, Huang C, Zhang H, Guo L, Jiang J, Xu C, Dai N, Zheng Y, Han J, Yang M, Xu T, Miao L (2022) Pilot study of a novel nanobody 68 Ga-NODAGA-SNA006 for instant PET imaging of CD8+ T cells. Eur J Nucl Med Mol Imaging 49(13):4394–4405
136. Maresca KP, Chen J, Mathur D, Giddabasappa A, Root A, Narula J, King L, Schaer D, Golas J, Kobylarz K, Rosfjord E, Keliher E, Chen L, Ram S, Pickering EH, Hardwick JS, Rejto PA, Hussein A, Ilovich O, Staton K, Wilson I, McCarthy TJ (2021) Preclinical evaluation of 89Zr-Df-IAB22M2C PET as an imaging biomarker for the development of the GUCY2C-CD3 bispecific PF-07062119 as a T cell engaging therapy. Mol Imaging Biol 23(6):941–951
137. Zhou H, Wang Y, Xu H, Shen X, Zhang T, Zhou X, Zeng Y, Li K, Zhang L, Zhu H, Yang X, Li N, Yang Z, Liu Z (2022) Noninvasive interrogation of CD8+ T cell effector function for monitoring early tumor responses to immunotherapy. J Clin Invest 132(16):e161065
138. Larimer BM, Wehrenberg-Klee E, Dubois F, Mehta A, Kalomeris T, Flaherty K, Boland G, Mahmood U (2017) Granzyme B PET imaging as a predictive biomarker of immunotherapy response. Cancer Res 77(9):2318–2327
139. Larimer BM, Bloch E, Nesti S, Austin EE, Wehrenberg-Klee E, Boland G, Mahmood U (2019) The effectiveness of checkpoint inhibitor combinations and administration timing can be measured by Granzyme B PET imaging. Clin Cancer Res 25(4):1196–1205
140. Zhao N, Bardine C, Lourenço AL, Wang YH, Huang Y, Cleary SJ, Wilson DM, Oh DY, Fong L, Looney MR, Evans MJ, Craik CS (2021) In vivo measurement of Granzyme proteolysis from activated immune cells with PET. ACS Cent Sci 7(10):1638–1649
141. Levi J, Perk T, Huynh L et al (2021) AI-assisted whole-body assessment of immunotherapy response using [18F]F-AraG, a PET agent for activated T cells. J Immuno Ther Cancer 9:A52

142. Ribas A, Benz MR, Allen-Auerbach MS, Radu C, Chmielowski B, Seja E, Williams JL, Gomez-Navarro J, McCarthy T, Czernin J (2010) Imaging of CTLA4 blockade-induced cell replication with (18)F-FLT PET in patients with advanced melanoma treated with tremelimumab. J Nucl Med 51:340–346
143. Majumder S, Katz S, Kontos D, Roshkovan L (2023) State of the art: radiomics and radiomics-related artificial intelligence on the road to clinical translation. BJR Open 6(1):tzad004
144. Maniaci A, Lavalle S, Gagliano C, Lentini M, Masiello E, Parisi F, Iannella G, Cilia ND, Salerno V, Cusumano G, La Via L (2024) The integration of Radiomics and artificial intelligence in modern medicine. Life (Basel) 14(10):1248
145. Sun R, Limkin EJ, Vakalopoulou M et al (2018) A radiomics approach to assess tumour-infiltrating CD8 cells and response to anti-PD-1 or anti-PD-L1 immunotherapy: an imaging biomarker, retrospective multicohort study. Lancet Oncol 19(9):1180–1191
146. Sun R, Sundahl N, Hecht M et al (2020) Radiomics to predict outcomes and abscopal response of patients with cancer treated with immunotherapy combined with radiotherapy using a validated signature of CD8 cells. J Immunother Cancer 8(2):e001429
147. Xue D, Li N, Yang J, Men K, Li L, Jiang H, Zhao X, Zhang S (2024) Sarcopenia predicts immune-related adverse events due to anti-PD-1/PD-L1 therapy in patients with advanced lung cancer. Front Oncol 14:1450020
148. Li S, Wang T, Tong G, Li X, You D, Cong M (2021) Prognostic impact of sarcopenia on clinical outcomes in malignancies treated with immune checkpoint inhibitors: a systematic review and meta-analysis. Front Oncol 11:726257
149. Deng Y, Zhao L, Huang X, Zeng Y, Xiong Z, Zuo M (2023) Contribution of skeletal muscle to cancer immunotherapy: a focus on muscle function, inflammation, and microbiota. Nutrition 105:111829
150. Roch B, Coffy A, Jean-Baptiste S, Palaysi E, Daures JP, Pujol JL, Bommart S (2020) Cachexia – sarcopenia as a determinant of disease control rate and survival in non-small lung cancer patients receiving immune-checkpoint inhibitors. Lung Cancer 143:19–26
151. Madeddu C, Busquets S, Donisi C, Lai E, Pretta A, López-Soriano FJ, Argilés JM, Scartozzi M, Macciò A (2023) Effect of cancer-related cachexia and associated changes in nutritional status, inflammatory status, and muscle mass on immunotherapy efficacy and survival in patients with advanced non-small cell lung cancer. Cancers (Basel) 15(4):1076
152. Castello A, Carbone FG, Rossi S, Monterisi S, Federico D, Toschi L, Lopci E (2020) Circulating tumor cells and metabolic parameters in NSCLC patients treated with checkpoint inhibitors. Cancers (Basel) 12(2):487
153. Yin H, Zhang M, Zhang Y, Zhang X, Zhang X, Zhang B (2025) Liquid biopsies in cancer. Mol Biomed 6(1):18
154. Castello A, Rossi S, Toschi L, Mansi L, Lopci E (2020) Soluble PD-L1 in NSCLC patients treated with checkpoint inhibitors and its correlation with metabolic parameters. Cancers (Basel) 12(6):1373
155. Connal S, Cameron JM, Sala A, Brennan PM, Palmer DS, Palmer JD, Perlow H, Baker MJ (2023) Liquid biopsies: the future of cancer early detection. J Transl Med 21(1):118
156. Fu SW, Tang C, Tan X, Srivastava S (2024) Liquid biopsy for early cancer detection: technological revolutions and clinical dilemma. Expert Rev Mol Diagn 24(10):937–955
157. Martins I, Ribeiro IP, Jorge J, Gonçalves AC, Sarmento-Ribeiro AB, Melo JB, Carreira IM (2021) Liquid biopsies: applications for cancer diagnosis and monitoring. Genes (Basel) 12(3):349
158. Shimada R, Iinuma H, Akahane T et al (2012) Prognostic significance of CTCs and CSCs of tumor drainage vein blood in dukes' stage B and C colorectal cancer patients. Oncol Rep 27:947–953
159. Pessoa LS, Heringer M, Ferrer VP (2020) ctDNA as a cancer biomarker: a broad overview. Crit Rev Oncol Hematol 155:103109
160. Kowal J, Arras G, Colombo M et al (2016) Proteomic comparison defines novel markers to characterize heterogeneous populations of extracellular vesicle subtypes. Proc Natl Acad Sci USA 113:E968–E977

161. Post CM, Ohaegbulam KC, Mitin T (2024) From planned neck dissection to PET response to circulating tumour DNA: changes in post-treatment assessment of HPV-driven oropharyngeal cancer†. J Med Radiat Sci 71(1):21–25
162. Zhang F, Wu X, Zhu J et al (2021) 18F-FDG PET/CT and circulating tumor cells in treatment-naive patients with non-small-cell lung cancer. Eur J Nucl Med Mol Imaging 48(10):3250–3259
163. Calabretta E, di Trani M, Corrado F et al (2024) Baseline circulating tumour DNA and interim PET predict response in relapsed/refractory classical Hodgkin lymphoma. Br J Haematol 204(2):514–524
164. Delfau-Larue MH, van der Gucht A, Dupuis J et al (2018) Total metabolic tumor volume, circulating tumor cells, cell-free DNA: distinct prognostic value in follicular lymphoma. Blood Adv 2(7):807–816
165. Ikeda D, Terao T, Oura M et al (2024) Analysis of baseline circulating tumor cells integrated with PET/CT findings in transplant-ineligible multiple myeloma. Blood Adv 8(1):37–46
166. Cabalag CS, Yates M, Corrales MB et al (2022) Potential clinical utility of a targeted circulating tumor DNA assay in esophageal adenocarcinoma. Ann Surg 276(2):e120–e126
167. Woff E, Kehagias P, Vandeputte C et al (2019) Combining 18F-FDG PET/CT-based metabolically active tumor volume and circulating cell-free DNA significantly improves outcome prediction in Chemorefractory metastatic colorectal cancer. J Nucl Med 60(10):1366–1372
168. Ramirez P, Sáenz L, Cascales-Campos PA et al (2016) Oncological evaluation by positron-emission tomography, circulating tumor cells and alpha fetoprotein in patients with hepatocellular carcinoma on the waiting list for liver transplantation. Transplant Proc 48(9):2962–2965
169. Marsavela G, McEvoy AC, Pereira MR et al (2022) Detection of clinical progression through plasma ctDNA in metastatic melanoma patients: a comparison to radiological progression. Br J Cancer 126(3):401–408
170. Schmidkonz C, Krumbholz M, Atzinger A et al (2020) Assessment of treatment responses in children and adolescents with Ewing sarcoma with metabolic tumor parameters derived from 18F-FDG-PET/CT and circulating tumor DNA. Eur J Nucl Med Mol Imaging 47(6):1613
171. Abrahamsson J, Aaltonen K, Engilbertsson H et al (2017) Circulating tumor cells in patients with advanced urothelial carcinoma of the bladder: association with tumor stage, lymph node metastases, FDG-PET findings, and survival. Urol Oncol 35(10):606.e9–606.e16

Advancements in Intraoperative Imaging for Enhanced Surgical Precision

31

Miles Pourbaghi, Feng Chen, Nabil Siddiqui, and Michelle Bradbury

Abbreviations

AI	Artificial Intelligence
AR	Augmented Reality
CE	Conformité Européenne
CLI	Cerenkov Luminescence Imaging
CT	Computed Tomography
cRGDY	cyclic Arginine-Glycine-Aspartic Acid-Tyrosine
Cy5	Cyanine 5 Dye
Cy5.5	Cyanine 5.5 Dye
EGFR	Epidermal Growth Factor Receptor
FGS	Fluorescence-Guided Surgery
FR	Folate Receptor
FRα	Folate Receptor-Alpha
FUS	Focused Ultrasound
HIFU	High-Intensity Focused Ultrasound
iCT	Intraoperative CT

M. Pourbaghi · F. Chen · N. Siddiqui
Molecular Imaging Innovations Institute, Department of Radiology, Weill Cornell Medicine, New York, NY, USA
e-mail: mip4021@med.cornell.edu; fec4008@med.cornell.edu; nas4031@med.cornell.edu

M. Bradbury (✉)
Molecular Imaging Innovations Institute, Department of Radiology, Weill Cornell Medicine, New York, NY, USA

Sandra & Edward Meyer Cancer Center, Weill Cornell Medicine, New York, NY, USA

Department of Radiation Oncology, Weill Cornell Medicine, New York, NY, USA
e-mail: msb2006@med.cornell.edu

O. Schober et al. (eds.), *Molecular Imaging in Oncology - Volume 2*, Recent Results in Cancer Research 225, https://doi.org/10.1007/978-3-032-21415-7_13

iUS	Intraoperative Ultrasound
iMRI	Intraoperative MRI
ICG	Indocyanine Green
IR700DX	Infrared Dye 700DX
IRDye800CW	Infrared Dye 800CW
IV	Intravenous
MR-HIFU	Magnetic Resonance-Guided High-Intensity Focused Ultrasound
MRI	Magnetic Resonance Imaging
MSKCC	Memorial Sloan Kettering Cancer Center
NIR	Near-Infrared
NIR-II	Second Near-Infrared Window
PET	Positron Emission Tomography
PIT	Photoimmunotherapy
PSMA	Prostate-Specific Membrane Antigen
RGS	Radioguided Surgery
SPECT	Single Photon Emission Computed Tomography
SPIONs	Superparamagnetic Iron Oxide Nanoparticles

31.1 Introduction

Image-guided intraoperative imaging has emerged as a pivotal advancement in surgical practice, offering real-time visualization and management of disease that significantly enhances the safety, precision, and outcome of procedures. This technology allows surgeons to visualize anatomic structures and pathological states with remarkable clarity, leading to more accurate and effective interventions. The integration of advanced imaging modalities into the surgical workflow represents a transformative shift in how surgeries are conducted, aligning with the broader trend toward precision medicine [1].

The evolution of intraoperative imaging can be traced back to the adaptation of foundational imaging technologies such as fluoroscopy, computed tomography (CT), and magnetic resonance imaging (MRI) for use in the operating room. These modalities have provided surgeons with critical anatomic and functional information that was previously unavailable during surgery, facilitating more thorough tumor removal and minimizing damage to surrounding healthy tissue, such as the eloquent cortex during neurosurgical procedures. Intraoperative MRI, for instance, has become a cornerstone in these procedures, allowing for real-time assessment of brain activity, tumor margins, and the extent of resection [2].

In addition to conventional imaging techniques, modalities such as fluorescence-guided surgery (FGS) and intraoperative ultrasound have allowed surgeons to visualize and characterize altered tissue morphologies, defining areas of abnormal perfusion and increased metabolic activity. The use of target-specific probes in this context improves diagnostic accuracy, aids identification of neural structures, such as during radical prostatectomy, and provides a strategic roadmap for directing targeted interventions to sites of nodal pathology, tumor margins, and residual disease.

Improved patient outcomes critically depend on implementing such oncologic approaches to facilitate more complete tumor resections [3]. Intraoperative ultrasound is particularly useful for dynamically guiding surgical assessments of liver and pancreatic cancers, where it can differentiate lesions from surrounding critical structures. The integration of imaging technologies with surgical procedures can enhance precision over that using traditional methods by providing on-the-fly adaptive guidance for treatment planning and ensuring that interventions are as targeted and as effective as possible. These capabilities are particularly valuable during complex procedures, where the ability to rapidly visualize and respond to findings in the surgical field can significantly impact patient outcomes.

Despite its many benefits, the implementation of intraoperative imaging is not without challenges. The high cost of imaging equipment and the need for specialized training can be barriers to widespread adoption. Additionally, the integration of imaging into the surgical workflow must be carefully managed to avoid disruptions and maintain the sterility of the operating environment. Nevertheless, ongoing advancements in imaging technology and the development of more user-friendly systems are expected to mitigate these challenges and expand the use of intraoperative imaging in clinical practice [4].

Looking ahead, the future of intraoperative imaging is poised to be shaped by emerging technologies such as artificial intelligence (AI) and augmented reality (AR). These innovations have the potential to further enhance the capabilities of intraoperative imaging by providing advanced image analysis and visualization tools that can assist surgeons in making more informed decisions. As these technologies continue to evolve, they are likely to play an increasingly important role in the surgical landscape, driving improvements in patient care and outcomes.

Finally, intraoperative imaging is a pivotal development in modern surgery, offering significant benefits in terms of precision, safety, and outcomes. As technology continues to advance, the integration of imaging into surgical practice is expected to become even more seamless and impactful, ultimately transforming the way surgeries are performed and enhancing the quality of care provided to patients.

31.2 Principles of Intraoperative Imaging

Intraoperative imaging is a transformative innovation in modern surgical practice, enabling real-time visualization and guidance during procedures. By integrating advanced imaging modalities into the surgical workflow, intraoperative imaging enhances precision, reduces complications, and improves patient outcomes [5]. The fundamental principles underlying this technology include adaptability to the surgical environment, seamless integration into workflows, and the provision of real-time feedback to guide decision-making [6].

Conventional imaging technologies such as CT, MRI, and ultrasound have undergone significant modifications to meet the unique demands of intraoperative applications [7]. For instance, intraoperative MRI (iMRI) systems are designed to operate within the confines of an operating room, featuring compact designs and specialized shielding to maintain sterility while minimizing electromagnetic interference. Similarly, intraoperative CT (iCT) scanners have been miniaturized and optimized for rapid image acquisition, allowing surgeons to assess surgical progress without interrupting the procedure. Intraoperative ultrasound (iUS), a portable and radiation-free modality, offers dynamic visualization of soft tissues and vascular structures, making it particularly useful in liver, pancreatic, and kidney surgeries. These adaptations ensure that imaging tools are not only effective, but also practical in the high-pressure environment of an operating theater. For example, mobile CT scanners provide immediate postsurgical imaging to verify implant placement or tumor resection before wound closure [7]. Additionally, innovations such as cone-beam CT and hybrid CT-MRI systems have improved imaging resolution and reduced radiation exposure, further enhancing their suitability for intraoperative use [8].

A critical principle of intraoperative imaging is its seamless integration into the surgical workflow. Advanced imaging systems are designed to be user-friendly and compatible with existing surgical tools. Software platforms enable real-time registration of imaging data with preoperative scans, allowing for precise navigation during surgery. For instance, AR overlays can project critical anatomical structures onto the surgical field, providing surgeons with a three-dimensional perspective that enhances spatial awareness [9]. Such integration minimizes disruptions while maintaining the sterile field. Moreover, clinical intraoperative imaging systems often incorporate advanced visualization technologies such as FGS. FGS requires fluorescent tracers to highlight pathological tissues in real time using specific excitation wavelengths of light [8]. This approach is particularly effective in oncologic surgeries for detecting nodal pathology, delineating tumor margins, and identifying residual disease [6]. Hybrid tracers combining fluorescence with radioisotopes further enhance precision by leveraging the strengths of both modalities—real-time visualization and deep tissue penetration [5].

The ability to provide immediate feedback is one of the most significant advantages of intraoperative imaging. Real-time visualization enables surgeons to adjust their techniques dynamically based on anatomical changes observed during the procedure [7]. This capability is especially valuable in complex surgeries such as neurosurgery and oncologic resections [6]. For example, iMRI allows neurosurgeons to detect brain shift—a phenomenon where brain tissues move during surgery—ensuring accurate resection of cancerous tissues while preserving critical functional areas [10]. iUS also exemplifies this principle by offering real-time assessment of vascular patency and perfusion during organ transplantation or tumor resection [11]. Its ability to detect additional lesions or characterize indeterminate findings can alter surgical plans mid-procedure, improving outcomes. Similarly, iCT provides rapid cross-sectional imaging that aids in verifying fracture reductions or implant positioning in orthopedic surgeries.

Recent advancements are expanding the capabilities of intraoperative imaging beyond traditional modalities. Molecular imaging techniques such as photoacoustic imaging and Raman spectroscopy have emerged as powerful tools for intraoperative diagnostics [12]. These technologies offer unparalleled specificity by targeting molecular markers associated with pathological tissues. For instance, photoacoustic imaging combines optical and ultrasound modalities to visualize deep tissue structures with high contrast [8]. AI-driven and machine learning algorithms are currently being integrated into intraoperative imaging systems to enhance decision-making [13]. AI algorithms can rapidly analyze large-scale imaging datasets in real time, identify subtle tissue abnormalities or characteristics, and predict surgical outcomes based on preoperative models. These innovations promise to make intraoperative imaging more efficient and precise.

The principles of adaptability, integration, and real-time feedback make intraoperative imaging indispensable across various surgical specialties. In neurosurgery, it facilitates safe resection of brain tumors while preserving neurological function. In oncology, it ensures complete tumor removal with negative margins by providing detailed visualization of tumor boundaries [6]. As these technologies continue to evolve, their role in personalized medicine is becoming increasingly evident. By combining diagnostic capabilities with therapeutic interventions—such as fluorescence-guided photodynamic therapy—surgeons can tailor treatments to individual patients' needs [6]. Indeed, the fundamental principles of intraoperative imaging—technological adaptation, workflow integration, and real-time feedback—form the foundation for its transformative impact on modern surgery. As emerging technologies further enhance its capabilities, intraoperative imaging is poised to redefine surgical precision and patient care.

31.3 Systemic Image-Guided Theranostic Applications for Patient Care

A major category of systemic theranostics aims to highlight tumor margins during surgery using intravenously (IV) administered agents that preferentially accumulate in cancerous tissue.

31.3.1 Fluorescence-Guided and Radio-Guided Surgery

EGFR-targeted agents Epidermal Growth Factor Receptor (EGFR), a transmembrane protein driving tumor growth, has served as an attractive clinical target as it is overexpressed by many epithelial tumors, including head and neck squamous cell carcinoma, non-small cell lung cancer, and colorectal cancer. Toward that end, monoclonal antibodies targeting EGFR and adapted with NIR fluorophores have served as delivery systems for image-guided detection and treatment. Cetuximab-IRDye800CW, for instance, an anti-EGFR antibody labeled with the 800 nm-excited fluorophore IRDye800CW, has been evaluated in Phase 1–3 trials (e.g., NCT05929456 Phase 1, NCT05499065 Phase 2, NCT03769506 Phase 3). These head and neck cancer trials showed that cetuximab-IRDye800CW safely and specifically highlights tumor tissue intraoperatively [14]. In fact, the fluorescence signal observed after cetuximab-IRDye800CW administration correlated with tumor location and enabled surgeons to identify cancerous margins undetectable by white light imaging. A recent Phase 3 trial of a related EGFR-targeted agent (cetuximab-IR700DX or ASP-1929) combined with phototherapy demonstrated improved locoregional disease control in recurrent head and neck cancer [15], underscoring the translational progress of EGFR-targeted fluorescence agents. The EGFR antibody, panitumumab, has been conjugated to IRDye800CW (NCT04511078 Phase 2), as well as to IRDye700DX, a bimodal agent used as a theranostic for both imaging and photodynamic therapy. These EGFR antibody platforms have reached advanced phase clinical trials, with ASP-1929 gaining approval in Japan for photoimmunotherapy (PIT), and cetuximab-IRDye800CW (Phase 3) for FGS [16]. These examples represent some of the most mature targeted IGS agents to date.

Folate receptor-targeted agents Folate receptor (FR) is another validated target. FR-alpha is overexpressed in ovarian cancer and several lung cancers. OTL38 (pafolacianine), a folate analog conjugated to the NIR dye S0456 (~788 nm excitation), was tested in a Phase 3 trial (NCT03180307) and subsequently approved by the Food and Drug Administration (FDA) as Cytalux™ for ovarian cancer surgery [17]. In the pivotal trial, pafolacianine enabled surgeons to detect 27% more malignant lesions that were missed by standard inspection [18]. Notably, these tumors were undetectable on preoperative scans and on gross inspection and were only identified by their emission under near-infrared illumination. These findings translated to significantly improved surgical outcomes given the reduction in residual disease. Cytalux was later also approved for the localization of lung nodules, making it the first targeted fluorescent drug in routine use. While earlier generation folate dyes, such as EC17, a fluorescein isothiocyanate (FITC)-conjugated folate (NCT01994369 Phase 1), were found to target tumors, they were often limited by poor tissue penetration and high autofluorescence due to the significant absorption of visible light by blood proteins, limiting their utility. The success of OTL38, which incorporates an 800 nm-range NIR dye, led to significantly enhanced intraoperative sensitivity by allowing deeper tissue penetration compared to visible light [18, 19].

PSMA-targeted agents Prostate-specific membrane antigen (PSMA)–targeted probes, developed as theranostic agents, integrate both fluorescence and radioactivity to enable dual-modality imaging, surgical guidance, and therapeutic assessments. PSMA is highly expressed in prostate cancer cells, as well as in the neovasculature of other solid tumors, making it an ideal target for radio-guided surgery (RGS). A systemically injected small-molecule PSMA inhibitor labeled with a gamma emitter (e.g., ^{99m}Tc-PSMA-I&S) has been used clinically for intraoperative localization of metastatic prostate cancer lesions. In a Phase 2/3 study (NCT05381103), ^{99m}Tc-PSMA-I&S RGS allowed surgeons to resect sub-centimeter nodal metastases that were detected by a handheld gamma probe. Sensitivity and specificity of PSMA RGS were 84% and 100%, respectively, in one analysis, and lesions as small as 3 mm could be successfully removed [20]. This approach is now entering routine practice for recurrent prostate cancer surgery. Building on these findings, additional PSMA-targeted fluorescence agents are in development, for example, a PSMA-targeting ligand linked to an indocyanine green (ICG)-like NIR dye (emission wavelength ~776 nm), referred to as "PSMA-Cytalux." Currently in Phase 2 clinical trials (NCT04832958), this probe enables real-time intraoperative visualization of prostatic tumor margins and/or occult tumor deposits, complementing preoperative PSMA Positron Emission Tomography (PET) imaging evaluations. Initial clinical studies have indeed shown that IV-injection of PSMA-targeted NIR dyes enables fluorescence imaging of PSMA-positive tumor foci and metastases in surgical specimens [21]. Multimodal PSMA agents incorporating an NIR fluorophore and radionuclide have also been developed and are being evaluated in early-phase trials, discussed below.

Enzyme-activated "smart" probes Beyond receptor targets, tumor-selective "activatable" or "smart" probes are being explored for FGS. Protease-activatable fluorescent agents remain inactive until cleaved by enzymes abundant in tumors, such as cathepsins and matrix metalloproteinases (MMP). LUM015 (pegulicianine), an IV-injected cathepsin-activated fluorescent imaging probe containing a Cy5 fluorophore (excitation wavelength ~650 nm), is activated following cleavage by cathepsins, yielding a fluorescence signal. In both Phase 1 (NCT01626066) and advanced phase (NCT02438358) breast cancer lumpectomy trials, the Lumicell™ system (i.e., LUM015) sensitively detected residual cancer within postsurgical cavity walls that was not otherwise detectable by the naked eye. A recent 400-patient pivotal trial reported that the investigational Lumicell™ device identified residual tumor in roughly 8% of patients after the surgeon believed that all cancerous foci were removed [22]. Notably, in the majority of cases, surgical margins were deemed negative by standard pathology, with fluorescent signal revealing tumor that pathology would have otherwise missed until recurrence. Furthermore, 14.5% of patients with initially positive margins were converted to negative margins intraoperatively by removing fluorescence-marked tissue, potentially sparing them a second surgery [22]. These results underscore the promise of enzyme-activated probes for achieving a more complete surgical resection. Another protease-activated Cy5 fluorescent agent, AVB-620, targeting MMP enzymes that mediate inflammation, remodeling, and repair, showed feasibility in a Phase 2 trial (NCT03113825) for assessing surgical margins in breast cancer patients, although detailed results are pending. Such broad-spectrum enzymatic targets serve as potential biomarkers across multiple tumor types and other diseases, unlike receptor-specific probes, but they must be tuned to avoid false positive results that may arise in the setting of inflammatory changes.

CEA-targeted agents Carcinoembryonic antigen (CEA) is a tumor marker targeted by SGM-101, a chimeric anti-CEA antibody labeled with a 700 nm fluorophore (BM104). Systemic SGM-101 has shown utility in colorectal cancer surgery. In a Phase 2/3 trial (NCT04642924), SGM-101 improved detection of peritoneal metastases and margins in colorectal and appendiceal cancers, and a Phase 3 trial (NCT05984810) in pancreatic cancer is presently underway. Early clinical use has shown that SGM-101 could safely highlight CEA-expressing tumors, influencing surgical decision-making in a significant fraction of patients [23]. Similarly, a CEA-targeted dual-modality agent, ^{111}In-DOTA-labetuzumab-IRDye800CW, has completed Phase 1 testing (NCT03699332) in colon cancer, enabling both preoperative Single Photon Emission Computed Tomography (SPECT) and intraoperative NIR imaging of CEA-positive lesions [24].

Overall trends in IV-injected theranostics, largely targeted to surgical margins, show progression from Phase 1 feasibility studies to larger Phase 2–3 trials, with regulatory approvals achieved for a few agents (i.e., pafolacianine, SGM-101 pending, etc.). Antibody-dye conjugates targeting EGFR or CEA, for instance, typically require dosing 2–4 days prior to surgery due to their slower uptake and clearance kinetics, whereas smaller-sized probes, such as small-molecule and ultrasmall particle tracers targeting folate, PSMA, and enzyme substrates, can be given within hours of the surgical procedure. Systemic approaches result in broad tumor exposure and can detect multifocal or occult disease. Many such agents have demonstrated that they can identify tumor deposits not detectable otherwise, thereby increasing complete resection rates. A key limitation, however, is the potential for off-target uptake, for instance, the binding of EGFR agents to skin or benign inflammatory tissues or the illumination of normal healthy folate-expressing tissues (i.e., kidneys, lungs) after administration of folate-targeting agents. This highlights the importance of selecting highly tumor-specific targets and optimizing dosing and clearance times.

31.3.2 Clinical Multimodal and Bimodal Systemic Approaches

A newer generation of theranostics combines distinct imaging capabilities into a single agent ("multimodal") or utilizes two agents of the same modality ("bimodal") to facilitate an integrated approach to treatment planning and intraoperative guidance. Multimodal probes generally combine preoperative PET imaging for localizing cancerous lesions with real-time fluorescence-guided surgery for precisely identifying optically active disease. Additionally, the application of dual-modality preoperative mapping of anatomic and functional disease by PET/CT or PET/MRI has also been performed, followed by fluorescence detection of the same probe for guiding tumor excision [25]. Such integrated imaging paradigms are transformative, as diagnostic and surgical treatment strategies have been integrated into a cohesive, seamless process. Below are several examples of systemically administered multimodal and bimodal agents designed to enhance disease evaluation that, in turn, inform clinical decision-making through enhanced sensitivity, precision, and specificity. Early results of representative Phase 1/2 clinical trials below highlight the feasibility of such approaches.

Multimodal theranostic probes Rapidly advancing multimodal probe developments are transforming cancer diagnostics and therapeutics. For instance, researchers in Europe reported a first-in-human trial in prostate cancer patients using ^{68}Ga-PSMA-11 conjugated to IRDye800CW, enabling detection of nodal metastases using preoperative PET and intraoperative fluorescence imaging guidance [20]. In both porcine and human studies, ^{68}Ga-PSMA-IRDye800 showed fluorescent localization to PSMA-expressing prostatic tissue within an hour of injection without significant background signal [26]. Similarly, a Phase 1 trial in malignant brain tumor patients (NCT03465618) utilized a systemically injected sub-8-nanometer multimodal integrin-targeting particle probe, Cornell prime dots (C′ dots), that bears PET radiolabels (e.g., iodine-124 (^{124}I)) and encapsulates far red/NIR dyes (i.e., Cy5/Cy5.5; excitation wavelengths ~650–678 nm) for aiding surgical management. As shown in Fig. 31.1, targeted delivery, penetration, and diffusion of this particle tracer were observed in a representative malignant brain tumor [27], confirmed by autoradiography and Cy5 fluorescence imaging of tumor tissue specimens. A second early-stage trial in advanced prostate cancer patients (NCT04167969) utilized the same particle designed to target PSMA, in addition to attaching zirconium-89 (^{89}Zr) to its surface, for preoperative PET mapping and detection and treatment of nodal metastases and/or residual disease along prostatectomy margins using FGS. In another example, colorectal cancers have been detected by the aforementioned multimodal probe ^{111}In-anti-CEA-IRDye800CW [24], while ^{111}In-girentuximab-IRDye800CW has been used to target carbonic anhydrase IX in clear-cell renal tumors (Phase 1, NCT02497599) [28]. In these cases, intraoperative guidance follows preoperative SPECT mapping of tumor deposits.

Cerenkov Luminescence Imaging Cerenkov luminescence imaging (CLI) leverages weak optical emissions emitted by certain PET tracers to guide real-time surgical management of tumors and assessment of margins. For example, in a Phase 2 breast cancer clinical trial (NCT05496101), optical emissions (i.e., Cerenkov light) from the IV-injected PET tracer, fluorodeoxyglucose (^{18}F-FDG), were detected by a CLI intraoperative camera system, enabling visualization of lumpectomy margins [29]. Moreover, coupling CLI findings with autoradiographic examination of breast lumpectomy specimens has emerged as a successful strategy for identifying positive tumor margins in breast lumpectomy specimens, potentially reducing re-excision rates [30]. Although not tumor-specific, positive ^{18}F-FDG-driven CLI results can serve as an imaging biomarker reflecting tumor presence, extent, and treatment response given the widespread use of ^{18}F-FDG for assessing glucose metabolism.

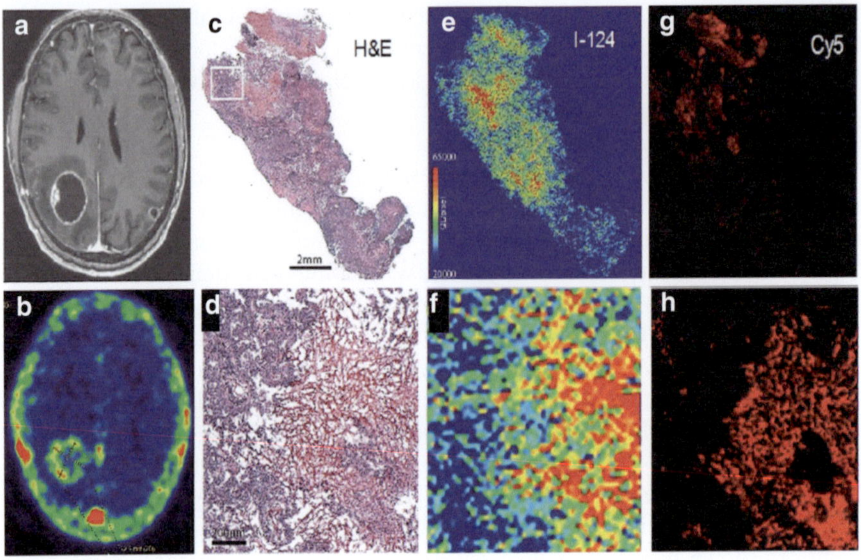

Fig. 31.1 Distribution and uptake of 124-I radiolabeled integrin-targeting C′ dots in a representative patient with metastatic breast cancer. (**a**) Contrast-enhanced brain MRI in a breast cancer patient showing a rim-enhancing cystic metastasis in the right occipital lobe. (**b**) Subsequent PET imaging 4 h after intravenously injected particle tracer, ^{124}I-cRGD-Cy5-C′ dots, was followed by surgical resection 24 h later. (**c–h**) Tumor tissue harvested from the patient during surgery underwent H&E staining (**c**, **d**), autoradiography (**e**, **f**), and fluorescence microscopy (**g**, **h**). Avid tracer uptake in both nodular and enhancing regions of the tumor on PET imaging corresponded with autoradiographic activity and Cy5 fluorescence of tumor tissue specimens. Findings are in keeping with particle uptake into the tumor and retention 24 h post-administration. Uptake in the leptomeninges on PET imaging is consistent with the expected particle distribution at this early time point [27]

Bimodal Fluorescence Imaging of brain tumors Bimodal fluorescence imaging approaches have been applied to the evaluation of malignant brain tumors to address challenges posed by the blood-brain barrier and the need to assess critical functional tissues during surgery and treatment (Fig. 31.2). In a pilot study (NCT02910804), patients with glioblastoma multiforme (GBM) were administered two probes—a dual-modality (PET-optical) bombesin (BBN)-receptor targeting tracer, ^{68}Ga-IRDye800CW-BBN, and 5-aminolevulinic acid (5-ALA; excitation/emission wavelength ~408 nm/635–710 nm), an approved tracer for fluorescence-guided neurosurgery [25]. Following confirmation of targeted tracer uptake with PET, patients received 5-ALA, and dual-channel fluorescence imaging was performed to visualize both spectrally distinct agents (i.e., IRDye800CW, 5-ALA) [25, 31]. Early results showed that infiltrative tumor (targeted tracer) could be distinguished from bulk high-grade tumor (5-ALA), and that integrating PET and dual-channel fluorescence imaging was feasible, as it enhanced the precise identification of residual tumor during resection with high sensitivity (~94%) and specificity (100%) [32].

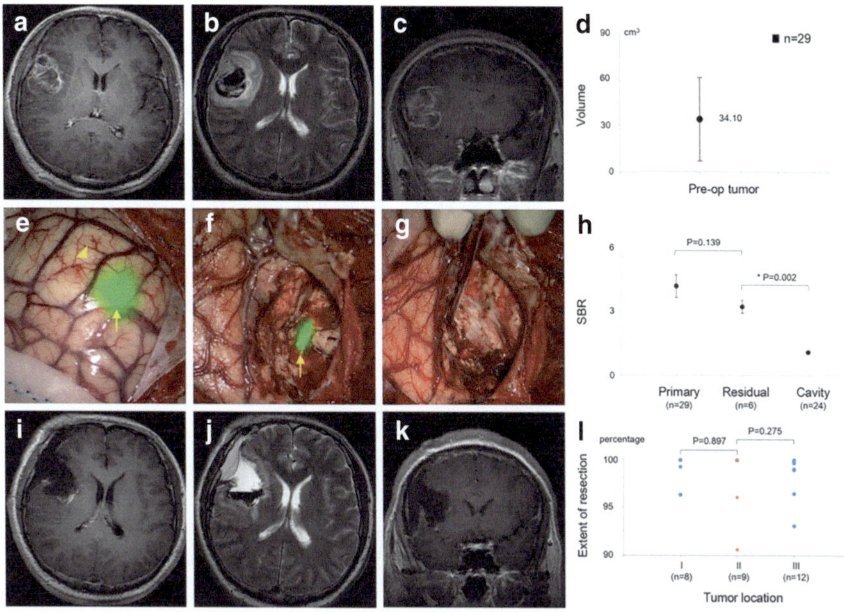

Fig. 31.2 Fluorescence-guided surgical resection of a glioblastoma multiforme (GBM) using IRDye800-BBN. (**a–c**) Right frontal lobe enhancing tumor on preoperative brain magnetic resonance imaging (MRI) is consistent with a GBM. (**d**) Plot of preoperative contrast-enhanced tumor volume. (**e**) Immediately after dural incision, a fluorescence signal was noted overlying the region of tumor (arrow); no fluorescence signal was seen to overlie normal cortical areas and the superficial vein (arrowhead). (**f**) Fluorescence signal at the site of residual tumor (arrow). (**g**) No fluorescence signal in the surgical cavity, indicating total resection. (**h**) Plot of signal-to-background ratio (SBR) values for primary tumor, residual disease, and surgical cavity. (**i–k**) Postoperative MRI confirmed no residual tumor. (**l**) Extent of resection at distinct tumor locations [31]

These findings highlight the utility of this bimodal approach, as targeted tracer was able to detect disease not visualized by 5-ALA.

The use of dual-modality (e.g., PET-MRI, PET-optical) imaging strategies with theranostic agents can enhance accuracy over that of single-modality agents. The combination of complementary techniques improves sensitivity, specificity, and disease localization that, in turn, reduces false positives/negatives and leads to better disease staging, surgical planning, and lesion characterization. Nuclear imaging, for instance, offers higher detection sensitivity than MRI but is associated with lower spatial resolution and specificity. In another case, suboptimal tissue penetration and lower sensitivity limit fluorescence imaging relative to nuclear imaging; however, its higher spatial resolution and specificity aids delineation of tumor boundaries not achievable with the latter. Indeed, radiodetection with a gamma probe can localize tumor, even when not detectable, but such deposits can be visualized and their extent better delineated along tumor margins with fluorescence imaging.

While the majority of systemic multimodal theranostics are currently in Phase 1–2 clinical trials, early findings suggest considerable promise for precision surgical applications. The fusion of such real-time imaging technologies with surgical intervention enables disease mapping (i.e., PET/SPECT) and precise excision (via fluorescence or CLI) with a single-dose administration. The translational maturity of these probes varies, with some being used at investigational stages, while others are used as approved agents (i.e., 5-ALA, ^{18}F-FDG), able to be repurposed and expected to reach clinical practice sooner. Challenges for these combinatorial products include regulatory complexity and logistical/scheduling issues. Yet, initial results of these studies underscore their safe use and clear benefit with respect to surgical outcomes.

31.3.3 Nontargeted Drug Delivery Systems

ThermoDox® ThermoDox® is a thermosensitive liposomal doxorubicin formulation that rapidly releases doxorubicin following exposure to heat (~40–43 °C). In the TARDOX Phase 1 study, patients with hepatic tumors received IV ThermoDox followed by MR-guided focused ultrasound (FUS) hyperthermia [33]. Doxorubicin delivery to heated tumors was markedly enhanced over unheated regions without serious adverse events beyond those induced by doxorubicin alone [33]. Incorporation of MRI tracers into liposomes confirmed high local drug release by MRI. A related ongoing trial (NCT04791228 Phase 2) is testing ThermoDox with MR-guided-high-intensity focused ultrasound (MR-HIFU) to precisely target and treat refractory solid tumors, with the goal of demonstrating improved tumor control after boosting intratumoral drug concentrations. This approach effectively utilizes imaging techniques (i.e., focused ultrasound) as a treatment tool to eradicate tissue through localized heat generation and controlled drug release with MR imaging guidance. A key advantage of this theranostic strategy is the spatiotemporal control of drug release to only sites of disease, achieving high local doses while minimizing systemic exposure. Limitations include its restriction to tumors accessible to FUS (e.g., liver, breast), in addition to requiring specialized MR-HIFU equipment.

AuroLase Therapy® AuroLase® therapy utilizes gold-silica nanoshells (GSN, AuroShell® particles) for ablating tumors. These IV-injected particles accumulate in tumors via the enhanced permeability and retention (EPR) effect [34] and, upon local exposure to an NIR laser, transform the energy into heat. In this way, particles are selectively activated by the laser at the precise target site, confining damage to the tumor. Gold nanoshell-mediated photothermal ablation has been demonstrated in preclinical models and an initial pilot in men with low-risk prostate cancer [34, 35] (Fig. 31.3). AuroShell particles are the first inorganic nanomaterial cleared by the FDA for photothermal therapy [34]. In a multisite clinical study (NCT02680535), the use of focal AuroLase ablative therapy resulted in complete ablation of 94% of treated tumors on follow-up biopsy with minimal side effects [36]; a pivotal trial

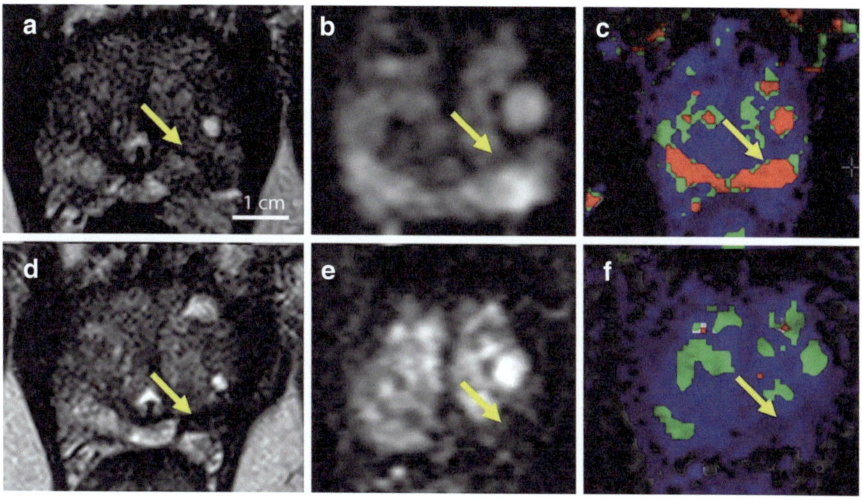

Fig. 31.3 Treatment of focal prostate cancer using GSN-directed laser excitation and ablation. Representative case of a 70-year-old man with prostate cancer successfully pretreated with laser excitation and ablation (**a**–**c**) and reevaluated 3 months (mo) posttreatment (**d**–**e**). A 3-mo follow-up biopsy was negative for cancer. (**a**) Axial T_2-weighted imaging demonstrates a left apex tumor Gleason 3+4 on targeted biopsy (arrow). (**b**) Diffusion-weighted image (DWI) for b = 2000 indicates restricted diffusion in tumor (hyperintensity relative to the normal peripheral zone). (**c**) Dynamic contrast-enhanced (DCE)-MRI parametric map (Ktrans/Ve) shows increased tumor enhancement. (**d**) Axial T_2-weighted imaging posttreatment shows contraction of the markedly hypointense ablation zone, compatible with hemorrhagic/necrotic changes. (**e**) DWI image for b = 2000 demonstrates resolution of restricted diffusion in the treated tumor (arrow). (**f**) DCE-MRI parametric map (Ktrans/Ve) shows resolution of abnormal enhancement in treated tumor (arrow) [35] (Scale bar: 1 cm)

(NCT04240639) is ongoing. In practice, AuroLase therapy utilizes MRI or ultrasound guidance for catheter placement and monitoring ablation zones. Integrating these technologies allows for highly targeted treatments beyond what is achievable with conventional lasers alone. Limitations include variations in particle uptake across solid tumors and the requirement of an unobstructed path for laser targeting. However, this platform underscores the successful translation of nanotechnology into a surgical adjunct, with ongoing studies exploring synergistic therapeutic strategies (e.g., salvage brachytherapy) for oncology [34].

NanoTherm® NanoTherm® therapy utilizes intratumorally injected superparamagnetic iron oxide nanoparticles (SPIONs) for magnetic hyperthermia, induced with an alternative magnetic field. In patients with recurrent GBM, a single-arm trial of NanoTherm therapy plus low-dose radiotherapy demonstrated a median overall survival of 13.4 months from recurrence without serious adverse events, comparing favorably to historical controls [37]. NanoTherm, which received a CE Mark in Europe for treating brain tumors, has aimed to further validate its efficacy in several clinical trials (e.g., MAGROT, NCT02250580, NCT06271421). During such procedures, MRI confirms the intratumoral distribution of particles and monitors edema. Its targeted activation via a magnetic field induces tissue heating with ensuing cell death. This approach guides targeting of infiltrative cells within the resection cavity that are otherwise difficult to excise, improving local tumor control. The invasiveness of the procedure is a limiting factor, which is best suited to fixed targets (i.e., brain tumors), and may justify a more localized approach given restrictive drug transport across the blood–brain barrier. Precise regulation of heating may be a challenge, but computer modeling and careful field calibration have made this safe, with only moderate side effects reported.

31.4 Local Image-Guided Theranostic Applications for Patient Care

Local administration of single-modality theranostics has been used to guide surgical treatment of locoregional disease spread involving draining lymph nodes for specific cancer types, such as breast cancer, melanoma, and head and neck cancers. Conventional methods often administer blue dyes (e.g., methylene blue, patent blue V) and/or a Single Photon Emission Computed Tomography (SPECT) tracer, technetium-99m (^{99m}Tc)-sulfur colloid, peritumorally for treating sentinel lymph nodes (SLNs), while newer dual-modality probes may combine ^{99m}Tc (half-life: 6 h) with an NIR dye (e.g., ICG) into a single hybrid tracer formulation, such as, ^{99m}Tc-nanocolloid. Following peritumoral injection, a gamma probe is typically used to detect SLN activity in deeper tissues, while fluorescence imaging permits real-time nodal visualization [19]. Specifically, radioguidance ensures nodes obscured by >1 cm of tissue are not missed, while fluorescence signal can generally only be observed through thin muscle or fat (up to ~0.5–1 cm depth) [19]. ICG-^{99m}Tc-nanocolloid, used clinically in Europe, has resulted in superior identification rates relative to blue dye alone using real-time optical imaging guidance, thus limiting the need for bulkier gamma cameras [38]. A more recent ongoing non-small cell lung cancer trial (NCT05555199) is also studying ICG-^{99m}Tc-nanocolloid for identifying and retrieving tumor-draining lymph nodes.

The use of macromolecular particle-based agents, such as Cy5.5-encapsulated C′ dots, can also be locally administered as theranostics for guiding nodal resection. For instance, following conjugation of multiple integrin-targeting peptides (cRGDY), cRGDY–Cy5.5 C-dots, targeted accumulation within lymphatic tissues was observed after intradermal injection about tumors. A Phase 1 trial (NCT02106598) in head and neck melanoma patients demonstrated that cRGDY–Cy5.5 C-dots are a high-sensitivity nodal detection platform for deep-tissue imaging (i.e., ~1.5–2.0 cm) and imaging of difficult-to-access anatomic sites, in some case, facilitating surgical excision of nodes through intact skin without extensive dissection of adjacent normal tissues (Fig. 31.4) [39]. Further surface labeling with iodine ^{124}I for PET imaging can also be conducted for preoperative evaluation.

In summary, local theranostic approaches are highly effective for regional nodal staging procedures. Many have been implemented into clinical practice. For

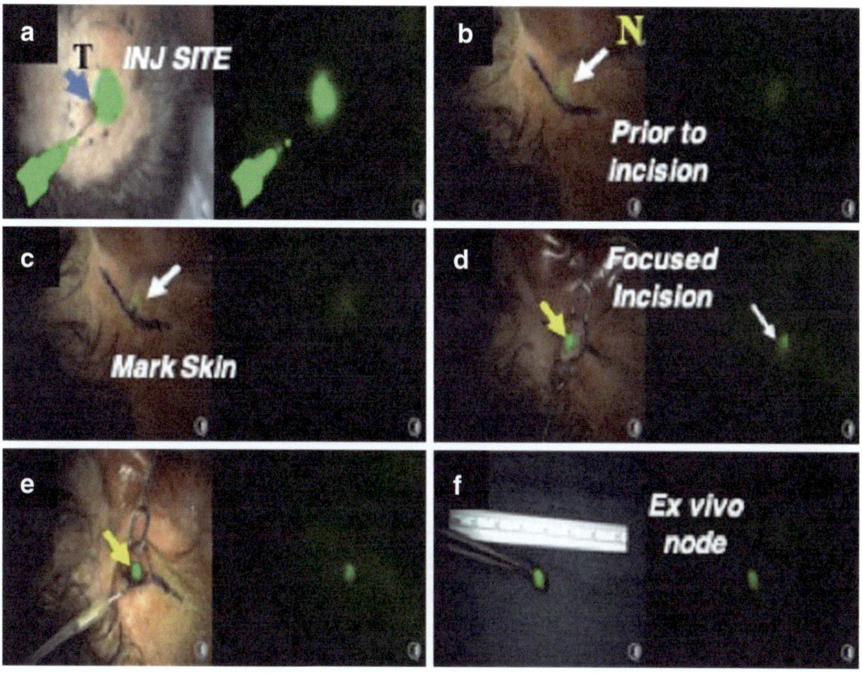

Fig. 31.4 Real-time Transcutaneous Visualization of a sentinel lymph node (SLN) using a fluorescent particle, C′ dots. A 54-year-old male with a scalp melanoma (T) was injected peritumorally with this targeted optical particle (green signal in (**a**)). A faint area of fluorescence was seen through the intact skin overlying a post-auricular SLN (N; arrow in (**b**)) using FGS for real-time optical imaging guidance. Limited extent of surgical dissection (short black line, arrow in (**c**)) and size of the resection cavity (**d**) relative to the planned area of dissection unaided (i.e., marked line in (**c**) is ~3 times larger than that actually drawn on the basis of the particle signal). Progressive dissection of the nodal bed with increasing fluorescent signal of the node (**e**). Ex vivo SLN (F) [39]

example, the use of ICG for treating SLNs in breast cancer patients is widespread, with studies showing it can equal or outperform detection rates with radiocolloids. The trend favors multimodal tracers that eliminate the need for two separate injections; a single injection yields optical and radioactive signals that improve surgical workflows and treatment accuracy. These agents have progressed significantly in clinical trials, with numerous Phase 3 and comparative studies, alongside real-world adoption of hybrid tracers in Europe and Asia.

31.5 Scientific and Clinical Implications

The advent of surgical theranostics is transforming oncology practice by enhancing precision, efficiency, and patient outcomes. First, by improving the clearance of disease along tumor margins and difficult-to-access nodes, they address a key predictor of patient outcomes: extent of tumor removal. For example, real-time imaging guidance of breast cancer lumpectomies has reduced the frequency of repeat surgical procedures. The use of Lumicell's Direct Visualization System led to the detection of residual breast cancer, which would have otherwise been missed in about 8% of patients following standard lumpectomy procedures [40]. In GBM, 5-ALA fluorescence guidance increased gross total resection rates from ~36% to 65% in a pivotal Phase 3 clinical trial, thereby prolonging overall survival [41]. The dual-modality GBM study further showed that integrating PET and optical imaging significantly improved resection margin visualization, while ensuring patient safety. In ovarian cancer, maximizing cytoreduction is crucial for improving treatment efficacy. With the introduction of pafolacianine, surgeons are able to better detect occult disease, directly impacting progression-free survival [42]. Essentially, these technologies are improving the surgeon's ability to achieve the oncologic ideal of "no tumor left behind," which should reduce local recurrence and improve survival in aggregate.

Molecular targeting also brings a level of precision that can spare healthy tissue in oncologic procedures. For example, EGFR-targeted probes should ideally highlight only EGFR-expressing tumor, not adjacent normal mucosa, enabling tighter excision margins and less normal tissue sacrifice. That said, an important consideration is tumor heterogeneity: not all tumor cells express a given target (e.g., an EGFR-negative subclone won't be seen by cetuximab-800CW). Therefore, a lack of fluorescence does not guarantee an absence of tumor; results must be interpreted in context. This has promoted significant interest in metabolic- (i.e., FDG, 5-ALA) and enzymatically (proteases) targeted probes visualizing biochemical activity in diseased tissues, which complement receptor-specific targets. Integrating agents (e.g., bimodal approaches) might offer a more comprehensive assessment of tumor biology, with one agent highlighting bulk tumor, and the other detecting missed disease. However, multi-agent use complicates workflows and regulatory approval, so the trend has shifted to using multifunctional single-agent theranostics.

The interplay between targeting moieties, cancer types, and imaging labels/modalities highlights the importance of precisely tailoring theranostic approaches to optimize diagnosis and treatment. Antibodies (e.g., anti-CEA, anti-EGFR) work well for intracavity surgeries (e.g., thoracic, abdominal), and are scheduled within days of agent injection to ensure maximum target-to-background ratios. Although their high specificity yields maximum contrast [14], the slow diffusion of such agents may miss active sites of disease. Small molecules (e.g., PSMA ligands) and macromolecular agents can be injected shortly before surgery, even intraoperatively, offering flexibility in timing and administration, making them useful for unpredictable surgical schedules. Yet, their faster kinetics may lead to quicker washout and potentially reduced signal intensity [43]. The choice of optical dyes is equally critical: IRDye800CW and other NIR-I dyes (700–800 nm range) typically exhibit penetration depths ranging from a few millimeters to 1 cm. These dyes are superior to visible dyes (e.g., FITC), as the latter results in lower penetration depths (i.e., 1–2 mm) [44]. NIR light emission (~700–1000 nm range) falls within the "tissue optical window" where biological absorption is low, allowing photons to travel farther. Thus, NIR dyes are optimal for detecting subsurface tumors or positive cavity margins. While deep-red dyes (e.g., Cy5) occupy the transition zone between visible and NIR imaging, resulting in less tissue penetration, they often exhibit higher quantum yields that yield greater fluorescence signal intensity. In practice, most clinical trials favor the use of ~700–800 nm dyes. An emerging area is the use of Second Near-Infrared Window (NIR-II) fluorophores (1000–1700 nm), which represent an exciting advancement in deep-tissue imaging. They offer greater penetration depths (i.e., up to 2 cm) due to reduced scattering, as evidenced by preclinical imaging of tumors beneath thick tissue sections [45]. NIR-II agents may overcome the depth limitations of FGS, provided they can be made clinically safe.

Radio-guided techniques serve as an essential complement to fluorescence imaging, enabling the detection of deep-seated tumors that optical methods may not identify. Gamma probes can effectively detect radioactive hotspots several centimeters deep. The high sensitivity of nuclear detection means even tiny tumor deposits can be found (down to milligrams of tissue). However, there is no real-time visualization of tumor boundaries. Rather, radioactively labeled regions simply aid in the localization of tumors and confirm their presence. Therefore, the integration of fluorescent signal or Cerenkov imaging can enhance radio-guided techniques by providing optical visualization of radiotracer distribution, adding significant value and enhancing surgical precision [46]. The complementary nature of these modalities reinforces the value of multimodal strategies, ensuring a more comprehensive approach to achieving surgical precision. Reports have echoed that sentiment, stating that a combined optical/nuclear probe "could be of additional value" since each modality's weaknesses are mitigated by the other.

Integrating such multimodal imaging strategies may have far-reaching effects on patient selection and personalized surgery, enabling interventions to be precisely tailored to individual tumor characteristics. Increasing availability of targeted tracers has paved the way for a more personalized approach to oncologic imaging, with tracer selection guided by specific biomarker assessments (e.g., EGFR, FRα, PSMA, etc.), the essence of personalized theranostics. Such biomarker-guided tracer selections need to be coordinated with nuclear medicine or radiopharmacy departments to ensure availability of suitable imaging agents. In the future, sequential administration of multiple tracers could enable targeting of different tumor subregions, in turn, offering insights into heterogeneity and biomarker distribution. However, challenges related to interpretation may require deconvolution by AI-powered image analysis.

Finally, these new advances will require the training of surgical staff. Real-time theranostics in the operating room represents a paradigm shift in surgical decision-making. Surgeons must integrate fluorescent or radioactive cues with anatomic knowledge and tailor resections accordingly. Early adopters have reported that fluorescence guidance changed their surgical planning in a significant subset of cases for the better. For example, surgeons removed additional tumor implants in 27% of ovarian cancer patients due to Cytalux's signal [42]. As confidence in these technologies grows with time, surgical oncology may routinely incorporate imaging feedback akin to how laparoscopic surgeons use a camera—here, the molecular camera becomes a standard extension of the surgeon's vision.

31.6 Strengths and Limitations of Approaches

Fluorescence-Guided Surgery The major strengths of FGS include visual confirmation of the tumor, enhanced discrimination of tissues, and potential for multimodal integration. FGS effectively highlights the tumor, allowing delineation of margins at the sub-millimeter level in real time [47, 48]. Modern NIR fluorescence camera systems can be integrated with surgical microscopes or laparoscopes, permitting surgeons to toggle between white-light and fluorescence views or see composite overlays. High-resolution mapping ensures that no small tumor cluster is left at the cut edge [47, 49]. FGS is relatively safe; the energy used (NIR light) is nonionizing and poses minimal risk to the patient and staff, and doses of imaging agents are typically very low (microdoses) compared to therapeutic levels. Another strength is speed, as feedback is instantaneous [47, 50]. If an area lights up, the surgeon can excise it and inspect for residual fluorescence signal, enabling iterative margin assessment for achieving a clean margin. The limitations of FGS include limited depth penetration of light (typically <10 mm), potential fluorescence quenching in very deep or large tumors, and the requirement that tumor uptake of fluorophore-bearing probes exceeds that of the background. Hemoglobin strongly absorbs light in the NIR spectrum, potentially reducing signal and obscuring visualization. However, in practice, careful suctioning and timing can mitigate this issue. Autofluorescence from surrounding tissues is usually low in NIR, but can sometimes cause unwanted background signal (e.g., baseline liver signal). Importantly, FGS only indicates presence, not viability, e.g., a necrotic tumor may or may not retain dye; some probes (like 5-ALA) actually highlight necrosis. Surgeons must interpret fluorescence in context (e.g., a nerve might appear dark, but absence of fluorescence does not mean it is safe to cut unless one knows its anatomy) [51]. Another limitation is that many current systems provide qualitative imaging. Quantitative fluorescence thresholds for malignancy are still being studied, and over-reliance can lead to removing benign tissue that lights up (false positives). Nevertheless, consensus statements now affirm that FGS is an effective and safe adjunct across various cancers, with evidence of improved outcomes [52]. Continued improvements in camera sensitivity and the move to NIR-II should further mitigate depth issues.

Radio-guided Surgery Radio-guided techniques using gamma probes or beta probes have the strength of sensitivity and depth. They can detect deeply seated radioactivity that no optical method can perceive. For example, SLNs behind a thick layer of muscle are located easily by a probe that can detect the ^{99m}Tc signal centimeters away [53]. RGS is also well-established—SLN biopsy with radiotracers has been routine in breast cancer and melanoma for decades, proving its reliability and benefit (i.e., reduced unnecessary nodal dissections). Gamma detection is semi-quantitative, as thresholding count rates is a key strategy to determine whether a tissue is radiotracer-positive (e.g., >10× background count) [54]. Limitations include the lack of a visual display, with only auditory feedback or numerical displays. In addition, spatial resolution is poor, often providing suboptimal discrimination of the signal source, which may impact disease localization [54]. Another consideration is radiation safety and logistics, as handling radioactive materials in RGS requires coordination with nuclear medicine, strict specimen management protocols, and measures to limit staff exposure. Some new RGS methods use beta-emitting tracers with probe detectors that only register signals when virtually touching the tissue; this improves localization. For example, the use of ^{18}F-FDG and a β-probe for assessing margins gives very localized readings, but requires direct contact scanning of the surface, which can be time-consuming [55]. Cerenkov imaging, as a camera-based RGS, offers an optical-like visualization of radionuclide distribution, helping to bridge the gap between conventional radioguidance and direct anatomical imaging. Its limitation is extreme faintness of the light, necessitating a dark room and a sensitive camera, typically only feasible on excised specimens or in open cavities after removing ambient light.

Multimodal and Bimodal Strategies Integrated hybrid strategies, such as a dual PET/fluorescence agent, permit whole-body nuclear imaging for depth and fluorescence for high-precision intraoperative visualization. Enabling multiscale imaging from the macro (whole body) to micro (cellular) level with a single agent is clearly a strength, as it simplifies both regulatory burdens and imaging logistics. During surgery, if lesion depth limits fluorescence detection, the surgeon can utilize a gamma probe with the same agent. Likewise, if a fluorescent margin is identified, but surgeons want to ensure that no deeper tumor deposits remain at the surgical site, they could perform intraoperative PET or a probe survey. Some groups have even integrated gamma probes into laparoscopic instruments and developed hybrid imaging systems (e.g., combined fluorescence–gamma cameras) [56]. The main limitation of multimodal agents is their relative complexity. Synthesizing a dual-labeled system is challenging, and given the possibility that one or more components can affect targeting or kinetics, regulatory approval must consider the safety of both components. Timing optimization is a crucial factor in dual PET/fluorescence imaging, as the ideal postinjection window for PET imaging may not align with the optimal fluorescence signal intensity for intraoperative visualization [57]. Some dual-modality probes may solve this issue by using a long-lived radionuclide (i.e., ^{111}In), so that imaging can be delayed until the fluorescence signal is optimized [58]. Bimodal optical agents leveraging spectrally distinct dyes can provide multi-layered tumor characterization, distinguishing high-grade from low-grade cancerous foci. However, this approach requires dual-channel imaging devices capable of wavelength discrimination to accurately differentiate signals. Neurosurgical assessments often use microscopes equipped with dual fluorescence capabilities in tumor visualization and precision resection (e.g., blue light for 5-ALA and NIR for antibody targeting) [59]. One limitation is that overlapping fluorescence signals may complicate interpretation when one tumor region takes up multiple agents. Careful agent selection can strategically enhance contrast, ensuring that one fluorophore highlights regions the other does not, reducing signal overlap and improving tumor characterization. Overall, multimodal strategies are powerful but require rigorous training and structured protocols to maximize benefit and avoid information overload.

31.7 Advanced Techniques Enhancing Theranostic IGS

AI is transforming surgical theranostics by aiding the design of smarter probes, real-time visualization, precision resection, and decision-making [60]. Machine learning models have been used to analyze large libraries of compounds and predict tumor-specific probes, for instance, the design of peptides or small molecules with optimal optical properties and binding [61]. Intraoperatively, AI can help distinguish true tumor fluorescence from background by analyzing intensity patterns in real-time video. An example is an "optical smart probe" system that utilizes a deep learning algorithm to quantify fluorescence, notifying the surgeon when fluorescence intensity surpasses a predefined malignancy threshold, ensuring real-time decision support [62]. Such a system was prototyped (OptiDX) to detect residual tumor in the surgical cavity, improving the objectivity of FGS interpretation. Another application involves augmented reality (AR) overlays, whereby preoperative imaging (CT, MRI, PET) data can be superimposed onto the surgeon's field-of-view through AR glasses or microscope displays, effectively "lighting up" where tumors or critical structures are behind tissue [63]. AI-driven deformable registration also plays a crucial role in matching preoperative imaging to real-time surgical anatomy, enabling precise spatial alignment despite tissue deformation [64]. In robotic surgery, efforts have been made to incorporate fluorescence imaging directly into the robotic system (e.g., the DaVinci robot incorporates Firefly© fluorescence imaging, utilizing ICG to enhance tissue visualization) and use AI-driven contrast optimization and camera adjustments to maximize fluorophore detection [65]. One study combining AI with fluorescence detection showed reduced false positives and allowed precise tumor margin mapping, yielding a new paradigm [66].

Combined MRI/FUS has been successfully used with ThermoDox. In addition, iMRI has become critical to neurosurgical practice, providing real-time imaging updates to ensure that no residual tumor is masked by anatomical shifts during resection [67]. HIFU is also being investigated, not only for drug release but also for direct ablation of inoperable tumor regions under imaging guidance. After removing safely resectable tissues, for example, MR-guided FUS could be used to ablate an infiltrative margin that cannot be excised. This concept of theranostic surgery goes beyond mechanical tumor resection; it integrates targeted imaging and therapeutic interventions to enhance local control and long-term oncologic outcomes [68]. We see similar combined modality use in prostate cancer, for instance, MR-guided laser ablation (i.e., biopsy- and MR-guided laser fiber placements), a form of image-guided therapy that complements surgical management of multifocal disease [69].

Another frontier focuses on quantitative imaging and feedback control. In HIFU drug delivery, MR thermometry provides a feedback loop to maintain temperatures in range, ensuring effective drug release without overheating. In photothermal particle therapy (AuroLase), real-time thermal cameras or MRI can ensure adequate heating at the target site, while preventing spread to adjacent tissues. Integration of these feedback mechanisms makes therapies safer and more reliable—essentially "closing the loop" between diagnostics and therapeutics in the surgical setting [70].

31.8 Future Directions

13.8.1 Targeted Fluorescence Agents

Future research will explore the development of new tumor-specific targets, such as ligands providing read-outs on metabolic activities or cancer stem cells, as well as higher performance fluorophores. NIR-II dyes and fluorescent nanoparticles are being investigated for deep-tissue imaging [45]. Ensuring biocompatibility and excretion of such probes is a priority for translation. Trifunctional theranostic platforms, particularly engineered antibodies, are being developed that seamlessly integrate imaging, tracking, and treatment in a single molecular system. Finally, PIT is an emerging theranostic approach utilizing IR700DX-based antibody conjugates and NIR light activation to selectively eliminate cancer cells. The success of ASP-1929, which combines cetuximab with IR700DX for treating head and neck cancer, suggests that future agents integrate low-intensity imaging for tumor localization with high-dose light activation for selective cytotoxicity [14]. Fine-tuning dosing and light delivery are critical to enhancing accuracy and maximizing treatment efficacy in PIT and light-activated theranostics.

31.8.2 Radio-Guided and Multimodal Agents

An important future direction involves the translation of promising dual-labeled probes to the clinic. This will involve conducting multicenter trials to demonstrate that, for example, a PET/optical PSMA tracer yields superior patient outcomes (e.g., higher lymph node yield, lower disease recurrence) relative to conventional methods. Comparing single- and dual-modality approaches is crucial to understanding the added value of integrating multiple imaging or therapeutic techniques. Also, engineering innovations are driving the creation of more universal multimodal platforms, for example, a chelator that attaches various radionuclides and a dye to *any* targeting moiety on demand. Such modular approaches simplify production and regulatory hurdles by having a single kit that can be customized for targeting different cancers by attaching the appropriate antibody or peptide. On the hardware side, development of hybrid imaging systems, for instance, a surgical gamma camera integrating fluorescence detection, is redefining real-time intraoperative visualization, as it allows surgeons to visualize both nuclear and optical signals simultaneously. Experimental devices, such as handheld PET probes or gamma cameras integrated into laparoscopes, have shown feasibility. Combined with AR, preoperative PET activity could be projected onto the surgical field in real time, guiding the surgeon's hand to expected sites of fluorescence signal, and refining precision in tumor resection. Multimodal image analysis software will also play a crucial role, providing surgeons with a comprehensive tumor map that surpasses individual modalities.

31.8.3 Smart Probes and Activatable Therapies

For enzyme-activated probes, future research aims to improve specificity, ensuring high-fidelity molecular targeting while minimizing off-target effects. Nanoparticle-based amplifying probes are also being tested; these are designed to dramatically enhance fluorescence signal upon enzymatic activation, making them valuable for detecting sparse or early-stage disease [71]. Some "smart" probes are being developed to not only signal tumor presence, but to locally deliver a toxin or immunotherapy once activated, thereby treating micrometastases in situ [72]. For instance, an enzyme-activated checkpoint inhibitor delivery system could revolutionize precision oncology, as it integrates surgical resection with localized immunotherapy at the microscopic level. While highly experimental, the convergence of surgical treatment with such adjuvant therapies is a logical extension of theranostics.

31.8.4 AI and Digital Surgery

Future directions include machine learning models that are trained on thousands of surgical cases to provide real-time decision support. For example, an AI-driven fluorescence intensity analysis algorithm could dramatically refine intraoperative decision-making, guiding surgeons on whether additional resection is warranted. In addition, AI-assisted fluorescence interpretation can significantly reduce user dependence and variability, thereby ensuring objective analyses. Efforts are also underway to develop standardized fluorescence quantitation, such as calibrated fluorescence thresholds, for improving tumor margin assessments [60]. Histopathology validation will be crucial for confirming the accuracy, reliability, and clinical utility of these methods. The vision of AI-guided surgical navigation—integrating preoperative MRI (or PET), intraoperative fluorescence, radioguidance, and real-time imaging—encapsulates the future of precision oncologic surgery, aiming to function like a surgical GPS to optimize tumor removal. AR visualization of these data, paired with holographic tumor mapping, has the potential to revolutionize and fundamentally change how surgery is performed in the next 10–20 years [73].

31.8.5 Thermal and Magnetic Therapies

For technologies such as HIFU-triggered drugs and NanoTherm, future research will focus on combining energy-based drug activation with chemotherapy and immunotherapy, for instance, to achieve enhanced tumor eradication. Combining NanoTherm hyperthermia with immunotherapy is intriguing, as thermal activation of tumors can induce antigen release, potentially converting "cold" tumors (which evade immune detection) into "hot" tumors that elicit a robust immune response. Trials combining local ThermoDox plus HIFU with checkpoint inhibitors may enhance systemic immune activation through the abscopal effect, with local therapy triggering diffuse tumor regression [74]. Miniaturizing magnetic field generators or

HIFU for intraoperative use would lead to new precision therapeutic approaches during, for instance, partial liver resection, enabling treatment of margins and satellite lesions. This would require portable and safe devices for open use. While intraoperative ultrasound ablation has become more accessible, MR-guided interventions remain largely confined to specialized suites due to technical issues.

31.8.6 Translation

In terms of translational maturity, we expect more Phase 3 trials over the next few years for front-runner agents that include EGFR-IRDye800CW for oral cancer [75], SGM-101 for colorectal cancer [76], and PSMA RGS for prostate cancer [76], given their strong Phase 2 results. Regulatory bodies are increasingly receptive to imaging adjuncts as data accrue that they improve patient outcomes. The FDA approval of pafolacianine and pegulicianine for breast cavity detection was a pivotal event that established a precedent for FGS and paved the way for next-generation agents. Future research needs to address cost-benefit analysis and the dissemination of training and prove that widespread adoption of these technologies is feasible and worth the investment for healthcare systems.

31.9 Conclusion

Surgical theranostics is the perfect convergence of molecular precision and surgical expertise, allowing surgeons to see beyond traditional anatomical structures and into the functional and biochemical profiles of cancer. Data from current trials and the use of systemically administered targeted agents against EGFR, FRα, PSMA, and CEA, for instance, are enabling more thorough resections across multiple cancer types, while enzymatically activated probes are providing a tumor-agnostic approach for visualizing cancerous tissue. Multimodal imaging agents are serving as the critical link between radiology and surgery, as they promote the integration of preoperative diagnostics with image-guided treatment. Importantly, the clinical trial landscape reflects a clear progression, ranging from molecular imaging and theranostic technologies (i.e., folate, EGFR, and CEA targeting) on the cusp of standard practice to others, such as multimodal particles and enzymatic probes in early-phase development with an eye toward product translation. Nontargeted drug delivery systems offer a broader therapeutic scope, allowing surgeons to not just cut what they see, but treat what they cannot cut. This foreshadows a future where surgery, imaging, and targeted therapy converge, creating a holistic, precision-driven approach in oncologic care.

To fully realize these innovations, continued interdisciplinary collaboration is essential. Surgical oncologists, nuclear medicine physicians, imaging scientists, and nanotechnology experts must work in concert to design next-generation clinical trials and refine surgical guidance approaches. The implementation of AI and advanced imaging paradigms will further augment surgeons' capabilities, potentially automating the detection of occult disease. Looking ahead, one can envision that a surgeon of the future, armed with a palette of theranostic agents, will merge precision imaging, AI-guided resection, and intraoperative therapy activation, creating an all-in-one biologically tailored intervention. This vision, while ambitious, is backed by rapid advancements in imaging, molecular science, and surgical innovation. Surgical theranostics are illuminating a more precise, biologically informed, and outcome-driven path forward for oncologic patients. The coming years of translational and clinical research will determine how well these potential technological breakthroughs can perform in oncologic practice, but the trajectory strongly points toward an era of molecularly informed precision surgery.

References

1. Dell'Oglio P et al (2022) Precision surgery: the role of intra-operative real-time image guidance - outcomes from a multidisciplinary European consensus conference. Am J Nucl Med Mol Imaging 12(2):74–80
2. Ogando-Rivas E et al (2022) Evolution and revolution of imaging technologies in neurosurgery. Neurol Med Chir (Tokyo) 62(12):542–551
3. Husarova T et al (2023) Intraoperative imaging in Hepatopancreatobiliary surgery. Cancers (Basel) 15:14
4. Zheng B, Cai X (2025) Fundamentals of digital surgery. Laparoscop Endoscop Robot Surg 8:115
5. Yaroslavsky AN, Feng X, Neel V (2017) Optical mapping of nonmelanoma skin cancers—a pilot clinical study. Lasers Surg Med 49(9):803–809
6. Belykh E et al (2016) Intraoperative fluorescence imaging for personalized brain tumor resection: current state and future directions. Front Surg 3:55
7. Kut C et al (2015) Detection of human brain cancer infiltration ex vivo and in vivo using quantitative optical coherence tomography. Sci Transl Med 7(292):292ra100
8. Yashin K et al (2022) OCT-guided surgery for gliomas: current concept and future perspectives. Diagnostics 12(2):335
9. Garcia M et al (2018) Bio-inspired imager improves sensitivity in near-infrared fluorescence image-guided surgery. Optica 5(4):413
10. Wu K et al (2021) Integration of microanatomy, neuronavigation, dynamic neurophysiologic monitoring, and intraoperative multimodality imaging for the safe removal of an insular glioma: 2-dimensional operative video. Oper Neurosurg 21(1):E28–E29
11. Almasian M et al (2019) Pilot feasibility study of in vivo intraoperative quantitative optical coherence tomography of human brain tissue during glioma resection. J Biophotonics 12(10):e201900037
12. Han JY, Lee DC, Lee SY (2018) Horizontal extraocular muscle and scleral anatomy in children: a swept-source anterior segment optical coherence tomography study. Korean J Ophthalmol 32(2):83
13. Tejedor P, Sagias F, Khan J (2020) The use of enhanced technologies in robotic surgery and its impact on outcomes in rectal cancer: a systematic review. Surg Innov 27(4):384–391
14. Bhandari C et al (2022) Towards photodynamic image-guided surgery of head and neck tumors: photodynamic priming improves delivery and diagnostic accuracy of Cetuximab-IRDye800CW. Front Oncol 12:853660
15. Biel MA et al (2019) A global phase III multicenter, randomized, double-arm, open label trial of ASP-1929 photoimmunotherapy versus physician's choice standard of care for the treatment of patients with locoregional, recurrent head and neck squamous cell carcinoma (rHNSCC). J Clin Oncol 37(15_suppl):TPS6094

16. Tahara M et al (2021) A phase I, single-center, open-label study of RM-1929 photoimmunotherapy in Japanese patients with recurrent head and neck squamous cell carcinoma. Int J Clin Oncol 26(10):1812–1821
17. Montaño AR et al (2025) Matrix-designed bright near-infrared fluorophores for precision peripheral nerve imaging. Biomaterials 319:123190
18. van Dam GM et al (2011) Intraoperative tumor-specific fluorescence imaging in ovarian cancer by folate receptor-α targeting: first in-human results. Nat Med 17(10):1315–1319
19. Vahrmeijer AL et al (2013) Image-guided cancer surgery using near-infrared fluorescence. Nat Rev Clin Oncol 10(9):507–518
20. Derks YHW et al (2019) PSMA-targeting agents for radio- and fluorescence-guided prostate cancer surgery. Theranostics 9(23):6824–6839
21. Kelderhouse LE et al (2013) Development of tumor-targeted near infrared probes for fluorescence guided surgery. Bioconjug Chem 24(6):1075–1080
22. Smith BL et al (2023) Intraoperative fluorescence guidance for breast cancer lumpectomy surgery. NEJM Evid 2(7):EVIDoa2200333
23. Boogerd LSF et al (2018) Safety and effectiveness of SGM-101, a fluorescent antibody targeting carcinoembryonic antigen, for intraoperative detection of colorectal cancer: a dose-escalation pilot study. Lancet Gastroenterol Hepatol 3(3):181–191
24. de Gooyer JM et al (2022) Multimodal CEA-targeted fluorescence and radioguided cytoreductive surgery for peritoneal metastases of colorectal origin. Nat Commun 13(1):2621
25. Li D et al (2018) First-in-human study of PET and optical dual-modality image-guided surgery in glioblastoma using (68)Ga-IRDye800CW-BBN. Theranostics 8(9):2508–2520
26. Baranski AC et al (2018) PSMA-11-derived dual-labeled PSMA inhibitors for preoperative PET imaging and precise fluorescence-guided surgery of prostate cancer. J Nucl Med 59(4):639–645
27. Juthani R et al (2020) Ultrasmall core-shell silica nanoparticles for precision drug delivery in a high-grade malignant brain tumor model. Clin Cancer Res 26(1):147–158
28. Hekman MC et al (2018) Tumor-targeted dual-modality imaging to improve intraoperative visualization of clear cell renal cell carcinoma: a first in man study. Theranostics 8(8):2161–2170
29. Intraoperative assessment of tumour excision margins using the lightpath imaging system for Cerenkov Luminescence Imaging (CLI) combined with Flexible Autoradiography (FAR) in women undergoing breast-conserving Surgery (BCS) (2022) Available from: https://clinicaltrials.gov/study/NCT05496101
30. Sinha A et al (2024) Cerenkov luminescence imaging and flexible autoradiography for specimen margin assessment during breast-conserving cancer surgery. Radiol Adv 1(2):umae015
31. He K et al (2021) Resection and survival data from a clinical trial of glioblastoma multiforme-specific IRDye800-BBN fluorescence-guided surgery. Bioeng Transl Med 6(1):e10182
32. Gautheron A et al (2024) 5-ALA induced PpIX fluorescence spectroscopy in neurosurgery: a review. Front Neurosci 18:1310282
33. de Maar JS et al (2020) Phase I feasibility study of magnetic resonance guided high intensity focused ultrasound-induced hyperthermia, Lyso-Thermosensitive liposomal doxorubicin and cyclophosphamide in de novo stage IV breast cancer patients: study protocol of the i-GO study. BMJ Open 10(11):e040162
34. Sung D, Sanchez A, Tward JD (2023) Successful salvage brachytherapy after infusion of Gold AuroShell Nanoshells for localized prostate cancer in a human patient. Adv Radiat Oncol 8(4):101202
35. Rastinehad AR et al (2019) Gold nanoshell-localized photothermal ablation of prostate tumors in a clinical pilot device study. Proc Natl Acad Sci 116(37):18590–18596
36. Kadria-Vili Y et al (2024) A detailed clinical case of localized prostate tumors treated with nanoparticle-assisted sub-ablative laser ablation. Nano 14(15):1261
37. Maier-Hauff K et al (2011) Efficacy and safety of intratumoral thermotherapy using magnetic iron-oxide nanoparticles combined with external beam radiotherapy on patients with recurrent glioblastoma multiforme. J Neuro-Oncol 103(2):317–324

38. Brouwer OR et al (2012) Comparing the hybrid fluorescent-radioactive tracer indocyanine green-99mTc-nanocolloid with 99mTc-nanocolloid for sentinel node identification: a validation study using lymphoscintigraphy and SPECT/CT. J Nucl Med 53(7):1034–1040
39. Zanoni DK et al (2021) Use of ultrasmall core-shell fluorescent silica nanoparticles for image-guided sentinel lymph node biopsy in head and neck melanoma: a nonrandomized clinical trial. JAMA Netw Open 4(3):e211936
40. Smith BL et al (2018) Real-time, intraoperative detection of residual breast cancer in lumpectomy cavity walls using a novel cathepsin-activated fluorescent imaging system. Breast Cancer Res Treat 171(2):413–420
41. Corns R et al (2015) 5-aminolevulinic acid guidance during awake craniotomy to maximise extent of safe resection of glioblastoma multiforme. BMJ Case Rep 2015:bcr2014208575
42. Tanyi JL et al (2023) A phase III study of Pafolacianine injection (OTL38) for intraoperative imaging of folate receptor-positive ovarian cancer (study 006). J Clin Oncol 41(2):276–284
43. Eder AC et al (2022) A new class of PSMA-617-based hybrid molecules for preoperative imaging and intraoperative fluorescence navigation of prostate cancer. Pharmaceuticals (Basel) 15(3):267
44. Zhu S et al (2018) Near-Infrared-II (NIR-II) bioimaging via off-peak NIR-I fluorescence emission. Theranostics 8(15):4141–4151
45. Zhao H et al (2024) Near-infrared II fluorescence-guided glioblastoma surgery targeting monocarboxylate transporter 4 combined with photothermal therapy. EBioMedicine 106:105243
46. Bugby SL, Lees JE, Perkins AC (2017) Hybrid intraoperative imaging techniques in radioguided surgery: present clinical applications and future outlook. Clin Translat Imaging 5(4):323–341
47. Fan X et al (2021) Nanoprobes-assisted multichannel NIR-II fluorescence imaging-guided resection and photothermal ablation of lymph nodes. Adv Sci 8(9):2003972
48. Gerber DA et al (2022) Indocyanine green as a navigational adjunct for laparoscopic ablation of liver tumors. Am Surg 89(11):4801–4805
49. Horgan CC et al (2021) Image-guided Raman spectroscopy probe-tracking for tumor margin delineation. J Biomed Opt 26(03):036002
50. Wang P et al (2018) NIR-II Nanoprobes in-vivo assembly to improve image-guided surgery for metastatic ovarian cancer. Nat Commun 9(1):2898
51. Paraboschi I et al (2021) Fluorescence imaging in pediatric surgery: state-of-the-art and future perspectives. J Pediatr Surg 56(4):655–662
52. Dip F et al (2022) Consensus conference statement on the general use of near-infrared fluorescence imaging and Indocyanine green guided surgery: results of a modified Delphi study. Ann Surg 275(4):685
53. Schottelius M et al (2015) [111In]PSMA-I&T: expanding the spectrum of PSMA-I&T applications towards SPECT and radioguided surgery. EJNMMI Res 5(1):68
54. Deus J et al (2015) Rescue Radioguided laparoscopy surgery for Meckel's Diverticulum. Medicine 94(25):e1017
55. Tyng CJ et al (2018) Computed tomography-guided preoperative localization of musculoskeletal lesions using the ROLL technique. Radiol Bras 51(3):147–150
56. Azargoshasb S et al (2021) The click-on gamma probe, a second-generation tethered robotic gamma probe that improves dexterity and surgical decision-making. Eur J Nucl Med Mol Imaging 48(13):4142–4151
57. Ariztia J et al (2022) Clickable C-Glycosyl Scaffold for the development of a dual fluorescent and [18F]fluorinated cyanine-containing probe and preliminary in vitro/vivo evaluation by fluorescence imaging. Pharmaceuticals 15(12):1490
58. Sano K et al (2019) Development of cancer-targeted single photon emission computed tomography/fluorescence dual imaging probe based on Polyoxazoline. ACS Appl Polym Mater 1(5):953–958
59. Valdés Olmos RA et al (2020) Sentinel node imaging and radioguided surgery in the era of SPECT/CT and PET/CT: toward new interventional nuclear medicine strategies. Clin Nucl Med 45(10):771

60. Ullah Z et al (2024) Fluorescence imaging-guided surgery: current status and future directions. Biomater Sci 12(15):3765–3804
61. Wang N et al (2021) Intelligent designs in nanophotonics: from optimization towards inverse creation. Photonix 2(1):22
62. Rasouli JJ et al (2020) Artificial intelligence and robotics in spine surgery. Glob Spine J 11(4):556–564
63. Haghighat A et al (2020) Applications of deep learning in intelligent transportation systems. J Big Data Anal Transp 2(2):115–145
64. Bu F et al (2021) A cloud-edge-aided incremental high-order possibilistic C-Means algorithm for medical data clustering. IEEE Trans Fuzzy Syst 29(1):148–155
65. Muhammad G, Alhussein M (2021) Convergence of artificial intelligence and Internet of Things in smart healthcare: a case study of voice pathology detection. IEEE Access 9:89198–89209
66. Liu X et al (2019) Secure Internet of Things (IoT)-based smart-world critical infrastructures: survey, case study and research opportunities. IEEE Access 7:79523–79544
67. Sun G et al (2011) Intraoperative MRI with integrated functional neuronavigation-guided resection of Supratentorial cavernous malformations in eloquent brain areas. J Clin Neurosci 18(10):1350–1354
68. Mehkri Y et al (2023) Surgical management of brain tumors with focused ultrasound. Curr Oncol 30(5):4990–5002
69. Westin C et al (2018) MRI findings after MRI-guided focal laser ablation of prostate cancer. Am J Roentgenol 211(3):595–604
70. Partanen A et al (2012) Mild hyperthermia with magnetic resonance-guided high-intensity focused ultrasound for applications in drug delivery. Int J Hyperth 28(4):320–336
71. Lu SB et al (2022) Recent advances in the enzyme-activatable organic fluorescent probes for tumor imaging and therapy. Chem Open 11(10):e202200137
72. Wang X et al (2022) Smart drug delivery systems for precise cancer therapy. Acta Pharm Sin B 12(11):4098–4121
73. Cheng H et al (2024) Illuminating the future of precision cancer surgery with fluorescence imaging and artificial intelligence convergence. NPJ Precis Oncol 8(1):196
74. Eranki A et al (2020) High-intensity focused ultrasound (HIFU) triggers immune sensitization of refractory murine neuroblastoma to checkpoint inhibitor therapy. Clin Cancer Res 26(5):1152–1161
75. Stone LD et al (2024) Interim phase II results using Panitumumab-IRDye800CW during Transoral robotic surgery in patients with oropharyngeal cancer. Clin Cancer Res 30(18):4016–4028
76. de Valk KS et al (2021) Dose-finding study of a CEA-targeting agent, SGM-101, for intraoperative fluorescence imaging of colorectal cancer. Ann Surg Oncol 28(3):1832–1844

Part IV

Image Guided Radiooncology

32 Molecular Imaging in Photon Radiotherapy

Sonja Adebahr, Jamina Tara Fennell, Eleni Gkika, and Anca L. Grosu

32.1 Brain Tumors

32.1.1 Gliomas

The standard imaging modality for the diagnosis of gliomas is MRI. T1 sequences with and without gadolinium contrast enhancement and T2/FLAIR sequences give a good indication of tumor spread and heterogeneity. While low-grade gliomas typically present themselves only as hypointense lesions in T1- and hyperintense lesions in FLAIR/T2-sequences, high-grade gliomas often have additional contrast enhancement in T1-sequences with central necrosis.

Because of the high sensitivity of these MRI sequences, the European Organization for Research and Treatment of Cancer (EORTC) and the Radiotherapy and Oncology Group (RTOG) recommend that target volume definition be based on them [1]. Unfortunately, this can result in large planning target volumes, increasing the risk of side effects like radionecrosis when curative doses are administered. Therefore, if critical structures like the optic nerves or brain stem are involved to any greater extent, the prescribed dose must be reduced even at the expense of local tumor control. However, at the same time, peritumoral edema, post-therapeutic gliosis, and radionecrosis have similar imaging characteristics as malignant tissue in

S. Adebahr · J. T. Fennell · A. L. Grosu (✉)
Department of Radiation Oncology, Medical Center-University of Freiburg, Faculty of Medicine, University of Freiburg, Freiburg, Germany
e-mail: Sonja.adebahr@uniklinik-freiburg.de; Jamina.tara.fennell@uniklinik-freiburg.de; anca.grosu@uniklinik-freiburg.de

E. Gkika
Department of Radiation Oncology, Medical Center Bonn, Bonn, Germany
e-mail: Eleni.Gkika@ukbonn.de

O. Schober et al. (eds.), *Molecular Imaging in Oncology - Volume 2*, Recent Results in Cancer Research 225, https://doi.org/10.1007/978-3-032-21415-7_14

the aforementioned MRI sequences, leading to a specificity of 50% and leaving considerable room for improvement [2].

Magnetic resonance spectroscopy (MRS) allows the comparison of chemical components between normal and abnormal brain tissue and thus offers information about the metabolism of the latter. Although MRS has only a low resolution, it has proven useful in distinguishing post-therapeutic tissue alterations from tumor recurrence [3]. Whether MRS should routinely be integrated into RT planning remains to be seen. Preliminary results are encouraging: a small phase II trial has shown dose escalation to areas of high choline/N-acetylaspartate ratio in patients with glioblastoma to be feasible and indicated an improved overall survival compared to a historic control [4]. In the United States, a pilot study investigating the possibility of MRS-guided dose escalation has been active since 2017 (NCT03137888). A large phase III trial in France with the same objective revealed that the MRS-guided boost was safe but did not result in a statistically significant improvement in OS or PFS [5].

Positron emission tomography (PET) is another way to increase the specificity of tumor detection. In case of gliomas, the most common PET tracers are the amino acids C11-methionine (MET) and 18F-(fluoroethyl)-L-tyrosine (FET). Comparative studies on patients with cerebral malignancies could not find a difference in uptake or tumor/brain ratio between the two tracers, and hence they are equivalent for clinical practice and RT planning [6, 7]. Both FET- and MET-PET were attributed superior specificity (75–95%) compared to MRI alone [8, 9]. The troublesome nature of this discovery is further illustrated by a study conducted on 39 high-grade glioma patients, who underwent MET-PET, MRI, and CT before receiving adjuvant RT, which showed that the GTV based on MET-PET corresponded only in 13% of cases to the GTV based on gadolinium contrast-enhanced MRI and exceeded in 50% even the hyperintense area in T2 [10]. In clinical practice, RT naïve patients receive FET- or MET-PET-based target volume definition only on a case-by-case basis, e.g., to decrease the high dose volume and spare healthy tissue (Fig. 32.1). Randomized trials, which prove that the use of PET in radiation planning translates into improved prognosis, are still lacking.

For treatment planning, updated EORTC guidelines recommend defining the clinical target volume (CTV) based on contrast-enhanced T1 MRI with isotropic margins and emphasize individualized planning based on image-guided radiotherapy (IGRT) protocols [11]. Regarding the role of PET imaging, amino acid PET is emphasized to be superior to FDG-PET and to provide valuable biological information that MRI often misses, supporting better tumor grading, distinguishing recurrence from treatment effects, guiding biopsies, and refining surgical and radiation planning [12]. Recent updated guidelines and reports emphasize the growing role of PET imaging, especially using radiolabeled amino acid tracers (e.g., FET, FDOPA, and MET), in the diagnosis, treatment planning, and monitoring of gliomas. The joint guidelines by EANM, SNMMI, EANO, and PET-RANO aim to standardize PET imaging practices across institutions, improve clinical care, and facilitate multicenter trials [13, 14].

Modern tools like spectroscopic MRI (sMRI) or the "Brain Imaging Collaboration Suite" (BrICS) platform—a cloud platform for integrating whole-brain sMRI into

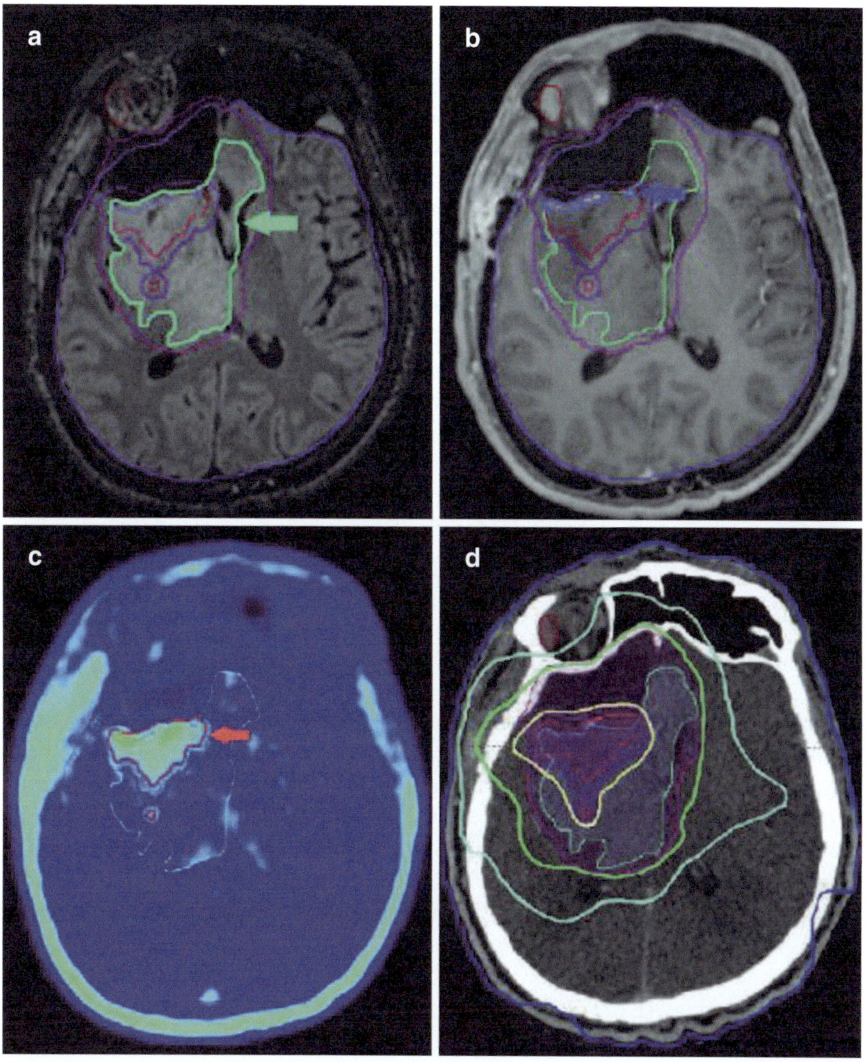

Fig. 32.1 Patient with oligodendroglioma WHO°III. After partial resection, imaging studies were performed for individual radiotherapy planning. (**a**) MRI-T2-weighted-fluid-attenuated inversion recovery (FLAIR) sequence: Gross tumor volume (GTV) according to FLAIR is highlighted in turquoise (->). (**b**) MRI-T1 sequence with gadolinium contrast enhancement (CE): GTV according to CE is highlighted in purple (->). (**c**) 18F-(fluoroethyl)-L-tyrosin positron emission tomography sequence (FET-PET): GTV according to FET-PET is highlighted in red (->). It is much larger than GTV-CE, but smaller than GTV-FLAIR, since it does not include edema. (**d**) Radiation plan using intensity-modulated radiotherapy (IMRT) with simultaneous integrated boost (SIB) to the GTV-FET; yellow: 95%-isodose (57 Gy), green: 76%-isodose (45.6 Gy), turquoise: 50%-isodose (30 Gy)

the RT-planning workflow—enable metabolic targeting and collaborative radiotherapy planning in multicenter trials [15]. Hybrid PET/MRI scanners may further enhance diagnostic precision, though initial studies suggest similar effectiveness between sequential and simultaneous imaging for routine clinical use [16].

In patients with high-grade glioma recurrence after RT who are eligible for re-irradiation, biological imaging is more commonly used, but again not systematically. A study of 44 patients with recurrence of high-grade glioma who received RT based on biological imaging, CT, and MRI showed improved overall survival compared to those patients whose RT relied only on CT and MRI [17]. While this small study offers promising results, the question of whether increased specificity of PET/CT translates into improved prognosis remains uncertain. To finally answer this question, the GLIAA trial, a prospective randomized multicenter phase II study, recruited patients with recurrent glioblastoma to treat them with re-irradiation either guided by PET/CT or by gadolinium enhancement on MRI (NCT01252459) [18]. The primary endpoint was progression-free survival after 6 months, and one of the secondary endpoints was overall survival. FET-PET-based target volume delineation for re-irradiation did not lead to a significant clinical benefit compared with T1MRI-based treatment [19].

32.2 Meningiomas

Similar to gliomas, MRI has been the imaging standard for the diagnosis of meningiomas because of its morphological precision. However, positron emission tomography (PET) imaging employing radiolabeled somatostatin receptor (SSTR) ligands as radiotracers plays an important role in the clinical management of meningiomas; in fact, the high tracer uptake of meningioma in SSTR-PET shows higher sensitivity than contrast-enhanced MRI alone [20, 21]. Recently published standardized guidelines provide recommendations for the application of PET imaging in patients with meningiomas and related somatostatin receptor (SSTR)-targeted peptide receptor radionuclide therapy [22]. According to the guidelines of the European Association of Neuro-Oncology (EANO), surgery remains the first-line treatment [23], but there are a considerable number of patients who are either ineligible for surgery or whose meningioma can only be partially surgically removed and therefore require either primary, adjuvant, or salvage RT. The most critical localization is the skull base, where any surgery has a considerable risk of neurological morbidity. Local tumor control after RT of skull base meningioma is excellent (86% after 10 years) [24]. However, the skull base is exactly the localization where precise meningioma demarcation in MRI reaches its limitations, especially around the cavernous sinus and the pituitary gland. Here, PET/CT with either MET or 68-Ga-labelled DOTA (0)-D-Phe (1)-Tyr (3)-Octreotide (DOTATOC) decreases interobserver variability, identifies portions of meningioma undetected by MRI and CT, and thereby significantly alters target volume definition [25–27]. For (68)Ga-labelled DOTA-Tyr3-octreotate (DOTATATE) PET/CT, standardized guidelines for PET-guided radiation treatment planning in resected meningiomas have recently been published to improve local control and reduce toxicity by enabling more precise and biomarker-informed radiation therapy [28]. Further, using [68Ga]-DOTATATE PET/MRI for radiation treatment planning and response assessment in meningiomas, a recent study revealed that DOTATATE PET/MR improves target delineation, leads to reduced radiation exposure to healthy tissue, and shows significant decreases in PET avidity post-radiosurgery (however, not clinically significant by RANO criteria) [29].

32.3 Head and Neck Cancer

Irradiating patients with head and neck squamous cell carcinoma (HNSCC) poses a multitude of challenges. Lymph drainage in the mouth, throat, and neck is rather complex; lymph nodes often are reactively enlarged due to inflammation or superinfection. RT is, in general, associated with considerable morbidity, and prognosis depends heavily on individual tumor characteristics. The introduction of IMRT has already significantly reduced the risk of developing long-term side effects like xerostomia through conformal radiation dose delivery without jeopardizing tumor control [30]. However, in order to balance the need for tumor control on the one hand and the effort to improve treatment tolerance on the other hand, dose prescription needs to be optimized according to individual risk stratification.

Diffusion-weighted MRI (DW-MRI), which visualizes areas of high cellularity, may present an easy and cost-effective way to increase the sensitivity of lymph node staging by MRI. Especially in cases of primary radiochemotherapy (RCT), the radiation oncologist has to rely on imaging to determine the extent of macroscopic tumor spread. T1 and T2 sequences offer morphological criteria whether or not a lymph node is involved, one of the most important criteria being a diameter larger than 1 cm. In a study of 33 patients with head and neck cancer, the histopathology of 301 lymph nodes was correlated with information obtained by DW-MRI. DW-MRI proved to be superior to anatomical MRI in predicting metastasis in lymph nodes smaller than 1 cm (sensitivity 76% vs. 7%, respectively) [31]. According to several small studies, low apparent diffusion coefficient values in DW-MRI during and near-term after RCT correlate with an unfavorable treatment response [32, 33] and are indicative of early recurrence with a reported accuracy of 90% [34]. Therefore, DW-MRI might be a useful monitoring tool to identify patients in need of early salvage therapy.

F18-fluorodeoxyglucose (FDG)-PET/CT may offer improved and new avenues to optimize target volume definition. A study, which compared target volume definition based on CT, MRI, and FDG-PET with surgical specimens, found that GTV definition based on FDG-PET to be the most accurate, while GTVs based on CT and MRI were larger than the actual tumor [35]. However, a recent review on imaging for target delineation in head and neck cancer pointed out that there is no solid evidence for which modality provides the most accurate illustration of the GTV tumor extension in all head and neck cancers, suggesting that the combined information provided by all modalities and the clinical examination could finally lead to the most correct contour [36].

Recent approaches aim at supporting the challenging accurate manual GTV definition for head and neck cancer by deep learning methods to enable autosegmentation of the GTV. Wang et al. showed encouraging results in transferability of the baseline models after facility-specific training [37].

Although the GTV receives in primary RCT a dose as high as 70 Gy, tumor recurrences occur most of the time in the high dose volume and even in 54% of cases inside the FDG-positive volume, indicating the tumor cells there to be highly radioresistant [38]. This may be overcome with dose escalation. In order to not increase treatment toxicity, investigators of a planning study used adaptive, voxel-by-voxel dose painting technology, so that only voxels with the highest FDG uptake would receive up to 86 Gy [39]. Obviously, this kind of methodology needs to be highly standardized in order to attempt any multicenter trials, which are necessary to evaluate the effect of these advanced treatment concepts on patient outcome [40].

A multicentric randomized controlled phase III trial of adaptive and FDG-PET-guided dose-redistribution in locally advanced head and neck squamous cell carcinoma (ARTFORCE) showed a trend for better locoregional control with FDG-PET-CT-based treatment planning and dose escalation, especially for patients with oropharyngeal carcinoma and patients with cN0/cN1 disease [41].

PET/CT may also identify nonresponders among patients with HNSCC treated with primary RCT through tumor hypoxia. The latter has proven to be a deciding factor for treatment resistance in a number of cancers but particularly in HNSCC [42, 43]. Using the PET-tracer fluoromisonidazole (FMISO), tumor hypoxia may be visualized noninvasively, which provides the possibility of monitoring hypoxia throughout RT [44]. Studies examining patients under RCT with serial FMISO-PET/CTs found that no hypoxia or hypoxia resolution early in therapy correlated with favorable outcomes [45, 46]. The hypoxic subvolume in patients with hypoxia persistence under RCT remains in the same topographical region [47]. The link between hypoxia and patient outcome prompted Lee et al. to de-escalate dose prescription to lymph nodes of patients with human papillomavirus-associated HNSCC if hypoxia measured by FMISO-PET/CT resolved after 1 week of RCT [48]. Thus, 30% of patients received 10 Gy less to the lymph nodes without affecting clinical outcome after 2 years of follow-up. While these endeavors pave the way to better treatment tolerance, simultaneously, efforts are being made to improve tumor control in patients with unfavorable prognosis through dose escalation to areas of hypoxia persistence during RCT. Doses of up to 80.5 Gy can be attained in hypoxic subvolumes without violating the dose constraints of healthy surrounding tissue [49]. However, the results of whether this strategy has a clinical benefit remain to be seen; a randomized phase II study is currently recruiting patients to escalate the dose in FMISO-positive subvolume to 77 Gy (NCT02352792).

Follow-up and the early detection of recurrence after RCT for HNSCC are very challenging because posttreatment alterations, scar tissue, and edema confound the sensitivity of CT and conventional MRI. Mehanna et al. could show that patients without residual activity in FDG-PET/CT 12 weeks after RCT could forego planned neck dissection without impact on clinical outcome [50]. FDG-PET has become an indispensable module of the diagnosis and treatment algorithm during follow-up of patients after RCT, according to the NCCN guideline [51].

32.4 Lung Cancer

Non-small cell lung cancer (NSCLC) is one of the most common forms of cancer and the leading cause of death among all tumor entities. Nowadays, the usefulness of FDG-PET/CT for initial staging of patients with NSCLS is universally accepted in the medical community and is mandatory prior to treatment. Already more than 20 years ago, radiation oncologists recognized the value of FDG-PET/CT for GTV definition of the primary tumor in case of atelectasis [52]. At the same time, FDG-PET/CT facilitates the identification of involved mediastinal lymph nodes [53].

PET/CT has significantly reduced interobserver variability and thus has contributed to further standardization of treatment [54–56]. The diagnostic accuracy of FDG PET/CT compared with historical CT imaging makes it possible to adapt the target volumes. Several retrospective and single-center analyses demonstrated an improvement in the inter-observer agreement for target volume delineation [52, 53, 57]. There have been efforts to even automate GTV segmentation by defining a standard uptake value (SUV) threshold, which is viewed very critically by experts since healthy tissue like myocardium or brown fat has a high SUV and necrosis has a low SUV [58]. Therefore, qualitative interdisciplinary analysis of the PET/CT images and manual editing of the automatically generated GTV remain indispensable [59, 60].

There are several pitfalls in the use of FDG-PET for RT planning. Most importantly, the duration between the FDG-PET scan and the start of radiation treatment should not be more than 3 weeks. Then, it is paramount to standardize window/level settings to avoid discrepancies in tumor size and maintain a low intra- and interobserver variability. Furthermore, FDG-PET-based volumes often appear a little larger than their counterparts in the CT scan due to respiratory motion during registration. Finally, FDG-PET/CT should be acquired in a radiation position to allow optimal starting conditions for RT planning [61].

Depending on tumor stage, there are two main ways to irradiate a patient with NSCLC: stereotactic body RT (SBRT) or conventionally fractionated radio(chemo) therapy. Patients with early-stage tumors without nodal involvement are eligible for SBRT. In order to define the internal target volume (ITV), which respects the position of the GTV in all breathing cycles, a 4D-CT is mandatory. While this may be absolutely sufficient in case of peripheral tumors, centrally localized NSCLCs are far less easily marked out (Fig. 32.2). Interobserver variability profits from 4D-FDG-PET/CT [62]. It was also employed for RT-planning in the LungTech trial (EORTC 22113-08113), which investigated outcomes after SBRT of centrally located NSCLCs [63].

Patients with locally advanced NSCLC are treated with radiochemotherapy (RCT). As mentioned above, PET/CT allows the distinction between atelectasis and tumor as well as reactive and involved lymph nodes. This harbors great potential for

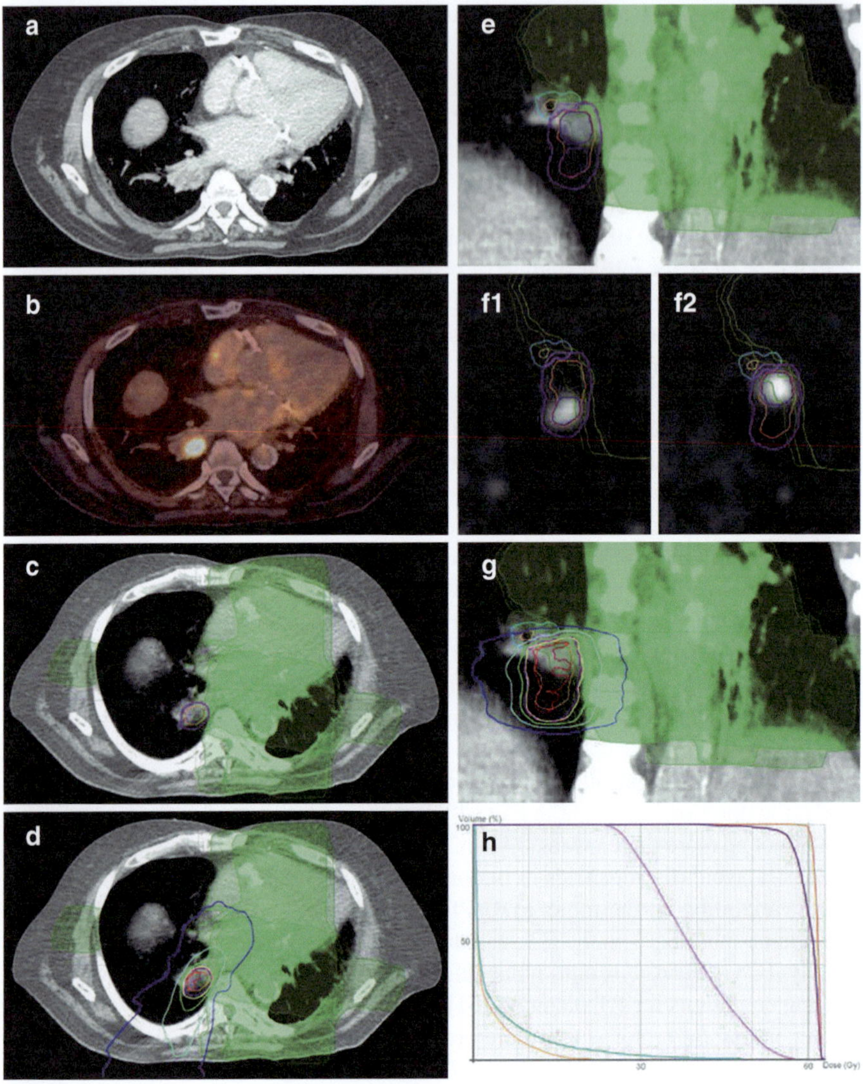
a
b
c
d
e
f1
f2
g
h
Volume (%)
100
50
30
60
Dose (Gy)

Fig. 32.2 Patient with non-small cell lung cancer (NSCLC) without lymph node or distant metastases. He was treated with neoadjuvant radiochemotherapy due to NSCLC of the contralateral lung 12 years ago with 50.4 Gy in 28 fractions. (**a**) Computer tomography (CT) with contrast enhancement (CE): right hilus is enlarged, but a precise distinction between tumor and blood vessel is not possible. (**b**) 18F-fluorodeoxyglucose positron emission tomography/CT (FDG-PET/CT): the tumor is now plainly demarcated, due to high FDG uptake. (**c**) Planning CT: integral tumor volume (ITV) is highlighted in orange; planning target volume (PTV) is highlighted in dark pink; isodoses of the previous irradiation are shown in green (30, 40, and 50 Gy). (**d**) Treatment plan for 55 Gy in 10 fractions: red: 112%-isodose (61.6 Gy); yellow: 100%-isodose (55 Gy); bright green: 80%-isodose (44 Gy); turquoise: 50%-isodose (27.5 Gy); dark blue: 20%-isodose (11 Gy). (**e**) Planning CT in sagittal plane with extremes of breathing cycle delineated: dark purple: gross tumor volume during different breathing positions; orange: ITV; ocher: right bronchus; bright blue: planning organ of risk volume (PRV) of the right bronchus; bright pink: SIP (simultaneous integrated protection volume [overlap between PTV and PRV]) (**f1/f2**) FDG-PET-scan with respiratory gating. (**g**) Treatment plan in sagittal plane: SIP will only receive 28 Gy in 10 fractions in order to not exceed the constraint to the right bronchus (34 Gy). (**g**) Treatment plan for 55 Gy in 10 fractions in sagittal plane: red: 112%-isodose (61.6 Gy); yellow: 100%-isodose (55 Gy); bright green: 80%-isodose (44 Gy); turquoise: 50%-isodose (27.5 Gy); dark blue: 20%-isodose (11 Gy). (**h**) Dose volume histogram: The right bronchus receives less than 30 Gy, while 95% of the ITV will receive at least 60 Gy

shrinking the radiation field and thereby allowing dose escalation. The results of the multicenter randomized phase II PET-Plan trial were published in 2020, showing noninferiority of FDG-PET/CT-based RT planning compared to conventional planning with a trend toward improved local control through isotoxic dose escalation [64]. In a secondary analysis of the PET-Plan trial, the use of additional invasive staging modalities (EBUS-TBNA and mediastinoscopy) in FDG-PET/CT-based target volume delineation for definitive RCT supported the use of endoscopic mediastinal staging in combination with molecular imaging [65]. Following up on the idea of the PET-Plan study, the prospective multicenter proof-of-principle phase II trial RTEP7-IFCT-1402 investigated the activity and safety of RT dose up to 74 Gy in a boost-volume given according to on-treatment FDG-PET results, presenting a promising local control rate without increasing toxicity [66].

Besides CT and PET/CT, PET/MRI seems to be a promising technique for lung cancer evaluation, combining metabolic PET information with anatomic and superior functional insights. It might especially be a useful tool for a better detection of metastases such as liver, brain, or adrenal glands. The potential value of the PET/MRI has recently been summarized by Alorfi et al. [67].

32.5 Esophageal Cancer

Esophageal cancer can be treated by RT either neoadjuvantly or primarily. Lymph node involvement significantly impacts target volume definition, since either mediastinal, cervical, or abdominal ones may be affected, depending on tumor location. Standard imaging consists of endoscopic ultrasound to evaluate locoregional lymph node metastases and mucosal tumor invasion, and CT scan to assess lymph nodes and distant metastases [68]. Furthermore, it has been demonstrated that PET/CT fused with MR achieved the highest agreement in identifying the primary tumor in ESCC. In addition, FDG-PET/CT is recommended for initial patient work-up according to international guidelines (NCCN, ESMO) [69], while the sensitivity and specificity of FDG-PET/CT for detecting locoregional lymph node metastases vary from study to study (30–93% and 79–100%, respectively) and equal endoscopic ultrasound (45–100% and 44–100%, respectively), it supersedes conventional CT scans in the detection of distant metastases [70–72]. Thus, patients who are eligible for surgery based on the local medical findings but were identified as having distant metastases in the FDG-PET/CT scan can be spared an invasive procedure. In case of oligometastatic disease, they may be eligible for an individualized treatment plan with RCT of the primary tumor and SBRT of the distant metastases. But even if there are no distant metastases detected, a study of 90 patients found that FDG-PET/CT leads to a change in the radiation treatment plan in around 50% of cases [73]. However, in the same study, PET/CT-based planning showed no benefit in terms of decreased locoregional recurrence.

There have been efforts to make FDG-PET/CT an even more integral part of esophageal cancer treatment. The MUNICON II trial subjected patients, who did not metabolically respond to neoadjuvant chemotherapy in FDG-PET/CT after 14 days to RCT of a total dose of 32 Gy. Unfortunately, that trial did not meet its primary endpoint of increased R0-resections, which may be due to the rather low total dose [74]. Another clinical trial evaluated the impact of dose escalation in patients who did not respond or only responded partially to RCT up to 50.4 Gy according to serial FDG-PET/CT scans. They found improved 2-year overall survival and local tumor control between the control and investigative group. Further analysis revealed that only the patient with partial treatment response had a significant benefit from dose escalation [75].

As molecular imaging with FDG-PET, despite all benefits, also faces some tracer-specific limitations, fibroblast activation protein inhibitor (FAPI) conjugated to [68Ga] seems to be a promising tracer in PET for diagnostic purposes and staging across different types of cancers. FAPI-PET in esophageal cancer shows improved tumor detection rates compared to FDG-PET/CT, a potential benefit for target volume definition, as well as a potential prognostic value to predict response to definitive RCT [76–78].

32.6 Prostate Cancer

RT is highly effective in patients with prostate cancer as primary therapy in localized disease with curative intent or for symptom control in a palliative setting [79]. Prostate cancer is the most common tumor entity among men. The current guidelines still recommend foregoing any imaging for low-risk patients, whereas intermediate patients may and high-risk patients absolutely should receive multiparametric MRI (mpMRI) and a bone scan to exclude metastatic disease. If conventional imaging is negative in high-risk patients, PSMA PET/CT can be considered to improve staging sensitivity [79–83].

32.6.1 Localized Prostate Cancer and Dose Escalation

Target definition in localized prostate cancer is dependent upon tumor stage. Moreover, several trials dating from 10 years ago have shown an improved biochemical progression-free survival after primary RT with dose escalation to 74–80 Gy [84–88], which was accompanied by greater urogenital and/or gastrointestinal early and late toxicity [84–87], as the dose was homogeneously prescribed to the whole prostate. Since the malignant tissue seldom encompasses the whole prostate, the next logical step is to limit the dose escalation only to the tumor, which would allow better protection for the bladder and rectum. The prerequisite for this approach is the ability to precisely identify malignant tumor tissue in an organ of around 25 ml.

MpMRI, which entails T1, T2, DW, and dynamic contrast-enhanced (DCE) sequences, has a good sensitivity (74–89%) and specificity (73–88%) for tumor detection [89, 90], and yet there is high interobserver variability in precise intraprostatic tumor delineation [91, 92] due partially to confounding factors like androgen deprivation therapy, previous biopsy, or fiducial implantation [93], lesions smaller than 0.5 ml [94] and benign prostate hyperplasia [95].The updated version of the Prostate Imaging Reporting and Data System (PI-RADSv2.1) endeavors to further standardize the evaluation of mpMRI and names the most significant sequences to detect malignant tissue in the different subregions of the prostate [96, 97].

Different PET tracers have been investigated in terms of their usefulness to stage prostate cancer. FDG has been proven unreliable because of similar uptake in benign prostate hyperplasia, prostate cancer, prostatitis, and normal prostate tissue [98]. Carbon-11-choline (11C-choline) has also failed to deliver reliable information about intraprostatic tumor spread [99, 100]. The rather new PET-tracer Prostate-specific membrane antigen (PSMA) has been shown to be more promising, especially in larger tumors [101]. ^{68}Ga-PSMA-PET provided valuable complementary information to mpMRI [102] and [^{18}F]PSMA-1007 PET identified more and larger intraprostatic tumor lesions than MRI and was able to detect a higher number of cT2c and cT3b stage tumors. Furthermore, PET demonstrated significantly better concordance in tumor laterality when compared to the surgical specimen, outperforming mpMRI and biopsy [103]. Convolutional neural network (CNN) trained on [^{18}F]PSMA-1007 PET [104] and ^{68}Ga-PSMA-PET [105], and were successfully used for automatic prostate cancer segmentation. Both[^{68}Ga]Ga-PSMA-11 and [^{18}F]PSMA-1007 PET imaging can identify variations in histological PSMA expression within prostate cancer lesions, enabling biologically guided radiotherapy [106]. A narrative review presented by Spohn and Grosu summarizes the impact of PSMA-PET on RT planning, highlighting its diagnostic performance and implications for RT treatment management [107]. Current data suggest that the combination of PSMA-PET/CT and mpMRI will result in the highest sensitivity and specificity in tumor tissue detection compared to histopathological analysis [108, 109]. Several planning studies have demonstrated that integrated dose escalation to the intraprostatic PSMA-uptake volume is feasible with nearly no increased risk of increased bladder and rectum toxicity [110, 111]. Similar results could be found for integrated dose escalation to a GTV based on PSMA-PET and mpMRI [112]. The feasibility phase II HypoFocal trial revealed low toxicity and perpetuation of quality of life after PSMA-PET- and MRI-based focal dose escalated radiotherapy for prostate cancer [113, 114]. The FLAME trial (NCT01168479) delivered an integrated boost to intraprostatic lesions of patients with localized intermediate- and high-risk prostate cancer and improved biochemical disease-free survival without impairing quality of life and safety [115]. Prospective SBRT focal-boost trials (the phase II hypo-FLAME trial with mpMRI-based boost [116] and phase II SPARC trial [CyberKnife-based SBRT] [117]) continue this line. The prospective multicenter phase III HypoFocal-SBRT trial investigating PSMA-PET and mpMRI-based SBRT versus moderate hypofractionated radiotherapy is still recruiting [118].

32.6.2 Lymph Node Metastases

Another important aspect in the target volume definition of localized prostate cancer is the identification of lymph node metastases. Unfortunately, conventional MRI sequences possess only low sensitivity (39%) with a specificity of 82% [119]. Sensitivity seems to be improving after consideration of DW-MRI (sensitivity 84.6% and specificity 89%) [120].

PSMA-PET/CT is also superior to conventional MRI sequences in detecting lymph node metastases. Sensitivity and specificity in studies have been 64–67% and 81–98.9%, respectively [121–123]. The proPSMA trial was the landmark prospective, randomized study demonstrating superior nodal detection accuracy of PSMA PET/CT compared to conventional staging in pretreatment of high-risk prostate cancer patients [124]. The precise identification of lymph node metastases allows the radiation oncologist to formulate individual treatment plans with enlarged para-aortal radiation fields and dose escalation to only PSMA-positive lymph nodes. Further, evaluation on outcomes of patients with PSMA-PET-based cN1 and/or cM1a PCa receiving primary radiotherapy and ADT revealed PSMA-PET as a potential prognostic factor. More than 2 PET-positive pelvic lymph nodes were associated with unfavorable biochemical recurrence-free survival, and high SUVmax values are associated with unfavorable metastasis-free survival [125].

32.6.3 Recurrence

RT is a common salvage therapy for patients with biochemical or macroscopic recurrence after primary treatment. An issue of contention is the PSA level, which warrants imaging diagnostics. Here, PSMA-PET/CT has proven to be valuable and significantly impacts the patient treatment plan in up to 50% of cases [126–128]. Currently, it may be performed at PSA levels as low as 0.2–0.5 ng/ml, although more recent data also show detectable results below 0.2 ng/ml [129]. However, the recommendation depends on the individual clinical setting, as of course, the likelihood of macroscopic tumor detection in PSMA-PET increases with absolute PSA value and PSA doubling time [130]. An analysis of 1007 patients with prostate cancer recurrence showed that in 79% of cases a macroscopic tumor could be detected [131].

Several retrospective analyses on large cohorts of patients with recurrent or persistent PSA after primary surgery have recently been published, addressing the outcome of salvage radiotherapy (sRT) with PSMA-PET guidance for PET-positive and PET-negative patient cohorts, supporting the current EAU recommendation to initiate sRT in a timely manner after detecting biochemical recurrence, even in PET negative patients [132–135]. To predict outcome after PSMA-PET-guided sRT, Spohn et al. developed a PSMA-PET + CT-based radiomic signature to predict biochemical recurrence, which might contribute to guide personalized treatment decisions [136].

32.6.4 Bone Metastases

Most of the distant metastases in prostate cancer are located in the bone. RT is indicated either in oligometastatic disease or in a palliative setting to maintain bone stability, manage pain or prevent, respectively, treat neurological symptoms due to spinal cord or nerve compression. The standard staging modality is a bone scan.

While a meta-analysis has shown a very high pooled sensitivity and specificity for the detection of bone metastases with MRI (96 and 98%), it can decidedly influence the treatment strategy in patients with high-risk prostate cancer [137, 138]. Depending on the country, it may be difficult and costly to scan all the body regions necessary to have a complete staging.

PSMA-PET/CT performed superiorly compared to a standard bone scan in an analysis of 126 patients (sensitivity 98.7–100% versus 86.7–89.3%, specificity 88.2–100% versus 60.8–96.1%) [139]. While still a costly imaging modality, PSMA-PET/CT has the added advantage of giving more information about bone stability due to the included CT scan and other metastases compared to bone scan and MRI. The prospective proPSMA trial confirmed that PSMA PET-CT is superior to the combined findings of CT and bone scanning in detecting bone metastases in high-risk prostate cancer patients [124]. A systematic review and network meta-analysis indicated that 68Ga-PSMA-PET/CT is superior to MRI [140]. Both ^{18}F-NaF PET/CT and ^{18}F-PSMA PET/CT demonstrate high diagnostic accuracy for identifying bone metastases in newly diagnosed high-risk prostate cancer patients. However, ^{18}F-PSMA PET/CT may reveal additional metastatic lesions not detected by ^{18}F-NaF PET/CT [141].

32.7 Uterine Cancer

32.7.1 Cervical Cancer

Cervical cancer is the second most common tumor entity among women, and RT is often used primarily or adjuvantly in a curative intent. Nevertheless, especially in the early stages, surgery presents the first-line approach. Therefore, traditionally, cervical cancer is classified by the International Federation of Gynecology and Obstetrics (FIGO) staging system, which is mainly based on clinical examination. But since risk factors like tumor size, stroma, or lymph node involvement have been identified to significantly impact prognosis, imaging with MRI and CT is now routinely performed. Additionally, FDG-PET/CT has proven to be more and more relevant in recent years, so much so that it has been introduced into the major NCCN and ESMO guidelines [142, 143].

During initial patient work-up, FDG-PET/CT does not perform better than MRI with regard to assessing tumor volume and parametric invasion, since the latter is unparalleled in depicting soft tissue contrast and resolution. But FDG-PET/CT has shown a high sensitivity and specificity for the detection of pelvic (65–90% and 96–99%, respectively) and para-aortal lymph node metastases (68–94% and 89–98%, respectively) as well as distant metastases [144]. This information directly affects radiation treatment planning and may result in an extended radiation field or dose escalation to lymph nodes with increased FDG uptake. In order to avoid increased toxicity during and after RT of lymph node metastases, intensity-modulated RT should be used [145]. Thus, a high local control rate may be achieved in the field, but, unfortunately, distant metastases are the most common failure site once there is lymph node involvement [146].

There are some studies exploring the feasibility of FDG-PET-guided HDR-brachytherapy, but the patient numbers are small, and there is no comparison to MRI-guided brachytherapy.

32.7.2 Endometrial Cancer

Surgery as primary therapy or for the purpose of staging is often the first procedure that patients with endometrial cancer have to undergo. Depending on individual risk factors, RT is mostly indicated adjuvantly, but is an option for primary treatment if the patient is inoperable [147]. Nevertheless, assessment of pelvic and para-aortal lymph node is indispensable for target definition. FDG-PET/CT presents an appropriate alternative for surgical staging with high sensitivity and specificity (73–85% and 91–98%, respectively) [148–151]. While current literature directly linking PET-guided RT in endometrial cancer is limited, several imaging biomarker and radiomics studies offer valuable insights into prognostication, therapy planning, and future theranostics perspectives, e.g., [152].

32.8 Conclusion and Outlook

Biological imaging is a useful tool of the radiation oncologist for tumor detection and identification of high-risk subvolumes. This makes it possible to further individualize treatment either through dose escalation or de-escalation.

A very promising prospect for future studies and clinical trials is radiomics, which may be the key to transcend the limitations of the human eye in the interpretation of imaging diagnostics and lead to improved treatment of cancer patients.

References

1. Zhao F, Li M, Kong L, Zhang G, Yu J (2016) Delineation of radiation therapy target volumes for patients with postoperative glioblastoma: a review. Onco Targets Ther 9:3197–3204
2. Weber WA, Grosu AL, Czernin J (2008) Technology Insight: advances in molecular imaging and an appraisal of PET/CT scanning. Nat Clin Pract Oncol 5:160–170
3. Nguyen ML, Willows B, Khan R, Chi A, Kim L, Nour SG, Sroka T, Kerr C, Godinez J, Mills M, Karlsson U, Altdorfer G, Nguyen NP, Jendrasiak G, International Geriatric Radiotherapy G (2014) The potential role of magnetic resonance spectroscopy in image-guided radiotherapy. Front Oncol 4:91
4. Einstein DB, Wessels B, Bangert B, Fu P, Nelson AD, Cohen M, Sagar S, Lewin J, Sloan A, Zheng Y, Williams J, Colussi V, Vinkler R, Maciunas R (2012) Phase II trial of radiosurgery to magnetic resonance spectroscopy-defined high-risk tumor volumes in patients with glioblastoma multiforme. Int J Radiat Oncol Biol Phys 84:668–674
5. Laprie A, Ken S, Filleron T, Lubrano V, Vieillevigne L, Tensaouti F, Catalaa I, Boetto S, Khalifa J, Attal J, Peyraga G, Gomez-Roca C, Uro-Coste E, Noel G, Truc G, Sunyach MP, Magne N, Charissoux M, Supiot S, Bernier V, Mounier M, Poublanc M, Fabre A, Delord JP, Cohen-Jonathan Moyal E (2019) Dose-painting multicenter phase III trial in newly diagnosed glioblastoma: the SPECTRO-GLIO trial comparing arm A standard radiochemotherapy to arm B radiochemotherapy with simultaneous integrated boost guided by MR spectroscopic imaging. BMC Cancer 19:167
6. Grosu AL, Astner ST, Riedel E, Nieder C, Wiedenmann N, Heinemann F, Schwaiger M, Molls M, Wester HJ, Weber WA (2011) An interindividual comparison of O-(2-[18F]fluoroethyl)-L-tyrosine (FET)- and L-[methyl-11C]methionine (MET)-PET in patients with brain gliomas and metastases. Int J Radiat Oncol Biol Phys 81:1049–1058
7. Weber WA, Wester HJ, Grosu AL, Herz M, Dzewas B, Feldmann HJ, Molls M, Stocklin G, Schwaiger M (2000) O-(2-[18F]fluoroethyl)-L-tyrosine and L-[methyl-11C]methionine uptake in brain tumours: initial results of a comparative study. Eur J Nucl Med 27:542–549
8. Dunet V, Rossier C, Buck A, Stupp R, Prior JO (2012) Performance of 18F-fluoro-ethyl-tyrosine (18F-FET) PET for the differential diagnosis of primary brain tumor: a systematic review and Metaanalysis. J Nucl Med 53:207–214
9. Grosu AL, Weber WA (2010) PET for radiation treatment planning of brain tumours. Radiother Oncol 96:325–327
10. Grosu AL, Weber WA, Riedel E, Jeremic B, Nieder C, Franz M, Gumprecht H, Jaeger R, Schwaiger M, Molls M (2005) L-(methyl-11C) methionine positron emission tomography for target delineation in resected high-grade gliomas before radiotherapy. Int J Radiat Oncol Biol Phys 63:64–74
11. Niyazi M, Andratschke N, Bendszus M, Chalmers AJ, Erridge SC, Galldiks N, Lagerwaard FJ, Navarria P, Munck Af Rosenschold P, Ricardi U, van den Bent MJ, Weller M, Belka C, Minniti G (2023) ESTRO-EANO guideline on target delineation and radiotherapy details for glioblastoma. Radiother Oncol 184:109663
12. Albert NL, Weller M, Suchorska B, Galldiks N, Soffietti R, Kim MM, la Fougere C, Pope W, Law I, Arbizu J, Chamberlain MC, Vogelbaum M, Ellingson BM, Tonn JC (2016) Response Assessment in Neuro-Oncology working group and European Association for Neuro-Oncology recommendations for the clinical use of PET imaging in gliomas. Neuro-Oncology 18:1199–1208
13. Law I, Albert NL, Arbizu J, Boellaard R, Drzezga A, Galldiks N, la Fougere C, Langen KJ, Lopci E, Lowe V, McConathy J, Quick HH, Sattler B, Schuster DM, Tonn JC, Weller M (2019) Joint EANM/EANO/RANO practice guidelines/SNMMI procedure standards for imaging of gliomas using PET with radiolabelled amino acids and [(18)F]FDG: version 1.0. Eur J Nucl Med Mol Imaging 46:540–557
14. Galldiks N, Niyazi M, Grosu AL, Kocher M, Langen KJ, Law I, Minniti G, Kim MM, Tsien C, Dhermain F, Soffietti R, Mehta MP, Weller M, Tonn JC (2021) Contribution of PET imag-

ing to radiotherapy planning and monitoring in glioma patients - a report of the PET/RANO group. Neuro-Oncology 23:881–893
15. Gurbani S, Weinberg B, Cooper L, Mellon E, Schreibmann E, Sheriff S, Maudsley A, Goryawala M, Shu HK, Shim H (2019) The Brain Imaging Collaboration Suite (BrICS): a cloud platform for integrating whole-brain spectroscopic MRI into the radiation therapy planning workflow. Tomography 5:184–191
16. Galldiks N, Lohmann P, Fink GR, Langen KJ (2023) Amino acid PET in neurooncology. J Nucl Med 64:693–700
17. Grosu AL, Weber WA, Franz M, Stark S, Piert M, Thamm R, Gumprecht H, Schwaiger M, Molls M, Nieder C (2005) Reirradiation of recurrent high-grade gliomas using amino acid PET (SPECT)/CT/MRI image fusion to determine gross tumor volume for stereotactic fractionated radiotherapy. Int J Radiat Oncol Biol Phys 63:511–519
18. Oehlke O, Mix M, Graf E, Schimek-Jasch T, Nestle U, Gotz I, Schneider-Fuchs S, Weyerbrock A, Mader I, Baumert BG, Short SC, Meyer PT, Weber WA, Grosu AL (2016) Amino-acid PET versus MRI guided re-irradiation in patients with recurrent glioblastoma multiforme (GLIAA) - protocol of a randomized phase II trial (NOA 10/ARO 2013-1). BMC Cancer 16:769
19. Grosu AL, Weber WA, Graf E, Mix M, Nestle U, Schimek-Jasch T, Wiehle R, Mader I, Würtemberger U, Langen KJ, Niyazi M, Paulsen F, König L, Giordano FA, Spehl I, Bernhardt D, Schymalla MM, Pöttgen C, Semrau S, Brunner T, Hültenschmidt B, Krause BJ, Ciernik IF, Beck J, Baumert BG, Meyer PT, Urbach H, Popp I, GLIAA Study Group (2026) O-(2-[18F]fluoroethyl)-L-tyrosine-PET-guided versus contrast-enhanced T1-weighted MRI-guided re-irradiation in patients with recurrent glioblastoma (GLIAA/NOA-10ARO2013-01): a multicentre, open-label, randomised trial. Lancet Oncol. 27(2):169–80. https://doi.org/10.1016/S1470-2045(25)00642-4
20. Afshar-Oromieh A, Wolf MB, Kratochwil C, Giesel FL, Combs SE, Dimitrakopoulou-Strauss A, Gnirs R, Roethke MC, Schlemmer HP, Haberkorn U (2015) Comparison of (6)(8) Ga-DOTATOC-PET/CT and PET/MRI hybrid systems in patients with cranial meningioma: initial results. Neuro-Oncology 17:312–319
21. Rachinger W, Stoecklein VM, Terpolilli NA, Haug AR, Ertl L, Poschl J, Schuller U, Schichor C, Thon N, Tonn JC (2015) Increased 68Ga-DOTATATE uptake in PET imaging discriminates meningioma and tumor-free tissue. J Nucl Med 56:347–353
22. Albert NL, Preusser M, Traub-Weidinger T, Tolboom N, Law I, Palmer JD, Guedj E, Furtner J, Fraioli F, Huang RY, Johnson DR, Deroose CM, Herrmann K, Vogelbaum M, Chang S, Tonn JC, Weller M, Wen PY, van den Bent MJ, Verger A, Ivanidze J, Galldiks N (2024) Joint EANM/EANO/RANO/SNMMI practice guideline/procedure standards for diagnostics and therapy (theranostics) of meningiomas using radiolabeled somatostatin receptor ligands: version 1.0. Eur J Nucl Med Mol Imaging 51:3662–3679
23. Goldbrunner R, Minniti G, Preusser M, Jenkinson MD, Sallabanda K, Houdart E, von Deimling A, Stavrinou P, Lefranc F, Lund-Johansen M, Moyal EC, Brandsma D, Henriksson R, Soffietti R, Weller M (2016) EANO guidelines for the diagnosis and treatment of meningiomas. Lancet Oncol 17:e383–e391
24. Combs SE, Farzin M, Boehmer J, Oehlke O, Molls M, Debus J, Grosu AL (2018) Clinical outcome after high-precision radiotherapy for skull base meningiomas: pooled data from three large German centers for radiation oncology. Radiother Oncol 127:274–279
25. Astner ST, Dobrei-Ciuchendea M, Essler M, Bundschuh RA, Sai H, Schwaiger M, Molls M, Weber WA, Grosu AL (2008) Effect of 11C-methionine-positron emission tomography on gross tumor volume delineation in stereotactic radiotherapy of skull base meningiomas. Int J Radiat Oncol Biol Phys 72:1161–1167
26. Grosu AL, Weber WA, Astner ST, Adam M, Krause BJ, Schwaiger M, Molls M, Nieder C (2006) 11C-methionine PET improves the target volume delineation of meningiomas treated with stereotactic fractionated radiotherapy. Int J Radiat Oncol Biol Phys 66:339–344
27. Milker-Zabel S, Zabel-du Bois A, Henze M, Huber P, Schulz-Ertner D, Hoess A, Haberkorn U, Debus J (2006) Improved target volume definition for fractionated stereotactic radio-

therapy in patients with intracranial meningiomas by correlation of CT, MRI, and [68Ga]-DOTATOC-PET. Int J Radiat Oncol Biol Phys 65:222–227

28. Perlow HK, Raleigh DR, Wang TJC, Pollom EL, Milano MT, Breen WG, Detsky J, Chang EL, Tom MC, Shiue KR, Lehrer EJ, Saeed H, Pike LRG, Lo SS, Mishra MV, Knisely JPS, Chao ST, Sahgal A, Palmer JD (2025) Consensus radiation treatment planning guidelines using (68)Ga-DOTATATE PET/CT for resected Meningiomas. Int J Radiat Oncol Biol Phys 122:150–158
29. Ivanidze J, Chang SJ, Haghdel A, Kim JT, Roy Choudhury A, Wu A, Ramakrishna R, Schwartz TH, Cisse B, Stieg P, Muller L, Osborne JR, Magge RS, Karakatsanis NA, Roytman M, Lin E, Pannullo SC, Palmer JD, Knisely JPS (2024) [Ga68] DOTATATE PET/MRI-guided radiosurgical treatment planning and response assessment in meningiomas. Neuro-Oncology 26:1526–1535
30. Marta GN, Silva V, de Andrade CH, de Arruda FF, Hanna SA, Gadia R, da Silva JL, Correa SF, Vita Abreu CE, Riera R (2014) Intensity-modulated radiation therapy for head and neck cancer: systematic review and meta-analysis. Radiother Oncol 110:9–15
31. Thoeny HC, De Keyzer F, King AD (2012) Diffusion-weighted MR imaging in the head and neck. Radiology 263:19–32
32. Dirix P, Vandecaveye V, De Keyzer F, Stroobants S, Hermans R, Nuyts S (2009) Dose painting in radiotherapy for head and neck squamous cell carcinoma: value of repeated functional imaging with (18)F-FDG PET, (18)F-fluoromisonidazole PET, diffusion-weighted MRI, and dynamic contrast-enhanced MRI. J Nucl Med 50:1020–1027
33. Vandecaveye V, Dirix P, De Keyzer F, de Beeck KO, Vander Poorten V, Roebben I, Nuyts S, Hermans R (2010) Predictive value of diffusion-weighted magnetic resonance imaging during chemoradiotherapy for head and neck squamous cell carcinoma. Eur Radiol 20:1703–1714
34. King AD, Mo FK, Yu KH, Yeung DK, Zhou H, Bhatia KS, Tse GM, Vlantis AC, Wong JK, Ahuja AT (2010) Squamous cell carcinoma of the head and neck: diffusion-weighted MR imaging for prediction and monitoring of treatment response. Eur Radiol 20:2213–2220
35. Daisne JF, Duprez T, Weynand B, Lonneux M, Hamoir M, Reychler H, Gregoire V (2004) Tumor volume in pharyngolaryngeal squamous cell carcinoma: comparison at CT, MR imaging, and FDG PET and validation with surgical specimen. Radiology 233:93–100
36. Jensen K, Al-Farra G, Dejanovic D, Eriksen JG, Loft A, Hansen CR, Pameijer FA, Zukauskaite R, Grau C (2021) Imaging for target delineation in head and neck cancer radiotherapy. Semin Nucl Med 51:59–67
37. Wang Y, Lombardo E, Huang L, Avanzo M, Fanetti G, Franchin G, Zschaeck S, Weingartner J, Belka C, Riboldi M, Kurz C, Landry G (2024) Comparison of deep learning networks for fully automated head and neck tumor delineation on multi-centric PET/CT images. Radiat Oncol 19:3
38. Due AK, Vogelius IR, Aznar MC, Bentzen SM, Berthelsen AK, Korreman SS, Loft A, Kristensen CA, Specht L (2014) Recurrences after intensity modulated radiotherapy for head and neck squamous cell carcinoma more likely to originate from regions with high baseline [18F]-FDG uptake. Radiother Oncol 111:360–365
39. Differding S, Sterpin E, Janssens G, Hanin FX, Lee JA, Gregoire V (2016) Methodology for adaptive and robust FDG-PET escalated dose painting by numbers in head and neck tumors. Acta Oncol 55:217–225
40. Gregoire V, Bol A, Geets X, Lee J (2006) Is PET-based treatment planning the new standard in modern radiotherapy? The head and neck paradigm. Semin Radiat Oncol 16:232–238
41. de Leeuw A, Giralt J, Tao Y, Benavente S, France Nguyen TV, Hoebers FJP, Hoeben A, Terhaard CHJ, Wai Lee L, Friesland S, Steenbakkers R, Tans L, Heukelom J, Kayembe MT, van Kranen SR, Bartelink H, Rasch CRN, Sonke JJ, Hamming-Vrieze O (2024) A multicentric randomized controlled phase III trial of adaptive and 18F-FDG-PET-guided dose-redistribution in locally advanced head and neck squamous cell carcinoma (ARTFORCE). Radiother Oncol 196:110281

42. Fleming IN, Manavaki R, Blower PJ, West C, Williams KJ, Harris AL, Domarkas J, Lord S, Baldry C, Gilbert FJ (2015) Imaging tumour hypoxia with positron emission tomography. Br J Cancer 112:238–250
43. Nordsmark M, Bentzen SM, Rudat V, Brizel D, Lartigau E, Stadler P, Becker A, Adam M, Molls M, Dunst J, Terris DJ, Overgaard J (2005) Prognostic value of tumor oxygenation in 397 head and neck tumors after primary radiation therapy. An international multi-center study. Radiother Oncol 77:18–24
44. Gagel B, Reinartz P, Dimartino E, Zimny M, Pinkawa M, Maneschi P, Stanzel S, Hamacher K, Coenen HH, Westhofen M, Bull U, Eble MJ (2004) pO(2) Polarography versus positron emission tomography ([(18)F] fluoromisonidazole, [(18)F]-2-fluoro-2′-deoxyglucose). An appraisal of radiotherapeutically relevant hypoxia. Strahlenther Onkol 180:616–622
45. Wiedenmann NE, Bucher S, Hentschel M, Mix M, Vach W, Bittner MI, Nestle U, Pfeiffer J, Weber WA, Grosu AL (2015) Serial [18F]-fluoromisonidazole PET during radiochemotherapy for locally advanced head and neck cancer and its correlation with outcome. Radiother Oncol 117:113–117
46. Zips D, Zophel K, Abolmaali N, Perrin R, Abramyuk A, Haase R, Appold S, Steinbach J, Kotzerke J, Baumann M (2012) Exploratory prospective trial of hypoxia-specific PET imaging during radiochemotherapy in patients with locally advanced head-and-neck cancer. Radiother Oncol 105:21–28
47. Bittner MI, Wiedenmann N, Bucher S, Hentschel M, Mix M, Weber WA, Grosu AL (2013) Exploratory geographical analysis of hypoxic subvolumes using 18F-MISO-PET imaging in patients with head and neck cancer in the course of primary chemoradiotherapy. Radiother Oncol 108:511–516
48. Lee N, Schoder H, Beattie B, Lanning R, Riaz N, McBride S, Katabi N, Li D, Yarusi B, Chan S, Mitrani L, Zhang Z, Pfister DG, Sherman E, Baxi S, Boyle J, Morris LG, Ganly I, Wong R, Humm J (2016) Strategy of using intratreatment hypoxia imaging to selectively and safely guide radiation dose de-escalation concurrent with chemotherapy for locoregionally advanced human papillomavirus-related oropharyngeal carcinoma. Int J Radiat Oncol Biol Phys 96:9–17
49. Grosu AL, Souvatzoglou M, Roper B, Dobritz M, Wiedenmann N, Jacob V, Wester HJ, Reischl G, Machulla HJ, Schwaiger M, Molls M, Piert M (2007) Hypoxia imaging with FAZA-PET and theoretical considerations with regard to dose painting for individualization of radiotherapy in patients with head and neck cancer. Int J Radiat Oncol Biol Phys 69:541–551
50. Mehanna H, Wong WL, McConkey CC, Rahman JK, Robinson M, Hartley AG, Nutting C, Powell N, Al-Booz H, Robinson M, Junor E, Rizwanullah M, von Zeidler SV, Wieshmann H, Hulme C, Smith AF, Hall P, Dunn J, Group P-NTM (2016) PET-CT surveillance versus neck dissection in advanced head and neck cancer. N Engl J Med 374:1444–1454
51. Pfister DG, Foote RL, Gilbert J, Gillison ML, Ridge JA, Rocco J (2018) NCCN guidelines index table of contents discussion 227
52. Nestle U, Walter K, Schmidt S, Licht N, Nieder C, Motaref B, Hellwig D, Niewald M, Ukena D, Kirsch CM, Sybrecht GW, Schnabel K (1999) 18F-deoxyglucose positron emission tomography (FDG-PET) for the planning of radiotherapy in lung cancer: high impact in patients with atelectasis. Int J Radiat Oncol Biol Phys 44:593–597
53. De Ruysscher D, Wanders S, van Haren E, Hochstenbag M, Geeraedts W, Utama I, Simons J, Dohmen J, Rhami A, Buell U, Thimister P, Snoep G, Boersma L, Verschueren T, van Baardwijk A, Minken A, Bentzen SM, Lambin P (2005) Selective mediastinal node irradiation based on FDG-PET scan data in patients with non-small-cell lung cancer: a prospective clinical study. Int J Radiat Oncol Biol Phys 62:988–994
54. Caldwell CB, Mah K, Ung YC, Danjoux CE, Balogh JM, Ganguli SN, Ehrlich LE (2001) Observer variation in contouring gross tumor volume in patients with poorly defined non-small-cell lung tumors on CT: the impact of 18FDG-hybrid PET fusion. Int J Radiat Oncol Biol Phys 51:923–931

55. Fox JL, Rengan R, O'Meara W, Yorke E, Erdi Y, Nehmeh S, Leibel SA, Rosenzweig KE (2005) Does registration of PET and planning CT images decrease interobserver and intraobserver variation in delineating tumor volumes for non-small-cell lung cancer? Int J Radiat Oncol Biol Phys 62:70–75
56. Hanna GG, McAleese J, Carson KJ, Stewart DP, Cosgrove VP, Eakin RL, Zatari A, Lynch T, Jarritt PH, Young VA, O'Sullivan JM, Hounsell AR (2010) (18)F-FDG PET-CT simulation for non-small-cell lung cancer: effect in patients already staged by PET-CT. Int J Radiat Oncol Biol Phys 77:24–30
57. Dwamena BA, Sonnad SS, Angobaldo JO, Wahl RL (1999) Metastases from non-small cell lung cancer: mediastinal staging in the 1990s—meta-analytic comparison of PET and CT. Radiology 213:530–536
58. Macmanus MP, Hicks RJ (2008) Where do we draw the line? Contouring tumors on positron emission tomography/computed tomography. Int J Radiat Oncol Biol Phys 71:2–4
59. Doll C, Duncker-Rohr V, Rucker G, Mix M, MacManus M, De Ruysscher D, Vogel W, Eriksen JG, Oyen W, Grosu AL, Weber W, Nestle U (2014) Influence of experience and qualification on PET-based target volume delineation. When there is no expert--ask your colleague. Strahlenther Onkol 190:555–562
60. MacManus M, Nestle U, Rosenzweig KE, Carrio I, Messa C, Belohlavek O, Danna M, Inoue T, Deniaud-Alexandre E, Schipani S, Watanabe N, Dondi M, Jeremic B (2009) Use of PET and PET/CT for radiation therapy planning: IAEA expert report 2006-2007. Radiother Oncol 91:85–94
61. Konert T, Vogel W, MacManus MP, Nestle U, Belderbos J, Gregoire V, Thorwarth D, Fidarova E, Paez D, Chiti A, Hanna GG (2015) PET/CT imaging for target volume delineation in curative intent radiotherapy of non-small cell lung cancer: IAEA consensus report 2014. Radiother Oncol 116:27–34
62. Chirindel A, Adebahr S, Schuster D, Schimek-Jasch T, Schanne DH, Nemer U, Mix M, Meyer P, Grosu AL, Brunner T, Nestle U (2015) Impact of 4D-(18)FDG-PET/CT imaging on target volume delineation in SBRT patients with central versus peripheral lung tumors. Multi-reader comparative study. Radiother Oncol 115:335–341
63. Levy A, Adebahr S, Hurkmans C, Ahmed M, Ahmad S, Guckenberger M, Geets X, Lievens Y, Lambrecht M, Pourel N, Lewitzki V, Konopa K, Franks K, Dziadziuszko R, McDonald F, Fortpied C, Clementel E, Fournier B, Rizzo S, Fink C, Riesterer O, Peulen H, Andratschke N, McWilliam A, Gkika E, Schimek-Jasch T, Grosu AL, Le Pechoux C, Faivre-Finn C, Nestle U (2024) Stereotactic body radiotherapy for centrally located inoperable early-stage NSCLC: EORTC 22113-08113 LungTech phase II trial results. J Thorac Oncol 19:1297–1309
64. Nestle U, Schimek-Jasch T, Kremp S, Schaefer-Schuler A, Mix M, Kusters A, Tosch M, Hehr T, Eschmann SM, Bultel YP, Hass P, Fleckenstein J, Thieme A, Stockinger M, Dieckmann K, Miederer M, Holl G, Rischke HC, Gkika E, Adebahr S, Konig J, Grosu AL, group PE-Ps (2020) Imaging-based target volume reduction in chemoradiotherapy for locally advanced non-small-cell lung cancer (PET-Plan): a multicentre, open-label, randomised, controlled trial. Lancet Oncol 21:581–592
65. Rimner A, Dejonckheere CS, Sahlmann J, Barth SA, Schimek-Jasch T, Adebahr S, Hecht M, Waller CF, Schmid S, Stolz D, Miederer M, Brose A, Binder H, Konig J, Grosu AL, Nestle U, Gkika E (2025) Impact of different mediastinal staging modalities on target volume delineation in locally advanced non-small cell lung cancer: a secondary analysis of the multicenter randomized PET-plan trial. Int J Radiat Oncol Biol Phys 122:1217–1226
66. Vera P, Thureau S, Le Tinier F, Chaumet-Riffaud P, Hapdey S, Kolesnikov-Gauthier H, Martin E, Berriolo-Riedinger A, Pourel N, Broglia JM, Boissellier P, Guillemard S, Salem N, Brenot-Rossi I, Le Pechoux C, Berthold C, Giroux-Leprieur E, Moreau D, Guillerm S, Benali K, Tessonnier L, Audigier-Valette C, Lerouge D, Quak E, Massabeau C, Courbon F, Moisson P, Larrouy A, Modzelewski R, Gouel P, Ghazzar N, Langlais A, Amour E, Zalcman G, Giraud P (2024) Adaptive radiotherapy (up to 74 Gy) or standard radiotherapy (66 Gy) for patients with stage III non-small-cell lung cancer, according to [(18)F]FDG-PET tumour

residual uptake at 42 Gy (RTEP7-IFCT-1402): a multicentre, randomised, controlled phase 2 trial. Lancet Oncol 25:1176–1187
67. Alorfi F, Bomanji J, Bertoletti L, Fraioli F (2025) PET/MRI in non-small cell lung cancer (NSCLC). Semin Nucl Med 55:234–239
68. Lordick F, Mariette C, Haustermans K, Obermannova R, Arnold D, Committee EG (2016) Oesophageal cancer: ESMO clinical practice guidelines for diagnosis, treatment and follow-up. Ann Oncol 27:v50–vv7
69. Ajani JA, Barthel JS, Bentrem DJ, D'Amico TA, Das P, Denlinger CS, Fuchs CS, Gerdes H, Glasgow RE, Hayman JA, Hofstetter WL, Ilson DH, Keswani RN, Kleinberg LR, Korn WM, Lockhart AC, Mulcahy MF, Orringer MB, Osarogiagbon RU, Posey JA, Sasson AR, Scott WJ, Shibata S, Strong VE, Varghese TK Jr, Warren G, Washington MK, Willett C, Wright CD, National Comprehensive Cancer N (2011) Esophageal and esophagogastric junction cancers. J Natl Compr Cancer Netw 9:830–887
70. Muijs CT, Beukema JC, Pruim J, Mul VE, Groen H, Plukker JT, Langendijk JA (2010) A systematic review on the role of FDG-PET/CT in tumour delineation and radiotherapy planning in patients with esophageal cancer. Radiother Oncol 97:165–171
71. van Vliet EP, Heijenbrok-Kal MH, Hunink MG, Kuipers EJ, Siersema PD (2008) Staging investigations for oesophageal cancer: a meta-analysis. Br J Cancer 98:547–557
72. van Westreenen HL, Westerterp M, Bossuyt PM, Pruim J, Sloof GW, van Lanschot JJ, Groen H, Plukker JT (2004) Systematic review of the staging performance of 18F-fluorodeoxyglucose positron emission tomography in esophageal cancer. J Clin Oncol 22:3805–3812
73. Muijs CT, Beukema JC, Woutersen D, Mul VE, Berveling MJ, Pruim J, van der Jagt EJ, Hospers GA, Groen H, Plukker JT, Langendijk JA (2014) Clinical validation of FDG-PET/CT in the radiation treatment planning for patients with oesophageal cancer. Radiother Oncol 113:188–192
74. zum Buschenfelde CM, Herrmann K, Schuster T, Geinitz H, Langer R, Becker K, Ott K, Ebert M, Zimmermann F, Friess H, Schwaiger M, Peschel C, Lordick F, Krause BJ (2011) (18)F-FDG PET-guided salvage neoadjuvant radiochemotherapy of adenocarcinoma of the esophagogastric junction: the MUNICON II trial. J Nucl Med 52:1189–1196
75. Ma J, Wang Z, Wang C, Chen E, Dong Y, Song Y, Wang W, You D, Jiang W, Zang R (2017) Individualized radiation dose escalation based on the decrease in tumor FDG uptake and normal tissue constraints improve survival in patients with esophageal carcinoma. Technol Cancer Res Treat 16:75–80
76. Liu H, Hu Z, Yang X, Dai T, Chen Y (2022) Comparison of [(68)Ga]Ga-DOTA-FAPI-04 and [(18)F]FDG uptake in esophageal cancer. Front Oncol 12:875081
77. Kroger K, Pepper NB, Ventura D, Troschel FM, Backhaus P, Rahbar K, Glasbrenner B, Bruwer M, Pascher A, Schafers M, Eich HT, Roll W (2025) FAPI-PET/CT guided radiotherapy for patients with esophageal cancer. Radiat Oncol 20:29
78. Hu X, Zhou T, Ren J, Duan J, Wu H, Liu X, Mu Z, Liu N, Wei Y, Yuan S (2023) Response prediction using (18)F-FAPI-04 PET/CT in patients with esophageal squamous cell carcinoma treated with concurrent chemoradiotherapy. J Nucl Med 64:625–631
79. Mohler JL, Lee RJ, Antonarakis ES, Higano CS, Richey S (2018) NCCN guidelines index table of contents. Prostate Cancer 151
80. Bekelman JE, Rumble RB, Freedland SJ (2018) Clinically localized prostate cancer: ASCO clinical practice guideline endorsement of an AUA/ASTRO/SUO guideline summary. J Oncol Pract 14:618–624
81. Mottet N, Bellmunt J, Bolla M, Briers E, Cumberbatch MG, De Santis M, Fossati N, Gross T, Henry AM, Joniau S, Lam TB, Mason MD, Matveev VB, Moldovan PC, van den Bergh RCN, Van den Broeck T, van der Poel HG, van der Kwast TH, Rouviere O, Schoots IG, Wiegel T, Cornford P (2017) EAU-ESTRO-SIOG guidelines on prostate cancer. Part 1: screening, diagnosis, and local treatment with curative intent. Eur Urol 71:618–629
82. NCCN Clinical Practice Guidelines in Oncology: Prostate Cancer, Version 2.2025
83. Cornford P, van den Bergh RCN, Briers E et al (2024) EAU-EANM-ESTRO-ESUR-ISUP-SIOG guidelines on prostate cancer (2024 update). Eur Urol 80(4):1–50

84. Dearnaley DP, Sydes MR, Graham JD, Aird EG, Bottomley D, Cowan RA, Huddart RA, Jose CC, Matthews JH, Millar J, Moore AR, Morgan RC, Russell JM, Scrase CD, Stephens RJ, Syndikus I, Parmar MK, collaborators RT (2007) Escalated-dose versus standard-dose conformal radiotherapy in prostate cancer: first results from the MRC RT01 randomised controlled trial. Lancet Oncol 8:475–487
85. Kuban DA, Levy LB, Cheung MR, Lee AK, Choi S, Frank S, Pollack A (2011) Long-term failure patterns and survival in a randomized dose-escalation trial for prostate cancer. Who dies of disease? Int J Radiat Oncol Biol Phys 79:1310–1317
86. Kuban DA, Tucker SL, Dong L, Starkschall G, Huang EH, Cheung MR, Lee AK, Pollack A (2008) Long-term results of the M. D. Anderson randomized dose-escalation trial for prostate cancer. Int J Radiat Oncol Biol Phys 70:67–74
87. Viani GA, Stefano EJ, Afonso SL (2009) Higher-than-conventional radiation doses in localized prostate cancer treatment: a meta-analysis of randomized, controlled trials. Int J Radiat Oncol Biol Phys 74:1405–1418
88. Zietman AL, DeSilvio ML, Slater JD, Rossi CJ Jr, Miller DW, Adams JA, Shipley WU (2005) Comparison of conventional-dose vs high-dose conformal radiation therapy in clinically localized adenocarcinoma of the prostate: a randomized controlled trial. JAMA 294:1233–1239
89. de Rooij M, Hamoen EH, Futterer JJ, Barentsz JO, Rovers MM (2014) Accuracy of multiparametric MRI for prostate cancer detection: a meta-analysis. AJR Am J Roentgenol 202:343–351
90. Woo S, Suh CH, Kim SY, Cho JY, Kim SH (2017) Diagnostic performance of prostate imaging reporting and data system Version 2 for detection of prostate cancer: a systematic review and diagnostic meta-analysis. Eur Urol 72:177–188
91. van Schie MA, Dinh CV, Houdt PJV, Pos FJ, Heijmink S, Kerkmeijer LGW, Kotte A, Oyen R, Haustermans K, van der Heide UA (2018) Contouring of prostate tumors on multiparametric MRI: evaluation of clinical delineations in a multicenter radiotherapy trial. Radiother Oncol 128:321–326
92. Steenbergen P, Haustermans K, Lerut E, Oyen R, De Wever L, Van den Bergh L, Kerkmeijer LG, Pameijer FA, Veldhuis WB, van der Voort van Zyp JR, Pos FJ, Heijmink SW, Kalisvaart R, Teertstra HJ, Dinh CV, Ghobadi G, van der Heide UA (2015) Prostate tumor delineation using multiparametric magnetic resonance imaging: inter-observer variability and pathology validation. Radiother Oncol 115:186–190
93. Barrett T, Gill AB, Kataoka MY, Priest AN, Joubert I, McLean MA, Graves MJ, Stearn S, Lomas DJ, Griffiths JR, Neal D, Gnanapragasam VJ, Sala E (2012) DCE and DW MRI in monitoring response to androgen deprivation therapy in patients with prostate cancer: a feasibility study. Magn Reson Med 67:778–785
94. Schmuecking M, Boltze C, Geyer H, Salz H, Schilling B, Wendt TG, Kloetzer KH, Marx C (2009) Dynamic MRI and CAD vs. choline MRS: where is the detection level for a lesion characterisation in prostate cancer? Int J Radiat Biol 85:814–824
95. Bonekamp D, Jacobs MA, El-Khouli R, Stoianovici D, Macura KJ (2011) Advancements in MR imaging of the prostate: from diagnosis to interventions. Radiographics 31:677–703
96. Weinreb JC, Barentsz JO, Choyke PL, Cornud F, Haider MA, Macura KJ, Margolis D, Schnall MD, Shtern F, Tempany CM, Thoeny HC, Verma S (2016) PI-RADS prostate imaging - reporting and data system: 2015, Version 2. Eur Urol 69:16–40
97. PI-RADS Prostate Imaging - Reporting and Data System: 2019, Version 2.1
98. Jadvar H (2011) Prostate cancer: PET with 18F-FDG, 18F- or 11C-acetate, and 18F- or 11C-choline. J Nucl Med 52:81–89
99. Bundschuh RA, Wendl CM, Weirich G, Eiber M, Souvatzoglou M, Treiber U, Kubler H, Maurer T, Gschwend JE, Geinitz H, Grosu AL, Ziegler SI, Krause BJ (2013) Tumour volume delineation in prostate cancer assessed by [11C]choline PET/CT: validation with surgical specimens. Eur J Nucl Med Mol Imaging 40:824–831
100. Grosu AL, Weirich G, Wendl C, Prokic V, Kirste S, Geinitz H, Souvatzoglou M, Gschwend JE, Schwaiger M, Molls M, Weber WA, Treiber U, Krause BJ (2014) 11C-Choline PET/

pathology image coregistration in primary localized prostate cancer. Eur J Nucl Med Mol Imaging 41:2242–2248
101. Giesel FL, Sterzing F, Schlemmer HP, Holland-Letz T, Mier W, Rius M, Afshar-Oromieh A, Kopka K, Debus J, Haberkorn U, Kratochwil C (2016) Intra-individual comparison of (68) Ga-PSMA-11-PET/CT and multi-parametric MR for imaging of primary prostate cancer. Eur J Nucl Med Mol Imaging 43:1400–1406
102. Spohn S, Jaegle C, Fassbender TF, Sprave T, Gkika E, Nicolay NH, Bock M, Ruf J, Benndorf M, Gratzke C, Grosu AL, Zamboglou C (2020) Intraindividual comparison between (68) Ga-PSMA-PET/CT and mpMRI for intraprostatic tumor delineation in patients with primary prostate cancer: a retrospective analysis in 101 patients. Eur J Nucl Med Mol Imaging 47:2796–2803
103. Marinescu IM, Spohn SKB, Kiefer S, Bronsert P, Ceci L, Holzschuh J, Sigle A, Jilg CA, Ruhle A, Sprave T, Nicolay NH, Winzer R, Rehm J, Kotzerke J, Holscher T, Grosu AL, Ruf J, Benndorf M, Zamboglou C (2022) Intraindividual comparison between [(18)F] PSMA-1007 PET/CT and multiparametric MRI for radiotherapy planning in primary prostate cancer patients. Front Oncol 12:880042
104. Holzschuh JC, Mix M, Ruf J, Holscher T, Kotzerke J, Vrachimis A, Doolan P, Ilhan H, Marinescu IM, Spohn SKB, Fechter T, Kuhn D, Bronsert P, Gratzke C, Grosu R, Kamran SC, Heidari P, Ng TSC, Konik A, Grosu AL, Zamboglou C (2023) Deep learning based automated delineation of the intraprostatic gross tumour volume in PSMA-PET for patients with primary prostate cancer. Radiother Oncol 188:109774
105. Kostyszyn D, Fechter T, Bartl N, Grosu AL, Gratzke C, Sigle A, Mix M, Ruf J, Fassbender TF, Kiefer S, Bettermann AS, Nicolay NH, Spohn S, Kramer MU, Bronsert P, Guo H, Qiu X, Wang F, Henkenberens C, Werner RA, Baltas D, Meyer PT, Derlin T, Chen M, Zamboglou C (2021) Intraprostatic tumor segmentation on PSMA PET images in patients with primary prostate cancer with a convolutional neural network. J Nucl Med 62:823–828
106. Waibel PMA, Glavynskyi I, Fechter T, Mix M, Kind F, Sigle A, Jilg CA, Gratzke C, Werner M, Schilling O, Bronsert P, Freitag MT, Zamboglou C, Grosu AL, Spohn SKB (2025) Can PSMA PET detect intratumour heterogeneity in histological PSMA expression of primary prostate cancer? Analysis of [(68)Ga]Ga-PSMA-11 and [(18)F]PSMA-1007. Eur J Nucl Med Mol Imaging 52:2023–2033
107. Spohn SKB, Grosu AL (2025) Impact of PSMA PET on radiation oncology planning. Semin Nucl Med 55:664
108. Eiber M, Weirich G, Holzapfel K, Souvatzoglou M, Haller B, Rauscher I, Beer AJ, Wester HJ, Gschwend J, Schwaiger M, Maurer T (2016) Simultaneous (68)Ga-PSMA HBED-CC PET/MRI improves the localization of primary prostate cancer. Eur Urol 70:829–836
109. Zamboglou C, Drendel V, Jilg CA, Rischke HC, Beck TI, Schultze-Seemann W, Krauss T, Mix M, Schiller F, Wetterauer U, Werner M, Langer M, Bock M, Meyer PT, Grosu AL (2017) Comparison of (68)Ga-HBED-CC PSMA-PET/CT and multiparametric MRI for gross tumour volume detection in patients with primary prostate cancer based on slice by slice comparison with histopathology. Theranostics 7:228–237
110. Thomas L, Kantz S, Hung A, Monaco D, Gaertner FC, Essler M, Strunk H, Laub W, Bundschuh RA (2018) (68)Ga-PSMA-PET/CT imaging of localized primary prostate cancer patients for intensity modulated radiation therapy treatment planning with integrated boost. Eur J Nucl Med Mol Imaging 45:1170–1178
111. Zamboglou C, Sachpazidis I, Koubar K, Drendel V, Wiehle R, Kirste S, Mix M, Schiller F, Mavroidis P, Meyer PT, Werner M, Grosu AL, Baltas D (2017) Evaluation of intensity modulated radiation therapy dose painting for localized prostate cancer using (68)Ga-HBED-CC PSMA-PET/CT: a planning study based on histopathology reference. Radiother Oncol 123:472–477
112. Zamboglou C, Thomann B, Koubar K, Bronsert P, Krauss T, Rischke HC, Sachpazidis I, Drendel V, Salman N, Reichel K, Jilg CA, Werner M, Meyer PT, Bock M, Baltas D, Grosu AL (2018) Focal dose escalation for prostate cancer using (68)Ga-HBED-CC PSMA PET/CT and MRI: a planning study based on histology reference. Radiat Oncol 13:81

113. Zamboglou C, Spohn SKB, Ruf J, Benndorf M, Gainey M, Kamps M, Jilg C, Gratzke C, Adebahr S, Schmidtmayer-Zamboglou B, Mix M, Bamberg F, Zschaeck S, Ghadjar P, Baltas D, Grosu AL (2022) PSMA-PET- and MRI-based focal dose escalated radiation therapy of primary prostate cancer: planned safety analysis of a nonrandomized 2-armed phase 2 trial (ARO2020-01). Int J Radiat Oncol Biol Phys 113:1025–1035
114. Spohn SKB, Zamboglou C, Burkle SL, Freitag MT, Brumberg J, Engel H, Gainey M, Kamps M, Toncheva P, Sprave T, Kirste S, Sigle A, Jilg C, Gratzke C, Adebahr S, Mix M, Bamberg F, Zschaeck S, Ghadjar P, Baltas D, Grosu AL (2025) Safety and quality of life of PSMA-PET- and MRI-based focal dose escalated radiotherapy for intermediate- and high-risk prostate cancer: primary endpoint analysis of the bi-centric phase II HypoFocal trial (ARO2020-01). Radiother Oncol 208:110883
115. Kerkmeijer LGW, Groen VH, Pos FJ, Haustermans K, Monninkhof EM, Smeenk RJ, Kunze-Busch M, de Boer JCJ, van der Voort van Zijp J, van Vulpen M, Draulans C, van den Bergh L, Isebaert S, van der Heide UA (2021) Focal boost to the intraprostatic tumor in external beam radiotherapy for patients with localized prostate cancer: results from the FLAME randomized phase III trial. J Clin Oncol 39:787–796
116. Draulans C, Haustermans K, Pos FJ, van der Heide UA, De Cock L, van der Voort van Zyp J, De Boer H, Smeenk RJ, Kunze-Busch M, Monninkhof EM, De Roover R, Isebaert S, Kerkmeijer LGW (2024) Stereotactic body radiotherapy with a focal boost to the intraprostatic tumor for intermediate and high risk prostate cancer: 5-year efficacy and toxicity in the hypo-FLAME trial. Radiother Oncol 201:110568
117. Yasar B, Suh YE, Chapman E, Nicholls L, Henderson D, Jones C, Morrison K, Wells E, Henderson J, Meehan C, Sohaib A, Taylor H, Tree A, van As N (2024) Simultaneous focal boost with stereotactic radiation therapy for localized intermediate- to high-risk prostate cancer: primary outcomes of the SPARC phase 2 trial. Int J Radiat Oncol Biol Phys 120:49–58
118. Zamboglou C, Spohn SKB, Adebahr S, Huber M, Kirste S, Sprave T, Gratzke C, Chen RC, Carl EG, Weber WA, Mix M, Benndorf M, Wiegel T, Baltas D, Jenkner C, Grosu AL (2021) PSMA-PET/MRI-based focal dose escalation in patients with primary prostate cancer treated with stereotactic body radiation therapy (HypoFocal-SBRT): study protocol of a randomized, multicentric phase III trial. Cancers (Basel) 13:5795
119. Hovels AM, Heesakkers RA, Adang EM, Jager GJ, Strum S, Hoogeveen YL, Severens JL, Barentsz JO (2008) The diagnostic accuracy of CT and MRI in the staging of pelvic lymph nodes in patients with prostate cancer: a meta-analysis. Clin Radiol 63:387–395
120. Vallini V, Ortori S, Boraschi P, Manassero F, Gabelloni M, Faggioni L, Selli C, Bartolozzi C (2016) Staging of pelvic lymph nodes in patients with prostate cancer: usefulness of multiple b value SE-EPI diffusion-weighted imaging on a 3.0 T MR system. Eur J Radiol Open 3:16–21
121. van Leeuwen PJ, Emmett L, Ho B, Delprado W, Ting F, Nguyen Q, Stricker PD (2017) Prospective evaluation of 68Gallium-prostate-specific membrane antigen positron emission tomography/computed tomography for preoperative lymph node staging in prostate cancer. BJU Int 119:209–215
122. Maurer T, Gschwend JE, Rauscher I, Souvatzoglou M, Haller B, Weirich G, Wester HJ, Heck M, Kubler H, Beer AJ, Schwaiger M, Eiber M (2016) Diagnostic efficacy of (68)Gallium-PSMA positron emission tomography compared to conventional imaging for lymph node staging of 130 consecutive patients with intermediate to high risk prostate cancer. J Urol 195:1436–1443
123. Obek C, Doganca T, Demirci E, Ocak M, Kural AR, Yildirim A, Yucetas U, Demirdag C, Erdogan SM, Kabasakal L, Members of Urooncology Association T (2017) The accuracy of (68)Ga-PSMA PET/CT in primary lymph node staging in high-risk prostate cancer. Eur J Nucl Med Mol Imaging 44:1806–1812
124. Hofman MS, Lawrentschuk N, Francis RJ, Tang C, Vela I, Thomas P, Rutherford N, Martin JM, Frydenberg M, Shakher R, Wong LM, Taubman K, Ting Lee S, Hsiao E, Roach P, Nottage M, Kirkwood I, Hayne D, Link E, Marusic P, Matera A, Herschtal A, Iravani A, Hicks RJ, Williams S, Murphy DG, pro PSGC (2020) Prostate-specific membrane antigen

PET-CT in patients with high-risk prostate cancer before curative-intent surgery or radiotherapy (proPSMA): a prospective, randomised, multicentre study. Lancet 395:1208–1216
125. Spohn SKB, Birkenmaier V, Ruf J, Mix M, Sigle A, Haehl E, Adebahr S, Sprave T, Gkika E, Ruhle A, Nicolay NH, Kirste S, Grosu AL, Zamboglou C (2022) Risk factors for biochemical recurrence after PSMA-PET-guided definitive radiotherapy in patients with De Novo Lymph node-positive prostate cancer. Front Oncol 12:898774
126. Habl G, Hatiboglu G, Edler L, Uhl M, Krause S, Roethke M, Schlemmer HP, Hadaschik B, Debus J, Herfarth K (2014) Ion Prostate Irradiation (IPI) - a pilot study to establish the safety and feasibility of primary hypofractionated irradiation of the prostate with protons and carbon ions in a raster scan technique. BMC Cancer 14:202
127. Shakespeare TP (2015) Effect of prostate-specific membrane antigen positron emission tomography on the decision-making of radiation oncologists. Radiat Oncol 10:233
128. Armstrong WR, Kishan AU, Booker KM, Grogan TR, Elashoff D, Lam EC, Clark KJ, Steinberg ML, Fendler WP, Hope TA, Nickols NG, Czernin J, Calais J (2024) Impact of prostate-specific membrane antigen positron emission tomography/computed tomography on prostate cancer salvage radiotherapy management: results from a prospective multicenter randomized phase 3 trial (PSMA-SRT NCT03582774). Eur Urol 86:52–60
129. Fendler WP, Calais J, Eiber M, Flavell RR, Mishoe A, Feng FY, Nguyen HG, Reiter RE, Rettig MB, Okamoto S, Emmett L, Zacho HD, Ilhan H, Wetter A, Rischpler C, Schoder H, Burger IA, Gartmann J, Smith R, Small EJ, Slavik R, Carroll PR, Herrmann K, Czernin J, Hope TA (2019) Assessment of 68Ga-PSMA-11 PET accuracy in localizing recurrent prostate cancer: a prospective single-arm clinical trial. JAMA Oncol 5:856–863
130. Verburg FA, Pfister D, Heidenreich A, Vogg A, Drude NI, Voo S, Mottaghy FM, Behrendt FF (2016) Extent of disease in recurrent prostate cancer determined by [(68)Ga]PSMA-HBED-CC PET/CT in relation to PSA levels, PSA doubling time and Gleason score. Eur J Nucl Med Mol Imaging 43:397–403
131. Afshar-Oromieh A, Holland-Letz T, Giesel FL, Kratochwil C, Mier W, Haufe S, Debus N, Eder M, Eisenhut M, Schafer M, Neels O, Hohenfellner M, Kopka K, Kauczor HU, Debus J, Haberkorn U (2017) Diagnostic performance of (68)Ga-PSMA-11 (HBED-CC) PET/CT in patients with recurrent prostate cancer: evaluation in 1007 patients. Eur J Nucl Med Mol Imaging 44:1258–1268
132. Solomonidou N, Germanou D, Strouthos I, Karagiannis E, Farolfi A, Koerber SA, Debus J, Peeken JC, Vogel ME, Vrachimis A, Spohn SKB, Shelan M, Aebersold D, Grosu AL, Ceci F, Kroeze SGC, Guckenberger M, Fanti S, Belka C, Hruby G, Scharl S, Wiegel T, Bartenstein P, Henkenberens C, Emmett L, Schmidt-Hegemann NS, Ferentinos K, Zamboglou C (2023) PSMA-PET/CT-guided salvage radiotherapy in recurrent or persistent prostate cancer and PSA < 0.2 ng/ml. Eur J Nucl Med Mol Imaging 50:2529–2536
133. Scharl S, Zamboglou C, Strouthos I, Farolfi A, Serani F, Lanzafame H, Giuseppe Morganti A, Trapp C, Koerber SA, Debus J, Peeken JC, Vogel MME, Vrachimis A, Spohn SKB, Ruf J, Grosu AL, Ceci F, Fendler WP, Bartenstein P, Kroeze SGC, Guckenberger M, Krafcsik M, Klopscheck C, Fanti S, Hruby G, Emmett L, Belka C, Stief C, Schmidt-Hegemann NS, Henkenberens C, Mayer B, Miksch J, Shelan M, Aebersold DM, Thamm R, Wiegel T (2023) Salvage radiotherapy is effective in patients with PSMA-PET-negative biochemical recurrence- results of a retrospective study. Radiother Oncol 184:109678
134. Adebahr S, Althaus A, Scharl S, Strouthos I, Farolfi A, Serani F, Lanzafame H, Trapp C, Koerber SA, Peeken JC, Vogel MME, Vrachimis A, Spohn SKB, Grosu AL, Kroeze SGC, Guckenberger M, Fanti S, Hruby G, Emmett L, Belka C, Schmidt-Hegemann NS, Henkenberens C, Aebersold DM, Wiegel T, Afshar-Oromieh A, Zamboglou C, Shelan M (2024) The prognostic significance of a negative PSMA-PET scan prior to salvage radiotherapy following radical prostatectomy. Eur J Nucl Med Mol Imaging 51:558–567
135. EAU Guidelines on Prostate Cancer (2023/2024)
136. Spohn SKB, Schmidt-Hegemann NS, Ruf J, Mix M, Benndorf M, Bamberg F, Makowski MR, Kirste S, Ruhle A, Nouvel J, Sprave T, Vogel MME, Galitsnaya P, Gschwend JE, Gratzke C, Stief C, Lock S, Zwanenburg A, Trapp C, Bernhardt D, Nekolla SG, Li M, Belka

C, Combs SE, Eiber M, Unterrainer L, Unterrainer M, Bartenstein P, Grosu AL, Zamboglou C, Peeken JC (2023) Development of PSMA-PET-guided CT-based radiomic signature to predict biochemical recurrence after salvage radiotherapy. Eur J Nucl Med Mol Imaging 50:2537–2547
137. Lecouvet FE, Geukens D, Stainier A, Jamar F, Jamart J, d'Othee BJ, Therasse P, Vande Berg B, Tombal B (2007) Magnetic resonance imaging of the axial skeleton for detecting bone metastases in patients with high-risk prostate cancer: diagnostic and cost-effectiveness and comparison with current detection strategies. J Clin Oncol 25:3281–3287
138. Woo S, Suh CH, Kim SY, Cho JY, Kim SH (2018) Diagnostic performance of magnetic resonance imaging for the detection of bone metastasis in prostate cancer: a systematic review and meta-analysis. Eur Urol 73:81–91
139. Pyka T, Okamoto S, Dahlbender M, Tauber R, Retz M, Heck M, Tamaki N, Schwaiger M, Maurer T, Eiber M (2016) Comparison of bone scintigraphy and (68)Ga-PSMA PET for skeletal staging in prostate cancer. Eur J Nucl Med Mol Imaging 43:2114–2121
140. Liu F, Dong J, Shen Y, Yun C, Wang R, Wang G, Tan J, Wang T, Yao Q, Wang B, Li L, Mi J, Zhou D, Xiong F (2021) Comparison of PET/CT and MRI in the diagnosis of bone metastasis in prostate cancer patients: a network analysis of diagnostic studies. Front Oncol 11:736654
141. Madsen C, Fuglo D, Pedersen M, Broholm R, Ostergren PB, Bisbjerg R, Kongsted P, Nielsen K, Haarmark C, Zacho H (2025) Prospective head-to-head comparison of (18)F-PSMA PET/CT and (18)F-NaF PET/CT for assessing bone metastases in 160 patients with newly diagnosed high-risk prostate cancer. J Nucl Med 66:223–229
142. Koh WJ, Abu-Rustum NR, Bean S, Bradley K, Campos SM, Cho KR, Chon HS, Chu C, Clark R, Cohn D, Crispens MA, Damast S, Dorigo O, Eifel PJ, Fisher CM, Frederick P, Gaffney DK, Han E, Huh WK, Lurain JR, Mariani A, Mutch D, Nagel C, Nekhlyudov L, Fader AN, Remmenga SW, Reynolds RK, Tillmanns T, Ueda S, Wyse E, Yashar CM, McMillian NR, Scavone JL (2019) Cervical cancer, Version 3.2019, NCCN clinical practice guidelines in oncology. J Natl Compr Cancer Netw 17:64–84
143. Marth C, Landoni F, Mahner S, McCormack M, Gonzalez-Martin A, Colombo N, Committee EG (2017) Cervical cancer: ESMO clinical practice guidelines for diagnosis, treatment and follow-up. Ann Oncol 28:iv72–iv83
144. Havrilesky LJ, Kulasingam SL, Matchar DB, Myers ER (2005) FDG-PET for management of cervical and ovarian cancer. Gynecol Oncol 97:183–191
145. Kidd EA, Siegel BA, Dehdashti F, Rader JS, Mutic S, Mutch DG, Powell MA, Grigsby PW (2010) Clinical outcomes of definitive intensity-modulated radiation therapy with fluorodeoxyglucose-positron emission tomography simulation in patients with locally advanced cervical cancer. Int J Radiat Oncol Biol Phys 77:1085–1091
146. Grigsby PW, Singh AK, Siegel BA, Dehdashti F, Rader J, Zoberi I (2004) Lymph node control in cervical cancer. Int J Radiat Oncol Biol Phys 59:706–712
147. Koh WJ, Abu-Rustum NR, Bean S, Bradley K, Campos SM, Cho KR, Chon HS, Chu C, Cohn D, Crispens MA, Damast S, Dorigo O, Eifel PJ, Fisher CM, Frederick P, Gaffney DK, George S, Han E, Higgins S, Huh WK, Lurain JR 3rd, Mariani A, Mutch D, Nagel C, Nekhlyudov L, Fader AN, Remmenga SW, Reynolds RK, Tillmanns T, Ueda S, Wyse E, Yashar CM, McMillian NR, Scavone JL (2018) Uterine neoplasms, Version 1.2018, NCCN clinical practice guidelines in oncology. J Natl Compr Cancer Netw 16:170–199
148. Antonsen SL, Jensen LN, Loft A, Berthelsen AK, Costa J, Tabor A, Qvist I, Hansen MR, Fisker R, Andersen ES, Sperling L, Nielsen AL, Asmussen J, Hogdall E, Fago-Olsen CL, Christensen IJ, Nedergaard L, Jochumsen K, Hogdall C (2013) MRI, PET/CT and ultrasound in the preoperative staging of endometrial cancer - a multicenter prospective comparative study. Gynecol Oncol 128:300–308
149. Crivellaro C, Signorelli M, Guerra L, De Ponti E, Pirovano C, Fruscio R, Elisei F, Montanelli L, Buda A, Messa C (2013) Tailoring systematic lymphadenectomy in high-risk clinical early stage endometrial cancer: the role of 18F-FDG PET/CT. Gynecol Oncol 130:306–311

150. Husby JA, Reitan BC, Biermann M, Trovik J, Bjorge L, Magnussen IJ, Salvesen OO, Salvesen HB, Haldorsen IS (2015) Metabolic tumor volume on 18F-FDG PET/CT improves preoperative identification of high-risk endometrial carcinoma patients. J Nucl Med 56:1191–1198
151. Signorelli M, Crivellaro C, Buda A, Guerra L, Fruscio R, Elisei F, Dolci C, Cuzzocrea M, Milani R, Messa C (2015) Staging of high-risk endometrial cancer with PET/CT and sentinel lymph node mapping. Clin Nucl Med 40:780–785
152. Li X, Shi W, Zhang Q, Lin X, Sun H (2025) A radiogenomics study on (18)F-FDG PET/CT in endometrial cancer by a novel deep learning segmentation algorithm. BMC Cancer 25:1006

The Role of Molecular Imaging in Ion Beam Therapy

33

Semi Harrabi and Jürgen Debus

33.1 Introduction

During the last decades, radiation oncology has undergone transformative technological advancements. The evolution from two-dimensional to computed tomography (CT)-based three-dimensional treatment planning laid the groundwork for increasingly sophisticated therapeutic strategies. The development of inverse treatment planning, enabled by advanced computer algorithms, allowed clinicians to optimize dose distributions while minimizing exposure to organs at risk. These innovations facilitated the clinical implementation of intensity-modulated radiotherapy, followed by stereotactic techniques such as radiosurgery using a Gamma Knife or specialized linear accelerators—collectively raising the level of precision in photon-based therapies.

In parallel with these developments in photon radiotherapy, ion beam therapy—most commonly using protons and carbon ions and more recently also helium ions—emerged as a high-precision treatment modality. Owing to its superior dose distribution and reduced integral dose to surrounding healthy tissue, ion beam therapy offers distinct physical and biological advantages. The unique inverse depth-dose profile of particle beams allows for low entrance doses, a sharp rise in dose deposition (the Bragg peak at the tumour site), and an abrupt fall-off beyond the target. Notably, carbon ions exhibit a narrower lateral dose profile (penumbra) than protons, enabling even more conformal dose delivery.

In terms of biological effectiveness, particle therapy exhibits significant variability. While protons have a relative biological effectiveness (RBE) similar to photons,

S. Harrabi · J. Debus (✉)
Heidelberg University Hospital, Department of Radiation Oncology, Heidelberg Ion Beam Therapy Centre (HIT), Heidelberg, Baden-Württemberg, Germany
e-mail: juergen.debus@med.uni-heidelberg.de

O. Schober et al. (eds.), *Molecular Imaging in Oncology - Volume 2*, Recent Results in Cancer Research 225, https://doi.org/10.1007/978-3-032-21415-7_15

carbon ions have a higher mass and charge that results in a higher linear energy transfer (LET) along the trajectory. High-LET radiation tends to cause more clustered DNA damage, which is more difficult for cells to repair, what leads to a 3–5-fold higher RBE of carbon ions compared to photons. Furthermore, RBE is also determined by dose and tissue type. Accurately modelling these effects requires complex biological models. In clinical practice, active beam delivery is favoured over passive scattering to minimize unwanted neutron production and enhance dose precision.

The combination of high local RBE and the high dose conformity makes carbon ion radiation therapy a powerful treatment option for tumours with higher resistance to radiation and in cases where critical healthy tissue is located adjacent to the target volume. Exploitation of the Bragg peak can expand the therapeutic range as in tumours at the skull base with close proximity to the optic system, brain stem, or spinal cord. Furthermore, ion beam therapy can be used in cases of reirradiation in which high radiation doses have already been applied and the surrounding normal structures show lower radiation tolerances than in the de novo case and would otherwise be dose-limiting.

Despite these physical advantages, the steep dose gradients of ion beams together with the increasing precision of treatment delivery impose the demand for accurate target volume delineation to reduce the risk of geographic miss; even small uncertainties in tumour definition could compromise therapeutic outcomes. Image guidance, especially when performed in treatment position prior to irradiation, is the method of choice to exploit the full potential of particle therapy.

Anatomical imaging alone, such as CT or MRI, often falls short—particularly when attempting to differentiate between viable tumour tissue and benign changes like fibrosis or post-treatment scar tissue. This challenge is especially pronounced in heterogeneous, infiltrative, or previously treated tumours.

Molecular imaging, particularly positron emission tomography (PET), provides valuable functional and biological information that complements morphological data. By visualizing metabolic activity, hypoxia, proliferation, or receptor expression, PET enables more confident and individualized tumour characterization.

33.2 Molecular Imaging in Treatment Planning

The integration of molecular imaging into radiotherapy planning has become increasingly significant, particularly for ion beam therapy, where the steep dose gradients and biological properties demand highly accurate tumour delineation. Modern high precision radiation techniques require exact targeting to avoid geographical misses but also to maximize the therapeutic ratio, e.g., by applying higher doses within a boost irradiation plan to regions within the target volume that is likely to exhibit increased radiation resistance.

Although molecular imaging also includes specialized MR imaging and certain rather novel techniques of functional MRI, such as protein-weighted MRI using chemical exchange saturation transfer or dynamic glucose-enhanced MRI has been applied for radiotherapy planning and response monitoring in the context of clinical studies, there is far more published evidence on PET in the context of ion beam therapy, and will therefore the focus of this article.

33.2.1 FDG-PET: Glucose Metabolism for Tumour Characterization

2-Fluor-2-deoxy-D-glucose (FDG) PET is the most widely used molecular imaging modality in oncology and plays a central role in radiation treatment planning. FDG is taken up by tumour cells due to their increased glycolytic activity and overexpression of glucose transporters. While FDG is not tumour-specific and is also taken up by inflammatory and some normal tissues, it has proven reliable in evaluating tumour burden, guiding biopsy, staging disease, and assessing treatment response.

In radiation oncology, and particularly in the context of ion beam therapy, FDG-PET provides critical functional data that enhances the accuracy of gross tumour volume (GTV) delineation [1]. This is particularly important in anatomically complex regions or after prior treatment, where conventional imaging may be confounded by post-therapeutic changes such as fibrosis or necrosis. FDG-PET can distinguish metabolically active tumour from such nonmalignant tissues, improving targeting precision and potentially reducing the volume of normal tissue exposed to high radiation doses.

In non-small cell lung cancer, FDG-PET/CT is now the standard of care for initial staging and is used routinely in defining GTVs for radiotherapy. This approach allows for accurate identification of involved lymph nodes and distant metastases, enabling proper stratification and exclusion of patients from local therapy when systemic disease is present [2]. In head and neck cancer, where tumours often infiltrate tissues and recur in previously irradiated fields, FDG-PET can differentiate viable tumour from post-treatment effects, thus guiding high-precision reirradiation strategies using protons or carbon ions.

In paediatric patients, FDG-PET is widely used for staging of tumours such as neuroblastoma (when Metaiodobenzylguanidine (MIBG)-negative), osteosarcoma, Ewing sarcoma, and rhabdomyosarcoma [3]. Its high sensitivity allows for accurate detection of nodal and distant metastases. Because children are particularly susceptible to the long-term effects of radiation, the role of FDG-PET in refining target volumes is crucial [4–6]. Proton therapy, with its reduced integral dose, is commonly used in this population to spare healthy tissue and reduce the risk of growth disturbances, hormonal deficiencies, and secondary malignancies. In this context, accurate tumour delineation via FDG-PET supports the use of proton therapy for maximal therapeutic benefit. A compelling application of FDG-PET in ion beam therapy is illustrated in a single-centre phase I/II trial evaluating combined ion-beam radiotherapy—using both protons and a carbon ion boost—in patients with inoperable osteosarcoma [7]. The trial included 20 patients with primarily pelvic or craniofacial disease, treated with 54 Gy RBE protons followed by an 18 Gy RBE carbon ion boost. FDG-PET/CT was used prior to therapy for diagnostic assessment and to identify metabolic activity as a potential prognostic factor. The study reported encouraging outcomes in this difficult-to-treat population, with a two-year overall survival of 68% and a local progression-free survival of 55%. Crucially, low FDG uptake and craniofacial tumour localization were both associated with improved survival. These findings underscore FDG-PET's role not only in target delineation but also in predicting therapeutic response and guiding dose escalation via carbon ion boost planning. Notably, outcomes appear even more favourable in patients with craniofacial osteosarcoma, where a separate cohort treated with carbon ion radiotherapy (CIRT) achieved a 5-year overall survival rate exceeding 80%, significantly higher than historical outcomes for this population [8]. This evidence supports the incorporation of FDG-PET into routine ion beam therapy planning for selected tumour types, particularly where aggressive biology or anatomical inoperability limit treatment options, enabling accurate target volume definition, biological characterization of tumours, and adaptive strategies that are essential for maximizing tumour control while minimizing toxicity in high-precision radiotherapy settings.

The value of FDG-PET extends beyond initial planning. Adaptive strategies based on interim PET imaging are increasingly used to inform treatment modifications. For example, the metabolic response to therapy can serve as a surrogate for radiosensitivity, allowing clinicians to escalate or de-escalate dose based on early treatment response. This has been particularly well-studied in lymphoma, where residual FDG uptake after chemotherapy can guide decisions regarding the use and extent of consolidation radiotherapy [9].

The utility of FDG-PET also extends into treatment response prediction. Studies in head and neck squamous cell carcinoma have shown that PET/CT performed approximately 12 weeks after radiotherapy can help differentiate between residual disease and post-treatment inflammation [10]. This can spare patients unnecessary surgeries, such as neck dissections, when PET shows a complete metabolic response. Such predictive use of FDG-PET may be particularly important in carbon ion reirradiation cases, where precision is critical and morphological imaging may be insufficient due to anatomical distortion from prior therapies [11].

Despite its many strengths, FDG-PET is prone to false positive signals due to uptake in areas of inflammation, infection, or physiologically active tissues like brain, brown fat, and bone marrow. Therefore, careful interpretation in conjunction with anatomical imaging and clinical context is essential. The need for standardized protocols, including uptake thresholds and segmentation methods, remains a subject of ongoing research.

In summary, FDG-PET is a foundational tool for personalized treatment planning in ion beam therapy, enabling accurate target volume definition, biological characterization of tumours, and adaptive strategies that are essential for maximizing tumour control while minimizing toxicity in high-precision radiotherapy settings.

33.2.2 FAPI-PET: Fibroblast Activation as a Target

The recent development of fibroblast activation protein inhibitor (FAPI) PET tracers represents a novel and promising approach to tumour imaging. FAPI binds to fibroblast activation protein, which is overexpressed by cancer-associated fibroblasts in the tumour microenvironment of various solid tumours, including breast, pancreatic, colorectal, and gastric cancers. Unlike traditional tracers such as FDG, FAPI-PET demonstrates minimal background uptake in normal tissues such as the brain, liver, and oral-laryngeal mucosa, offering superior tumour-to-background contrast in these anatomical regions [12, 13].

A key advantage of FAPI-PET is its patient convenience, as it does not require fasting and can be performed without a delay following tracer injection. This makes it a more flexible tool in routine clinical workflows. However, FAPI is not without limitations. Similar to FDG, it can accumulate in areas of inflammation, which may limit its specificity in certain clinical contexts. Nevertheless, its potential utility in radiation oncology—particularly in ion beam therapy—is considerable.

One of the most compelling clinical applications of FAPI-PET is in the treatment planning of pancreatic cancer, a malignancy characterized by late diagnosis, poor prognosis, and a highly desmoplastic stroma. This tumour microenvironment leads to poor perfusion, hypoxia, and resistance to conventional therapies. The dense stromal content can represent up to 90% of the tumour mass, making it an ideal target for FAPI-based imaging. Conventional imaging techniques such as FDG-PET have shown limited sensitivity and specificity in pancreatic cancer, particularly for nodal staging and assessment of treatment response [14–17].

In this context, carbon ion therapy has emerged as a promising treatment modality due to its superior dose conformity and higher RBE, which are particularly beneficial in overcoming the radio-resistance associated with pancreatic tumours. The Japan Carbon-ion Radiation Oncology Study Group has reported encouraging outcomes using carbon ion therapy with concomitant gemcitabine chemotherapy for patients with inoperable pancreatic ductal adenocarcinoma, demonstrating a median overall survival of over 21 months [18, 19]. These results suggest that biologically effective dose escalation is feasible and beneficial in this setting.

FAPI-PET/CT has the potential to further enhance these outcomes by improving target volume delineation, especially in cases where tumour margins are poorly defined on CT or MRI. It can also support biological dose painting, identifying subvolumes within the tumour that may benefit from LET- or RBE-guided escalation using carbon ions. Additionally, FAPI-PET may assist in treatment response assessment, helping to distinguish viable tumour tissue from fibrosis or inflammation, which is particularly challenging in post-treatment pancreatic cancer patients.

As research progresses, FAPI-PET may become an indispensable tool in the management of desmoplastic tumours. For ion beam therapy, which demands high spatial precision and benefits most from biologically informed planning, the use of FAPI-based imaging could significantly improve patient outcomes through more accurate targeting, dose escalation in resistant regions, and better patient selection for high-cost modalities like carbon ion therapy. Currently, the role is investigated in the prospective phase II trial PACK [20].

33.2.3 DOTATOC-PET: Receptor Imaging in Skull Base Meningioma

^{68}Ga-DOTATOC PET/CT is a somatostatin receptor-targeted imaging modality that plays a significant role in the management of skull base meningiomas, particularly when tumours are inoperable or histological confirmation is not available. These tumours frequently arise in anatomically complex regions such as the sphenoidal wing, petroclival area, or cavernous sinus, where surgical resection carries a high risk of morbidity. In such cases, radiation therapy—especially ion beam therapy—has emerged as a crucial therapeutic option, offering high local control while sparing adjacent critical structures.

DOTATOC-PET is highly sensitive for meningioma detection due to the overexpression of somatostatin receptor subtype 2 (SSTR2) in these tumours. Compared to MRI, it provides superior tumour-to-background contrast, particularly in regions adjacent to the falx cerebri or skull base, where conventional imaging may be ambiguous. This makes DOTATOC-PET particularly useful for both diagnosis and target volume delineation.

Edotreotide or (DOTA(0)-Phe(1)-Tyr(3))octreotide (DOTATOC)-PET helps identify tumour borders more clearly than MRI alone, which can struggle to differentiate tumour from postoperative scar tissue or surrounding anatomical structures. Accurate GTV definition is critical, as benign meningiomas typically have no additional clinical target volume expansion, and geographic misses could result in treatment failure. A recent study involving 47 patients—including 30 with meningioma—demonstrated that the integration of DOTA-PET/CT into treatment planning improved interobserver consistency and enhanced the detection of tumour volumes not visible on MRI [21]. In several cases, PET/CT identified additional tumour areas that were critical for radiation planning, underscoring the value of DOTATOC-PET in ensuring comprehensive and accurate target volume delineation for highly conformal ion beam therapy. In this context, the potential clinical integration of helium ions represents an exciting development [22]. Helium ions combine the favourable depth-dose characteristics of protons with even sharper distal and lateral dose gradients and a more favourable RBE profile. In-silico treatment planning studies using Monte Carlo-based engines have shown that helium ions provide comparable target coverage with improved sparing of surrounding critical structures, particularly in tumours adjacent to organs-at-risk such as brain and ocular meningiomas [23]. When combined with precise molecular imaging such as DOTATOC-PET, helium ion therapy could further reduce radiation-induced side effects and represents a promising modality for treating tumours in highly conformal, anatomically complex regions.

Clinical experience has shown that DOTATOC-PET is valuable not only for initial planning but also for reirradiation strategies and treatment of atypical meningiomas, where treatments with carbon ions are currently being investigated [24]. These approaches aim to leverage the higher LET and RBE of carbon ions to improve tumour control in more aggressive subtypes. Recent clinical evidence from a prospective phase II trial has shown that bimodal radiotherapy, consisting of a carbon ion boost (18 Gy RBE) combined with photon RT (50 Gy), yields promising results in patients with subtotal resection of grade 2 meningiomas [25]. With a median follow-up of 42 months, the study reported 3-year progression-free survival and overall survival rates of over 80% and 89%, respectively. These outcomes suggest a potential therapeutic advantage over standard photon regimens.

33.3 In-Vivo Range Verification and Beam Monitoring

High-precision ion beam therapy relies heavily on accurate beam delivery and precise targeting of the tumour. While the unique physical and biological properties of ion beams—such as the Bragg peak and increased RBE—enable superior tumour conformity and sparing of normal tissue, they also demand advanced monitoring strategies to mitigate uncertainties that arise from tissue characteristics and positioning accuracies. In particular, knowledge of the actual beam range within the patient is critical to ensure the intended dose distribution.

Traditionally, range prediction is based on converting X-ray computed tomography (CT) images into stopping power ratios, which estimate the ion beam penetration in tissue compared to water. However, this semiempirical conversion introduces inherent range uncertainties of approximately 3%, compounded further by inter-fractional anatomical changes and patient positioning inaccuracies [26]. Consequently, safety margins must be conservatively applied, often at the cost of optimal normal tissue sparing. Reducing these uncertainties is central to realizing the full therapeutic potential of ion beam therapy, especially in hypofractionated treatments or reirradiation scenarios.

To address this challenge, several in-vivo treatment monitoring techniques have been explored, including PET, prompt gamma imaging, and charged secondary ion detection. These modalities aim to provide real-time or near-real-time feedback on the actual beam path and range within the patient.

33.3.1 Range Verification by Positron Emission Tomography (PET)

PET-based range monitoring exploits the production of positron-emitting isotopes such as ^{11}C and ^{10}C during nuclear interactions of the ion beam with patient tissue. These isotopes decay with half-lives of approximately 20 min, respectively, emitting positrons that annihilate into two 511 keV photons. By detecting these photons, PET systems can reconstruct the spatial distribution of activated tissue and compare it to the expected dose deposition.

This method has been successfully implemented at carbon ion centres, demonstrating the capability to detect misalignments or deviations in dose delivery with sub-millimetre accuracy [27, 28]. Despite its promise, PET range verification remains limited by the low amount of activation signal, differences in biological washout, and logistical challenges associated with online acquisition and image reconstruction. While offline PET has seen early clinical use in carbon ion radiotherapy [29], more recent efforts at facilities such as National Center of Oncological Hadrontherapy (CNAO) in Italy have led to the development and clinical trial use of online PET systems [30].

33.3.2 Prompt Gamma Imaging (PGI)

Prompt gamma imaging (PGI) is a real-time method for in vivo range verification during particle therapy. It detects high-energy gamma photons (2–10 MeV) emitted within nanoseconds of inelastic nuclear interactions between therapeutic ion beams and tissue. Unlike PET, PGI does not suffer from biological washout and offers immediate feedback, making it especially promising for adaptive treatment strategies [31].

Several PGI systems are under development:

- Slit cameras use collimated detectors to produce one-dimensional range profiles. Clinical prototypes have demonstrated range shift detection with ~2 mm accuracy during proton therapy.
- Fast scintillator systems such as prompt gamma spectroscopy and prompt gamma timing measure energy and time-of-flight to deduce beam range with high precision.
- Compton cameras (CC) reconstruct 3D emission profiles using gamma scattering events and are advancing toward clinical testing.

Despite these advances, PGI remains technically challenging in carbon ion radiotherapy (CIRT) due to the significantly lower prompt gamma yield—about 20 times less than in protons—resulting in poor signal-to-noise ratios. In summary, PGI offers a noninvasive, real-time range verification method with strong potential in proton therapy [32]. For CIRT, alternative approaches such as PET and secondary ion tracking currently remain more practical.

33.3.3 Charged Secondary Ion Detection

An emerging technique with substantial potential involves detecting charged nuclear fragments—predominantly protons and helium ions—that are emitted during ion-tissue nuclear interactions. These secondary ions provide a distinct advantage for range verification, as they are emitted along the beam path with minimal background signal. By measuring their origins and trajectories, it is possible to infer variations in patient anatomy or positioning with high specificity [33].

Despite their promise, secondary ions undergo multiple Coulomb scattering within tissue, leading to angular deviations that can affect spatial resolution. Nevertheless, the overwhelming forward emission and lack of background particles make this method especially appealing. The Innovative Solutions for Dosimetry in Hadrontherapy (INSIDE) collaboration at CNAO has already demonstrated its feasibility in clinical trials using a detector composed of scintillating fibres and silicon photomultipliers [30]. More recently, a monitoring system based on Timepix3 pixel detectors has been developed and implemented in the InViMo clinical trial at the Heidelberg Ion Beam Therapy Centre (HIT), specifically targeting skull base tumours [33, 34].

33.4 Emerging Technologies and Future Directions

33.4.1 Hypoxia-Guided Treatment Personalization

Tumour hypoxia is a well-established mechanism of radioresistance, posing a major limitation for conventional photon-based radiotherapy. Hypoxic tumours are less susceptible to indirect DNA damage caused by free radicals generated through ionizing radiation due to the lack of molecular oxygen, which stabilizes DNA damage. However, carbon ion radiotherapy offers an important biological advantage through its high LET. LET-optimization in CIRT has emerged as a promising strategy to enhance tumour control while preserving normal tissue safety—especially in the context of radioresistant or hypoxic tumours. Unlike conventional photon or even proton therapy, carbon ions inherently possess high LET near the Bragg peak, leading to densely clustered and irreparable DNA damage. However, the LET distribution within a tumour is not uniform, and clinical evidence increasingly suggests that regions with insufficient LET—particularly in hypoxic tumour sub-volumes—may limit therapeutic efficacy [35].

Recent studies have shown that the minimum dose-averaged LET within the GTV is a significant predictor of local control in various malignancies [36–38]. This insight has led to the development of LET painting—a technique designed to modulate beam delivery to increase LET in specific tumour regions without exceeding clinical dose constraints to organs at risk. In head and neck cancers, LET painting has demonstrated the ability to raise minimum LETd by 8–24 keV/μm while maintaining homogeneous RBE-weighted dose coverage [39].

Innovative delivery approaches, such as multifield optimization and arc-based carbon beam scanning (e.g., Spot-Scanning Hadron Arc (SHArc)), have further expanded the possibilities for LET optimization, achieving LETd values above 70 keV/μm in complex tumour geometries. Importantly, these advances have been validated in both phantom experiments and early-phase clinical trials, showing promising tumour response rates with acceptable toxicity profiles [39–41].

Molecular imaging of tumour hypoxia using radiolabelled PET tracers such as ^{18}F-fluoromisonidazole (^{18}F-FMISO), ^{18}F-fluoroazomycin-arabinoside (^{18}F-FAZA), and ^{18}F-HX4 has enabled non-invasive detection and quantification of hypoxia. These tracers accumulate in hypoxic but viable tumour regions, and increased uptake has been shown to correlate with poorer treatment outcomes.

A randomized phase II trial in locally advanced head-and-neck cancer confirmed the prognostic relevance of tumour hypoxia using dynamic ^{18}F-FMISO PET/CT. Among 53 patients, 74% had hypoxic tumours. Those without hypoxia had excellent 5-year local control (LC) of 100%, compared to 74% in hypoxic cases ($p = 0.039$). Patients with hypoxia were randomized to standard radiochemotherapy (70 Gy) or functional dose escalation to 77 Gy within the hypoxic subvolume. The dose escalation group showed improved 5-year LC (84% vs. 59%), though not statistically significant due to small sample size ($p = 0.150$). Importantly, toxicity was not increased with dose escalation, supporting its feasibility. While limited by complexity and early trial closure, the study suggests that hypoxia-guided dose painting is safe and may enhance tumour control in selected patients [42].

Standardization of hypoxia imaging protocols and quantification strategies will be essential to enable integration into multicentre trials and facilitate its role in personalized radiotherapy planning. As hypoxia remains one of the main biological targets for improvement in cancer radiotherapy, the combination of LET-optimized CIRT and hypoxia-guided imaging represents a promising frontier.

33.4.2 Challenges and Future Directions

Molecular imaging, particularly positron emission tomography (PET), provides valuable functional and biological information that complements morphological data. By visualizing metabolic activity, hypoxia, proliferation, or receptor expression, PET enables more confident and individualized tumour characterization. However, clinical integration remains complex. Partial volume effects, limited spatial resolution, and dependence on tracer uptake thresholds (e.g., standardized uptake value) pose challenges for accurate segmentation. While automated contouring is generally more reproducible than visual interpretation, a universally accepted segmentation strategy has yet to be established.

Ion beam therapy currently remains a resource-intensive modality due to technological complexity, size, and cost of the building and operating ion beam therapy centres—especially those offering multi-ion species. Thus, its availability remains limited. As of 2025, approximately 116 proton therapy centres are in operation globally, compared to only sixteen carbon ion facilities (Particle Therapy Co-Operative Group, PTCOG 2025). This restricted access underscores the importance of maximizing the therapeutic benefit of ion beam therapy through personalized treatment strategies, where molecular imaging plays a central role—not only in initial target volume delineation but also in guiding biologically tailored planning, adaptation, and response assessment.

References

1. Farina E, Ferioli M, Castellucci P, Farina A, Rambaldi GZ, Cilla S, Cammelli S, Fanti S, Morganti AG (2017) 18F-Fdg-PET-guided planning and re-planning (adaptive) radiotherapy in head and neck cancer: current state of art. Anticancer Res 37(12):6523–6532
2. Brose A, Miederer I, König J, Gkika E, Sahlmann J, Schimek-Jasch T, Schreckenberger M, Nestle U, Kappes J, Miederer M (2024) Prognostic value of metabolic tumor volume on [(18) F]FDG PET/CT in addition to the TNM classification system of locally advanced non-small cell lung cancer. Cancer Imaging 24(1):171
3. Chambers G, Frood R, Patel C, Scarsbrook A (2019) ^{18} F-FDG PET-CT in paediatric oncology: established and emerging applications. Br J Radiol 92(1094):20180584
4. Gatta G, Botta L, Rossi S, Aareleid T, Bielska-Lasota M, Clavel J, Dimitrova N, Jakab Z, Kaatsch P, Lacour B, Mallone S, Marcos-Gragera R, Minicozzi P, Sánchez-Pérez M-J, Sant M, Santaquilani M, Stiller C, Tavilla A, Trama A, Visser O, Peris-Bonet R (2014) Childhood cancer survival in Europe 1999–2007: results of EUROCARE-5—a population-based study. Lancet Oncol 15(1):35–47
5. Merchant TE, Rose SR, Bosley C, Wu S, Xiong X, Lustig RH (2011) Growth hormone secretion after conformal radiation therapy in pediatric patients with localized brain tumors. J Clin Oncol 29(36):4776–4780
6. Vatner RE, Niemierko A, Misra M, Weyman EA, Goebel CP, Ebb DH, Jones RM, Huang MS, Mahajan A, Grosshans DR, Paulino AC, Stanley T, MacDonald SM, Tarbell NJ, Yock TI (2018) Endocrine deficiency as a function of radiation dose to the hypothalamus and pituitary in pediatric and young adult patients with brain tumors. J Clin Oncol 36(28):2854–2862
7. Seidensaal K, Mattke M, Haufe S, Rathke H, Haberkorn U, Bougatf N, Kudak A, Blattmann C, Oertel S, Kirchner M, Buesch C, Kieser M, Herfarth K, Kulozik A, Debus J, Uhl M, Harrabi SB (2021) The role of combined ion-beam radiotherapy (CIBRT) with protons and carbon ions in a multimodal treatment strategy of inoperable osteosarcoma. Radiother Oncol 159:8–16
8. Seidensaal K, Dostal M, Liermann J, Adeberg S, Weykamp F, Schmid MP, Freudlsperger C, Hoffmann J, Hompland I, Herfarth K, Debus J, Harrabi SB (2022) Inoperable or incompletely resected craniofacial osteosarcoma treated by particle radiotherapy. Front Oncol 12:927399
9. Freeman CL, Savage KJ, Villa DR, Scott DW, Srour L, Gerrie AS, Brown MJ, Slack GW, Farinha P, Skinnider B, Morris J, Bénard F, Aquino-Parsons C, Lo A, Pickles T, Wilson DC, Tonseth P, Connors JM, Sehn LH (2021) Long-term results of PET-guided radiation in patients with advanced-stage diffuse large B-cell lymphoma treated with R-CHOP. Blood 137(7):929–938
10. Mehanna H, Wong W-L, McConkey CC, Rahman JK, Robinson M, Hartley AGJ, Nutting C, Powell N, Al-Booz H, Robinson M, Junor E, Rizwanullah M, Von Zeidler SV, Wieshmann H, Hulme C, Smith AF, Hall P, Dunn J (2016) PET-CT surveillance versus neck dissection in advanced head and neck cancer. N Engl J Med 374(15):1444–1454
11. Held T, Lang K, Regnery S, Weusthof K, Hommertgen A, Jäkel C, Tonndorf-Martini E, Krisam J, Plinkert P, Zaoui K, Freudlsperger C, Moratin J, Krauss J, Harrabi SB, Herfarth K, Debus J, Adeberg S (2020) Carbon ion reirradiation compared to intensity-modulated re-radiotherapy for recurrent head and neck cancer (CARE): a randomized controlled trial. Radiat Oncol 15(1):190
12. Giesel FL, Kratochwil C, Lindner T, Marschalek MM, Loktev A, Lehnert W, Debus J, Jäger D, Flechsig P, Altmann A, Mier W, Haberkorn U (2019) ^{68} Ga-FAPI PET/CT: biodistribution and preliminary dosimetry estimate of 2 DOTA-containing FAP-targeting agents in patients with various cancers. J Nucl Med 60(3):386–392
13. Loktev A, Lindner T, Mier W, Debus J, Altmann A, Jäger D, Giesel F, Kratochwil C, Barthe P, Roumestand C, Haberkorn U (2018) A tumor-imaging method targeting cancer-associated fibroblasts. J Nucl Med 59(9):1423–1429
14. Wang Z (2013) FDG-PET in diagnosis, staging and prognosis of pancreatic carcinoma: a meta-analysis. World J Gastroenterol 19(29):4808

15. Zhang Z, Guo S, Su W, Pan G, Cao K, Jiang H, Zhang L, Cheng C, Jin G, Zuo C (2025) Preoperative assessment of pancreatic cancer with [(68)Ga]Ga-DOTA-FAPI-04 PET/MR versus [(18)F]-FDG PET/CT plus contrast-enhanced CT: a prospective preliminary study. Eur J Nucl Med Mol Imaging 52(3):1017–1027
16. Yun WG, Gil J, Choi H, Han Y, Jung HS, Cho YJ, Suh M, Kwon W, Lee YS, Cheon GJ, Jang JY (2024) Prospective comparison of [(18)F]FDG and [(18)F]AIF-FAPI-74 PET/CT in the evaluation of potentially resectable pancreatic ductal adenocarcinoma. Mol Imaging Biol 26(6):1068–1077
17. Li X, Lu N, Sun K, Shi F, Lin L, Chen Y, Wang Y, Wang M, Sun K, Xue X, Xiao W, Su X, Bai X, Liang T (2025) [(18)F]FAPI- 04 PET/CT for pathologic response assessment in pancreatic cancer patients with systemic treatment. Eur J Nucl Med Mol Imaging:3938
18. Kawashiro S, Yamada S, Okamoto M, Ohno T, Nakano T, Shinoto M, Shioyama Y, Nemoto K, Isozaki Y, Tsuji H, Kamada T (2018) Multi-institutional study of carbon-ion radiotherapy for locally advanced pancreatic cancer: Japan Carbon-ion Radiation Oncology Study Group (J-CROS) study 1403 pancreas. Int J Radiat Oncol Biol Phys 101(5):1212–1221
19. Shinoto M, Yamada S, Terashima K, Yasuda S, Shioyama Y, Honda H, Kamada T, Tsujii H, Saisho H, Asano T, Yamaguchi T, Amano H, Ishihara T, Otsuka M, Matsuda M, Kainuma O, Funakoshi A, Furuse J, Nakagori T, Okusaka T, Ishii H, Nagakawa T, Takahashi S, Hishinuma S, Nakamura M, Saito H, Ohara K, Ohkawa S, Hiraoka M (2016) Carbon ion radiation therapy with concurrent gemcitabine for patients with locally advanced pancreatic cancer. Int J Radiat Oncol Biol Phys 95(1):498–504
20. Liermann J, Naumann P, Hommertgen A, Pohl M, Kieser M, Debus J, Herfarth K (2020) Carbon ion radiotherapy as definitive treatment in non-metastasized pancreatic cancer: study protocol of the prospective phase II PACK-study. BMC Cancer 20(1):947
21. Lutgendorf-Caucig C, Wieland P, Hug E, Flechl B, Tubin S, Galalae R, Georg P, Fossati P, Mumot M, Harrabi S, Pradler I, Pelak MJ (2024) The value of PET/CT in particle therapy planning of various tumors with SSTR2 receptor expression: comparative interobserver study. Cancers (Basel) 16(10):1877
22. Mairani A, Mein S, Blakely E, Debus J, Durante M, Ferrari A, Fuchs H, Georg D, Grosshans DR, Guan F, Haberer T, Harrabi S, Horst F, Inaniwa T, Karger CP, Mohan R, Paganetti H, Parodi K, Sala P, Schuy C, Tessonnier T, Titt U, Weber U (2022) Roadmap: helium ion therapy. Phys Med Biol 67(15)
23. Tessonnier T, Mairani A, Chen W, Sala P, Cerutti F, Ferrari A, Haberer T, Debus J, Parodi K (2018) Proton and helium ion radiotherapy for meningioma tumors: a Monte Carlo-based treatment planning comparison. Radiat Oncol 13(1):2
24. Li JY, Li JW, Jin YC, Li MX, Guo LP, Bing ZT, Zhang QN, Bai F, Wang XH, Li XX, Yang KH (2021) The efficacy and safety of carbon ion radiotherapy for Meningiomas: a systematic review and meta-analysis. Front Oncol 11:620534
25. Deng MY, Maas SLN, Hinz F, Karger CP, Sievers P, Eichkorn T, Meixner E, Hoegen-Sassmannshausen P, Hörner-Rieber J, Lischalk JW, Seidensaal K, Bernhardt D, Jungk C, Unterberg A, Wick A, Wick W, von Deimling A, Sahm F, Combs S, Herfarth K, Debus J, König L (2024) Efficacy and toxicity of bimodal radiotherapy in WHO grade 2 meningiomas following subtotal resection with carbon ion boost: prospective phase 2 MARCIE trial. Neuro-Oncology 26(4):701–712
26. Paganetti H (2012) Range uncertainties in proton therapy and the role of Monte Carlo simulations. Phys Med Biol 57(11):R99–117
27. Enghardt W, Crespo P, Fiedler F, Hinz R, Parodi K, Pawelke J, Pönisch F (2004) Charged hadron tumour therapy monitoring by means of PET. Nucl Instrum Methods Phys Res, Sect A 525(1):284–288
28. Paganetti H (2025) Proton therapy physics, 3rd edn. Boca Raton, Florida, USA; CRC Press
29. Bauer J, Unholtz D, Sommerer F, Kurz C, Haberer T, Herfarth K, Welzel T, Combs SE, Debus J, Parodi K (2013) Implementation and initial clinical experience of offline PET/CT-based verification of scanned carbon ion treatment. Radiother Oncol 107(2):218–226

30. Kraan AC, Susini F, Moglioni M, Battistoni G, Bersani D, Carra P, Cerello P, De Gregorio A, Ferrero V, Fiorina E, Franciosini G, Morrocchi M, Muraro S, Patera V, Pennazio F, Retico A, Rosso V, Sarti A, Schiavi A, Sportelli G, Traini G, Vischioni B, Vitolo V, Bisogni MG (2024) In-beam PET treatment monitoring of carbon therapy patients: results of a clinical trial at CNAO. Phys Med 125:104493
31. Paganetti H, Beltran C, Both S, Dong L, Flanz J, Furutani K, Grassberger C, Grosshans DR, Knopf A-C, Langendijk JA (2021) Roadmap: proton therapy physics and biology. Phys Med Biol 66(5):05RM1
32. Krimmer J, Dauvergne D, Létang JM, Testa É (2018) Prompt-gamma monitoring in hadrontherapy: a review. Nucl Instrum Methods Phys Res, Sect A 878:58–73
33. Kelleter L, Marek L, Echner G, Ochoa-Parra P, Winter M, Harrabi S, Jakubek J, Jäkel O, Debus J, Martisikova M (2024) An in-vivo treatment monitoring system for ion-beam radiotherapy based on 28 Timepix3 detectors. Sci Rep 14(1):15452
34. Schweins L, Kirchgässner R, Ochoa-Parra P, Winter M, Harrabi S, Mairani A, Jäkel O, Debus J, Martišíková M, Kelleter L (2025) Detection of an internal density change in an anthropomorphic head phantom via tracking of charged nuclear fragments in carbon-ion radiotherapy. Med Phys 52(4):2399–2411
35. Sokol O, Durante M (2023) Carbon ions for hypoxic tumors: are we making the most of them? Cancers (Basel) 15(18):4494
36. Hagiwara Y, Bhattacharyya T, Matsufuji N, Isozaki Y, Takiyama H, Nemoto K, Tsuji H, Yamada S (2020) Influence of dose-averaged linear energy transfer on tumour control after carbon-ion radiation therapy for pancreatic cancer. Clin Transl Radiat Oncol 21:19–24
37. Matsumoto S, Lee SH, Imai R, Inaniwa T, Matsufuji N, Fukahori M, Kohno R, Yonai S, Okonogi N, Yamada S, Kanematsu N (2020) Unresectable chondrosarcomas treated with carbon ion radiotherapy: relationship between dose-averaged linear energy transfer and local recurrence. Anticancer Res 40(11):6429–6435
38. Morelli L, Parrella G, Molinelli S, Magro G, Annunziata S, Mairani A, Chalaszczyk A, Fiore MR, Ciocca M, Paganelli C, Orlandi E, Baroni G (2023) A Dosiomics analysis based on linear energy transfer and biological dose maps to predict local recurrence in sacral Chordomas after carbon-ion radiotherapy. Cancer 15(1):33
39. Kohno R, Koto M, Ikawa H, Lee SH, Sato K, Hashimoto M, Inaniwa T, Shirai T (2024) High-linear energy transfer irradiation in clinical carbon-ion beam with the linear energy transfer painting technique for patients with head and neck cancer. Adv Radiat Oncol 9(1):101317
40. Mein S, Tessonnier T, Kopp B, Schömers C, Harrabi S, Abdollahi A, Debus J, Haberer T, Mairani A (2022) Biological dose optimization for particle arc therapy using helium and carbon ions. Int J Radiat Oncol Biol Phys 114(2):334–348
41. Baltazar F, Longarino FK, Stengl C, Liermann J, Mein S, Debus J, Tessonnier T, Mairani A (2025) Investigating LETd optimization strategies in carbon ion radiotherapy for pancreatic cancer: a dosimetric study using an anthropomorphic phantom. Med Phys 52(3):1746–1757
42. Welz S, Paulsen F, Pfannenberg C, Reimold M, Reischl G, Nikolaou K, La Fougère C, Alber M, Belka C, Zips D, Thorwarth D (2022) Dose escalation to hypoxic subvolumes in head and neck cancer: a randomized phase II study using dynamic [18F]FMISO PET/CT. Radiother Oncol 171:30–36

Internal Radiation Therapy

34

Uwe Haberkorn, Clemens Kratochwil, Eduards Mamlins, Yuriko Mori, and Frederik L. Giesel

Internal radiation therapy or endoradiotherapy of tumors refers to a localized introduction of radioactively labeled particles or molecules with therapeutically usable radiation. This can be done either by invasive methods in which radiolabeled nontumor-affine particles are brought directly to the tissue to be treated (nonspecific method) or by the administration of tumor affinity molecules that selectively accumulate in the tumor after intravenous administration (specific method). An advantage of endoradiotherapy with specific ligands over traditional therapies or immunotherapy is the cross-fire effect induced by the β-particles emanating from

U. Haberkorn
Department of Nuclear Medicine, University Hospital Heidelberg, Heidelberg, Germany

Clinical Cooperation Unit Nuclear Medicine, German Cancer Research Center (DKFZ), Heidelberg, Germany

Translational Lung Research Center Heidelberg (TLRC), German Center for Lung Research (DZL), Heidelberg, Germany
e-mail: uwe.haberkorn@med.uni-heidelberg.de

C. Kratochwil
Department of Nuclear Medicine, University Hospital Heidelberg, Heidelberg, Germany
e-mail: clemens.kratochwil@med.uni-heidelberg.de

E. Mamlins · Y. Mori
Department of Nuclear Medicine, Medical Faculty and University Hospital Duesseldorf, Heinrich-Heine-University Duesseldorf, Duesseldorf, Germany
e-mail: eduards.mamlins@med.uni-duesseldorf.de; yuriko.mori@med.uni-duesseldorf.de

F. L. Giesel (✉)
Department of Nuclear Medicine, Medical Faculty and University Hospital Duesseldorf, Heinrich-Heine-University Duesseldorf, Duesseldorf, Germany

Institute for Radiation Sciences, Osaka University, Osaka, Japan
e-mail: frederik.giesel@med.uni-duesseldorf.de

O. Schober et al. (eds.), *Molecular Imaging in Oncology - Volume 2*, Recent Results in Cancer Research 225, https://doi.org/10.1007/978-3-032-21415-7_16

the binding site. These particles lead to the destruction of multiple cells in the vicinity of the receptor-positive cell and can, therefore, partially compensate for heterogenic expression of the target structure in the tumor. This cannot be achieved with nonradioactive methods, because only those cells are destroyed which bind the molecule used therapeutically. A further increase in the therapeutic effect is achieved by the radiation-induced bystander effect (RIBE). RIBE describes the situation in which cells that are not directly exposed to ionizing radiation behave like exposed cells: these cells die or show chromosomal instabilities. Although the exact mechanism of RIBE is not yet fully understood, there is evidence that chemical signaling leads to deleterious information from exposed cells to adjacent cells.

34.1 Nonspecific Therapy

34.1.1 Selective Internal Radiotherapy (SIRT)

The SIRT radionuclides are introduced into the tumor or metastases via the blood supplying arterial vessels after coupling to glass or resin beads (microspheres). The isotopes used for SIRT are ^{90}Y, ^{131}I, and ^{188}Re, with the current focus on the commercially available ^{90}Y microspheres. TheraSpheres® are nondegradable glass microspheres incorporating ^{89}Y, which is converted to ^{90}Y by neutron bombardment in a reactor. The SIR-Spheres® are synthetic resin particles with the radionuclide bound on their surface. TheraSphere® has a significantly higher activity per particle than the SIR-Spheres®. Therefore, SIR-Spheres requires significantly more particles than TheraSpheres. The increased number of particles and the larger diameter of the SIR-Spheres® usually result in embolization of the tumor and its afferent vessels. ^{90}Y emits β particles with an energy of 2.24 MeV and has a half-life of 64 h. The β particles have an average range of 2.5–3.5 mm in the tissue. The SIRT therapy is used either for the treatment of liver metastases or hepatocellular carcinoma (HCC). Therapy of HCC with ^{90}Y microspheres is based on the strong arterial hypervascularization of these tumors. Since the arterially injected microspheres are deposited in proportion to the perfusion and the tumors usually are highly perfused, this leads to a higher concentration as compared to the liver and thus a higher radiation dose in the tumor. Important prerequisites in addition to the proof of hypervascularization are verified tumor diagnosis, adequate liver function, missing extrahepatic metastases, no or correctable visceral shunt, a shunt-related lung dose below 30 Gy, no other vascular anatomic contraindications, and a missing portal vein thrombosis (only SIR-Spheres) [1] (Table 34.1).

So far, only nonrandomized studies are available for HCC and liver metastases. However, despite their heterogeneity in patient populations and tumor stage, many open-label phase 2 studies have demonstrated a positive effect on survival and quality of life. Similarly, these studies demonstrate that the toxicity of therapy can be minimized with optimal preparation of the patient [2–4]. A multivariate analysis of prognostic factors revealed that a dose of >104 Gy, a tumor in Okuda stage I, and a tumor-to-liver ratio of >2 correlated significantly with improved survival in terms of

Table 34.1 Contraindications for SIRT

Absolute contraindications
Not correctable gastrointestinal shunt
Lung dose > 30 Gy
Contraindications against angiography of the liver artery
Severe liver and lung dysfunction
Relative contraindications
Thrombosis of the portal vein (only SIR-Spheres®)
Bilirubin > 2 mg/dL
Infiltrative tumor growth
Tumor volume > 70% of the target volume
Transaminases > 5 ULN
Extrahepatic metastases
Situation after papillotomy of the papilla vater and/or biliary stent insertion

According to [1]

microsphere distribution [2]. Median survival is reported in several larger studies for Okuda I patients with 628–649 days and Okuda II patients with 302–324 days, which are significantly better than the 244- and 64-day historical control. A comparison with chemoembolization with respect to postembolization (PES) effects such as fever, nausea, and abdominal pain showed a better radiological tumor response after SIRT and that the PES occurred after treatment with ^{90}Y microspheres about four times less often than after chemoembolization [5, 6]. Several studies addressed the treatment of liver metastases showing also positive results [7, 8]. In a large recent study, Sato et al. performed 225 therapeutic treatments in 137 patients. The primary tumors in these patients were colon, breast, neuroendocrine tumors, pancreas, lung, cholangiocarcinoma, melanoma, kidney, esophagus, ovary, adenocarcinoma of unknown origin, lymphoma, stomach, duodenum, bladder, angiosarcoma, thyroid, adrenal, and parotid. The mean number of therapies was 1.6 and the mean activity and dose were 1.83 GBq and 112.8 Gy. Side effects included fatigue (56%), abdominal pain (26%), and nausea (23%). Further follow-up showed a response in 42.8% of the patients (2.1% complete, 40.7% partial). The median survival in all patients was 300 days (1-year survival 47.8%, 2-year survival 30.9%). In patients with colorectal tumors, median survival was 457 days, in patients with neuroendocrine tumors even 776 days [9].

34.1.2 Radiopharmaceuticals with Accumulation in Areas of Bone Remodeling

Patients in late stages of their disease often have bone metastases with severe pain. In these patients, radionuclide therapy with bone-searching molecules has great potential. The procedure is used when multiple lesions with associated pain symptoms are shown in the bone scintigraphy. The anionic bone-seeking substances, mostly based on organic phosphates, are incorporated into the bone matrix. Rhenium and samarium phosphonates accumulate specifically at the site of the osseous conversion zones. In this case, the γ-portion of the radiation allows post-therapeutic imaging or follow-up when several cycles are given. Initially, this therapy was more likely to be used in late stages. However, it is now believed that earlier use could also lead to an increase in survival. Absolute contraindications are pregnancy and breastfeeding; relative contraindications are low hematological parameters, i.e., values for platelets $<1 \times 10^5/\mu l$, leukocytes $<3 \times 10^3/\mu l$, red blood cells $<3 \times 10^6/\mu l$, hemoglobin <12 g/l, or hematocrit <30. Some randomized studies showed a significant improvement in the pain symptoms for rhenium and samarium versus placebo with pain reduction in over 80%. In 30–60%, there was a complete disappearance of the pain. A short-term increase of pain known as flare phenomenon can be observed in less than 10% of cases, which usually occurs on day 2 or 3 and disappears after 1 week. The reduction in pain can last up to a year. Furthermore, it can lead to a stabilization or even regression of the lesions. Decrease of tumor markers and prolonged survival up to 1 year have been described as further effects, especially in case of early use.

The hematological toxicity is usually low and only transient with a normalization within 3 months. The nadir with a drop of 25–30% is reached after about 2–6 weeks. Factors that influence the extent and duration of toxicity are dose and concomitant chemo or radiotherapy. Even repeated treatment with ^{153}Sm-EDTMP in patients with metastatic prostate cancer did not lead to pronounced and long-lasting hematological effects. Radionuclide therapy with rhenium or samarium has so far only been used to a limited extent by oncological colleagues, despite its known effect and low side effects. All the more surprising is the acceptance of radium-223 chloride (Xofigo). Radium-223 is an alpha emitter with a half-life of 11.4 days and a penetration distance of 80–90 microns. A multinational phase III study ALpharadin in SYMPtomatic Prostate CAncer (ALSYMPCA trial) evaluated the efficacy and side effects of Xofigo in patients with metastatic, castration-resistant prostate cancer versus a placebo group [10–13]. Therapy with Ra-223 prolonged the median survival by about 3 months with minor hematological and nonhematological (diarrhea) side effects. There was also a delay of osseous complications and pain reduction in at least 50% of patients. A controlled study investigating the therapeutic potential of rhenium or samarium compounds over radium ^{223}Ra would be desirable.

34.2 Specific Procedures

Specific methods use transport molecules that specifically bind to target structures. These transport molecules can be coupled with chemotherapeutic agents or radioactive isotopes. In most cases, antibodies are used against tumor antigens or peptides that bind to overexpressed receptors.

34.2.1 Peptide Receptor Radionuclide Therapy (PRRT)

Peptides are useful molecules for the targeted delivery of radionuclides to the desired localization in an organism. If the corresponding receptor is overexpressed in a tumor, therapeutically relevant doses can be achieved in tumor lesions with low or moderate side effects. Depending on the isotopes used, radioactively labeled peptides additionally allow imaging. The attractive feature here is that first the peptide can be labeled with a γ or positron emitter and used to identify those patients who can benefit from a PRRT, i.e., those patients showing a high accumulation in tumor lesions. Then, the same molecule can be labeled with an α or β emitter and used for therapy.

34.2.2 Somatostatin Receptor Ligands

Imaging and therapy with somatostatin receptor ligands can be seen as a paradigm for a whole range of possible methods based on the use of peptides. The high affinity of the peptides for the receptor as well as the internalization of the receptor–peptide complex facilitates the retention of the radiation source in receptor-positive tumors, while the relatively small size enables a quick clearance from the blood. Somatostatin receptors are overexpressed by a variety of tumors such as neuroendocrine tumors of the pancreas and intestine, pituitary adenoma, pheochromocytoma, paraganglioma, small cell lung carcinoma, neuroblastoma, medullary thyroid carcinoma, and meningioma (Table 34.2). Due to their high receptor density, gastroenteropancreatic neuroendocrine tumors, pheochromocytomas, paragangliomas, and bronchial carcinoids are promising candidates for PRRT. In some cases, small cell lung and medullary thyroid carcinomas or a small proportion of nonoperable meningiomas, neuroblastomas, thyroid carcinomas, renal cell carcinomas, or breast cancers can be treated. Various peptides have already been labeled for therapeutic use with the following radionuclides: ^{111}In, ^{90}Y, and ^{177}Lu. The physical properties of isotopes that may possibly be used for endoradiotherapy are shown in Table 34.3. Due to the high particle energy and relatively short half-life, ^{90}Y-labeled molecules result in a higher tumor cell dose per peptide and a better cross-fire effect. This feature is particularly needed for the treatment of larger tumors and tumors with heterogeneous receptor expression. In contrast, the lower energy and smaller particle range of ^{177}Lu lead to better absorption in smaller tumors. Furthermore, the γ radiation of ^{177}Lu can be used in addition to therapy for imaging and dosimetry. Preclinical studies on tumor-bearing animals confirmed these properties by showing excellent antitumor effects and the expected influence of tumor size. Therefore, a combination of both radionuclides has been proposed for the treatment of tumors of different sizes and inhomogeneous distribution of receptor expression [15].

Many of the available reports suffer somewhat from the heterogeneity of patient populations and the use of different isotopes, peptides, and nonstandardized doses. In contrast to antibodies in radioimmunotherapies, no evidence of immunogenicity of the peptides was found. Initial studies with high doses (cumulative doses between 20 and >100 GBq) of the Auger electron-emitting ^{111}In-DTPA0 octreotide in patients with metastatic neuroendocrine tumors and in poor clinical condition have shown positive symptom-related effects, but few partial remissions [16]. Toxicity was mainly observed in the form of bone marrow suppression. ^{90}Y-DOTA0, Tyr3 octreotide (DOTATOC), binds to the somatostatin receptor subtype 2 with an approximately 10-fold higher affinity than ^{111}In-DTPA0 octreotide. Therefore, some phase

Table 34.2 Peptide receptor expression in different tumors

Tumor	Receptors
Carcinoid (intestine)	SSTR2 > SSTR1, SSTR5, VIP, GRP/Bombesin (NMB-R), CCK (CCK1)
Gastrinoma	SSTR2, VIP, GRP-R
Insulinoma	SSTR, VIP, CCK (CCK2)
Paraganglioma	SSTR2, VIP (PAC1), CRF1
Pheochromocytoma	SSTR2, VIP (PAC1)
C-cell carcinoma	SSTR, NTR1, CCK (CCK2), NK1
SCLC	SSTR2, VIP, GRP/Bombesin (BB3), CCK (CCK2), NK1
NSCLC	VIP (VPAC1)
Meningioma	SSTR2, VIP, NTR1, CCK (CCK1)
Neuroblastoma	SSTR2, VIP (PAC1), CCK (CCK1)
Medulloblastoma	SSTR2, VIP, NTR1
Astrocytoma	SSTR, VIP (PAC1), NTR1, CCK (CCK2), NK1
Glioblastoma	VIP (PAC1), NK1
Exocrine pancreatic cancer	VIP (VPAC1), NTR1
Colorectal carcinoma	VIP (VPAC1)
Gastric cancer	SSTR, VIP (VPAC1)
Hepatocellular carcinoma	SSTR, VIP (VPAC1)
Esophageal carcinoma	VIP (VPAC1)
Renal cell carcinoma	SSTR, VIP (VPAC1), GRP/Bombesin
Prostate carcinoma	SSTR1, VIP (VPAC1), GRP/Bombesin
Bladder cancer	VIP (VPAC1)
Breast cancer	SSTR, VIP (VPAC1), GRP/Bombesin (GRP-R), NK1, NPY-R (Y1)
Ovarian cancer	SSTR, VIP (VPAC1)
Lymphoma	SSTR, VIP
Ewing sarcoma	NTR1
Leiomyoma	SSTR, VIP (VPAC2)
GIST	BB2, CCK2, VIP2

Modified according to [14]

BB2 and BB3 bombesin receptor subtypes 2 and 3, *CCK1 and CCK2* cholecystokinin receptor subtypes 1 and 2, *CRF1 and CRF2* corticotropin-releasing factors 1 and 2, *GRP* gastrin-releasing peptide, *NK1* neurokinin receptor subtype 1, *NPY* neuropeptide Y, *NTR1* neurotensin receptor subtype 1, *PAC1* PACAP receptor subtype 1, *SSTR1, SSTR2, and SSTR5* somatostatin receptor subtypes 1, 2, and 5, *VIP* vasoactive intestinal peptide, *VPAC1 and VPAC2* VIP receptor subtypes 1 and 2, *Y1* NPY receptor subtype 1

1 and phase 2 PRRT studies were performed with this molecule. Initial therapies with doses of 6 and 7.4 GBq given over four cycles showed a general response rate of 24 or 33% with administration of 7.4 GBq in two cycles [17]. A dose escalation of up to 5.6 GBq/cycle did not result in severe acute reactions and in reversible grade 3 hematologic toxicity in 43% of patients after administration of 5.2 GBq. This dose was then defined as the maximum tolerated dose per cycle. The proportion of partial (PR) and complete remissions (CR) was 28% in 87 patients [18].

Table 34.3 Physical properties of isotopes with possible application for radionuclide therapy

Isotope	Emission	Half-life (*d*)	Max β energy (keV)	Max distance (mm)
^{90}Y	β−	2.7	2270	12
^{177}Lu	γ, β−	6.7	497	2.1
^{131}I	γ, β−	8	606	2.4
^{64}Cu	β−, β+	0.5	570	2.5
^{67}Cu	γ, β−	2.5	40; 480; 580	0.4
^{166}Ho	β−	1.1	711; 1850	8.7
^{188}Re	β−	0.7	1960; 2120	11
^{211}At	α	7.2 h	5.867; 7.450	<0.1
^{213}Wi	α	45 min	8.380	<0.1

Modified according to [14]

Other studies report similar results with a median interval to clinical progression of 33 months [19]. In summary, despite differences in protocols, CRs and PRs were at 10–30% with ^{90}Y-DOTA0, Tyr3 octreotide in most of these studies, higher than those obtained with ^{111}In-DTPA0 octreotide.

Replacement of the C-terminal threoninol by threonine at the C-terminus of DOTATOC results in DOTA0, Tyr3 octreotate (DOTATATE), which results in a further increase (9-fold) in affinity to DOTATOC [20]. The ^{177}Lu DOTATATE complexes showed a higher affinity than the ^{90}Y complexes. Preclinical studies with tumor-bearing rats revealed improved tumor regression and survival of the animals with the ^{177}Lu compound. ^{177}Lu-DOTATATE was comparable to ^{111}In-DTPA0 octreotide in terms of its accumulation in kidney, spleen, and liver, but showed a 3–4-fold higher accumulation in tumors [21]. Therefore, ^{177}Lu-DOTA0, Tyr3 octreotate represents an interesting development as it results in higher absorbed tumor doses at comparable doses for potentially dose-limiting organs. Therapy of patients with gastroenteropancreatic neuroendocrine tumors with ^{177}Lu-DOTA0, Tyr3 octreotate resulted in complete or partial remissions in 30%, metabolic response in 12%, stable disease in 40%, and progression in 18% of 76 patients. Figure 34.1 shows an example of a patient with metastasized NET receiving four doses of ^{177}Lu-labeled DOTATOC. The tumor regression was positively correlated to a higher uptake observed in OctreoScan® scintigraphy, a limited hepatic tumor mass, and a high Karnofsky index. Adverse events were rare and transient, mainly as low-to-moderate bone marrow suppression. In summary, improvements in symptoms after therapy with somatostatin analogs have been observed, with better results for tumor regression after therapy with ^{90}Y-DOTA0, Tyr3 octreotide and ^{177}Lu-DOTA0, Tyr3 octreotate. Renal toxicity could be reduced by the simultaneous infusion of lysine and arginine solutions. Further side effects of this therapy were only mild. The duration of therapy response was more than 2 years for both radiopharmaceuticals. Differences in therapeutic efficacy are most likely caused by the already mentioned variations in doses, regimens of therapy (dose-escalating versus fixed dose), and patient populations. A critical point here is the proper selection of patients who can benefit from treatment. Criteria for successful application are the level of uptake in

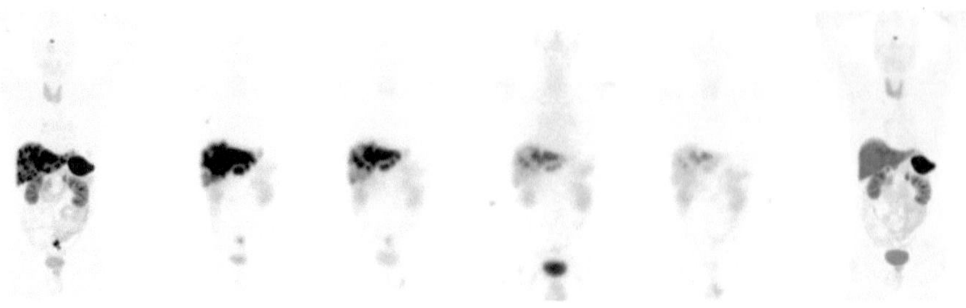

10/17 MIP (PET) Ga-68 Dotatoc | 12/17 7.4 GBq Lu-177 Dotatoc | 03/18 7.4 GBq Lu-177 Dotatoc | 05/18 7.4 GBq Lu-177 Dotatoc | 08/18 7.4 GBq Lu-177 Dotatoc | 10/18 MIP (PET) Ga-68 Dotatoc

Fig. 34.1 Patient with metastasized NET with multiple lesions in the liver and one lesion in the lower abdomen as shown in the DOTATOC-PET/CT from 10/2017 (MIP). The patient got four doses of 7.4 GBq ^{177}Lu-DOTATOC until 8/2018. The corresponding scintigraphic images (images 2–5 from the left) during therapy demonstrated a decline in number and intensity of the lesions. Finally, the DOTATOC-PET taken in 10/2018 revealed only a few remaining metastases in the liver

pretherapeutic imaging (i.e., receptor density), total tumor burden, and the extent of liver and kidney accumulation.

Recently, the Neuroendocrine Tumors Therapy trial (NETTER), a randomized multicenter study evaluating ^{177}Lu-DOTATATE therapy in 229 patients with advanced progressive, somatostatin-receptor-positive midgut neuroendocrine tumors was published. In this study, the patients were randomized to receive either four doses of 7.4 GBq ^{177}Lu-DOTATATE every 8 weeks and best supportive care including i.m. 30 mg octreotide long-acting repeatable (LAR) or 60 mg octreotide LAR alone every 4 weeks (control group).

The estimated rate of progression-free survival at month 20 was 65.2% in the ^{177}Lu-DOTATATE group and 10.8% in the control group. In addition, the response rate was 18% in the ^{177}Lu-DOTATATE group versus 3% in the control group ($P < 0.001$). During that period, 14 deaths occurred in the ^{177}Lu-DOTATATE group and 26 in the control group ($P = 0.004$). Grade 3 or 4 neutropenia, thrombocytopenia, and lymphopenia occurred in 1%, 2%, and 9%, respectively, of patients in the ^{177}Lu-Dotatate group as compared with no patients in the control group. No evidence of renal toxicity was seen [22]. A second evaluation determined the impact of ^{177}Lu-DOTATATE treatment on time to deterioration in health-related quality of life. Patients completed the European Organisation for Research and Treatment of Cancer quality-of-life questionnaires QLQ C-30 and G.I.NET-21 at baseline and every 12 weeks until tumor progression. The analysis showed that the time to quality-of-life deterioration (TTD) was significantly longer in the ^{177}Lu-DOTATATE group versus the control group with respect to global health status (hazard ratio [HR], 0.406), physical functioning (HR, 0.518), role functioning (HR, 0.580), fatigue (HR, 0.621), pain (HR, 0.566), diarrhea (HR, 0.473), disease-related worries (HR, 0.572), and body image (HR, 0.425). Differences in median TTD were clinically significant with 28.8 months versus 6.1 months for global health status and 25.2 months versus 11.5 months for physical functioning [23].

Improvement of therapeutic efficacy can be obtained by changing the administration route of the tracer. This was first evaluated in 15 patients with gastroenteropancreatic neuroendocrine tumors where intravenous and intra-arterial administration of ^{68}Ga-DOTATOC was compared and quantified using PET [24]. Compared with i.v. infusion, the i.a. infusion resulted in an increased SUV in 117 of 122 (96%) liver metastases. The average increase in SUV was 3.75-fold higher for the i.a. administration. The increase in uptake of primary tumors was dependent on the selectivity of the catheter placement with increases in SUV after i.a. injection which were between 1.44- and 7.8-fold higher. Consequently, the therapeutic effectiveness of arterial administered DOTATOC, labeled with ^{90}Y and ^{177}Lu, was evaluated in 15 patients with liver metastases from gastroenteropancreatic neuroendocrine tumors (GEP-NETs) [25]. Response was assessed using DOTATOC-PET, multiphase contrast-enhanced computed tomography, magnetic resonance imaging, and chromogranin A values. Complete remission was obtained in one (7%) patient and partial remission in eight (53%) patients, and six patients were classified as stable (40%). Furthermore, there was a correspondence of the decrease of chromogranin A and the radiologic response. The median time to progression was not reached within a mean follow-up period of 20 months. Receptor saturation and redistribution effects were identified as limiting factors for i.a. DOTATOC therapy. The high rate of objective radiologic response in these NET patients treated with arterial infusion of ^{90}Y-/^{177}Lu-DOTATOC compared favorably with systemic chemotherapy and intravenous radiopeptide therapy.

Another interesting group of radioactively labeled peptides is somatostatin receptor antagonists. DOTA coupled to [NH2-CO-c (DCys-Phe-Tyr-DAgl8 (Me, 2-naphthoyl)-Lys-Thr-Phe-Cys)-OH (DOTA-sst3-ODN-8) and [4-NO2-Phe-c (DCys-Tyr-DTrp-Lys-Thr-Cys)-DTyr-NH2] (DOTA-sst2-ANT)] showed high sst3 and sst2 binding affinity after complexing with 111In [26]. The uptake and persistence of both peptides in ST3- or sst2-receptor-transfected HEK293 cells and tumor transplants were surprisingly high. This effect was explained by more than 10-fold higher number of binding sites on the receptor compared to the agonist. Whether these promising properties can also be used on human tumors and within the framework of a PRRT remains to be clarified. In addition to combinations of peptide analogs labeled with different radionuclides, future activities could use several strategies: upregulation of somatostatin receptor expression of tumors, early diagnosis with PET tracers could identify patients with a low tumor burden and higher chance of response, peptides with binding to multiple receptors or receptor subtypes and combination with radiosensitizers, surgery, chemotherapy, immunotherapy, and radiotherapy.

34.2.3 Cholecystokinin (CCK) Receptor Ligands

These receptors show increased expression in medullary thyroid carcinomas, gastroenteropancreatic neuroendocrine tumors, small-cell lung cancer (SCLC), ovarian carcinomas, and also in gastrointestinal stromal tumors. Therefore, various cholecystokinin (CCK)-A and CCK-B/gastrin-related peptides have been developed and evaluated in preclinical studies [27]. The human heptadecapeptide gastrin-I and ^{111}In-DOTA/DTPA-CCK-B analogs [28] showed biological half-lives of several hours, a predominantly renal excretion and a specific uptake both in CCK-B-expressing organs and in medullary thyroid carcinomas with values up to 9% ID/g 1 h after administration of the tracer. Since medullary thyroid carcinomas express CCK2 receptors in almost all cases, a first clinical study was performed in patients with these tumors. A DTPA-D-Glu-modified minigastrin labeled with ^{90}Y was used. Unfortunately, this first attempt had to be stopped because of kidney and hematotoxicity [29]. The situation changed with the development of new CCK analogs with lower renal uptake and improved affinity for the target structure. These new ligands were obtained by removing four glutamic acid residues from a minigastrin analog and showed a 5-fold higher binding affinity for the CCK2 receptor (0.2 nM) and a 25-fold lower renal uptake [29]. In a European collaboration as part of a COST action, the in vitro stability of a series of peptides binding to the CCK2 receptor was compared [30]. Twelve different 1,4,7,10-tetraazacyclododecane-N,N′,N″,N‴-tetraacetic acid (DOTA)-minigastrin/CCK conjugates were radiolabeled with 177Lu and the in vitro stability was tested in fresh human serum. In these compounds, a variable stability in human serum was found with half-lives between 4.5 ± 0.1 and 198 ± 0.1 h. In urine of normal mice, only metabolized peptide fragments were detected even at short times after injection for all peptides. Matrix-assisted laser desorption/ionization time of flight mass spectrometry (MALDI-TOF MS) revealed a major cleavage site of all minigastrin derivatives between Asp and Phe-NH(2) at the C-terminal end.

34.2.4 Vasoactive Intestinal Peptide (VIP) Receptor Ligands

Since VIP receptors are overexpressed in a variety of tumors including gastrointestinal adenocarcinomas and carcinoids, studies to develop diagnostic tracers were first performed by labeling VIP with ^{123}I [31] or its TP-3654 analogs with ^{99m}Tc [32]. Unfortunately, these compounds showed a rapid degradation in the blood. Furthermore, VIP is pharmacologically highly potent with the potential for toxic effects at submicrogram doses, requiring preparations with high specific activity. These disadvantages limited the clinical application of VIP-derived tracers to a few studies reporting imaging in selected patients [33, 34]. In these studies, ^{123}I-VIP was used as a nonspecific molecule for the receptor subtypes VIP-pituitary adenylate cyclase-activating polypeptide 1 and 2 (VPAC1 and 2). Targeting of subtype 1, despite its expression in many tumors, does not appear promising because the receptor is ubiquitously expressed. In contrast, VPAC2 shows low expression in normal tissues and could be used as a target in patients with VPAC2-expressing tumors such as GIST.

34.2.5 Bombesin (BN) Receptor Ligands

Bombesin receptors belong to the group of G-protein-coupled receptors and are overexpressed in common tumors such as prostate and breast cancers [35]. Therefore, some bombesin-based radioligands have been developed and evaluated in preclinical and clinical studies [36, 37]. One of the first molecules, ^{99m}Tc-BN (7-14), showed a high specific binding to rat cortex membranes in the nanomolar range (IC50 0.8 nM) [38]. Preliminary clinical results showed good tumor demarcation in prostate cancer patients. Some of these new bombesin-based radiopeptides were conjugated to DOTA and labeled with ^{68}Ga. ^{67}Ga or ^{68}Ga-DOTA-PEG2-[D-Tyr6, βAla11, Thi13, Nle14] bombesin (6–14) showed in a pancreatic carcinoma model (AR42J) high affinity and rapid internalization in vitro with more than 85% internalized activity after 1 h. The tumor uptake in vivo at 1 h p.i. was between 5.5 and 11% ID/g depending on the amount of injected peptide and with a biological half-life of 15 h. Scintigraphic images after 1 h p.i. showed a high specific accumulation in the tumor, kidneys, intestine, and pancreas [39], which was confirmed by biodistribution and competition studies. Since internalization has been described for the DTPA-coupled BN agonists, these molecules are of interest not only for diagnostic but also for PRRT, as the chelator also allows labeling with ^{90}Y or ^{177}Lu. Nevertheless, the pharmacological activity of the BN derivative could limit therapeutic application of these peptides.

The gastrin-releasing peptide (GRP) receptor is overexpressed in a variety of tumors such as carcinoma of the lung, breast, prostate, and pancreas. GRP receptor heterogeneity often occurs in breast cancer and may be a problem for GRP receptor radiotherapy. On the other hand, Gastrointestinal stromal tumors (GISTs) are exceptionally well suited for a PRRT because of their extremely high GRP receptor density [40]. Prostate carcinomas represent another interesting field of application, especially because overexpression of GRP receptors is seen in invasive or advanced tumors. Although the 14-amino acid neuropeptide bombesin (BN) has a high binding affinity for GRP receptors, various derivatives of this molecule showed suboptimal hepatobiliary clearance with a correspondingly difficult interpretation of the abdomen due to high background activity. However, a BN derivative with low liver and intestinal uptake has been synthesized [41].

In addition to agonists, also antagonists have been developed [42–46]. These have been used for mono- or combined therapy with rapamycin of prostate cancer. The antagonist ^{177}Lu-RM2 was applied alone and in combination with rapamycin in tumor cells and tumor-bearing animals. Monotherapy with ^{177}Lu-RM2 was effective at doses of 72 and 144 MBq with complete tumor remission in 60% of the treated mice. However, combination therapy with 37 MBq ^{177}Lu-RM2 and rapamycin resulted in a significantly longer survival than with either agent alone without treatment-related toxicity [42]. Since the gastrin-releasing peptide receptor is also overexpressed in breast cancer, ^{68}Ga-labeled RM2 was used for an imaging study in 15 patients with breast cancer [46]. In 13 of 15 tumors, a high tracer uptake was found, whereas normal breast tissue showed interindividually and intraindividually variable and moderate tracer accumulation. The uptake in other organs was considerably less except in the pancreas. The implication of these findings for radiopeptide therapy of breast cancer has to be determined.

34.2.6 Glucagon-Like Peptide 1 (GLP1) Receptor Ligands

A high density of GLP1 receptors has been reported in insulinomas and gastrinomas, suggesting the use of GLP1 analogs for the PRRT of these tumors [14]. A GLP1 analog [Lys40 (Ahx-DTPA-^{111}In) NH2] exendin-4 was presented in 2006 [47] which is now in clinical use for imaging. The molecule showed a high binding affinity (IC50 = 2.1 nM) and specific tumor targeting in biodistribution experiments (up to 290% ID/g). Furthermore, an exclusively renal metabolism and a short plasma half-life were observed, with a simultaneous long retention in transgenic Rip1Tag2 mice developing tumors originating from pancreatic β-cells. The high uptake and the long tumor retention are good prerequisites for a PRRT.

34.2.7 Neurotensin (NT) Receptor Ligands

A subgroup of ductal pancreatic tumors is considered to be good candidates for a PRRT as they have a high density of NT receptors. Various ^{99m}Tc and ^{111}In-DTPA/DOTA-labeled neurotensin derivatives were, therefore, evaluated in preclinical and clinical studies, unfortunately with the result of rapid degradation in vivo [14]. Nevertheless, several ^{111}In-labeled NT analogs with better serum stability and rapid internalization after binding to the NT receptor could be found and recently promising new tracers have been developed [48]. Biodistribution experiments revealed evidence of high potential for efficient tumor targeting [49]. Other tumors with NT receptor expression are meningiomas and Ewing sarcomas.

34.3 Other Targets

Other possible target structures are located on the membranes of endothelial cells, such as z-B. αv integrins (αvβ3, αvβ5), vascular endothelial growth factor (VEGF) receptors, and fibroblast growth factor (FGF) receptors. ^{123}I-labeled VEGF165 and VEGF121 have been used in animal experiments, as well as in initial clinical trials, and demonstrated binding to a variety of human tumor cells or tissues and a 58% detection rate in a study of 40 patients with gastrointestinal tumors [50]. Furthermore, some other peptides are considered, e.g., for CXCR4 [51, 52], melanocortin receptors [53–55], endoglin (CD105), epidermal growth factor, or αvβ6 ligands [56, 57].

Future developments of PRRT are the transfer of this therapeutic approach from somatostatin receptors to other target structures, as many tumors, including mammary, prostate, colon, pancreatic, and brain tumors overexpress various other peptide receptors (see above and Table 34.2). Since tumors can simultaneously express multiple peptide receptors, combinations of two or more peptides represent a promising option. This approach should result in a higher tumor dose and a more homogeneous distribution of the radioactivity in the tumors. Tumors that are good targets for multireceptor targeting are breast cancers (GRP and NPY receptors) and GISTs (GRP, CCK2, and VPAC2 receptors) [40, 58].

34.4 Prostate-Specific Membrane Antigen

The prostate-specific membrane antigen (PSMA) is an ideal membrane-bound structure for imaging and targeted therapy of prostate cancer: as a transmembrane protein with glutamate-carboxypeptidase activity and its active site located extracellularly, it can be addressed by rational design of inhibitors mimicking the binding of the natural substrates, for example, the peptidic neurotransmitter NAAG. Furthermore, after binding of a ligand, internalization occurs via clathrin-coated pits and subsequent endocytosis. This results in enhanced uptake and retention in the tumor, which are prerequisites for a high contrast in imaging and a high local dose deposit obtained in therapeutic applications. Finally, the protein shows high expression in most tumors and low expression in normal tissues. Possible ligands for PSMA are antibodies like J591 and small molecule inhibitors. Both have been used for imaging as well as for therapy and, therefore, are candidates for in vivo theranostics. With respect to the influence of PSMA ligand imaging on the planning of therapies other than endoradiotherapy, several studies showed changes in up to 63% of the cases in the setting of biochemical relapse and approximately in 25% in the primary situation [59–62]. On the other hand, the attractive feature of endoradiotherapy is that patients may first be identified as possible candidates for this treatment after labeling of the carrier molecule with a beta or positron emitter. Upon positive findings, the same molecule can be used for therapy by labeling with an α- or β-emitting isotope. In addition, a pretherapeutic dosimetry is possible.

34.5 Endoradiotherapy with Antibodies and Small Molecules

Although phase I and II studies with ^{90}Y- or ^{177}Lu-labeled J591 revealed benefits with respect to survival and stabilization of PSA and manageable side effects [63–65], small molecule radiopharmaceuticals have some advantages over antibodies such as better tumor penetration, fast blood clearance, and low background activity. This should result in a lower dose for normal organs. Dosimetry with the compound ^{124}I-MIP-1095 revealed that the organs receiving the highest absorbed doses after administration of ^{131}I-MIP-1095 are the salivary glands (mean dose 4.6 mGy/MBq), the liver (1.5 mGy/MBq), and the kidneys (1.5 mGy/MBq). The mean total whole body absorbed dose was 0.38 mGy/MBq resulting in 0.76 to 2.7 Gy based on the injected activities. Due to faster kinetics, the PSMA-targeted small molecule ^{131}I-MIP-1095 showed a better therapeutic range in comparison to J591 with PSA responses after one therapeutic dose (mean activity 4.8 GBq) in 17/28 patients [66].

Since ^{177}Lu has a better beta-to-gamma ratio as compared to ^{131}IPSMA, ligands coupled to more universal chelates were developed such as PSMA-617 [67, 68].

Doses obtained with ^{177}Lu-PSMA-617 were even lower with 1.4 mGy/MBq for the salivary glands, 0.1 mGy/MBq for the liver, 0.75 mGy/MBq for the kidneys, and 0.03 mGy/MBq for the red marrow. These dosimetric data were found independently by four centers [61, 62, 69–71]. Consequently, side effects with respect to bone marrow were mild to moderate. Diffuse bone marrow involvement was a risk factor for higher grade myelosuppression but could be identified by PSMA imaging in advance. A therapy response as measured by a decrease in PSA as well as lesion number and size was seen in approximately 70% for both ^{131}I-MIP1095 and ^{177}Lu-PSMA-617 [61, 62, 66]. Furthermore, pain relief was obtained in almost all patients. Another chelator-coupled tracer, ^{177}Lu-DOTAGA-(I-y)fk(Sub-KuE), resulted in high absorbed tumor doses (median 3.3 Gy/GBq) as compared to normal organs of 0.8 Gy/GBq for kidneys or 1.3 Gy/GBq for salivary glands. Furthermore, a high rate of overall PSA responders without the presence of severe acute toxicity was seen [72]. However, the first reports suffered from variations of dose and schedule as well as from heterogeneity of the patient population.

Ahmadzadehfar et al. [73] reported therapeutic effects in 24 patients receiving two doses ^{177}Lu-PSMA-617 (mean dose 6 GBq per cycle). Although the PSA response after the first dose was approximately 80%, some patients presented with early relapse and in only 70% of the patients the PSA response lasted until 8–10 weeks after the first dose. Kratochwil et al. [61, 62] found in 30 patients receiving up to 3 doses ^{177}Lu-PSMA-617 given bimonthly at a dose of 6 GBq a PSA response (any decline of PSA at week-8) in 70% of the patients after the first dose. Figures 34.2 and 34.3 show examples of a varying response after treatment with multiple doses of ^{177}Lu-PSMA-617. However, the duration of response was also limited and only 40% of the patients presented with ongoing response until 6 months after initiation of treatment. In both analyses, few patients died early after therapy by tumor progression, and only grade-1/2 hematologic toxicities were seen as well as sporadically mild xerostomia and fatigue.

Furthermore, the >50% PSA decline rate at week-8 was similar with 41.6% [73] and 43.3% [61, 62]. Another analysis in patients treated with 7.4 GBq ^{177}Lu-PSMA-I&T reported a >50% PSA response rate of 33% at 8 weeks after therapy [74]. In summary, independent of the PSMA ligand applied, all centers reported that the treatment was well tolerated with no or only few grade-3/4 toxicities. However, a further common finding was that 20–40% of the patients were refractory to treatment with ^{177}Lu-PSMA ligands despite a high tracer uptake in the pretherapeutic PSMA ligand PET/CT. Patients with a diffuse infiltration of the red marrow have to be considered as patients at risk for the development of higher grade hematotoxicity [61, 62].

A multicenter retrospective analysis in Germany was performed for 145 patients with metastatic castration-resistant prostate cancer (mCRPC) receiving 1–4 therapy cycles with 2–8 GBq ^{177}Lu-PSMA-617. Nineteen patients died during the observation period. Grade 3–4 hematotoxicity occurred in 18 patients: 10%, 4%, and 3% of the patients experienced anemia, thrombocytopenia, and leukopenia, respectively. Xerostomia occurred in 8%. The overall biochemical response rate was 45% after all therapy cycles, whereas 40% of patients already responded after a single cycle [75].

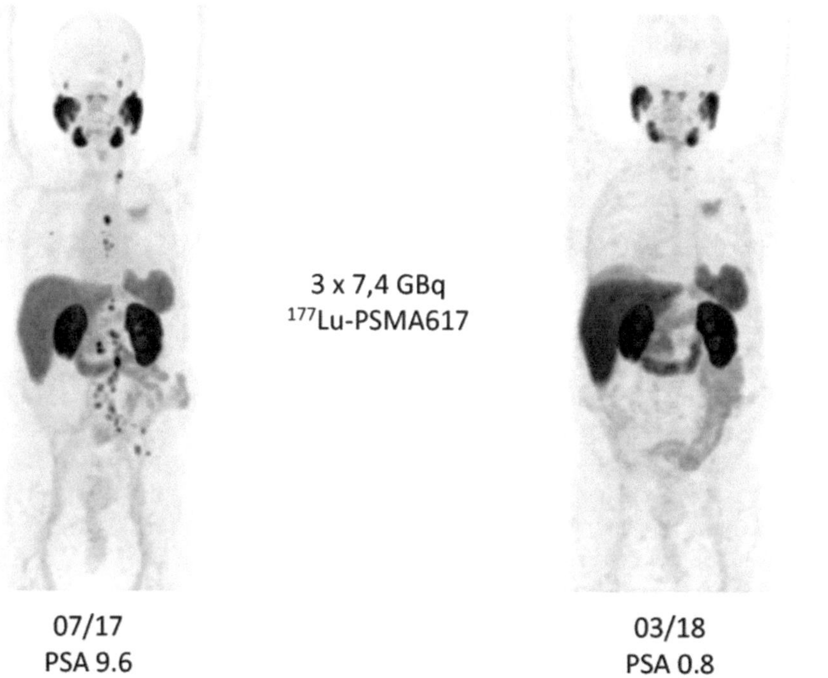

Fig. 34.2 PSMA ligand PET/CT (MIP) of a patient with metastasized prostate cancer prior (left) and after (right) three doses of 7.4 GBq ^{177}Lu-PSMA-617. The PSA value decreased from 9.6 to 0.8 indicating a partial response. Imaging revealed a substantial decrease in the number of lesions

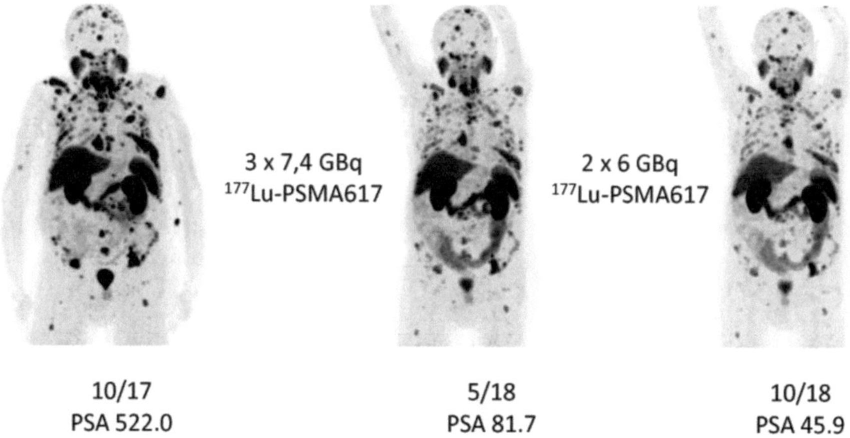

Fig. 34.3 PSMA ligand PET/CT (MIP) of a patient with metastasized prostate cancer prior (left) and three doses of 7.4 GBq ^{177}Lu-PSMA-617 (middle) and after two additional doses of 6 GBq ^{177}Lu-PSMA-617 (right). The PSA value decreased from 522 to 81.7 and 45.9 after three doses and five doses of ^{177}Lu-PSMA-617, respectively. Imaging showed a corresponding decrease in number and intensity of the tumor lesions

In recent years, numerous international studies have been conducted on therapy with ^{177}Lu-PSMA-617, providing extended insights into the safety and efficacy of the treatment. Notably, the phase III study by Sartor et al., known as VISION trial [76], led to the approval of ^{177}Lu-PSMA-617 (Pluvicto ®) in the USA (FDA 03/2022) and Europe (12/2022). The study investigated the efficacy of ^{177}Lu-PSMA-617 in patients with advanced metastatic castration-resistant prostate cancer (mCRPC) who had already undergone at least one androgen receptor pathway inhibitor therapy, such as enzalutamide, and one or two taxane-based chemotherapies (e.g., docetaxel or cabazitaxel). Inclusion criteria required the presence of PSMA-positive lesions on ^{68}Ga-PSMA PET imaging, with lesion uptake greater than that of liver tissue. Patients were randomized into two groups in a 2:1 ratio, with the larger group receiving ^{177}Lu-PSMA-617 therapy along with standard of care (excluding chemotherapy, immunotherapy, or ^{223}Ra therapy), and the control group receiving standard of care alone.

The results showed significant advantages of ^{177}Lu-PSMA-617 therapy. Firstly, there was a longer median overall survival in patients with ^{177}Lu-PSMA-617 of 15.3 months, compared to 11.3 months in the control group. Secondly, there was an improved progression-free survival (median 8.7 months in the ^{177}Lu-PSMA group vs. 3.4 months in the control group). Additionally, patients in the experimental group experienced later symptomatic or fatal osseous events (11.5 months vs. 6.8 months in the control group), and the proportion of patients with a PSA reduction of at least 50% was higher in the ^{177}Lu-PSMA-617 group compared to the control group. Overall, ^{177}Lu-PSMA therapy not only prolonged survival but also provided superior disease control.

A further phase III multicenter study investigated the efficacy of ^{177}Lu-PSMA-617 therapy in mCRPC patients who had progressed on androgen receptor pathway inhibitors (ARPI) therapy but had not yet received taxane-based chemotherapy [77]. The study compared the efficacy of ^{177}Lu-PSMA-617 with a change in ARPI. ^{177}Lu-PSMA-617 significantly extended radiographic progression-free survival and slowed the progression of prostate specific antigen (PSA) and symptomatic osseous events. Thus, Pluvicto® reduced the risk of disease progression or death by 59% compared to change in ARPI treatment. The median radiographic progression-free survival time doubled from 5.6 months to 11.6 months. Additionally, PSMA therapy had a favorable safety profile, with the most common side effects being dry mouth (61%), fatigue (53%), nausea (32%), and constipation (22%). Therapy with ^{177}Lu-PSMA-617 did not affect the patients' ability to receive subsequent chemotherapy. This study led to an expanded indication for Pluvicto® by the FDA in early 2025. The therapeutic agent can now be used earlier in the treatment sequence, specifically after treatment with an androgen receptor pathway inhibitor and prior chemotherapy in patients with PSMA-positive metastatic castration-resistant prostate cancer. This change in indication increases the number of potential patients threefold.

Replacement of beta emitters by alpha emitters such as ^{225}Ac is one option to address resistance to beta irradiation as well as diffuse involvement of the bone marrow. In a first approach, a dosimetry estimate was calculated on the basis of time-activity curves derived from serially obtained ^{177}Lu-PSMA-617 scans extrapolated to the physical half-life of ^{225}Ac, assuming instant decay of unstable daughter nuclides. This revealed mean doses of 2.3 Sv for salivary glands, 0.7 Sv for kidneys, and 0.05 Sv for red marrow. Thereafter, therapy was initiated in final stage patients with 50, 100, 150, and 200 kBq/kg of ^{225}Ac-PSMA-617. Severe xerostomia was identified as the dose-limiting toxicity for therapeutic doses greater than 100 kBq/kg per dose. With 100 kBq/kg, the duration of a decrease in PSA was less than 4 months. However, repeated bimonthly administration resulted in additive antitumor effects. Significant antitumor activity measured as radiologic response and/or decrease of PSA was seen in 9 of 11 patients [78]. A further analysis was done in 40 patients after treatment with three 100 kBq/kg doses of ^{225}Ac-PSMA-617 at 2-mo intervals [79]. The median duration of tumor control after ^{225}Ac-PSMA-617 last-line therapy was 9 months; 5 patients had a long-lasting response of more than 2 years. Since all patients were final-stage patients, this compares favorably with the tumor control rates associated with medications given at earlier stages of the disease such as abiraterone (10 months), docetaxel (6.5 months), enzalutamide (6.5 months), and cabazitaxel (6 months), respectively. Xerostomia was the main reason for discontinuation of therapy and was in the same dimension as nonresponse. According to these preliminary experiences, there is a clear benefit of ^{225}Ac over ^{177}Lu in prostate cancer patients with disseminated late-stage disease in the bone marrow. This relates to antitumor effects as well as to hematologic side effects. However, effects as well as side effects are a matter of radionuclide, dose, and time. Although more efficient with respect to tumor cell killing α emitters will destroy the salivary glands with a reduction of quality of life. For this reason, strategies need to be developed which reduce the tracer accumulation in these organs.

Another radionuclide that can be used for targeted alpha therapy is Astatine-211 (^{211}At). In contrast to ^{225}Ac, ^{211}At can be produced in larger quantities using a cyclotron. It also has a shorter physical half-life of 7.2 h and does not generate alpha-emitting daughter isotopes, which may offer safety advantages. Watabe et al. [80] labeled various ligands with ^{211}At and tested them in mouse xenograft models. Among the compounds evaluated, ^{211}At-PSMA5 demonstrated the most favorable properties, showing high tumor retention and no significant damage to the salivary glands, spleen, or stomach. Mild toxicity was observed in the kidneys. In a first-in-human study, ^{211}At-PSMA5 showed high tumor uptake, which was visualized via SPECT/CT imaging and strongly correlated with tracer accumulation observed using ^{18}F-PSMA-1007 PET/CT. The physiological biodistribution of ^{211}At-PSMA5 was also similar to that of ^{18}F-PSMA-1007, with tracer uptake in the salivary glands, liver, spleen, small intestine, and kidneys, but no urinary excretion via the bladder [81]. This suggests that ^{18}F-PSMA-1007 PET imaging may serve as an ideal phenotyping tool prior to ^{211}At-PSMA therapy.

Another aspect to be considered in terms of PSMA-targeted therapies is the obvious heterogeneity of PSMA expression in primary tumors and metastases. This heterogeneity may lead to the selection of clones with low or even no PSMA expression and, therefore, to resistance to endoradiotherapy with PSMA ligands. In the latter case, new biological targets and new radiopharmaceuticals have to be identified and developed for clinical application.

34.6 Fibroblast Activation Protein (FAP)

Fibroblast activation protein (FAP) has emerged as a promising oncological target in recent years in the context of stroma targeting. FAP is a membrane-bound protein located on the surface of the so-called cancer-associated fibroblasts (CAFs), which constitute a large proportion of the tumor stroma of epithelial tumors and are detectable in over 90% of cancers of epithelial origin [82]. FAP targeting has thus emerged as a potential "pan-tumor" strategy, which, among other potential targets, aims at epithelial tumors largely independently of tumor entities and metabolic processes, but also addresses several individual tumor cells that express FAP, e.g., ovarian, pancreatic cancer, or sarcoma [83]. This shift of focus from the tumor cell to the tumor microenvironment or "soil" of malignancy is important in the theranostic point of view, because in the tumor environment CAFs among other cellular and noncellular components coexist with tumor cells, providing the paracrine/immunological niche and nutrients that are needed for tumors to grow [84]. Breaking this contact via therapeutic agent /alpha- or beta-emitters leads to the interruption of cellular and noncellular cross-linking, which presumably causes fundamental damage to the tumor growth. Furthermore, several by-effects of therapeutic emitters, e.g., cross-fire and bystander effect, contribute to the additional destruction of the vital scaffold for malignant maintenance. In alpha-therapy, it has been suggested that the DNA-double strand break via alpha-emitting particles leads to the stimulation and migration of immune cells, enhancing the antitumor effect [85].

34.7 FAP Targeting and the RLT with FAPI

FAP as a target structure is a membrane-anchored glycoprotein, chemically classified as a typ II serine protease of 97 kDa with larger extracellular domain, which allows the selective binding of ligands [86]. Early clinical translations of FAP-tracers occurred as early as in the 1990s using antibodies, without substantial success beyond clinical phase II [87]. The essential step toward theranostic approach, with conceptual combination of diagnostic and therapeutic emitters in a specific tracer, began with the implementation of small molecule FAP-enzyme inhibitors (FAPI) in 2018 [88]. The majority of the developed FAPI compounds contain DOTA-chelators potentially capable of theranostic use (radiolabeling with Ga-68, Y-90, Lu-177, Ac-225). From the 15 different FAPI tracers synthesized in the early phase of tracer development, FAPI-04 was initially identified as the most suitable for the potential theranostic tracer [89]. Analog to its precursor FAPI-02, FAPI-04 demonstrated rapid tracer internalization into FAP-positive tumoral lesions as well as fast clearance from the blood pool [90]. The intravenous application of the compound resulted in the fast accumulation in the tumor with favorable tumor-to-background ratio. Moreover, the effective tumor uptake after 24 h was considerably higher for FAPI-04 than for FAPI-02, which provided the great advantage for the therapeutic application [90]. The first therapeutic in-human administration of FAPI compound was 2.9 GBq of Y-90-FAPI-04 (24 nmol/GBq) in a patient with metastasized breast cancer after a preceding diagnostic FAPI-PET, showing a substantial intratumoral uptake [91]. The application of rather low therapeutic dose led to a significant reduction in pain medication in this patient with clinical tolerability. The bremsstrahlung images showed persistent accumulation of the tracer at 3 h and 1 d after administration in the tumoral lesions, confirming the sustaining therapeutic effect (Fig. 34.4).

From further developed FAPI compounds (FAPI-20 to FAPI-55), FAPI-46 was identified as the most promising derivative displaying considerably longer retention in the FAP-expressing cells [92]. In the biodistribution study, FAPI-46 was excreted much slowly in comparison to FAPI-04, retaining other favorable properties in regard to target binding and pharmacokinetic profile [92].

After the publication of the above-mentioned work of Heidelberger group, FAPI-46 has begun to be widely used in the theranostic setting. For example, Assadi et al. have administered Lu-177-FAPI-46 in 18 patients with advanced cancers. The tumor entities include ovarian, colon, and breast cancer [93]. The treatment included escalating doses of Lu-177-FAPI-46 (median injected dose 3.7 GBq) per cycle with intervals of 4–6 weeks between the cycles. Overall, 36 therapy cycles were performed, with the median number of 2 cycles per patient. The dosimetric analysis revealed median absorbed doses of 0.026, 0.136, 0.886, and 0.02 mGy/MBq for the

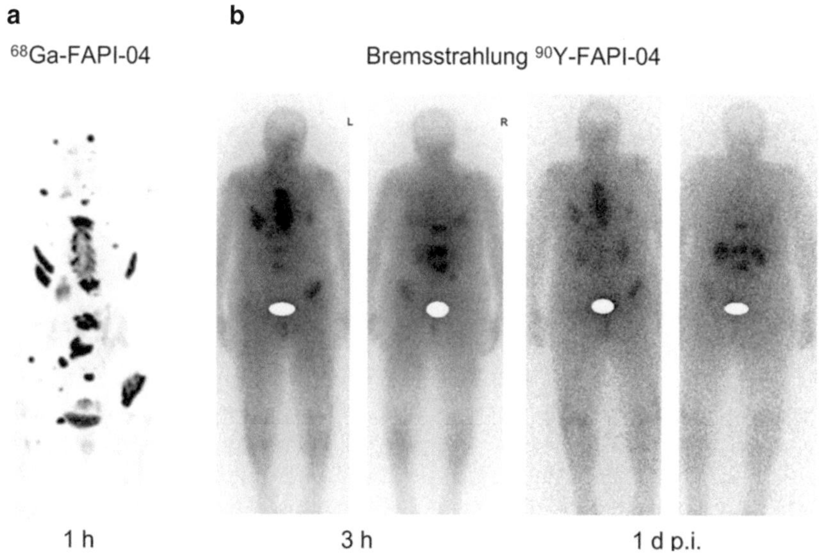

Fig. 34.4 (**a**) PET maximum-intensity projection of a patient with metastasized breast cancer 1 h after administration of 270 MBq of 68Ga-FAPI-04. Robust uptake is seen in metastases. (**b**) Bremsstrahlung images showing uptake at 3 h and even 1 d after treatment with 90Y-FAPI-04 in the same patient. (Reprinted, with permission, from Ref. [91])

whole body, liver, kidneys, and spleen, respectively. The therapy showed good tolerability in almost all patients, except one patient who suffered low-grade thrombocytopenia and leukopenia and an additional mild anemia. Overall, the therapy resulted in 12 cases of stable disease and 6 cases of progressive disease [93].

Ferdinandus et al. used Y-90-FAPI-46 in 9 patients either with metastatic soft-tissue or bone sarcoma or with pancreatic cancer, who showed both an exhaustion of all approved therapies [94]. Patients received a median of 3.8 GBq for the first cycle, and 3 patients received subsequent cycles with a median of 7.4 GBq. Overall, 13 therapy cycles were performed, with 1–3 cycles for each patient. Posttreatment Y-90-FAPI-46 bremsstrahlung scintigraphy demonstrated persistent Y-90-FAPI-46 uptake in tumor lesions in 7 of 9 patients (78%). The dosimetric analysis revealed median absorbed doses of 0.52 Gy/GBq in the kidney, 0.04 Gy/GBq in bone marrow, and less than 0.26 Gy/GBq in the lung and liver. Measured tumor lesions showed up to 2.28 Gy/GBq (median, 1.28 Gy/GBq). In this study, G3 or G4 hematological toxicities were noted in 4 patients (44%, 2 patients with thrombocytopenia only, 2 patients with new onset of thrombocytopenia and anemia). Overall, the therapy resulted in 4 cases of stable disease and 4 cases of progressive disease [94].

A combinational use of therapeutics has been reported by Kratochwil et al. in a patient with lung metastasized soft tissue sarcoma, who received 3 cycles with cumulative 20 GBq of Sm-153- and 8 GBq of Y-90-FAPI-46 [95]. The patient had a progressive metastatic disease after surgery, external-beam radiotherapy, and succeeding multiple oncological therapies in the later stage including cyclophosphamide and pazopanib. The experimental FAPI-RLT was thus considered a promising option for the possible subsequent immunotherapy. Here, the RLT with FAPI-46 was well tolerated and the patient achieved stable disease for 8 months. The subsequent immunotherapy with pembrolizumab, experimentally enhanced with oncolytic parvovirus, and nab-paclitaxel led to the disease progression after only 3 months [95].

34.8 RLT with Other FAP Ligands

A new peptide conjugate FAP-2286 was introduced in 2021, which selectively binds to FAP with low off-target activity [96]. FAP-2286 is coupled with DOTA chelator and thus can be radiolabeled with emitters with theranostic purposes. The first-in-human application of FAP-2286 was performed in 11 patients with metastasized pancreatic, breast, rectal, and ovarian cancer [97] (Fig. 34.5). The mean administered dose was 5.8 GBq for each patient. 1–3 therapy cycles were performed per patient with overall 22 therapies. The whole-body effective dose was 0.07 ± 0.02 Gy/GBq. Higher uptake with longer tumor retention was observed in bone metastases. The therapy was well tolerated and no grade 4 adverse events were observed. The major reported events were grade 3 events occurred in 3 patients with pancytopenia, leukocytopenia, and pain flare-up. Posttherapy evaluation in all patients at 6–8 weeks after the first therapy revealed stable disease in 2 patients and progression in the

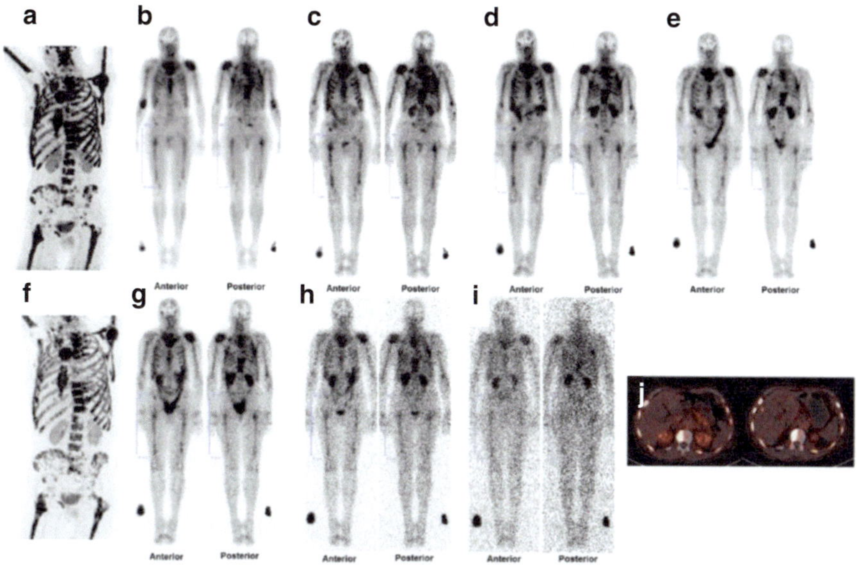

Fig. 34.5 (**a**) Patient 6, with breast cancer, presented predominantly with diffuse FAP-positive bone and bone marrow metastases (but also lymph node metastases) on ^{68}Ga-FAP-2286 PET/CT. (**b–i**) Serial whole-body scintigraphy in anterior and posterior views at 3 h (**b**), 20 h (**c**), 44 h (**d**), 68 h (**e**), 92 h (**g**), 7 d (**h**), and 10 d (**i**) after PTRT using 2.4 GBq of ^{177}Lu-FAP-2286 demonstrated uptake and retention in metastases. (**f**) ^{68}Ga-FAP-2286 PET/CT after 8 wk demonstrated mixed response: regression of bone and bone marrow lesions but overall progressive disease with new evidence of liver metastases. (**j**) Axial ^{68}Ga-FAP-2286 PET/CT images before (left) and after (right) PTRT show FAP-positive metastases in ribs and vertebrae, and occurrence of a new liver metastasis on the right side. (Reprinted, with permission, from Ref. [97])

other 9 patients. This finding was in concordance with serum tumor marker level and with Ga-68-FAP-2286 PET/CT findings [97].

DOTA.SA.FAPi is another FAP targeting compound, introduced in 2021 [98]. The critical subunits are the squaramide linker unit coupled with the DOTA chelators and a FAP inhibitor targeting moiety. The thus synthesized SA.FAPi monomer showed a high tumor affinity, but early washout of the radiotracer, which was completely eliminated by 48 h p.i [98]. To encounter this problem and to prolong tumor retention, the same group further constructed the homodimer DOTAGA.(SA.FAPi)$_2$ [99]. The homodimeric structure significantly increased tumor uptake and tumor retention. The background uptake was also lower at 24 h p.i. compared to the monomer. Both SA.FAPi monomer and DOTAGA.(SA.FAPi)$_2$ were well tolerated in patients and showed minimal toxicities. The first application of Ga-68-guided Lu-177-DOTA.SA.FAPi therapy was performed in patients with advanced stage breast cancer15. Three patients were injected with 2.96 GBq (median cumulative activity) of Lu-177-DOTA.SA.FAPi as one treatment cycle. In the Lu-177-DOTAGA.(SA.FAPi)$_2$ group, seven patients with various cancer entities (thyroid cancer, breast cancer, paraganglioma) were injected with a median dose of 1.48 GBq at the first cycle of treatment. Two cycles of treatment at a median interval of 2 months were performed in this group. The therapy was well tolerated and none of the patients showed any early adverse events. Overall, grade III and grade I anemia and thrombocytopenia were reported with no other grade III/IV toxicities noted [99].

34.9 Future Challenges

FAP-targeted RLT is an attractive oncological strategy, since FAP tracers selectively bind to cancer-associated fibroblasts (CAFs) in tumor stroma in a variety of solid tumors with an excellent target-to-background ratio. The first reported results are promising, revealing a partial response or stable disease in the majority of cases with well patient tolerability. Limitations may result from the fact that patients who received FAP-RLT are basically end-stage cancer patients after exhaustion of available therapy options. This might have led to a heterogeneity of reported cases with limited possibility of comparison to allow a general statement. For the future implementation of theranostic regime, well-designed larger clinical studies as well as further optimization of ligands may be pivotal. In a future compound development, several aspects should be considered: 1) prolonged tumor retention time, 2) correct selection of the suitable radionuclide to match the physiological and biological half-life of the tracer; these should be done while considering also the potential heterogeneity of the target mass and minimizing radiation toxicity.

FAP ligand development is in this regard a still ongoing, dynamic process. The advancement of radiochemistry with new compound development, increasing use of alpha emitters and a clinical synergistic combination with nonradioactive cancer therapeutics including immunotherapeutics are emerging trends and might suggest the future direction.

References

1. Hilgard P, Müller S, Hamami M, Sauerwein WS, Haberkorn U, Gerken G, Antoch G (2009) Selektive interne Radiotherapie (Radioembolisation) und Strahlentherapie beim HCC - Stand und Perspektiven. Z Gastroenterol 47:37–54
2. Dancey JE, Shepherd FA, Paul K, Sniderman KW, Houle S, Gabrys J et al (2000) Treatment of nonresectable hepatocellular carcinoma with intrahepatic ^{90}Y-microspheres. J Nucl Med 41:1673–1681
3. Goin JE, Salem R, Carr BI, Dancey JE, Soulen MC, Geschwind JF et al (2005) Treatment of unresectable hepatocellular carcinoma with intrahepatic yttrium 90 microspheres: factors associated with liver toxicities. J Vasc Interv Radiol 16:205–213
4. Salem R, Thurston KG, Carr BI, Goin JE, Geschwind JF (2002) Yttrium-90 microspheres: radiation therapy for unresectable liver cancer. J Vasc Interv Radiol 13:S223–S229
5. Carr BI (2004) Hepatic arterial ^{90}Yttrium glass microspheres (Therasphere) for unresectable hepatocellular carcinoma: interim safety and survival data on 65 patients. Liver Transpl 10:S107–S110

6. Geschwind JF, Salem R, Carr BI, Soulen MC, Thurston KG, Goin KA et al (2004) Yttrium-90 microspheres for the treatment of hepatocellular carcinoma. Gastroenterology 127(5 Suppl 1):S194–S205
7. Herba MJ, Thirlwell MP (2002) Radioembolization for hepatic metastases. Semin Oncol 29:152–159
8. Lewandowski RJ, Thurston KG, Goin JE et al (2005) ^{90}Y microsphere (TheraSphere) treatment for unresectable colorectal cancer metastases of the liver: response to treatment at targeted doses of 135–150 Gy as measured by [^{18}F] fluorodeoxyglucose positron emission tomography and computed tomographic imaging. J Vasc Interv Radiol 16:1641–1651
9. Sato KT, Lewandowski RJ, Mulcahy MF, Atassi B, Ryu RK, Gates VL, Nemcek A, Barakat O, Benson A III, Mandal R, Talamonti M, Wong CY, Miller FH, Newman SB, Shaw JM, Thurston KG, Omary KA, Salem R (2008) Unresectable chemorefractory liver metastases: radioembolization with 90Y microspheres—safety, efficacy, and survival. Radiology 247:507–515
10. Hoskin P, Sartor O, O'Sullivan JM et al (2014) Efficacy and safety of radium-223 dichloride in patients with castration-resistant prostate cancer and symptomatic bone metastases, with or without previous docetaxel use: a prespecified subgroup analysis from the randomised, double-blind, phase 3 ALSYMPCAtrial. Lancet Oncol 15:1397–1406
11. Parker CC, Coleman RE, Sartor O et al (2017) Three-year safety of radium-223 dichloride in patients with castration-resistant prostate cancer and symptomatic bone metastases from phase 3 randomized alpharadin in symptomatic prostate cancer trial. Eur Urol pii:S0302-2838(17)30516-X. https://doi.org/10.1016/j.eururo.2017.06.021
12. Saad F, Carles J, Gillessen S et al (2016) Radium-223 and concomitant therapies in patients with metastatic castration-resistant prostate cancer: an international, early access, open-label, single-arm phase 3b trial. Lancet Oncol 17:1306–1316
13. Sartor O, Coleman R, Nilsson S et al (2014) Effect of radium-223 dichloride on symptomatic skeletal events in patients with castration-resistant prostate cancer and bone metastases: results from a phase 3, double-blind, randomised trial. Lancet Oncol 15:738–746
14. Haberkorn U, Eisenhut M, Altmann A, Mier W (2008) Endoradiotherapy with peptides—status and future development. Curr Med Chem 15:219–234
15. Dejong M, Breeman WAP, Valkema R, Bernard BF, Krenning EP (2005) Combination radionuclide therapy using ^{177}Lu- and ^{90}Y-labeled somatostatin analogs. J Nucl Med 46:13S–17S
16. Valkema R, de Jong M, Bakker WH, Breeman WA, Kooij PP, Lugtenburg PJ, DeJong FH, Christiansen A, Kam BL, DeHerder WW, Stridsberg M, Lindemans J, Ensing G, Krenning EP (2002) Phase I study of peptide receptor radionuclide therapy with [In-DTPA]octreotide: the Rotterdam experience. Semin Nucl Med 32:110–122
17. Waldherr C, Pless M, Maecke HR, Haldemann A, Mueller-Brand J (2001) The clinical value of [^{90}Y-DOTA]-D-Phe1-Tyr3-octreotide (90Y-DOTATOC) in the treatment of neuroendocrine tumours: a clinical phase II study. Ann Oncol 12:941–945
18. Chinol M, Bodei L, Cremonesi M, Paganelli G (2002) Receptor-mediated radiotherapy with Y-DOTA-DPhe-Tyr-octreotide: the experience of the European Institute of Oncology Group. Semin Nucl Med 32:141–147
19. Bodei L, Cremonesi M, Zoboli S, Grana C, Mazzetta C, Rocca P, Caracciolo M, Mäcke HR, Chinol M, Paganelli G (2003) Receptor-mediated radionuclide therapy with 90Y-DOTATOC in association with amino acid infusion: a phase I study. Eur J Nucl Med Mol Imaging 30:207–216
20. Reubi JC, Schar JC, Waser B, Wenger S, Heppeler A, Schmitt JS, Mäcke HR (2000) Affinity profiles for human somatostatin receptor subtypes SST1-SST5 of somatostatin radiotracers selected for scintigraphic and radiotherapeutic use. Eur J Nucl Med 27:273–282
21. Kwekkeboom DJ, Bakker WH, Kooij PP, Konijnenberg MW, Srinivasan A et al (2001) [^{177}Lu-DOTAOTyr3]octreotate: comparison with [^{111}In-DTPAo]octreotide in patients. Eur J Nucl Med 28:1319–1325
22. Strosberg J, El-Haddad G, Wolin E, the NETTER-1 Trial Investigators (2017) Phase 3 trial of ^{177}Lu dotatate for midgut neuroendocrine tumors. N Engl J Med 376:125–135

23. Strosberg J, Wolin E, Chasen B, the NETTER-1 Study Group (2018) Health-related quality of life in patients with progressive midgut neuroendocrine tumors treated with ^{177}Lu-dotatate in the phase III NETTER-1 trial. J Clin Oncol 36:2578–2584
24. Kratochwil C, Giesel FL, López-Benítez R et al (2010) Intraindividual comparison of selective arterial versus venous ^{68}Ga-DOTATOC PET/CT in patients with gastroenteropancreatic neuroendocrine tumors. Clin Cancer Res 16:2899–2905
25. Kratochwil C, Lopez-Benıtez R, Mier W et al (2011) Hepatic arterial infusion enhances DOTATOC radiopeptide therapy in patients with neuroendocrine liver metastases. Endocr Relat Cancer 18:595–602
26. Ginj M, Zhang H, Waser B, Cescato R, Wild D, Wang X, Erchegyi J, Rivier J, Maecke HR, Reubi JC (2006) Radiolabeled somatostatin receptor antagonists are preferable to agonists for in vivo peptide receptor targeting of tumors. Proc Natl Acad Sci USA 103:16436–16441
27. de Jong M, Bakker WH, Bernard BF, Valkema R, Kwekkeboom DJ, Reubi JC et al (1999) Preclinical and initial clinical evaluation of ^{111}In-labeled nonsulfated CCK8 analog: a peptide for CCK-B receptor-targeted scintigraphy and radionuclide therapy. J Nucl Med 40:2081–2087
28. Reubi JC, Waser B, Schaer JC, Laederach U, Erion J, Srinivasan A, Schmidt MA, Bugai JE (1998) Unsulfated DTPA- and DOTA-CCK analogs as specific high-affinity ligands for CCK-B receptor-expressing human and rat tissues in vitro and in vivo. Eur J Nucl Med 25:481–490
29. Behr TM, Béhé M (2002) Cholecystokinin-B/gastrin receptor-targeting peptides for staging and therapy of medullary thyroid cancer and other cholecystokinin-B receptor-expressing malignancies. Semin Nucl Med 32:97–107
30. Ocak M, Helbok A, Rangger C et al (2011) Comparison of biological stability and metabolism of CCK2 receptor targeting peptides, a collaborative project under COST BM0607. Eur J Nucl Med Mol Imaging 38:1426–1435
31. Raderer M, Kurtaran A, Leimer M, Angelberger P, Niederle B, Vierhapper H, Vorbeck F, Hejna MH, Scheithauer W, Pidlich J, Virgolini I (2000) Value of peptide receptor scintigraphy using (123)I-vasoactive intestinal peptide and (111)In-DTPA-D-Phe1-octreotide in 194 carcinoid patients: Vienna University Experience, 1993 to 1998. J Clin Oncol 18:1331–1336
32. Thakur ML, Marcus CS, Saeed S, Palella V, Minami C, Diggles L, Le Pham H, Ahdoot R, Kalinowski EA (2000) ^{99m}Tc-labeled vasoactive intestinal peptide analog for rapid localization of tumors in humans. J Nucl Med 41:107–110
33. Hessenius C, Bäder M, Meinhold H, Bohmig M, Faiss S, Reubi JC, Wiedenmann B (2000) Vasoactive intestinal peptide receptor scintigraphy in patients with pancreatic adenocarcinomas or neuroendocrine tumours. Eur J Nucl Med 27:1684–1693
34. Virgolini I, Raderer M, Kurtaran A, Angelberger P, Yang Q, Radosavlejvic M et al (1996) ^{123}I-vasoactive intestinal peptide (VIP) receptor scanning: update of imaging results in patients with adenocarcinomas and endocrine tumors of the gastrointestinal tract. Nucl Med Biol 23:685–692
35. Maecke HR, Hofmann M, Haberkorn U (2005) Gallium-68 labeled peptides in tumor imaging. J Nucl Med 46:172–178
36. Breeman WA, de Jong M, Erion JL, Bugaj JE, Srinivasan A, Bernard BF, Kwekkeboom DJ, Visser TJ, Krenning E (2002) Preclinical comparison of (111)In-labeled DTPA- or DOTA-bombesin analogs for receptor-targeted scintigraphy and radionuclide therapy. J Nucl Med 43:1650–1656
37. Scopinaro F, De Vincentis G, Varvarigou AD, Laurenti C, Iori F, Remediani S, Chiarini S, Stella S (2003) ^{99m}Tc-bombesin detects prostate cancer and invasion of pelvic lymph nodes. Eur J Nucl Med Mol Imaging 30:1378–1382
38. Baidoo KE, Lin KS, Zhan Y, Finley P, Sheffel U, Wagner HN Jr (1998) Design, synthesis, and initial evaluation of high-affinity technetium bombesin analogues. Bioconjug Chem 9:218–225
39. Schuhmacher J, Zhang H, Doll J, Mäcke HR, Matys R, Hauser H, Henze M, Haberkorn U, Eisenhut M (2005) GRP receptor-targeted PET of a rat pancreas carcinoma xenograft in nude mice with a ^{68}gallium labeled bombesin (6-14) analog. J Nucl Med 4:691–699

40. Reubi JC, Korner M, Waser B, Mazzucchelli L, Guillou L (2004) High expression of peptide receptors as a novel target in gastrointestinal stromal tumours. Eur J Nucl Med Mol Imaging 31:803–810
41. Lin KS, Luu A, Baidoo KE, Hashemzadeh-Gargari H, Chen MK, Brenneman K et al (2005) A new high affinity technetium-99 m-bombesin analogue with low abdominal accumulation. Bioconjug Chem 16:43–50
42. Dumont RA, Tamma M, Braun F et al (2013) Targeted radiotherapy of prostate cancer with a gastrin-releasing peptide receptor antagonist is effective as monotherapy and in combination with rapamycin. J Nucl Med 54:762–769
43. Gourni E, Mansi R, Jamous M et al (2014) N-terminal modifications improve the receptor affinity and pharmacokinetics of radiolabeled peptidic gastrin-releasing peptide receptor antagonists: examples of ^{68}Ga- and ^{64}Cu-la beled peptides for PET imaging. J Nucl Med 55:1719–1725
44. Mansi R, Abiraj K, Wang X et al (2015) Evaluation of three different families of bombesin receptor radioantagonists for targeted imaging and therapy of gastrin releasing peptide receptor (GRP-R) positive tumors. J Med Chem 58:682–691
45. Popp I, Del Pozzo L, Waser B et al (2017) Approaches to improve metabolic stability of a statine-based GRP receptor antagonist. Nucl Med Biol 45:22–29
46. Stoykow C, Erbes T, Maecke HR et al (2016) Gastrin-releasing peptide receptor imaging in breast cancer using the receptor antagonist (68)Ga-RM2 and PET. Theranostics 6:1641–1650
47. Wild D, Béhé M, Wicki A, Storch D, Waser B, Gotthardt M, Keil B, Christofori G, Reubi JC, Mäcke HR (2006) [Lys40(Ahx-DTPA-111In)NH2]exendin-4, a very promising ligand for glucagon-like peptide-1 (GLP-1) receptor targeting. J Nucl Med 47:2025–2033
48. Maschauer S, Prante O (2018) Radiopharmaceuticals for imaging and endoradiotherapy of neurotensin receptor-positive tumors. J Label Compd Radiopharm 61:309–325
49. de Visser M, Janssen PJJM, Srinivasan A, Reubi JC, Waser B, Erion JL, Schmidt MA, Krenning EP, de Jong M (2003) Stabilised 111In-labelled DTPA- and DOTA-conjugated neurotensin analogues for imaging and therapy of exocrine pancreatic cancer. Eur J Nucl Med 30:1134–1139
50. Li S, Peck-Radosavljevic M, Kienast O, Preitfellner J, Hamilton G, Kurtaran A, Pirich C, Angelberger P, Dudczak R (2003) Imaging gastrointestinal tumours using vascular endothelial growth factor-165 (VEGF165) receptor scintigraphy. Ann Oncol 14:1274–1277
51. Lapa C, Herrmann K, Schirbel A et al (2017) CXCR4-directed endoradiotherapy induces high response rates in extramedullary relapsed multiple myeloma. Theranostics 7:1589–1597
52. Walenkamp AME, Lapa C, Herrmann K, Wester HJ (2017) CXCR4 ligands: the next big hit? J Nucl Med 58:77S–82S
53. Martin ME, Sue O'Dorisio M, Leverich WM, Kloepping KC, Walsh SA, Schultz MK (2013) "Click"-cyclized (68)Ga-labeled peptides for molecular imaging and therapy: synthesis and preliminary in vitro and in vivo evaluation in a melanoma model system. Recent Results Cancer Res 194:149–175
54. Rosenkranz A, Slastnikova TA, Durymanov MO, Sobolev AS (2013) Malignant melanoma and melanocortin 1 receptor A. Biochem Mosc 7:1228–1237
55. Zhang C, Zhang Z, Lin KS, Lau J, Zeisler J, Colpo N, Perrin DM, Bénard F (2018) Melanoma imaging using ^{18}F-labeled α-melanocyte-stimulating hormone derivatives with positron emission tomography. Mol Pharm 15:2116–2122
56. Altmann A, Sauter M, Roesch S, Mier W, Warta R, Debus J, Dyckhoff G, Herold-Mende C, Haberkorn U (2017) Identification of a novel ITGαvβ6-binding peptide using protein separation and phage display. Clin Cancer Res 23:4170–4180
57. Roesch S, Lindner T, Sauter M, Loktev A, Flechsig P, Müller M, Mier W, Warta R, Dyckhoff G, Herold-Mende C, Haberkorn U, Altmann A (2018) Comparative study of the novel RGD motif-containing αvβ6 integrin binding peptides SFLAP3 and SFITGv6 for diagnostic application in HNSCC. J Nucl Med pii:jnumed.118.210013. https://doi.org/10.2967/jnumed.118.210013

58. Reubi JC, Gugger M, Waser B (2002) Co-expressed peptide receptors in breast cancer as a molecular basis for in vivo multireceptor tumour targeting. Eur J Nucl Med 29:855–862
59. Haberkorn U, Eder M, Kopka K, Babich JW, Eisenhut M (2016) New strategies in prostate cancer: prostate- specific membrane antigen (PSMA) ligands for diagnosis and therapy. Clin Cancer Res 22:9–15
60. Haberkorn U, Kopka K, Giesel F, Kratochwil C (2016) Future trends in prostate cancer theranostics with PSMA ligands. Clin Translat Imaging 4:487–489
61. Kratochwil C, Afshar-Oromieh A, Kopka K et al (2016) Current status of prostate-specific membrane antigen targeting in nuclear medicine: clinical translation of chelator containing prostate-specific membrane antigen ligands into diagnostics and therapy for prostate cancer. Semin Nucl Med 46:405–418
62. Kratochwil C, Giesel FL, Stefanova M, Benešová M, Bronzel M, Afshar-Oromieh A, Mier W, Eder M, Kopka K, Haberkorn U (2016) PSMA-targeted radionuclide therapy of metastatic castration-resistant prostate cancer with Lu-177 labeled PSMA-617. J Nucl Med 57:1170–1176
63. Bander NH, Milowsky MI, Nanus DM, Kostakoglu L, Vallabhajosula S, Goldsmith SJ (2005) Phase I trial of ^{177}lutetium-labeled j591, a monoclonal antibody to prostate-specific membrane antigen, in patients with androgen-independent prostate cancer. J Clin Oncol 23:4591–4601
64. Milowsky MI, Nanus DM, Kostakoglu L et al (2007) Vascular targeted therapy with anti-prostate-specific membrane antigen monoclonal antibody J591 in advanced solid tumors. J Clin Oncol 25:540–547
65. Vallabhajosula S, Nikolopoulou A, Jhanwar YS et al (2016) Radioimmunotherapy of metastatic prostate cancer with ^{177}Lu-DOTAhuJ591 anti prostate specific membrane antigen specific monoclonal antibody. Curr Radiopharm 9:44–53
66. Zechmann CM, Afshar-Oromieh A, Armor T et al (2014) Radiation dosimetry and first therapy results with a ^{124}I/^{131}I-labeled small molecule (MIP-1095) targeting PSMA for prostate cancer therapy. Eur J Nucl Med Mol Imaging 41:1280–1292
67. Benešová M, Schäfer M, Bauder-Wüst U, Afshar-Oromieh A, Kratochwil C, Mier W et al (2015) Preclinical evaluation of a tailor-made DOTA-conjugated PSMA inhibitor with optimized linker moiety for imaging and endoradiotherapy of prostate cancer. J Nucl Med 56:914–920
68. Benešová M, Bauder-Wüst U, Schäfer M et al (2016) Linker modification strategies to control the prostate-specific membrane antigen (PSMA)-targeting and pharmacokinetic properties of DOTA-conjugated PSMA inhibitors. J Med Chem 59:1761–1775
69. Delker A, Fendler WP, Kratochwil C et al (2016) Dosimetry for ^{177}Lu-DKFZ-PSMA-617: a new radiopharmaceutical for the treatment of metastatic prostate cancer. Eur J Nucl Med Mol Imaging 43:42–51
70. Hohberg M, Eschner W, Schmidt M et al (2016) Lacrimal glands may represent organs at risk for radionuclide therapy of prostate cancer with ^{177}LuDKFZ-PSMA-617. Mol Imaging Biol 18(3):437–445
71. Kabasakal L, AbuQbeitah M, Aygün A et al (2015) Pre-therapeutic dosimetry of normal organs and tissues of ^{177}Lu-PSMA-617 prostate-specific membrane antigen (PSMA) inhibitor in patients with castration-resistant prostate cancer. Eur J Nucl Med Mol Imaging 42:1976–1983
72. Baum RP, Kulkarni HR, Schuchardt C, Singh A, Wirtz M, Wiessalla S, Schottelius M, Mueller D, Klette I, Wester HJ (2016) Lutetium-177 PSMA radioligand therapy of metastatic castration-resistant prostate cancer: safety and efficacy. J Nucl Med 57:1006–1013
73. Ahmadzadehfar H, Eppard E, Kürpig S, Fimmers R, Yordanova A, Schlenkhoff CD, Gärtner F, Rogenhofer S, Essler M (2016) Therapeutic response and side effects of repeated radioligand therapy with ^{177}Lu-PSMA-DKFZ-617 of castrate-resistant metastatic prostate cancer. Oncotarget 7:12477–12488
74. Heck MM, Retz M, Alessandria D, Rauscher I, Scheidhauer K, Maurer T, Storz E, Janssen F, Schottelius M, Wester HJ, Gschwend JE, Schwaiger M, Tauber R, Eiber M (2016) Systemic radioligand therapy with ^{177}Lu-PSMA-I&T in patients with metastatic castration-resistant prostate cancer. J Urol 196:382–391

75. Rahbar K, Ahmadzadehfar H, Kratochwil C et al (2017) German multicenter study investigating ^{177}Lu-PSMA-617 radioligand therapy in advanced prostate cancer patients. J Nucl Med 58:85–90
76. Sartor O, de Bono J, Chi KN et al (2021) Lutetium-177–PSMA-617 for metastatic castration-resistant prostate cancer. N Engl J Med 385:1091–1103
77. Morris MJ, Castellano D, Herrmann K et al (2024) 177Lu-PSMA-617 versus a change of androgen receptor pathway inhibitor therapy for taxane-naive patients with progressive metastatic castration-resistant prostate cancer (PSMAfore): a phase 3, randomised, controlled trial. Lancet 404:1227–1239
78. Kratochwil C, Bruchertseifer F, Rathke H et al (2017) Targeted α-therapy of metastatic castration-resistant prostate cancer with ^{225}Ac-PSMA-617: dosimetry estimate and empiric dose finding. J Nucl Med 58:1624–1631
79. Kratochwil C, Bruchertseifer F, Rathke H et al (2018) Targeted a-therapy of metastatic castration-resistant prostate cancer with ^{225}Ac-PSMA-617: swimmer-plot analysis suggests efficacy regarding duration of tumor control. J Nucl Med 59:795–802
80. Watabe T, Kaneda-Nakashima K, Shirakami Y et al (2023) Targeted α-therapy using astatine (211At)-labeled PSMA1, 5, and 6: a preclinical evaluation as a novel compound. Eur J Nucl Med Mol Imaging 50:849–858
81. Watabe T, Hatano K, Naka S et al (2024) First-in-human SPECT/CT imaging of [211At]PSMA-5: targeted alpha therapy in a patient with refractory prostate cancer. Eur J Nucl Med Mol Imaging 52:2253
82. Scanlan MJ, Raj BKM, Calvo B et al (1994) Molecular cloning of fibroblast activation protein alpha, a member of the serine protease family selectively expressed in stromal fibroblasts of epithelial cancers. Proc Natl Acad Sci USA 91:657–5661
83. Dohi O, Ohtani H, Hatori M et al (2009) Histogenesis-specific expression of fibroblast activation protein and Dipeptidylpeptidase-IV in human bone and soft tissue tumours. Histopathology 55:432–440
84. Koustoulidou S, Hoorens MWH, Dalm SU et al (2021) Cancer-associated fibroblasts as players in cancer development and progression and their role in targeted radionuclide imaging and therapy. Cancers (Basel) 13(5):1100
85. Claesson AK, Stenerlöw B, Jacobsson L, Elmroth K (2007) Relative biological effectiveness of the alpha-particle emitter (211)At for double-strand break induction in human fibroblasts. Radiat Res 167(3):312–318
86. Zi F, He J, He D, Li Y, Yang L, Cai Z (2015) Fibroblast activation protein α in tumor microenvironment: recent progression and implications. Mol Med Rep 11:3203–3211
87. Hofheinz RD, al-Batran SE, Hartmann F et al (2003) Stromal antigen targeting by a humanised monoclonal antibody: an early phase II trial of sibrotuzumab in patients with metastatic colorectal cancer. Onkologie 26(1):44–48
88. Mori Y, Dendl K, Cardinale J, Kratochwil C, Giesel FL, Haberkorn U (2023) FAPI PET: fibroblast activation protein inhibitor use in oncologic and nononcologic disease. Radiology 306(2):e220749
89. Loktev A, Lindner T, Mier W, Debus J, Altmann A, Jager D et al (2018) A tumor-imaging method targeting cancer-associated fibroblasts. J Nucl Med 59(9):1423–1429
90. Giesel FL, Kratochwil C, Lindner T et al (2019) 68Ga-FAPI PET/CT: biodistribution and preliminary dosimetry estimate of 2 DOTA-containing FAP-targeting agents in patients with various cancers. J Nucl Med 60(3):386–392
91. Lindner T, Loktev A, Altmann A, Giesel F, Kratochwil C, Debus J et al (2018) Development of Quinoline-based Theranostic ligands for the targeting of fibroblast activation protein. J Nucl Med 59(9):1415–1422
92. Loktev A, Lindner T, Burger EM, Altmann A, Giesel F, Kratochwil C et al (2019) Development of fibroblast activation protein-targeted radiotracers with improved tumor retention. J Nucl Med 60(10):1421–1429
93. Assadi M, Rekabpour SJ, Jafari E, Divband G, Nikkholgh B, Amini H et al (2021) Feasibility and therapeutic potential of 177Lu-fibroblast activation protein Inhibitor-46

for patients with relapsed or refractory cancers: a preliminary study. Clin Nucl Med 46(11):e523–ee30

94. Ferdinandus J, Fragoso Costa P, Kessler L, Weber M, Hirmas N, Kostbade K et al (2021) Initial clinical experience with (90)Y-FAPI-46 radioligand therapy for advanced stage solid tumors: a case series of nine patients. J Nucl Med. https://doi.org/10.2967/jnumed.121.262468
95. Kratochwil C, Giesel FL, Rathke H, Fink R, Dendl K, Debus J et al (2021) [(153)Sm]Samarium-labeled FAPI-46 radioligand therapy in a patient with lung metastases of a sarcoma. Eur J Nucl Med Mol Imaging 48(9):3011–3013
96. Zboralski D, Hoehne A, Bredenbeck A et al (2022) Preclinical evaluation of FAP-2286 for fibroblast activation protein targeted radionuclide imaging and therapy. Eur J Nucl Med Mol Imaging 49(11):3651–3667
97. Baum RP, Schuchardt C, Singh A et al (2022) Feasibility, biodistribution, and preliminary dosimetry in peptide-targeted radionuclide therapy of diverse adenocarcinomas using (177) Lu-FAP-2286: first-in-humans results. J Nucl Med 63(3):415–423
98. Moon ES, Ballal S, Yadav MP, Bal C, Rymenant YV, Stephan S, Bracke A, der Veken PV, Meester ID, Roesch F (2021) Fibroblast activation protein (FAP) targeting homodimeric FAP inhibitor radiotheranostics: a step to improve tumor uptake and retention time. Am J Nucl Med Mol Imaging 11:476
99. Ballal S, Yadav MP, Moon ES, Kramer VS, Roesch F, Kumari S, Bal C (2021) First-in-human results on the biodistribution, pharmacokinetics, and dosimetry of [177Lu]Lu-DOTA.SA.FAPi and [177Lu]Lu-DOTAGA.(SA.FAPi)2. Pharmaceuticals (Basel) 14(12):1212

35 Clinical Applications of Theranostics

Jonathan Kuten, Lisa Bodei, and Jason S. Lewis

35.1 Introduction

The term theranostics means the integrated use of targeted diagnostic tests and therapeutic interventions. Radiotheranostics specifically combines molecular imaging (PET or SPECT) with targeted radionuclide therapy. This approach allows clinicians to “see” the tumor with a radiolabeled imaging agent and treat it with the same agent radiolabeled with a therapeutic isotope. By verifying the presence of a molecular target in a patient’s tumor via imaging and then delivering radiation precisely to those cancer cells, radiotheranostics epitomizes personalized medicine—we can treat what we see and monitor the response in real time. Theranostics offers several advantages over conventional treatments, including the ability to visualize the target in real time, a feature that is not possible during chemotherapy or radiation therapy, and the ability to treat patients systematically, which is not feasible with external beam radiotherapy [1, 2].

Radiotheranostics has rapidly expanded in recent years and is becoming an increasingly important modality in oncology. Several radiotheranostic agents are now clinically available, transforming care for diseases like neuroendocrine tumors and prostate cancer. The appeal of theranostics lies in its high specificity and the dual role of radiopharmaceuticals: providing diagnostic information (extent of disease, uptake, heterogeneity) and delivering therapy if the target is appropriately

J. Kuten · L. Bodei
Department of Radiology, Memorial Sloan Kettering Cancer Center, New York, NY, USA
e-mail: kutenj@mskcc.org; bodeil@mskcc.org

J. S. Lewis (✉)
Department of Radiology, Memorial Sloan Kettering Cancer Center, New York, NY, USA

Molecular Pharmacology, Sloan Kettering Institute, New York, NY, USA
e-mail: lewisj2@mskcc.org

O. Schober et al. (eds.), *Molecular Imaging in Oncology - Volume 2*, Recent Results in Cancer Research 225, https://doi.org/10.1007/978-3-032-21415-7_17

expressed. This chapter provides a comprehensive overview of radiotheranostics in oncology, including its historical development, key milestones, mechanisms of action, and current clinical applications with evidence from major trials, as well as challenges and future directions [2–4].

35.2 Mechanism of Action

Radiotheranostic agents generally consist of a vector (such as a small molecule, peptide, or monoclonal antibody) that binds to a tumor-associated target, paired with a radioisotope (Tables 35.1 and 35.2).

For imaging, the isotope emits γ-rays or positrons detectable by SPECT (e.g., ^{111}In) or PET (e.g., ^{68}Ga, ^{18}F), whereas for therapy, it emits cytotoxic radiation (commonly beta or alpha particles). The same vector can often be labeled with either a diagnostic or therapeutic radioisotope—thus constituting a "theranostic pair." For example, a somatostatin analog can be labeled with ^{68}Ga for PET imaging of neuroendocrine tumors and with ^{177}Lu (a β-emitter) for therapy. Similarly, prostate-specific membrane antigen (PSMA) ligands can be labeled with ^{68}Ga or ^{18}F for PET scanning and with ^{177}Lu for radiopharmaceutical therapy. Some radiopharmaceuticals—e.g., sodium iodide-131—allow both imaging and therapy at once. Many radiopharmaceuticals are labeled with metallic radionuclides and need a linked chelator that allows stable binding of the radiometal to the radiopharmaceutical during its transit in the body to the target lesion. The imaging step confirms that the tumor expresses the target, and that the radiopharmaceutical localizes to tumor sites, thereby identifying patients likely to benefit. Once the target expression is visualized, the therapeutic radioisotope is administered to deliver radiation specifically to those cancer cells (Fig. 35.1).

This strategy also incorporates dosimetry, quantification of radiotracer uptake to determine the radiation dose absorbed by the tumor and normal organs, thus increasing efficacy and safety. Treatment is often divided into cycles, and interim imaging can be performed to evaluate response and assess any change in target expression and extent of disease [2, 4].

Therapeutic isotopes emit ionizing radiation that can kill cells primarily by inducing DNA damage. Beta (β) emitters (e.g., ^{177}Lu, ^{90}Y) have millimeter-range penetration and medium energy, causing predominantly single-strand DNA breaks. Their longer range can kill adjacent tumor cells via the *crossfire effect*. Alpha (α) emitters (e.g., ^{223}Ra, ^{225}Ac) release high-energy helium nuclei with a very short range (50–100 microns) but densely ionizing tracks that cause predominantly double-strand DNA breaks; thus, α-radiation is more lethal per track. Auger electron emitters (e.g., ^{111}In) cause very short-range damage and are more efficient when intercalated into the DNA molecule [2, 4].

An ideal radiopharmaceutical should accumulate rapidly in tumors, relatively spare normal organs, and be excreted rapidly from nontarget tissues. Internalization of the agent into tumor cells is desirable as it may enhance its cytotoxicity. Possible vectors in clinical use include small molecules, peptides, low molecular weight

Table 35.1 Approved radiopharmaceuticals for radionuclide therapy

Radiopharmaceutical	Indication	Approval year	Companion diagnostic
^{131}I-NaI	Differentiated thyroid carcinoma	1971 (FDA)	^{131}I-NaI
90Y-ibritumomab tiuxetan	Relapsed/refractory low-grade or follicular B-cell NHL; previously untreated follicular non-Hodgkin lymphoma with a partial or complete response to first-line chemotherapy	2002 (FDA)	111In-ibritumomab
^{131}I-tositumomab	CD20+ relapsed and refractory low-grade, follicular, or transformed NHL following disease progression during or after treatment with rituximab	2003 (FDA, EMA)	^{131}I-tositumomab
^{223}Ra-dichloride	Castration-resistant prostate cancer with bone metastases and no known visceral metastases	2013 (FDA, EMA)	Technetium-99m bone scan
^{177}Lu-DOTATATE	Gastroenteropancreatic neuroendocrine tumors	2018 (FDA, EMA)	^{68}Ga-DOTATATE, 64Cu-DOTATATE
^{177}Lu-PSMA-617	Metastatic castration-resistant prostate cancer following disease progression on androgen receptor inhibitors and taxane-based chemotherapy	2022 (FDA)	^{68}Ga-PSMA-11
^{131}I-MIBG	Unresectable metastatic pheochromocytoma/paraganglioma	2018 (FDA)	^{123I}-MIBG
^{153}Sm-EDTMP	Palliation of bone pain in skeletal metastases	1997 (FDA, EMA)	^{99m}Tc-bone scan
^{89}SrC12	Palliation of bone pain in skeletal metastases	1993 (FDA, EMA)	^{99m}Tc-bone scan
^{90}Y-microspheres	Unresectable metastatic liver tumors from primary colorectal cancer with adjuvant intrahepatic artery chemotherapy of floxuridine	2002 (FDA, EMA)	Technetium-99m hepatic artery shunt scan
^{90}Y-Glass microspheres	Unresectable hepatocellular carcinoma	2021 (FDA)	Technetium-99m hepatic artery shunt scan

EMA European Medicines Agency, *FDA* Food and Drug Administration

proteins, and monoclonal antibodies. The latter have longer biological residence time (days). The paired imaging radionuclide is chosen to match the targeting molecule; for example, short-lived nuclides for small molecules such as ^{68}Ga and long-lived nuclides for slowly excreted agents such as ^{89}Zr [4].

The *therapeutic index* refers to the goal of maximizing tumor dose while minimizing normal organ dose. Radiotheranostics uniquely allows real-time assessment

Table 35.2 Selected isotopes used in radiotheranostics, their half-lives, production pathway, and roles

Isotope	Half-life	Common production pathway	Role in radiotheranostics
^{131}I	8.0 days	Fission product in nuclear reactors	Therapy (thyroid cancer), Imaging
^{177}Lu	6.7 days	Neutron activation of 176Lu in nuclear reactors	Therapy (NETs, prostate cancer), Imaging
^{223}Ra	11.4 days	Decay of 227Ac (actinium-227)	Therapy (bone metastases in prostate cancer)
^{90}Y	64.1 h	Neutron activation of 89Y in nuclear reactors	Therapy (lymphoma, liver tumors)
^{68}Ga	67.7 min	Generator-based from ^{68}Ge decay	Imaging (PET for neuroendocrine and prostate cancer)
^{18}F	109.8 min	Cyclotron-produced from 18O(p,n)18F reaction	Imaging (PET for various cancers)
^{153}Sm	46.3 h	Neutron activation of 152Sm in nuclear reactors	Therapy (palliative bone pain relief)
^{89}Sr	50.5 days	Neutron activation of 88Sr in nuclear reactors	Therapy (palliative bone pain relief)
^{225}Ac	9.9 days	Cyclotron-produced from 226Ra irradiation or decay of 229Th	Therapy (prostate cancer, neuroendocrine tumors)
^{111}In	2.8 days	Cyclotron-produced via proton irradiation of cadmium targets	Imaging (SPECT), Auger therapy
^{64}Cu	12.7 h	Cyclotron-produced from 64Ni(p,n)64Cu reaction	Imaging (PET), Therapy (emerging theranostics)
^{188}Re	17.0 h	Generator-based from tungsten-188 decay	Therapy (bone metastases)
^{186}Re	3.7 days	Neutron activation of rhenium-185	Therapy (bone metastases)
^{212}Pb	10.6 h	Generator-based from 224Ra decay	Therapy (targeted alpha therapy, emerging applications)
^{213}Bi	45.6 min	Generator-based from 225Ac decay	Therapy (targeted alpha therapy, emerging applications)

(continued)

Table 35.2 (continued)

Isotope	Half-life	Common production pathway	Role in radiotheranostics
^{227}Th	18.7 days	Decay of 235U, typically sourced from nuclear reactors	Therapy (bone metastases, prostate cancer)
^{211}At	7.2 h	Cyclotron bombardment of bismuth-209	Therapy (targeted alpha therapy, emerging applications)
^{203}Pb	51.9 h	Cyclotron production via lead-204(p,n) reaction	Imaging (SPECT for targeted radiotherapy planning)
^{47}Sc	3.4 days	Cyclotron production from titanium-48 irradiation	Therapy (beta therapy, emerging applications)
^{161}Tb	6.9 days	Neutron activation in nuclear reactors	Therapy (beta therapy, emerging applications)
^{86}Y	14.7 h	Cyclotron-produced from strontium-86	Imaging (PET for dosimetry planning in Y-90 therapies)
^{89}Zr	78.4 h	Cyclotron-produced from 89Y(p,n)89Zr reaction	Imaging (PET for monoclonal antibody-based therapies)

of drug distribution and dosimetry by using the emissions of a therapy isotope, usually γ emissions, sometimes brehsmsstrahlung (X ray) radiation or positron emission for imaging (e.g., in treatment with ^{90}Y); thus, one can confirm drug delivery to tumors and estimate doses to organs such as kidney or bone marrow. In practice, fixed activities are often administered empirically, but patient-specific dosimetry may enable optimizing dosing per individual. This may be especially important in cases of retreatment; i.e., for patients who already received a large cumulative dose, or in patients with reduced marrow or renal reserve, in which the therapeutic index is narrow. Typically, radiotheranostic treatments cause mild to moderate side effects including early effects such as nausea and fatigue, midterm effects like transient cytopenias, or long-term effects such as rare instances of myelodysplastic syndrome or xerostomia in the case of PSMA-targeting treatments. However, higher doses or repeated treatments can lead to dose-limiting organ toxicities (e.g., renal injury from peptides cleared by kidneys, salivary gland damage from radioiodine or PSMA agents, and bone marrow suppression for the majority). For example, severe salivary gland fibrosis and xerostomia occur in a subset of patients treated with ^{177}Lu-PSMA (mild in ~8%), and much more frequently with ^{225}Ac-PSMA therapy (xerostomia in >80%, severe in ~10%). Long term, a small risk of therapy-related myelodysplasia or leukemia exists after high cumulative doses (e.g., after extensive ^{131}I or ^{90}Y therapy, ~1.5–2% incidence). Therefore, the treatment team must balance efficacy and safety—escalating the dose will increase tumor kill but also normal

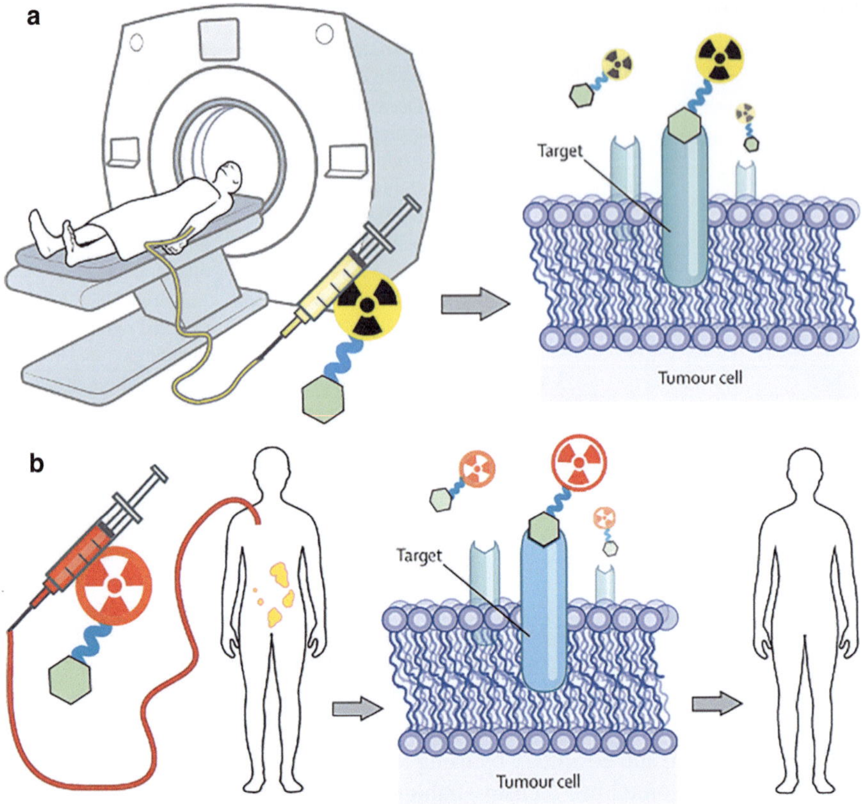

Fig. 35.1 Principles of theranostics. This figure illustrates the distinct roles of diagnostic (**a**) and therapeutic (**b**) radiopharmaceuticals in theranostics. (**a**) Diagnostic agents containing a radionuclide for imaging (e.g., PET/CT) hone to specific targets on tumor cells. (**b**) Therapeutic agents, carrying a cytotoxic radionuclide, bind to the same targets for localized radiation delivery and tumor cell destruction

tissue exposure. The use of radioprotective measures, such as amino acid infusions to protect kidneys during peptide therapy and administering personalized doses, aims to improve this balance [2].

35.3 Patient Selection

One of the fundamentals of theranostics, if not the most important one, is selecting patients who express sufficient amounts of the therapeutic target. Before therapy, a diagnostic scan is performed—e.g., a PET scan with ^{68}Ga-PSMA-11 in metastatic prostate cancer or ^{68}Ga-DOTATATE in neuroendocrine tumors—and only patients with sufficient uptake in neoplastic lesions proceed to therapy. This is evaluated on the paired diagnostic scan by comparing tumor uptake to reference organs, for example, in the case of PSMA or DOTATATE. Uptake greater than liver background is considered adequate. Clinical trials have adopted this approach; the VISION trial, for instance, required PSMA PET-positive disease for enrollment. Patients are also evaluated for suitability based on disease stage, overall well-being and organ function (e.g., bone marrow reserve, since marrow is often the dose-limiting organ), and renal function [2, 5].

35.4 Radioiodine

The roots of theranostics in oncology can be traced back to 1936 when Massachusetts General Hospital physician Dr. Saul Hertz hypothesized that a radioactive form of iodine could be used to both diagnose and treat thyroid disorders. Iodide-131 is a β particle-emitting radiohalogen with a half-life of 8.02 days. Thyroid follicular cells and differentiated follicular thyroid cancer cells concentrate iodine via a sodium-iodide symporter. In 1941, Hertz and colleagues used the radioisotope iodine-131 (^{131}I) to treat patients with hyperthyroidism, the first therapeutic use of a radionuclide in medicine [6]. In 1946, Seidlin et al. reported a case of a patient with thyroid cancer successfully treated with ^{131}I, marking the first published clinical application of a radiotheranostic paradigm. And so, ^{131}I was established as the prototype theranostic agent. In the following decades, ^{131}I became the standard of care for differentiated thyroid carcinoma and by 1971, it was formally approved in the U.S. Pre-therapy imaging is possible with either ^{123}I or ^{124}I. Treatment of differentiated thyroid cancer (DTC) with radioiodine has excellent outcomes—it can eradicate residual thyroid tissue in ~92% of low-risk cases and in metastatic thyroid cancer, about 59% of patients show uptake on radioiodine scans and many can have prolonged survival with repeated ^{131}I treatments [2, 7]. Treatment is well tolerated and side effects include transient neck pain or swelling, xerostomia, and, rarely, secondary malignancies (e.g., leukemia) at high cumulative activities. Patients must also follow radiation safety precautions for a few days after treatment. Over time, some DTCs lose the ability to uptake iodine (de-differentiation). In these radioiodine-refractory cases, there is growing interest in redifferentiation therapy; i.e., administering drugs such as mitogen-activated protein kinase (MAPK) pathway inhibitors (e.g., selumetinib) to restore radioiodine uptake before ^{131}I treatment. MAPK signaling inhibits the expression of thyroid hormone biosynthesis genes, including the sodium-iodide symporter and thyroid peroxidase, which facilitate iodine uptake and organification, respectively. By inhibiting MAPK downstream signaling, tumors regain the ability to trap radioiodine [8].

After the introduction of radioiodine, the field of nuclear medicine advanced mainly on the diagnostic front, with the development of new imaging tracers and gamma cameras, but therapeutic applications lagged for some time. Isotopes such as strontium-89 and phosphorus-32 were used in the mid-twentieth century for bone metastases and blood disorders, but these lacked a diagnostic counterpart and were not targeted to specific tumor biomarkers.

35.5 Anti-CD20 Radioimmunotherapy

The next major milestone in theranostics came with radiolabeled antibodies. Monoclonal antibodies against cancer antigens were developed and conjugated with radionuclides, giving rise to *radioimmunotherapy*. A landmark was the targeting of the CD20 antigen on B-cells in lymphoma. This culminated in the FDA approval of ^{90}Y-ibritumomab tiuxetan (Zevalin) in 2002, which incorporated an imaging step using ^{111}In-ibritumomab to first confirm biodistribution. In clinical trials, ^{90}Y-ibritumomab produced higher response rates than antibody therapy alone and a head-to-head trial against rituximab in relapsed low-grade non-Hodgkin's lymphoma showed that Zevalin improved both overall response rate (80% vs. 56%) and complete response rate (30% vs. 16%) [9]. This was followed by the approval of ^{131}I-tositumomab (Bexxar) in 2003, another anti-CD20 antibody with theranostic capability, which used the same ^{131}I-labeled antibody for both imaging dosimetry and therapy [10]. Clinically, these radioimmunotherapies were largely confined to second-line or later therapy in patients who had failed chemotherapy and rituximab. Zevalin was shown to significantly prolong progression-free survival (PFS) as a consolidation treatment after first remission in follicular lymphoma. Other than infusion-related reactions, the major toxicity was bone marrow suppression with predictable transient cytopenia about 4–6 weeks after injection. Treatment was usually not performed if the patient had low marrow reserve due to marrow involvement or after prior extensive chemotherapy. There was also a small risk (~2–3%) of late secondary myelodysplasia or acute leukemia [2].

Despite their clinical effectiveness and limited toxicity profile, both Zevalin and Bexxar struggled commercially with declining use in favor of convenient non-radioactive treatments (such as rituximab and CAR T-cell therapy). Bexxar's manufacturer withdrew it in 2014 and Zevalin was discontinued in some markets by 2021 and is rarely utilized in practice. Factors that led to this commercial failure included complex administration, logistical challenges (coordination between oncology and nuclear medicine, referral patterns), limited patient populations, high cost, lack of widespread physician adoption, lack of knowledge of theranostics and the theranostics principle, and competition from non-radioactive alternatives. Nonetheless, these pioneering therapies proved that targeted radiotherapy could be delivered systemically and safely, and lessons learned have informed the development of next-generation radioimmunotherapies [11].

35.6 Somatostatin Analogs

Another important development was the use of radiolabeled *peptides*. Following the discovery of somatostatin receptors (SSRs) overexpressed in neuroendocrine tumors, Eric P. Krenning at Erasmus University in Rotterdam succeeded in radiolabeling octreotide with ^{123}I. The first 10 patients studied with ^{123}I-Tyr3-octreotide were announced in 1989 as proof of principle of the value of SSR imaging. Iodinated octreotide, however, had some disadvantages including difficult radiolabeling, high cost, scarce availability of ^{123}I, and predominant biliary excretion with substantial accumulation in the intestines. This led to the replacement of ^{123}I with ^{111}In, which required using the chelating group DTPA. ^{111}In-pentetreotide, or OctreoScan (Mallinckrodt) had predominant renal excretion and a longer half-life. The first 26 patients studied were published in the seminal article "Somatostatin Receptor Scintigraphy with Indium-111-DTPA-D-Phe-1-Octreotide in Man: Metabolism, Dosimetry and Comparison with Iodine-123-Tyr-3-Octreotide" in 1992. It received FDA approval in 1994 [12].

High-dose ^{111}In-pentetreotide was also used for therapy utilizing its Auger electrons; however, efficacy was limited (objective response up to ~8%). Despite the disappointing initial results, the concept of treating tumors with targeted radiopharmaceuticals based on the distribution of the diagnostic counterpart was developed. Subsequently, higher energy and longer range β-emitting isotopes were used—first, yttrium-90 (^{90}Y) and then lutetium-177 (^{177}Lu). Although yttrium-90 DOTATOC (DOTA-Tyr3-octreotide) has been largely replaced by ^{177}Lu-DOTATATE, it was the workhorse of peptide receptor radionuclide therapy (PRRT) for many years. The main advantage of ^{90}Y is its higher β particle energy (Eβmax = 2.28 MeV vs. 0.497 MeV for ^{177}Lu) leading to a larger range (maximum tissue range of ~11 mm vs. ~2.5 mm for ^{177}Lu), making it more suitable for larger tumors. On the other hand, ^{90}Y has several disadvantages that led to it falling out of favor, including higher renal toxicity due to the higher energy, lack of in-treatment imaging, and logistical issues related to large-scale availability of ^{90}Y [13].

DOTA-TATE (DOTA0-Tyr3-Thr8-octreotate) differs from DOTA-TOC (DOTA-Tyr3-octreotide) in their C-terminal, resulting in a ~9-fold enhancement in affinity for SSTR2 of DOTATATE compared to DOTA-TOC, leading to a ~4–5 times enhancement in tumor uptake and correspondingly enhanced radiation-absorbed dose [13]. The development of a new octreotide derivative, DOTA-octreotate (DOTA0-Tyr3-Thr8-octreotide), led to the use of ^{177}Lu-DOTA-octreotate (also known as ^{177}Lu-DOTATATE or ^{177}Lu-octreotate; *Lutathera*) with higher affinity for SSR2, easier manageability, lower dosimetric burden in the kidneys, and the possibility of obtaining scintigraphic images and dosimetric studies at the same time, given the gamma photon co-emission of ^{177}Lu, optimal for gamma camera imaging [13].

By the early 2000s, clinical studies of ^{90}Y- and ^{177}Lu-labeled peptides showed significantly improved tumor response rates in patients with metastatic neuroendocrine tumors. Among these, ^{177}Lu-DOTATATE emerged as a preferred agent due to its ability to be imaged via γ emission and its favorable safety profile. This approach, known as peptide receptor radionuclide therapy (PRRT), represented a major advancement. PRRT with ^{177}Lu-DOTATATE, as we know it today, is indicated for unresectable or metastatic gastroenteropancreatic neuroendocrine tumors (NETs) (regardless of grade in the US, and only for G1 and G2 in Europe) that demonstrate SSR expression on imaging. It is typically given as four cycles (administered every 8 weeks). Patient selection is based on histological confirmation, somatostatin-analog positivity on molecular imaging, and safety measures per pretherapy labs.

Fluorodeoxyglucose (^{18}F) (FDG) PET/CT can serve as a prognostic parameter but is not universally included as a stratification factor [13].

The NETTER-1 trial (initiated in 2012), a randomized phase 3 study in advanced grade 1–2 midgut neuroendocrine tumors (NET), showed significant improvement in PFS (28.4 vs. 8.5 months) with ^{177}Lu-DOTATATE therapy compared to high-dose octreotide long-acting release (LAR), along with improved health-related quality of life. This study also showed a relatively safe toxicity profile of PRRT; treatment-related serious adverse events of grade 3 or worse were recorded in 3 of 111 (2.7%) patients in the ^{177}Lu-DOTATATE group. Two patients developed myelodysplastic syndrome, one of whom died 33 months after randomization (the only reported treatment-related death). Long-term follow-up did not show statistically significant survival benefit, although there was a meaningful 11.2-month gain; however, this was likely due to crossover of patients from the control group to the PRRT arm and other confounders [14, 15].

Based on the NETTER-1 and other studies, in 2018, ^{177}Lu-DOTATATE gained FDA approval for the treatment of gastroenteropancreatic (GEP) NETs, about 25 years after the initial somatostatin imaging agent was introduced. The FDA also simultaneously approved ^{68}Ga-DOTATATE PET for selecting patients, solidifying the theranostic concept in routine care [2].

More recently, NETTER-2, a phase 3 clinical trial, evaluated the efficacy and safety of first-line ^{177}Lu-DOTATATE therapy in patients with newly diagnosed, advanced high-grade 2 (Ki-67 > 10%) and grade 3 well-differentiated GEP NETs. The study enrolled 226 patients across 45 centers in North America, Europe, and Asia. Participants were randomly assigned to receive either ^{177}Lu-DOTATATE combined with octreotide LAR 30 mg or high-dose octreotide LAR 60 mg alone. The results demonstrated significant improvement in PFS for the ^{177}Lu-DOTATATE group, with a median PFS of 22.8 months compared to 8.5 months in the control group. This translates to a 72% reduction in the risk of disease progression or death (hazard ratio 0.276; $p < 0.0001$). Adverse events were comparable between the two groups, with no treatment-related deaths reported during the study period. Although the comparator arm represented a low bar in terms of realistic management of high-grade well-differentiated NETs, these findings suggest that ^{177}Lu-DOTATATE, in combination with octreotide LAR, should be considered a new standard of care for first-line treatment in this patient population [16]. Results from the ongoing COMPOSE trial, which randomizes the same population to either receive six cycles of ^{177}Lu-DOTATOC vs. standard-of-care treatment including chemotherapy, will lead to more practical insights from this clinical scenario in this advanced disease (NCT04919226).

PRRT is generally well tolerated. The main side effects are transient hematologic suppression—about 9% of patients have grade 3–4 neutropenia or thrombocytopenia during treatment, which is usually reversible. Nausea and fatigue can occur around the infusion days. Significant kidney damage is uncommon thanks to concomitant renal-protective amino acid infusions (long-term grade 4 renal toxicity in ~2–3%). Rarely (~2%), patients may develop therapy-related myelodysplastic syndrome months to years after treatment, especially if heavily pretreated or after multiple PRRT courses. Clinical risk factors have been shown to be of limited value in predicting toxicity. Toxicity could thus represent individual susceptibility, based on an intrinsic genomic susceptibility in addition to residual reserve from previous treatments [17].

Eventually, most patients will show progression of disease after PRRT. Approximately 15–30% of patients treated with PRRT will have disease progression during therapy, and another 10–15% of patients will progress early (i.e., in 6 months to 1 year). The NETTER-1 study evaluated several factors as possible predictors of outcome, such as Ki-67, grading or secretory markers such as CgA and NSE; however, none were significantly associated with patient outcome. Bodei et al. have shown the integration of gene expression and tumor grade using logistic regression modeling, known as PRRT predictive quotient (PPQ), to be an efficacious pretreatment predictive biomarker of the efficacy of PRRT and later validated in further studies [18–20].

Retreatment with a second course of PRRT is a topic of interest, as many patients have limited therapeutic options and tolerate their first course of PRRT well. A meta-analysis of 13 studies evaluating retreatment with ^{177}Lu-DOTATATE (7 studies) or mixed ^{90}Y-PRRT and ^{177}Lu-DOTATATE had shown encouraging median PFS in patients with NETs with a safety profile similar to initial PRRT, although these results are somewhat limited due to the heterogeneity of available studies. Studies varied in inclusion criteria and treatment protocol, with treatments ranging between 1 and 6 cycles, usually with 7.4 GBq per cycle. Some studies required a minimum period of PFS from first treatment with PRRT to be included in a retreatment trial; for example, at least 18 months in a study by Van der Zwan et al. [21]. For retreatment with ^{177}Lu-DOTATATE, the median PFS was 12.52 months, median overall survival was 26.78 months, and disease control rate was 71%. Grade 3/4 adverse events occurred in 5% of patients, with very low occurrence of severe renal toxicity (one reported case) and a pooled incidence of 0% for secondary hematologic malignancies (four cases reported) [22, 23].

Some data exist on the potential role of PRRT in the neoadjuvant setting. In one study with a small noncontrolled cohort, ^{177}Lu-DOTATATE converted 15 of 57 (26.3%) unresectable primary GEP NETs into resectable ones [24].

Studies have evaluated therapy using other somatostatin receptors (SSTR)-radiolabeled agonists, such as ^{177}Lu-edotreotide, using the labeled somatostatin analog DOTATOC, which has shown better tumor-to-background ratio in vivo. For example, the ongoing prospective, randomized, open-label multicenter phase 3 COMPETE trial (NCT03049189) aimed to evaluate the safety and efficacy of no carrier added (i.e., higher specific activity) ^{177}Lu-edotreotide compared to everolimus in patients with grade 1 and 2 pancreatic NETs and gastroenteric NETs. Uniquely, patients may be included as first-line therapy. The primary endpoint is PFS with key secondary endpoints including safety and tolerability, dosimetry, objective response rate, overall survival, and quality of life. This study and its compound have evolved into the COMPOSE study, mentioned above.

A topic of considerable interest is the need to improve the efficacy and tolerability of PRRT. Several strategies have been investigated, including combinations, new SSR-targeting molecules, and α therapy.

35.7 Combinations of Therapy

Therapeutic combinations such as PRRT with immunotherapy (e.g., NCT04525638), and particularly the use of PRRT with radiosensitizer chemotherapy agents such as capecitabine-temozolomide, have been investigated. In one prospective phase 2 single-center study, 30 patients with advanced progressive grade 1 or 2 pancreatic NETs were treated with this combination and followed up for up to 4 years. The treatment was well tolerated with no dose-limiting toxicities. The overall response rate was 80%, with 13% complete remission. Median overall survival had not been reached at a median follow-up of 33 months [25]. The Australian CONTROL NET trial randomized 75 patients with pancreatic and midgut NETs to a combination of PRRT and capecitabine-temozolomide vs. control groups of PRRT (midgut NETs) or capecitabine-temozolomide (pancreatic NETs). The study met its primary endpoint target of PFS of 12 months in pancreatic and 15 months in midgut NETs, with higher response rates in both combination therapy groups, but with higher hematologic toxicity in the treated midgut NET group [26]. It should be noted that combining PRRT with chemotherapy (CAP or CAPTEM) more than doubled the rate of myelodysplastic syndromes or acute leukemia to over 4.8% [27].

Combining ^{177}Lu- and ^{90}Y-based PRRT is of interest, as the hypothesis is that the higher maximum energy and longer-range β particles of ^{90}Y make it theoretically better suited for treating large-volume disease, whereas ^{177}Lu is more beneficial for smaller lesions. Studies in which this combination therapy was administered in sequential cycles or as a cocktail infusion show that it is feasible and may improve treatment outcomes, although it is associated with more toxicity [28]. Concerns for increased nephrotoxicity, however, limited the expansion of this approach [17].

35.8 Improved SSR-Targeting Molecules

Radiolabeled antagonists to SSTR-2 are another treatment approach under investigation. Compared to agonists that only bind to active SSTR, despite reduced internalization of the SSTR compared with agonists, antagonists show higher tumor uptake and retention, owing to more receptor binding sites and slower dissociation [29–32], which translates into better image contrast and higher lesion detection [33].

Krebs et al. compared tumor uptake of ^{68}Ga-DOTA-JR11 and ^{177}Lu-satoreotide tetraxetan (^{177}Lu-DOTA-JR11) in 95 lesions in 20 patients with NETs. In this study, the lesion uptake ratio for ^{177}Lu-satoreotide tetraxetan vs. ^{68}Ga-DOTA-JR11 was high, suggesting that these can be used as a theranostic pair. Uptake was high even in those with low uptake on ^{68}Ga-DOTA-JR11 PET/CT, suggesting the potential for treating tumors with a relatively lower expression of SSTR2 [34].

A phase 1 study from the same group that included 20 heavily treated patients with advanced SSTR2-positive NETs showed promise for treatment with 7.4 GBq of ^{177}Lu-satoreotide tetraxetan, with high radiation dose to tumors and a favorable tumor-to-normal organ dose ratio. A median PFS of 21 months and disease control rate of 85% were achieved. Interestingly, an unexpected high rate of grade 4 hematologic toxicity was observed after the second cycle, suggesting that a reduced treatment dose may be warranted for this agent [35]. In a phase 1/2 study by Wild et al., 40 patients with previously treated progressive NETs were treated with ^{177}Lu-satoreotide tetraxetan. Based on their findings, the authors recommend a dose of 4.5 GBq per cycle given for three cycles, to avoid severe hematologic toxicity while achieving a therapeutic benefit comparable to that of PRRT agonists but in fewer cycles and dose (94.7% disease control rate in this cohort). In the same study, there was a 5% incidence of treatment-associated myeloid malignancies, which is comparable to that seen with agonist PRRT; however, long-term follow-up is needed to evaluate the true risk [36].

Given the relatively narrow therapeutic window due to hematologic toxicity, a new generation of SSR antagonists has been developed. Baum et al. treated 51 patients with advanced metastatic NETs with the antagonist ^{177}Lu-DOTA-LM3 ((DOTA-p-Cl-Phe-c[d-Cys-Tyr-d-Aph(Cbm)-Lys-Thr-Cys]-d-Tyr-NH2)) while using ^{68}Ga-NODAGA-LM3 PET/CT for patient selection and follow-up. Higher uptake and a longer effective half-life were found compared to ^{177}Lu-DOTATOC in normal organs and tumors, which led to a disease control rate of 85.1%. Treatment was well tolerated, with thrombocytopenia occurring in only a few patients. In this study, no grade 4 hematologic toxicities were reported; however, the rate of severe hematologic toxicity was higher than reported for PRRT agonists, which might be related to the patients undergoing retreatment after prior PRRT. Of note, despite the higher renal absorbed dose seen with SSTR antagonists, no nephrotoxicity was observed [37].

35.9 Improved Strategies

Intra-arterial delivery of PRRT exploits the first-pass effect absorption of the radiopharmaceutical with increased uptake in the liver lesions. The LUTIA study aimed to enhance liver metastases uptake via intra-arterial administration of ^{177}Lu-DOTATATE through the hepatic artery [38]. Twenty-seven patients with grade 1–2 GEP NETs and bilobar liver metastases were randomized to receive intra-arterial PRRT in the left or right liver lobe for four consecutive cycles with the other lobe serving as control. Intra-arterial therapy was shown to be safe but did not lead to clinically significantly improved tumor uptake, probably due to the randomness of intra-arterial delivery, regardless of the distribution of the disease inside the liver.

35.10 Alpha Therapy

Another area of ongoing research is the use of α emitters such as ^{225}Ac-labeled SSR agonists, which have higher energy deposited over a shorter range and might lead to improved outcomes in patients with neuroendocrine neoplasms [4]. For example, the ongoing ALPHAMEDIX02 trial (NCT05153772) is evaluating treatment with ^{212}Pb-DOTATATE and the ongoing ACTION-1 trial (NCT05477576) is treating patients with GEP NETs who had progression after ^{177}Lu somatostatin analog therapy with ^{225}Ac-DOTATATE.

35.11 Other Diseases

PRRT is used to treat pheochromocytomas/paragangliomas, as these tumors often express SSRs. Studies have shown its efficacy in treating these tumors, controlling hypertension, significantly increasing PFS, and improving response to treatment compared to ^{131}I-MIBG, with lower risk of toxicity, particularly hematological [39]. A recent meta-analysis assessing the efficacy of PRRT in 213 patients affected by pheochromocytomas/paragangliomas found a pooled disease control rate of 83% and 76% for ^{177}Lu-DOTATATE and ^{90}Y-DOTATOC treatments, respectively, with a good toxicity profile [40].

PRRT has also been used for the treatment of SSTR-expressing meningiomas, with a special interest in treating progressive/refractory tumors, leading to disease stabilization [41–43].

35.12 ^{223}Ra-Dichloride

A key milestone was the advent of α particle therapy for bone metastases using radium-223 dichloride (^{223}Ra) (Xofigo), an α emitter that mimics calcium and localizes to bone. The phase 3 ALSYMPCA trial in 2013 showed improved overall survival in men with metastatic castration-resistant prostate cancer and bone metastases treated with ^{223}Ra. Although ^{223}Ra was not paired with a diagnostic equivalent, it reinforced the theranostic principle of targeting a specific metastatic niche (i.e., the bone microenvironment) with a systemic radionuclide. ^{223}Ra extended median survival by over 3 months vs. placebo (14.9 vs. 11.3 months, HR 0.70) and reduced skeletal morbidity, leading to FDA approval in 2013 [44]. Its success also marked the decline of older β-emitting bone agents such as strontium-89 and samarium-153, which, while used for pain palliation, had not shown a survival benefit. Of note, the ERA 223 trial, combining ^{223}Ra-dichloride with abiraterone, an androgen receptor signaling inhibitor (ARSI), revealed an increased rate of symptomatic skeletal events, leading to premature unblinding [45]. Now, typically ^{223}Ra is administered alongside bone-protective agents such as zoledronic acid or denosumab.

Currently, treatment with ^{223}Ra-dichloride is under investigation for various cancers with bone metastases, including nonsmall cell lung cancer (NCT02283749), renal cell carcinoma (NCT04071223), and breast cancer (NCT02366130 and NCT02258451) [4].

35.13 PSMA-Targeting Agents

In parallel with PRRT, in the 2010s, PSMA-targeted molecular imaging transformed the management of prostate cancer. PSMA is a cell-surface protein highly expressed in most prostate cancers, especially in advanced hormone-resistant disease, making it an attractive theranostics target [46].

The diagnostic component is PSMA-targeted PET imaging, performed with tracers such as ^{68}Ga-PSMA-11 or ^{18}F-DCFPyL, both now FDA-approved for patients with prostate cancer with suspected metastases who are candidates for initial definitive therapy and for those with suspected disease recurrence based on an elevated serum prostate-specific antigen (PSA) level. ^{68}Ga-PSMA PET was shown to detect metastases with unprecedented sensitivity and is also used to select patients for PSMA therapy [5, 47].

Therapeutic radioligands labeled with ^{177}Lu soon followed and showed impressive anti-tumor activity in early studies of metastatic castration-resistant prostate cancer (mCRPC). The phase 3 VISION trial in 2021 reported that ^{177}Lu-PSMA-617 plus standard care significantly prolonged survival in mCRPC patients compared to standard care alone (median overall survival 15.3 vs. 11.3 months; HR 0.62, $P < 0.001$). It also improved radiographic PFS (8.7 vs. 3.4 months; HR ~0.40) and delayed symptomatic skeletal complications. About 46% of men on ^{177}Lu-PSMA achieved a ≥50% decline in PSA levels, vs. 7% in the control arm. Based on this, ^{177}Lu-PSMA-617 (commercial name *Pluvicto*) was approved by the FDA in March 2022 for treatment of PSMA-positive mCRPC after androgen receptor (AR) pathway inhibitor and chemotherapy. As in the VISION trial, therapy is typically given as four to six doses every 6 weeks [5] (Fig. 35.2).

The toxicity profile of ^{177}Lu-PSMA is favorable relative to chemotherapy. Nausea and fatigue are possible side effects and the main toxicities are hematologic (around 10% grade 3–4 thrombocytopenia or anemia in VISION), and xerostomia may be seen in ~40% of patients, mostly grade 1–2. Severe bone marrow suppression or renal impairment are infrequent, given appropriate patient selection [5].

Multiple studies are investigating the role of ^{177}Lu-PSMA in earlier phases of disease. The phase 2 TheraP study compared ^{177}Lu-PSMA-617 to chemotherapy (cabazitaxel) in men with mCRPC who had progressed after docetaxel. TheraP showed higher PSA response rates (66% vs. 37%) and longer PFS with ^{177}Lu-PSMA than with second-line chemo [48]. The PSMAfore trial, a phase 3 randomized, controlled trial conducted at 74 sites across Europe and North America, aimed to evaluate the efficacy and safety of ^{177}Lu-PSMA in taxane-naïve patients with mCRPC who had progressed once on a previous androgen receptor pathway inhibitor (ARPI). Patients were either treated with ^{177}Lu-PSMA or with a different ARPI. Crossover from ARPI change to ^{177}Lu-PSMA-617 was allowed after centrally confirmed radiographic progression. Treatment with ^{177}Lu-PSMA prolonged

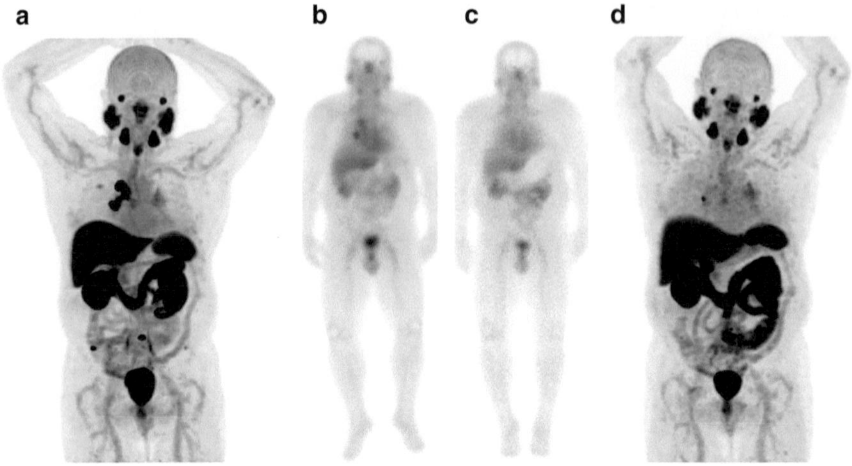

Fig. 35.2 Example of theranostics in prostate cancer. 72-year-old male with mCRPC, PSA 2.33 ng/ml, pre-therapy PSMA PET/CT (**a**) shows PSMA-avid lung, bone, and nodal metastases. The patient underwent treatment with six cycles of ^{177}Lu-PSMA-617, cumulative dose of 1178.86 mCi. Anterior planar images from post-therapy rapid scans taken in cycles 1 (**b**) and 6 (**c**). Post-treatment PSA was 0.06 ng/ml; restaging PSMA PET/CT (**d**) showed decreased and resolved PSMA-avid metastases in all locations

radiographic PFS relative to ARPI change (the primary endpoint), 11.60 vs. 5.59 months (HR 0.49), with a favorable safety profile [49].

Based on these results, the FDA has extended the label to include chemotherapy-naïve patients, as of April 2025. The ongoing PSMAddition trial aims to compare ^{177}Lu-PSMA with standard of care vs. standard of care alone in patients with newly diagnosed metastatic hormone-sensitive prostate cancer (NCT04720157). The LuTectomy trial aims to evaluate treatment with ^{177}Lu-PSMA-617 in the neoadjuvant setting prior to prostatectomy in high-risk localized prostate cancer. In the cohort of 20 men, 1–2 cycles of ^{177}Lu-PSMA delivered high levels of targeted radiation doses with few toxicities and did not compromise surgical safety. Surgical pathology revealed evidence of treatment effect in the majority of patients; however, none of the patients achieved a complete pathological response. Long-term follow-up to evaluate oncological benefit is pending [50].

The Australian UpFrontPSMA study, a multicenter, open-label randomized phase 2 trial, evaluated treatment with ^{177}Lu-PSMA-617 prior to chemotherapy in patients with PSMA-avid de-novo high-volume metastatic hormone-sensitive prostate cancer. Patients were randomly assigned to either treatment with two cycles of 7.5 GBq ^{177}Lu-PSMA followed by six cycles of docetaxel vs. docetaxel alone. Treatment with ^{177}Lu-PSMA followed by docetaxel improved antitumor activity without increased toxic effects; 41% of patients had undetectable PSA levels at 48 weeks compared with 16% in the chemotherapy-only group [51].

Other strategies under investigation are combination therapies such as ARPIs, which upregulate PSMA expression, with ^{177}Lu-PSMA; e.g., combining

^{177}Lu-PSMA-617 with enzalutamide improved PSA PFS vs. enzalutamide alone in the Enza-p trial [52].

Multiple studies have shown enhanced anti-tumor activity from combined PARPi and radiotherapy. Based on these, LuPARP is an ongoing phase 1 trial set to evaluate the combination therapy of ^{177}Lu-PSMA and olaparib, a PARP inhibitor, in PSMA-positive mCRPC after progression on ARSI and possible prior treatment with docetaxel [53, 54].

Combining radiotheranostics with immunotherapy is an interesting approach in tumors characterized by a prominent immune modulation, as can be seen in some metastatic prostate cancers. Radiation is presumed to sensitize tumors to immune checkpoint inhibitors by inducing immunogenic cell death and triggering the release of pro-inflammatory cytokines. An interim report of the phase 1b/2 PRINCE trial (NCT03658447) combining ^{177}Lu-PSMA with pembrolizumab for mCRPC found a PSA decline of ≥50% in about 75% among 37 patients. Seven of 9 patients with measurable disease exhibited partial response [54].

Several clinical trials are studying treatment of mCRPC with α emitters (e.g., NCT06402331 making use of 225Ac-PSMA-I&T for patients post 177Lu-PSMA); the most studied thus far is ^{225}Ac-PSMA-617, which can be effective in patients resistant to ^{177}Lu-PSMA, but leads to higher rates of xerostomia. ^{225}Ac has a half-life of about 10 days and its decay chain to stable ^{209}Bi results in the release of four different α particles, which increases its therapeutic efficacy [4]. Preliminary results of the ongoing TATCIST trial evaluating treatment with ^{225}Ac-PSMA-I&T in patients with mCRPC, including patients previously treated with ^{177}Lu-PSMA, showed a PSA decline of ≥50% in 50% of patients. Adverse effects were mostly grade 1–2 with some grade 3 anemia and thrombocytopenia [55].

Several studies are evaluating radiotheranostics for prostate cancer using alternative ligands or isotopes; e.g., the ongoing ECLIPSE (NCT05204927) and SPLASH (NCT04647526) trials are evaluating treatment with ^{177}Lu-PSMA-I&T. The ongoing VIOLET trial is investigating treatment with ^{161}Tb-PSMA-I&T, which has similar physical characteristics to ^{177}Lu; however, it has abundant emission of Auger and conversion electrons that deposit their energy over a shorter distance with higher linear energy transfer than β electrons, resulting in greater cell death and thus higher radiation doses to single tumor cells and micrometastases [56]. The ongoing ProstACT GLOBAL trial (NCT04876651) is evaluating the benefit of treatment with a PSMA-targeted antibody, ^{177}Lu-DOTA-rosopatamab (^{177}Lu-DOTA-TLX591 (m17)) [57].

No systematic data is currently available regarding the feasibility of radiotheranostic therapy with ^{177}Lu-PSMA beyond the usual six cycles. The prospective REALITY study (NCT04833517) aimed to evaluate the benefit of retreating patients who had partial response to initial treatment, and later progression. Over half (57.4%) of patients had at least 50% decline in PSA levels after one cycle. The median PFS was 8.7 months and the median OS was 22.7 months, with longer OS in patients with ≥50% PSA decline (27.3 months). Most patients who continued to second and third retreatment cycles responded. A favorable safety profile was seen with most events being of mild-to-moderate severity [58]. A multicenter retrospective analysis evaluated 111 patients who had continuous, extended, or rechallenge therapy. Retreatment was not associated with increased grade 3–4 toxicity. Patients had a favorable median survival of 31.3 months from the first administration and efficacy was also seen in the rechallenge group [59]. In a study evaluating ^{177}Lu-PSMA in mCRPC with long-term follow-up, a subgroup of 15 patients was retreated at progression after prior response, with higher response rates compared to patients treated with other systemic therapies [60].

35.14 MIBG

The theranostic pair of ^{123}I-MIBG and ^{131}I-MIBG for imaging and therapy, respectively, utilizes the ligand metaiodobenzylguanidine (MIBG), an analog of norepinephrine, taken up by tumor cells through the neuronal uptake-1 transporter. ^{131}I-MIBG is one of the oldest theranostic radiopharmaceuticals, introduced in the 1980s by a group in Ann Arbor [61]. It was designed for pheochromocytomas, paragangliomas, and neuroblastomas, as well as NETs—entities considered rare at that time, thus precluding its wider implementation. ^{131}I-MIBG was FDA-approved for imaging in 1994 and later, in 2008, ^{123}I-MIBG was approved for imaging pediatric neuroblastoma. Treatment with ^{131}I-MIBG is given as either monotherapy or as part of combination therapy; e.g., with radiosensitizing chemotherapy and supported by autologous stem cell rescue, in high-risk refractory or relapsed neuroblastoma with high response rates. Treatment has also been shown to improve bone pain. Despite its benefit, disadvantages include limited supply, possible undertreatment with weight-based or fixed doses rather than dosimetry-based doses and low specific activity in commercial preparations [62]. More recently, in 2018, ^{131}I-MIBG was FDA-approved for treatment of unresectable metastatic pheochromocytoma/paraganglioma in patients aged 12 and older. In the randomized study that led to FDA approval, 25% of patients achieved sustained blood pressure control and 92% had partial response or stable disease [63]. Hematologic toxicity can occur, especially in neuroblastoma regimens where doses are higher. Other side effects include nausea, transient hypertension during infusion (from catecholamine release), and, long term, a small risk of secondary malignancies. Thyroid protection with potassium iodide is needed to block free radioiodine.

35.15 SIRT

A different form of theranostics is selective internal radiation therapy (SIRT), also called trans-arterial radioembolization (TARE). Here, the “targeting” is done by catheter-directed delivery into the hepatic artery feeding a liver tumor. Microscopic beads loaded with a radionuclide (usually Yttrium-90 in glass or resin microspheres, or Holmium-166 microspheres) are infused, delivering high-dose local radiation. Post-^{90}Y therapy imaging can be done via bremsstrahlung SPECT or PET scanning to visualize activity distribution and confirm that the tumor received an adequate dose. Pretherapy imaging is done with diagnostic angiography and 99mTc MAA scans to simulate distribution and evaluate extra-hepatic activity and lung shunting. The safety of radioembolization is linked to patient selection and technique. A pre-treatment 99mTc-MAA scan can ensure there is no significant extra-hepatic activity or shunting to the lungs that would preclude the procedure due to risk of radiation pneumonitis or GI ulceration. The main side effects are post-embolization syndrome (fatigue, mild fever, abdominal pain) and transient liver enzyme elevations. Radiation-induced liver disease is a rare complication seen when large liver volumes receive high radiation; personalization of dosimetry can reduce this risk [64].

SIRT is used for unresectable primary liver cancers (hepatocellular carcinoma, or HCC) and for liver-dominant metastatic disease (e.g., colorectal metastases). Until recently, evidence was mostly from non-randomized studies that showed tumor control and downstaging prior to surgery in some cases. In 2021, the EPOCH randomized trial showed that adding ^{90}Y radioembolization to second-line chemotherapy in metastatic colorectal cancer improved both overall and hepatic PFS (median hepatic PFS 9.1 vs. 7.2 months, HR 0.59, median overall PFS 8.0 vs. 7.2 months, HR 0.69), although it did not significantly improve overall survival [65].

The SARAH and SIRveNIB trials compared ^{90}Y microspheres to sorafenib in locally advanced HCC and showed similar survival outcomes [66, 67]. The DOSISPHERE-01 trial showed that compared with standard dosimetry, personalized dosimetry significantly improved the objective response rate in locally advanced HCC treated with TARE [68]. In a post-hoc long-term analysis of OS, significant improvement in survival was seen in the personalized dosimetry group, with dramatic improvement in the patients who were downstaged toward resection [69].

35.16 Current Challenges and Future Prospects

Despite successful clinical outcomes, the widespread implementation of theranostics faces several challenges. These span from practical issues related to production and delivery, workforce and infrastructure limitations, and regulatory and financial hurdles to biological considerations. While these challenges must be addressed, the future of theranostics looks bright with expanded therapies, new indications, and novel agents.

35.16.1 Production and Availability of Radioisotopes

The field of nuclear medicine has experienced significant growth in recent years, driven by regulatory approvals of novel diagnostic and therapeutic agents, increased use of PET and SPECT imaging, and the expansion of theranostics, particularly in NETs and prostate cancer. This surge in demand necessitates the enhanced production of both established and emerging radionuclides.

Many theranostic therapies are concentrated in certain centers or countries. A 2020 SNMMI global survey highlighted inequities: While ^{131}I therapy was available in 94% of surveyed countries, newer agents like ^{177}Lu-DOTATATE and ^{177}Lu-PSMA were available in fewer than 20% of those countries at that time [2].

^{177}Lu is generated through neutron irradiation of isotopically enriched ^{176}Lu (or ^{176}Yb) targets, followed by processing of the irradiated material. The continued reliance on aging reactor infrastructure for production presents a significant challenge. According to the International Atomic Energy Agency's research reactor database, approximately 60 research reactors worldwide contribute to radionuclide production, with only 8 to 10 serving as the primary producers of medical radionuclides. Recent disruptions in reactor functionality and supply chain challenges, exacerbated by events such as the COVID-19 pandemic, have highlighted vulnerabilities in the supply system.

Increased demand for radiopharmaceuticals has also placed additional strain on cyclotron, radiochemical, and imaging scanner infrastructure. In response, cyclotron installations for routine medical radionuclide production have increased around the world. However, establishing new PET centers and expanding infrastructure remain complex, time-intensive, and costly.

^{225}Ac is obtained from the decay of Thorium-229 (^{229}Th), which itself originates from the decay of Uranium-233 (^{233}U). Given the past sporadic issues with supply, and the projected increase in future demand, research efforts are ongoing to explore alternative production pathways for this α emitter and others, including accelerator-based techniques such as proton irradiation of ^{232}Th, electron accelerators, and medium-energy cyclotrons [4].

35.16.2 Regulatory and Reimbursement Considerations

Regulatory bodies like the FDA and EMA demand robust evidence of safety and efficacy before approving a new theranostic agent, which requires large multicenter trials. Historically, many theranostics were developed at academic centers under compassionate or single-site protocols and translating these into industry-sponsored multicenter trials has been challenging. A lack of harmonization between regulatory agencies can cause significant delays; for instance, ^{177}Lu-DOTATATE was approved in Europe months before the U.S., and each approval required separate reviews despite similar data. Even after approval, not all countries quickly reimbursed or adopted these therapies due to local regulatory or resource issues [2].

Currently, numerous pharmaceutical companies have ventured into the field of theranostics, capitalizing on the recent surge in success and demand for these drugs. The wealth of clinical trials available is an achievement in its own right (Table 35.3). Nevertheless, this has resulted in an overwhelming array of similar drugs targeting the same conditions, which can create a quandary in choosing the most promising trial.

Theranostic drugs are expensive, often costing tens of thousands of dollars per dose, similar to other nonradioactive drugs in the same clinical setting. This is a major change for the nuclear medicine community from the days of routine use of radioiodine and MIBG, which are relatively low priced. Reimbursement policies for

Table 35.3 Key trials in theranostics

Trial name	Year	Main findings	Reference (PMID/NCT)
ALSYMPCA	2013	Radium-223 significantly prolonged overall survival and time to skeletal complications in men with mCRPC with bone metastases. Led to first FDA approval of an alpha-emitting radiotherapeutic.	23863050
NETTER-1	2017	^{177}Lu-DOTATATE showed a marked improvement in progression-free survival in midgut NETs, with a 5-fold reduction in disease progression risk compared to high-dose octreotide.	28076709
DOSISPHERE-01	2021	Personalized dosimetry with 90Y radioembolization significantly increased objective response rates in locally advanced hepatocellular carcinoma.	33166497
EPOCH	2021	EPOCH trial demonstrated that adding 90Y radioembolization to second-line chemotherapy in metastatic colorectal cancer improved both overall and hepatic progression-free survival.	34541864

(continued)

Table 35.3 (continued)

Trial name	Year	Main findings	Reference (PMID/ NCT)
TheraP	2021	^{177}Lu-PSMA-617 outperformed cabazitaxel chemotherapy in mCRPC, with superior progression-free survival and improved quality-of-life measures.	33581798
VISION	2021	VISION trial demonstrated that ^{177}Lu-PSMA-617 plus standard care significantly improved overall survival in advanced PSMA-positive mCRPC, leading to FDA approval.	34161051
NETTER-2	2024	NETTER-2 aims to evaluate ^{177}Lu-DOTATATE in first-line treatment of aggressive neuroendocrine tumors to determine its efficacy in earlier-stage disease.	38851203
PSMAfore	2024	Treatment with ^{177}Lu-PSMA prolonged radiographic progression-free survival relative to ARPI change in taxane-naive patients with mCRPC who had progressed once on a previous ARPI	39293462

(continued)

Table 35.3 (continued)

Trial name	Year	Main findings	Reference (PMID/NCT)
UpFrontPSMA	2024	^{177}Lu-PSMA followed by docetaxel improves antitumor activity in patients with de-novo high-volume metastatic hormone-sensitive prostate cancer compared with docetaxel alone, without increased toxic effects	39293461
LuTectomy	2024	LuTectomy is investigating the use of ^{177}Lu-PSMA-617 as neoadjuvant therapy before prostatectomy in high-risk localized prostate cancer.	37891072; NCT04430192
PSMAddition	Ongoing	PSMAddition is assessing the efficacy of ^{177}Lu-PSMA-617 in metastatic hormone-sensitive prostate cancer (mHSPC) to determine its role in earlier treatment settings.	NCT04720157
LuPARP	Ongoing	LuPARP is studying the combination of ^{177}Lu-PSMA-617 with PARP inhibitors in mCRPC to assess synergy between DNA damage repair inhibition and radioligand therapy.	NCT03874884

nuclear imaging agents and radiotherapeutics vary across different countries and healthcare systems. Despite these challenges, the demonstrated success of radio-theranostics in NETs and prostate cancer has led to increased investment by the pharmaceutical industry and regulatory support from agencies like the FDA.

Dosimetry for radiopharmaceutical therapy is another reimbursement issue as it remains underdeveloped and lacks standardization, as opposed to external beam radiotherapy, for which dosimetry is routinely covered. Appropriate reimbursement structures are needed [4].

35.16.3 Advances in Chelators

The development of new radiometals for imaging and therapy has led to the creation of stable chelators tailored to specific isotopes. However, designing and synthesizing novel chelators remains a resource-intensive process. As a result, commonly used chelators such as DOTA and NOTA continue to be employed, despite their limitations. For instance, DOTA provides a suboptimal coordination environment for radiocopper. The ongoing development of more specialized chelators remains an important research area; for instance, new macrocyclic chelators for actinium and novel linker technologies (e.g., Evans blue modifications for albumin binding, to increase circulating time and tumor uptake) [2, 4].

35.16.4 Expanding Applications and Dose Optimization

As mentioned, ongoing clinical trials are investigating the potential of radiotheranostics in earlier stages of disease. For example, ^{177}Lu-DOTATATE as a first-line therapy for advanced NETs, while ^{177}Lu-PSMA is being evaluated for chemo-naïve mCRPC and hormone-sensitive disease. Research is also exploring new indications, including the use of ^{177}Lu-DOTATATE for pheochromocytoma/paraganglioma and meningiomas, as well as various ^{223}Ra-dichloride applications for cancers with bone metastases. Efforts are also underway to investigate the effects of increased administration cycles and dose escalation. These initiatives are accompanied by advancements in dosimetry, incorporating quantitative imaging techniques to enhance accuracy. Along with the anticipation for clinical benefit, these will also contribute to the increased demand for radiopharmaceutical production [4].

35.16.5 Biological Challenge

Response rates of current radiotheranostics range from roughly 30–60%, and median PFS is on the order of months to a couple of years depending on tumor type. These are influenced by heterogeneous target expression in tumor tissues, low tumor uptake, and radioresistance/radiosensitivity of the tumor and normal organs. Methods to overcome tumor resistance include the "crossfire" effect of β emitters, better understanding the tumor microenvironment, which can modulate the radiopharmaceutical, as well as strategies under investigation such as combination therapies and therapy with α-emitting agents [2].

35.16.6 Combination Therapies

Resistance to radiopharmaceutical therapies, potentially due to cancer cell populations with low or absent target expression, highlights the necessity for combination therapies [70]. As detailed above, trials are currently evaluating the synergistic effects of radiotheranostics alongside immunotherapy, DNA repair inhibitors (e.g., poly ADP-ribose polymerase inhibitors) (NCT03317392 and NCT04375267), and chemotherapy. Preclinical and clinical data suggest that radiotherapy may enhance the immune response by promoting neoantigen release and reducing immunosuppressive cell populations within the tumor microenvironment [4] (Fig. 35.3).

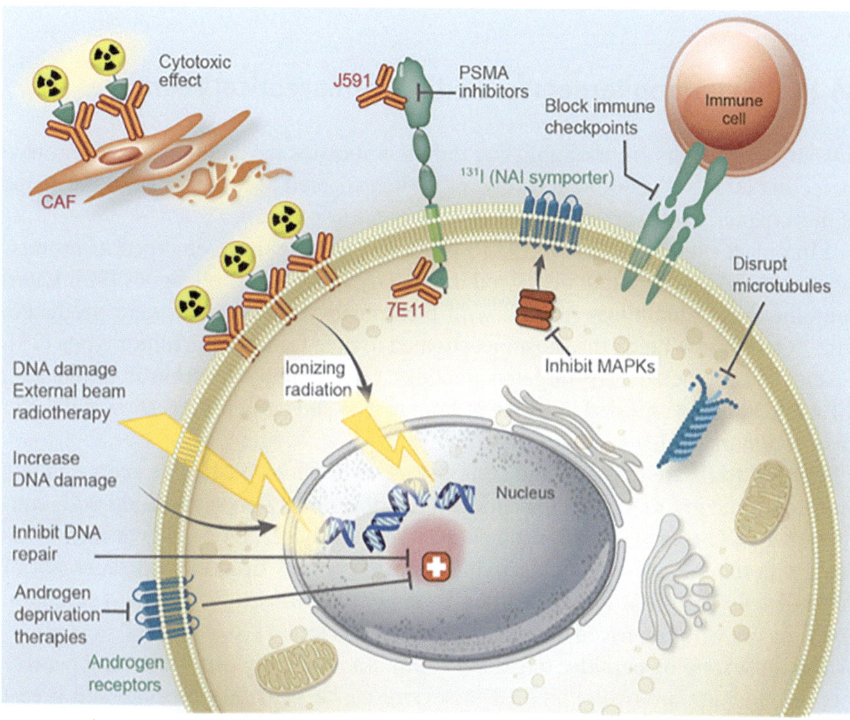

Fig. 35.3 Synergistic approaches to potentiate theranostics and radiotherapy. Various molecular and cellular interactions can be leveraged to enhance the effectiveness of theranostics. Direct cytotoxic effects from targeted radiopharmaceuticals (e.g., via PSMA, NAI symporter, or antibody conjugates) are depicted here, along with strategies to sensitize cells to radiation, such as inhibiting DNA repair, modulating androgen receptors, or disrupting signaling pathways (MAPKs). The figure also highlights methods to influence the tumor microenvironment through immune checkpoint blockade and targeting cancer-associated fibroblasts, underscoring the multifactorial approach to improving radiation-based cancer treatments

35.16.7 Targeted α Emitter Therapy

Alpha emitters possess high linear energy transfer (LET), leading to increased double-strand DNA damage and a more potent antitumor effect compared to β emitters. Several α-emitting isotopes are being tested in clinical trials. Actinium-225's decay chain emits four α particles with a cumulative energy of approximately 28 MeV, making it a highly potent radionuclide. Clinical trials are investigating the sequential administration of ^{225}Ac following ^{177}Lu therapy in patients exhibiting disease progression. Additionally, dual-isotope approaches combining ^{177}Lu- and ^{225}Ac-labeled radiopharmaceuticals are under evaluation. Similarly, Astatine-211 (^{211}At) and Lead-212 (^{212}Pb) are under investigation for therapeutic applications, though their complex chemistry and short half-lives pose distribution challenges [71].

35.16.8 Emerging Targets for Radiopharmaceutical Therapy

Encouraging results from established radiotheranostics have driven interest in new molecular targets. A complete review of all investigated agents is beyond the scope of this chapter; however, we will elaborate on a few of them.

Fibroblast activation protein (FAP) inhibitors (FAPIs) have emerged as promising agents. FAPIs were first described in 2014 by Jansen and colleagues [72]. Later, quinoline-based inhibitors labeled with theranostic radionuclides were produced, with ^{68}GaFAPI-04 being the most investigated to date for multiple tumor types [73]. Several ^{177}Lu-labeled FAP-targeted peptides are currently in clinical trials; e.g., ^{177}Lu-FAP-2286 was tested in a first-in-human trial and early reports show uptake in diverse tumors [74].

Clinical trials are ongoing and demonstrate that, while Ga-FAPI tracers enabled improved imaging of several cancers that are notoriously poorly imaged with conventional FDG (e.g., GI malignancies, pancreatic cancer, and breast cancer), treatment with the therapeutic counterpart (Lu-FAPI) suffers from early detachment of the molecule from the target, leading to suboptimal doses [75]. New-generation FAPI tracers with improved stability are being developed [76].

Bombesin analog peptides target the G protein-coupled gastrin-releasing peptide receptors, which are overexpressed in several cancers, mainly prostate and breast cancer [77, 78]. Several studies have evaluated the use of bombesin agonists for imaging and therapy [79]. However, issues with symptoms related to receptor activation and poor plasma stability have led to the investigation of bombesin antagonists with superior targeting properties such as ^{68}Ga-RM2, ^{68}Ga-RM26, and ^{68}Ga-NeoBOMB1 for imaging and therapy with ^{177}Lu-NeoBOMB1 and ^{177}Lu-RM2 [78]. The dosimetry of the GRPR antagonist ^{177}Lu-RM2 was recently studied in patients with mCRPC, showing high tumor doses with rapid clearance from normal organs [80].

Another interesting target for imaging and therapy is C-X-C motif chemokine receptor 4 (CXCR4), which is upregulated in a variety of cancers. Imaging of this target using ^{68}Ga-Pentixa has been shown to be useful in tumors such as adrenocortical carcinoma and small-cell lung cancer, as well as hematologic malignancies including multiple myeloma, marginal zone lymphoma, and mantle cell lymphoma. ^{177}Lu- and ^{90}Y-based radiotheranostics targeting CXCR4 have been investigated as well with good response rates; e.g., in relapsed myeloma [81, 82].

Delta-like protein 3 (DLL3) is a Notch ligand found in NET cells, including in more than 80% of small cell lung cancer and other high-grade NECs (e.g., lung, ovarian, prostate, bladder) with minimal to no expression in normal tissue. Radiolabeled antibodies against DLL3 (^{177}Lu-SC16) have achieved high tumor uptake and even complete tumor responses in preclinical models of small cell lung cancer in mice [83]. More recently, a first-in-human trial showed that ^{89}Zr-labeled DLL3 imaging of patients with neuroendocrine cancers is safe and feasible [84].

35.16.9 Integration of Artificial Intelligence

Artificial intelligence (AI) is poised to revolutionize nuclear medicine by enhancing imaging analysis, lesion detection, and dosimetry. AI-based quantification of PSMA PET/CT has already received FDA approval, with systems like PYLARIFY AI, enabling standardized quantitation and reporting of PSMA PET/CT to improve accuracy. As AI algorithms continuously evolve and improve, future developments may incorporate AI-driven risk stratification and treatment response prediction, thereby enhancing accuracy for disease staging and monitoring, tumor burden quantification, and internal radiation dosimetry, further optimizing patient management [4, 85].

35.16.10 Personalized Dosimetry and Imaging Technologies

Advancements in PET and SPECT imaging, including whole-body PET scanners and digital SPECT, are improving dosimetry accuracy. These innovations facilitate serial quantitative imaging and time-integrated activity measurements, paving the way for personalized radiopharmaceutical therapy, allowing for safer dose escalation and re-treatment in clinical trials, which may lead to better outcomes [4].

35.16.11 Training Needs

A Lancet Oncology Commission report in 2024 revealed an international shortage of nuclear medicine specialists [86]. A well-trained workforce, including nuclear medicine physicians, radiochemists, technologists, medical physicists, nurses, and radiopharmacists is essential to support the field's growth. These individuals need to be properly trained in theranostics, possibly via specialized fellowship training programs. Multidisciplinary training programs that integrate nuclear medicine, radiation oncology, and medical physics will be critical in ensuring safe and effective radiopharmaceutical therapy administration [2–4, 70, 87–89].

35.16.12 Overcoming Clinician Hesitance and Public Perception Challenges

Beyond logistical and technical hurdles, public perception of radiation-based treatments remains a significant barrier. Efforts to educate both healthcare professionals and patients about the safety and efficacy of radiotheranostics will be crucial in fostering broader acceptance and adoption of these innovative therapies [4].

35.17 Conclusion

The historical trajectory—from radioiodine to modern radioligand therapies, owing to innovations in chemistry and imaging technology—has greatly facilitated the advancement of theranostics, while maintaining the key concept of "treat what you see and see what you treat" by pairing diagnostic imaging to guide radionuclide therapy, as envisioned decades ago (Fig. 35.4).

The future of oncologic theranostics will likely be marked by greater personalization, more targets, and combination treatment strategies. Treatments will move from a last-resort therapy to an earlier, even first-line option in some types of cancer. Diagnostic scans will not only identify candidates, but guide dosing and combinations, and dosimetry may allow for dose escalation as part of a more personalized regimen. Data on long-term benefits and risks will further optimize treatments.

As theranostics expands from a niche to a widely accessible routine oncologic treatment, challenges will need to be overcome, including adequate radionuclide production and supply chains, worldwide availability of agents, enhanced facilities and technology, and increased training for personnel. Furthermore, regulatory and reimbursement issues must be addressed, public opinion must be improved, and multidisciplinary collaborations must be cultivated. Given the strong momentum of ongoing clinical trials in combination with the accumulating clinical evidence from key studies and regulatory approvals, theranostics is poised to become an indispensable pillar of cancer care in the coming decades, embodying the ideals of precision medicine.

Ultimately, to ensure that these pharmaceuticals remain integral to the treatment armamentarium of multiple cancer types and that further advancements are made, it is crucial to implement the theranostic principle in their delivery. Consequently, it is imperative that theranostics are administered by professionals with specialized knowledge and clinical skills, capable of working alongside oncological teams.

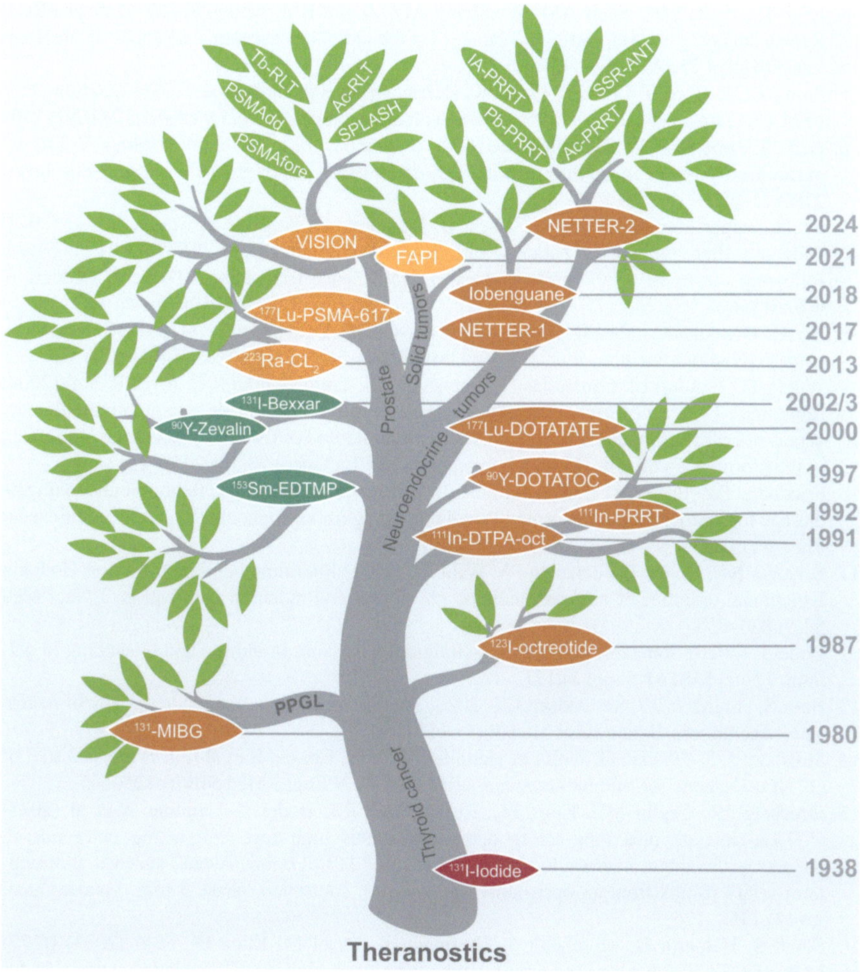

Fig. 35.4 Theranostics tree: evolution and key milestones. The historical development of theranostics, with different disease applications and the emergence of key radiopharmaceuticals over time, is shown here. Clinical trials: PSMAfore, PSMAddition, SPLASH; RLT radioligand therapy, IA intra-arterial, SSR-ANT somatostatin receptor antagonists

References

1. Jadvar H, Chen X, Cai W, Mahmood U (2018) Radiotheranostics in cancer diagnosis and management. Radiology 286(2):388–400
2. Bodei L, Herrmann K, Schöder H, Scott AM, Lewis JS (2022) Radiotheranostics in oncology: current challenges and emerging opportunities. Nat Rev Clin Oncol 19(8):534–550
3. Herrmann K, Schwaiger M, Lewis JS, Solomon SB, McNeil BJ, Baumann M et al (2020) Radiotheranostics: a roadmap for future development. Lancet Oncol 21(3):e146–ee56

4. Lapi SE, Scott PJH, Scott AM, Windhorst AD, Zeglis BM, Abdel-Wahab M et al (2024) Recent advances and impending challenges for the radiopharmaceutical sciences in oncology. Lancet Oncol 25(6):e236–ee49
5. Sartor O, de Bono J, Chi KN, Fizazi K, Herrmann K, Rahbar K et al (2021) Lutetium-177-PSMA-617 for metastatic castration-resistant prostate cancer. N Engl J Med 385(12):1091–1103
6. Hertz S, Roberts A (1942) Radioactive iodine as an indicator in thyroid physiology. V. The use of radioactive iodine in the differential diagnosis of two types of graves' disease. J Clin Invest 21(1):31–32
7. Schlumberger M, Leboulleux S, Catargi B, Deandreis D, Zerdoud S, Bardet S et al (2018) Outcome after ablation in patients with low-risk thyroid cancer (ESTIMABL1): 5-year follow-up results of a randomised, phase 3, equivalence trial. Lancet Diabetes Endocrinol 6(8):618–626
8. Ho AL, Grewal RK, Leboeuf R, Sherman EJ, Pfister DG, Deandreis D et al (2013) Selumetinib-enhanced radioiodine uptake in advanced thyroid cancer. N Engl J Med 368(7):623–632
9. Witzig TE, Gordon LI, Cabanillas F, Czuczman MS, Emmanouilides C, Joyce R et al (2002) Randomized controlled trial of yttrium-90-labeled ibritumomab tiuxetan radioimmunotherapy versus rituximab immunotherapy for patients with relapsed or refractory low-grade, follicular, or transformed B-cell non-Hodgkin's lymphoma. J Clin Oncol 20(10):2453–2463
10. Friedberg JW, Fisher RI (2004) Iodine-131 tositumomab (Bexxar): radioimmunoconjugate therapy for indolent and transformed B-cell non-Hodgkin's lymphoma. Expert Rev Anticancer Ther 4(1):18–26
11. Schaefer NG, Huang P, Buchanan JW, Wahl RL (2011) Radioimmunotherapy in non-Hodgkin lymphoma: opinions of nuclear medicine physicians and radiation oncologists. J Nucl Med 52(5):830–838
12. Bodei L (2020) Somatostatin receptor scintigraphy: blazing in indium and quenching in gallium. J Nucl Med 61(Suppl 2):121s–122s
13. Basu S, Parghane RV, Kamaldeep CS (2020) Peptide receptor radionuclide therapy of neuroendocrine tumors. Semin Nucl Med 50(5):447–464
14. Strosberg J, El-Haddad G, Wolin E, Hendifar A, Yao J, Chasen B et al (2017) Phase 3 trial of (177)Lu-Dotatate for Midgut neuroendocrine tumors. N Engl J Med 376(2):125–135
15. Strosberg JR, Caplin ME, Kunz PL, Ruszniewski PB, Bodei L, Hendifar A et al (2021) (177)Lu-Dotatate plus long-acting octreotide versus high-dose long-acting octreotide in patients with midgut neuroendocrine tumours (NETTER-1): final overall survival and long-term safety results from an open-label, randomised, controlled, phase 3 trial. Lancet Oncol 22(12):1752–1763
16. Singh S, Halperin D, Myrehaug S, Herrmann K, Pavel M, Kunz PL et al (2024) [(177)Lu]Lu-DOTA-TATE plus long-acting octreotide versus high-dose long-acting octreotide for the treatment of newly diagnosed, advanced grade 2-3, well-differentiated, gastroenteropancreatic neuroendocrine tumours (NETTER-2): an open-label, randomised, phase 3 study. Lancet 403(10446):2807–2817
17. Bodei L, Kidd M, Paganelli G, Grana CM, Drozdov I, Cremonesi M et al (2015) Long-term tolerability of PRRT in 807 patients with neuroendocrine tumours: the value and limitations of clinical factors. Eur J Nucl Med Mol Imaging 42(1):5–19
18. Bodei L, Schöder H, Baum RP, Herrmann K, Strosberg J, Caplin M et al (2020) Molecular profiling of neuroendocrine tumours to predict response and toxicity to peptide receptor radionuclide therapy. Lancet Oncol 21(9):e431–ee43
19. Bodei L, Kidd M, Modlin IM, Severi S, Drozdov I, Nicolini S et al (2016) Measurement of circulating transcripts and gene cluster analysis predicts and defines therapeutic efficacy of peptide receptor radionuclide therapy (PRRT) in neuroendocrine tumors. Eur J Nucl Med Mol Imaging 43(5):839–851
20. Bodei L, Kidd MS, Singh A, van der Zwan WA, Severi S, Drozdov IA et al (2018) PRRT genomic signature in blood for prediction of (177)Lu-octreotate efficacy. Eur J Nucl Med Mol Imaging 45(7):1155–1169

21. van der Zwan WA, Brabander T, Kam BLR, Teunissen JJM, Feelders RA, Hofland J et al (2019) Salvage peptide receptor radionuclide therapy with [(177)Lu-DOTA,Tyr(3)]octreotate in patients with bronchial and gastroenteropancreatic neuroendocrine tumours. Eur J Nucl Med Mol Imaging 46(3):704–717
22. Strosberg J, Leeuwenkamp O, Siddiqui MK (2021) Peptide receptor radiotherapy re-treatment in patients with progressive neuroendocrine tumors: a systematic review and meta-analysis. Cancer Treat Rev 93:102141
23. Sitani K, Parghane R, Talole S, Basu S (2022) The efficacy, toxicity and survival of salvage retreatment PRRT with (177)Lu-DOTATATE in patients with progressive NET following initial course of PRRT. Br J Radiol 95(1137):20210896
24. Parghane RV, Bhandare M, Chaudhari V, Ostwal V, Ramaswamy A, Talole S et al (2021) Surgical feasibility, determinants, and overall efficacy of neoadjuvant (177)Lu-DOTATATE PRRT for locally advanced unresectable gastroenteropancreatic neuroendocrine tumors. J Nucl Med 62(11):1558–1563
25. Claringbold PG, Turner JH (2016) Pancreatic neuroendocrine tumor control: durable objective response to combination 177Lu-Octreotate-Capecitabine-Temozolomide radiopeptide chemotherapy. Neuroendocrinology 103(5):432–439
26. Pavlakis N, Ransom DT, Wyld D, Sjoquist KM, Wilson K, Gebski V et al (2022) Australasian Gastrointestinal Trials Group (AGITG) CONTROL NET study: ^{177}Lu-DOTATATE peptide receptor radionuclide therapy (PRRT) and capecitabine plus temozolomide (CAPTEM) for pancreas and midgut neuroendocrine tumours (pNETS, mNETS)-final results. J Clin Oncol 40(16_suppl):4122
27. Goncalves I, Burbury K, Michael M, Iravani A, Ravi Kumar AS, Akhurst T et al (2019) Characteristics and outcomes of therapy-related myeloid neoplasms after peptide receptor radionuclide/chemoradionuclide therapy (PRRT/PRCRT) for metastatic neuroendocrine neoplasia: a single-institution series. Eur J Nucl Med Mol Imaging 46(9):1902–1910
28. La Salvia A, Espinosa-Olarte P, Riesco-Martinez MDC, Anton-Pascual B, Garcia-Carbonero R (2021) Targeted cancer therapy: what's new in the field of neuroendocrine neoplasms? Cancers (Basel) 13(7):1701
29. Cescato R, Schulz S, Waser B, Eltschinger V, Rivier JE, Wester HJ et al (2006) Internalization of sst2, sst3, and sst5 receptors: effects of somatostatin agonists and antagonists. J Nucl Med 47(3):502–511
30. Eychenne R, Bouvry C, Bourgeois M, Loyer P, Benoist E, Lepareur N (2020) Overview of Radiolabeled somatostatin analogs for cancer imaging and therapy. Molecules 25(17):4012
31. Ginj M, Zhang H, Waser B, Cescato R, Wild D, Wang X et al (2006) Radiolabeled somatostatin receptor antagonists are preferable to agonists for in vivo peptide receptor targeting of tumors. Proc Natl Acad Sci USA 103(44):16436–16441
32. Perrin MH, Sutton SW, Cervini LA, Rivier JE, Vale WW (1999) Comparison of an agonist, urocortin, and an antagonist, astressin, as radioligands for characterization of corticotropin-releasing factor receptors. J Pharmacol Exp Ther 288(2):729–734
33. Wild D, Fani M, Behe M, Brink I, Rivier JE, Reubi JC et al (2011) First clinical evidence that imaging with somatostatin receptor antagonists is feasible. J Nucl Med 52(9):1412–1417
34. Krebs S, O'Donoghue JA, Biegel E, Beattie BJ, Reidy D, Lyashchenko SK et al (2020) Comparison of (68)Ga-DOTA-JR11 PET/CT with dosimetric (177)Lu-satoreotide tetraxetan ((177)Lu-DOTA-JR11) SPECT/CT in patients with metastatic neuroendocrine tumors undergoing peptide receptor radionuclide therapy. Eur J Nucl Med Mol Imaging 47(13):3047–3057
35. Reidy-Lagunes D, Pandit-Taskar N, O'Donoghue JA, Krebs S, Staton KD, Lyashchenko SK et al (2019) Phase I trial of well-differentiated neuroendocrine tumors (NETs) with radiolabeled somatostatin antagonist (177)Lu-Satoreotide Tetraxetan. Clin Cancer Res 25(23):6939–6947
36. Wild D, Grønbæk H, Navalkissoor S, Haug A, Nicolas GP, Pais B et al (2023) A phase I/II study of the safety and efficacy of [(177)Lu]Lu-satoreotide tetraxetan in advanced somatostatin receptor-positive neuroendocrine tumours. Eur J Nucl Med Mol Imaging 51(1):183–195
37. Baum RP, Zhang J, Schuchardt C, Müller D, Mäcke H (2021) First-in-humans study of the SSTR antagonist (177)Lu-DOTA-LM3 for peptide receptor radionuclide therapy in patients

with metastatic neuroendocrine neoplasms: dosimetry, safety, and efficacy. J Nucl Med 62(11):1571–1581

38. Ebbers SC, Barentsz MW, de Vries-Huizing DMV, Versleijen MWJ, Klompenhouwer EG, Tesselaar MET et al (2024) Intra-arterial peptide-receptor radionuclide therapy for neuroendocrine tumour liver metastases: an in-patient randomised controlled trial (LUTIA). Eur J Nucl Med Mol Imaging 51(4):1121–1132
39. Bracigliano A, Marretta AL, Guerrera LP, Simioli R, Clemente O, Granata V et al (2024) The management of Phaeochromocytomas and Paragangliomas in the era of precision medicine: where are we now? evidence-based systemic treatment options and future cluster oriented perspectives. Pharmaceuticals (Basel) 17(3):354
40. Marretta AL, Ottaiano A, Iervolino D, Bracigliano A, Clemente O, Di Gennaro F et al (2023) Response to peptide receptor radionuclide therapy in Pheocromocytomas and Paragangliomas: a systematic review and meta-analysis. J Clin Med 12(4):1494
41. Bartolomei M, Bodei L, De Cicco C, Grana CM, Cremonesi M, Botteri E et al (2009) Peptide receptor radionuclide therapy with (90)Y-DOTATOC in recurrent meningioma. Eur J Nucl Med Mol Imaging 36(9):1407–1416
42. Hartrampf PE, Hänscheid H, Kertels O, Schirbel A, Kreissl MC, Flentje M et al (2020) Long-term results of multimodal peptide receptor radionuclide therapy and fractionated external beam radiotherapy for treatment of advanced symptomatic meningioma. Clin Transl Radiat Oncol 22:29–32
43. Mair MJ, Tabouret E, Johnson DR, Sulman EP, Wen PY, Preusser M, Albert NL (2024) Radioligand therapies in meningioma: evidence and future directions. Neuro-Oncology 26(Supplement_9):S215–s28
44. Parker C, Nilsson S, Heinrich D, Helle SI, O'Sullivan JM, Fosså SD et al (2013) Alpha emitter radium-223 and survival in metastatic prostate cancer. N Engl J Med 369(3):213–223
45. Smith M, Parker C, Saad F, Miller K, Tombal B, Ng QS et al (2019) Addition of radium-223 to abiraterone acetate and prednisone or prednisolone in patients with castration-resistant prostate cancer and bone metastases (ERA 223): a randomised, double-blind, placebo-controlled, phase 3 trial. Lancet Oncol 20(3):408–419
46. Eder M, Schäfer M, Bauder-Wüst U, Hull WE, Wängler C, Mier W et al (2012) 68Ga-complex lipophilicity and the targeting property of a urea-based PSMA inhibitor for PET imaging. Bioconjug Chem 23(4):688–697
47. Hofman MS, Lawrentschuk N, Francis RJ, Tang C, Vela I, Thomas P et al (2020) Prostate-specific membrane antigen PET-CT in patients with high-risk prostate cancer before curative-intent surgery or radiotherapy (proPSMA): a prospective, randomised, multicentre study. Lancet 395(10231):1208–1216
48. Hofman MS, Emmett L, Sandhu S, Iravani A, Joshua AM, Goh JC et al (2021) [(177) Lu]Lu-PSMA-617 versus cabazitaxel in patients with metastatic castration-resistant prostate cancer (TheraP): a randomised, open-label, phase 2 trial. Lancet 397(10276):797–804
49. Morris MJ, Castellano D, Herrmann K, de Bono JS, Shore ND, Chi KN et al (2024) (177) Lu-PSMA-617 versus a change of androgen receptor pathway inhibitor therapy for taxane-naive patients with progressive metastatic castration-resistant prostate cancer (PSMAfore): a phase 3, randomised, controlled trial. Lancet 404(10459):1227–1239
50. Eapen RS, Buteau JP, Jackson P, Mitchell C, Oon SF, Alghazo O et al (2024) Administering [(177)Lu]Lu-PSMA-617 prior to radical prostatectomy in men with high-risk localised prostate cancer (LuTectomy): a single-Centre, single-arm, phase 1/2 study. Eur Urol 85(3):217–226
51. Azad AA, Bressel M, Tan H, Voskoboynik M, Suder A, Weickhardt AJ et al (2024) Sequential [(177)Lu]Lu-PSMA-617 and docetaxel versus docetaxel in patients with metastatic hormone-sensitive prostate cancer (UpFrontPSMA): a multicentre, open-label, randomised, phase 2 study. Lancet Oncol 25(10):1267–1276
52. Emmett L, Subramaniam S, Crumbaker M, Nguyen A, Joshua AM, Weickhardt A et al (2024) [(177)Lu]Lu-PSMA-617 plus enzalutamide in patients with metastatic castration-resistant prostate cancer (ENZA-p): an open-label, multicentre, randomised, phase 2 trial. Lancet Oncol 25(5):563–571

53. Marchetti A, Rosellini M, Nuvola G, Tassinari E, Mollica V, Rizzo A et al (2022) PARP inhibitors and radiometabolic approaches in metastatic castration-resistant prostate cancer: what's now, what's new, and what's coming? Cancers (Basel) 14(4):907
54. Sandhu S, Joshua AM, Emmett L, Crumbaker M, Bressel M, Huynh R et al (2023) LuPARP: Phase 1 trial of 177Lu-PSMA-617 and olaparib in patients with metastatic castration resistant prostate cancer (mCRPC). J Clin Oncol 41(16_suppl):5005
55. Delpassand ES, Hashmi MJ, Kazakin J, Nawaz O, Garufi G, Schindler J, Nordquist L (2024) Abstract CT224: preliminary efficacy and safety results from the (TATCIST) trial: a PSMA-directed targeted alpha therapy with FPI-2265 (225Ac-PSMA-I&T) for the treatment of metastatic castration-resistant prostate cancer (mCRPC). Cancer Res 84(7_Supplement):CT224-CT
56. Buteau JP, Kostos L, Alipour R, Jackson P, McInstosh L, Emmerson B et al (2024) Clinical trial protocol for VIOLET: a single-Center, phase I/II trial evaluation of Radioligand treatment in patients with metastatic castration-resistant prostate cancer with [(161)Tb]Tb-PSMA-I&T. J Nucl Med 65(8):1231–1238
57. Tagawa ST, Thomas C, Sartor AO, Sun M, Stangl-Kremser J, Bissassar M et al (2024) Prostate-specific membrane antigen-targeting alpha emitter via antibody delivery for metastatic castration-resistant prostate cancer: a phase I dose-escalation study of (225)Ac-J591. J Clin Oncol 42(7):842–851
58. Rosar F, Schuler J, Burgard C, Blickle A, Bartholomä M, Maus S et al (2024) Efficacy and safety of rechallenge [(177)Lu]Lu-PSMA-617 RLT after initial partial remission in patients with mCRPC: evaluation of a prospective registry (REALITY study). Eur J Nucl Med Mol Imaging 51(13):4151–4162
59. Seifert R, Telli T, Lapa C, Desaulniers M, Hekimsoy T, Weber WA et al (2024) Safety and efficacy of extended therapy with [(177)Lu]Lu-PSMA: a German multicenter study. J Nucl Med 65(6):909–916
60. Violet J, Sandhu S, Iravani A, Ferdinandus J, Thang SP, Kong G et al (2020) Long-term follow-up and outcomes of retreatment in an expanded 50-patient single-center phase II prospective trial of (177)Lu-PSMA-617 Theranostics in metastatic castration-resistant prostate cancer. J Nucl Med 61(6):857–865
61. Von Moll L, McEwan AJ, Shapiro B, Sisson JC, Gross MD, Lloyd R et al (1987) Iodine-131 MIBG scintigraphy of neuroendocrine tumors other than pheochromocytoma and neuroblastoma. J Nucl Med 28(6):979–988
62. Fabozzi F, Villani MF, Del Bufalo F, Altini C, Cannatà V, Davide C et al (2025) (131)I-mIBG therapy in relapsed/refractory neuroblastoma: a weapon from the future past. Crit Rev Oncol Hematol 207:104606
63. Pryma DA, Chin BB, Noto RB, Dillon JS, Perkins S, Solnes L et al (2019) Efficacy and safety of high-specific-activity (131)I-MIBG therapy in patients with advanced Pheochromocytoma or Paraganglioma. J Nucl Med 60(5):623–630
64. Weber M, Lam M, Chiesa C, Konijnenberg M, Cremonesi M, Flamen P et al (2022) EANM procedure guideline for the treatment of liver cancer and liver metastases with intra-arterial radioactive compounds. Eur J Nucl Med Mol Imaging 49(5):1682–1699
65. Mulcahy MF, Mahvash A, Pracht M, Montazeri AH, Bandula S, Martin RCG et al (2021) Radioembolization with chemotherapy for colorectal liver metastases: a randomized, open-label, International, Multicenter, Phase III Trial. J Clin Oncol 39(35):3897–3907
66. Vilgrain V, Pereira H, Assenat E, Guiu B, Ilonca AD, Pageaux GP et al (2017) Efficacy and safety of selective internal radiotherapy with yttrium-90 resin microspheres compared with sorafenib in locally advanced and inoperable hepatocellular carcinoma (SARAH): an open-label randomised controlled phase 3 trial. Lancet Oncol 18(12):1624–1636
67. Chow PKH, Gandhi M, Tan SB, Khin MW, Khasbazar A, Ong J et al (2018) SIRveNIB: selective internal radiation therapy versus Sorafenib in Asia-Pacific patients with hepatocellular carcinoma. J Clin Oncol 36(19):1913–1921
68. Garin E, Tselikas L, Guiu B, Chalaye J, Edeline J, de Baere T et al (2021) Personalised versus standard dosimetry approach of selective internal radiation therapy in patients with locally

advanced hepatocellular carcinoma (DOSISPHERE-01): a randomised, multicentre, open-label phase 2 trial. Lancet Gastroenterol Hepatol 6(1):17–29
69. Garin E, Tselikas L, Guiu B, Chalaye J, Rolland Y, de Baere T et al (2024) Long-term overall survival after selective internal radiation therapy for locally advanced hepatocellular carcinomas: updated analysis of DOSISPHERE-01 trial. J Nucl Med 65(2):264–269
70. Sgouros G, Bodei L, McDevitt MR, Nedrow JR (2020) Radiopharmaceutical therapy in cancer: clinical advances and challenges. Nat Rev Drug Discov 19(9):589–608
71. Jang A, Kendi AT, Johnson GB, Halfdanarson TR, Sartor O (2023) Targeted alpha-particle therapy: a review of current trials. Int J Mol Sci 24(14):11626
72. Jansen K, Heirbaut L, Cheng JD, Joossens J, Ryabtsova O, Cos P et al (2013) Selective inhibitors of fibroblast activation protein (FAP) with a (4-Quinolinoyl)-glycyl-2-cyanopyrrolidine Scaffold. ACS Med Chem Lett 4(5):491–496
73. Kratochwil C, Flechsig P, Lindner T, Abderrahim L, Altmann A, Mier W et al (2019) (68) Ga-FAPI PET/CT: tracer uptake in 28 different kinds of cancer. J Nucl Med 60(6):801–805
74. Baum RP, Schuchardt C, Singh A, Chantadisai M, Robiller FC, Zhang J et al (2022) Feasibility, biodistribution, and preliminary dosimetry in peptide-targeted radionuclide therapy of diverse adenocarcinomas using (177)Lu-FAP-2286: first-in-humans results. J Nucl Med 63(3):415–423
75. Juneau D, Kavan P, Metser U, Abikhzer G, Bodei L, Liberman M et al (2024) FRONTIER: FAPi Radioligand OpeN-label, phase 1 study to evaluate safety, Tolerability and dosImetry of [Lu-177]-PNT6555; a dose Escalation study for tReatment of patients with select solid tumors. J Nucl Med 65(supplement 2):241162
76. Greifenstein L, Gunkel A, Hoehne A, Osterkamp F, Smerling C, Landvogt C et al (2023) 3BP-3940, a highly potent FAP-targeting peptide for theranostics - production, validation and first in human experience with Ga-68 and Lu-177. iScience 26(12):108541
77. Jensen RT, Battey JF, Spindel ER, Benya RV, International Union of Pharmacology. LXVIII (2008) Mammalian bombesin receptors: nomenclature, distribution, pharmacology, signaling, and functions in normal and disease states. Pharmacol Rev 60(1):1–42
78. Baratto L, Jadvar H, Iagaru A (2018) Prostate cancer theranostics targeting gastrin-releasing peptide receptors. Mol Imaging Biol 20(4):501–509
79. Bodei LFM, Nunn A, Llull J, Cremonesi M, Martano L, Laurora G, Scardino E, Tiberini S, Bufi G, Eaton S, de Cobelli O, Paganelli G (2007) Lu-177-AMBA Bombesin analogue in hormone refractory prostate cancer patients: a phase i escalation study with single-cycle administrations. Eur J Nucl Med Mol Imaging 34:S221-S
80. Kurth J, Krause BJ, Schwarzenböck SM, Bergner C, Hakenberg OW, Heuschkel M (2020) First-in-human dosimetry of gastrin-releasing peptide receptor antagonist [(177)Lu]Lu-RM2: a radiopharmaceutical for the treatment of metastatic castration-resistant prostate cancer. Eur J Nucl Med Mol Imaging 47(1):123–135
81. Buck AK, Serfling SE, Lindner T, Hänscheid H, Schirbel A, Hahner S et al (2022) CXCR4-targeted theranostics in oncology. Eur J Nucl Med Mol Imaging 49(12):4133–4144
82. Lapa C, Herrmann K, Schirbel A, Hänscheid H, Lückerath K, Schottelius M et al (2017) CXCR4-directed endoradiotherapy induces high response rates in extramedullary relapsed Multiple Myeloma. Theranostics 7(6):1589–1597
83. Tully KM, Tendler S, Carter LM, Sharma SK, Samuels ZV, Mandleywala K et al (2022) Radioimmunotherapy targeting Delta-like Ligand 3 in small cell lung cancer exhibits antitumor efficacy with low toxicity. Clin Cancer Res 28(7):1391–1401
84. Tendler S, Dunphy MP, Agee M, O'Donoghue J, Aly RG, Choudhury NJ et al (2024) Imaging with [89Zr]Zr-DFO-SC16.56 anti-DLL3 antibody in patients with high-grade neuroendocrine tumours of the lung and prostate: a phase 1/2, first-in-human trial. Lancet Oncol 25(8):1015–1024
85. Belge Bilgin G, Bilgin C, Burkett BJ, Orme JJ, Childs DS, Thorpe MP et al (2024) Theranostics and artificial intelligence: new frontiers in personalized medicine. Theranostics 14(6):2367–2378

86. Scott AM, Zeglis BM, Lapi SE, Scott PJH, Windhorst AD, Abdel-Wahab M et al (2024) Trends in nuclear medicine and the radiopharmaceutical sciences in oncology: workforce challenges and training in the age of theranostics. Lancet Oncol 25(6):e250–e2e9
87. Abdel-Wahab M, Giammarile F, Carrara M, Paez D, Hricak H, Ayati N et al (2024) Radiotherapy and theranostics: a Lancet Oncology Commission. Lancet Oncol 25(11):e545–ee80
88. Giammarile F, Paez D, Zimmermann R, Cutler CS, Jalilian A, Korde A et al (2024) Production and regulatory issues for theranostics. Lancet Oncol 25(6):e260–e2e9
89. Czernin J, Calais J (2020) Nuclear medicine, molecular imaging, and theranostics: the future is bright. J Nucl Med Technol 48(Suppl 1):82s–83s

Part V

Future Challenges

Future Challenges of Molecular Imaging in Oncology

36

Otmar Schober, Fabian Kiessling, and Jürgen Debus

36.1 Understanding the Future Challenges

The challenges facing molecular imaging in oncology reflect both practical needs and scientific ambitions. At their core, these challenges are rooted in a commitment to improving patient care while being driven by the intrinsic curiosity that promotes scientific discovery. The future evolves from the foundations of the past and the realities of the present—often incrementally, but sometimes through supposedly sudden breakthroughs or so-called "quantum leaps" in research. The previous chapters have repeatedly shown the transition from current practice to future applications in oncology. This concluding chapter is intended as an outlook, expressing both expectations of development and hopes for progress: sapere aude, dare to know (Kant, 1784).

In summary, molecular imaging in oncology is a challenging but promising frontier at the interface of science, humanities, research, and patient care. It is a crucial building block for a better future of medicine, the humanities, and knowledge. Building on this promise, several driving factors will shape the trajectory of molecular imaging in oncology and beyond:

O. Schober (✉)
Department of Nuclear Medicine, University of Münster, Münster, Northrhein-Westphalia, Germany
e-mail: otmar.schober@uni-muenster.de

F. Kiessling
Institute for Experimental Molecular Imaging, University Hospital, RWTH Aachen University, Northrhein-Westphalia, Germany
e-mail: fkiessling@ukaachen.de

J. Debus
Department of Radiation Oncology, Heidelberg University Hospital, Heidelberg, Germany
e-mail: juergen.debus@med.uni-heidelberg.de

O. Schober et al. (eds.), *Molecular Imaging in Oncology - Volume 2*, Recent Results in Cancer Research 225, https://doi.org/10.1007/978-3-032-21415-7_18

1. **Opportunities (*Gaude*)**

The overarching motivations behind molecular imaging include:

- Advancing scientific knowledge (basic research)
- Translating discoveries into practice (technology development)
- Improving patient outcomes (clinical care)

Achieving these goals requires the ability to perceive, understand, and integrate complex biological information. Altogether, these arguments underscore the urgent need for reliable imaging biomarkers in cancer. Significant advancements include:

- "Quantum leaps" in temporospatial resolution
- The development of question-oriented and innovative biomarkers and imaging techniques
- Coregistration of independent and complementary imaging techniques

Chronobiology: Time as a Parameter in the Kinetics of Biological and Biochemical Processes

Without time, there is no life—no lifetime.

Imaging typically occurs at discrete time points, capturing snapshots of ongoing biological processes, from initial diagnostics to long-term clinical follow-up. However, a comprehensive understanding of these processes requires knowledge of their kinetics across different scales, particularly in molecular biology and oncology. Despite its importance, the temporal dimension is often underappreciated in the development and application of imaging technologies.

For deeper tissues, transmission and emission-based imaging methods are constrained by technical limitations and patient burden. An exception, to some extent, is ultrasound imaging, which allows real-time monitoring without radiation exposure.

Accurately quantifying dynamic biological processes depends on the understanding of their kinetics, yet this remains a neglected area. Techniques such as compartmental analysis are crucial for modeling interactions within the tumor microenvironment—the immediate histological and biochemical context surrounding tumor cells—but remain challenging to implement. Precise quantification may also require knowledge of the biomarker's input function, while both the temporal and spatial resolution of imaging data must meet high-quality standards to ensure meaningful interpretation.

However, several practical factors influence the feasibility of acquiring kinetic data: the complexity and duration of imaging procedures (e.g., in MRI), radiation exposure (as in CT), the invasiveness of the method, availability of resources, cost-effectiveness, and the expertise of the personnel involved.

On the other hand, molecular imaging offers a key advantage over histology that harbors a huge potential for novel insights into the individual dynamics of disease: the ability to perform repeated, noninvasive scans. This enables precise monitoring of therapy-related responses over time and allows timely therapeutic adjustments—an essential component of personalized, adaptive treatment strategies.

2. **Risk (*Cave*)**

To avoid the pitfall of misguided tool-driven research, imaging methods must be selected and developed based on well-defined scientific or clinical needs—not convenience or technological availability. A major risk lies in allowing imaging techniques to dictate the scientific or clinical question, rather than the other way around.

As Abraham H. Maslow famously noted:

> *If the only tool you have is a hammer, it is tempting to treat everything as if it were a nail.* (*The Psychology of Science*, 1966).

The *Law of the Instrument*, also known as *Maslow's Hammer*, is a cognitive bias in which individuals tend to over-rely on a familiar tool or method—even when more appropriate alternatives are available.

In science and medicine, the underlying scientific and clinical questions must lead the way. These questions drive the search for appropriate biomarkers and, in turn, determine which measurement techniques and technologies are most suitable or have to be developed.

Emerging technologies—such as optical imaging, total-body positron emission tomography (PET), and super-resolution ultrasound—are expected to significantly transform diagnostics and therapy. However, their adoption requires standardized scan protocols and reporting practices. For instance, while metrics like SUVmax (Standardized Uptake Value maximum) are relatively robust, ensuring cross-comparability of measurements remains a persistent challenge.

Artificial intelligence (AI), particularly deep learning, is poised to enrich all the domains discussed here. One of its strengths lies in the integration of data across multiple disciplines and domains. However, its critical application depends on a clear understanding of data sources and the algorithms used.

This interdisciplinary integration is already widely practiced in research and has become the norm in many collaborative projects. In clinical practice, a key challenge remains: ensuring that patient individuality is respected. Professional responsibility also includes recognizing the limits of one's own expertise when applying AI-based tools.

AI applications have already shown substantial benefits—for example, in large-scale screening programs for common diseases and in diagnosing rare or orphan diseases at the individual level. Continued advancements are both expected and needed.

3. **Barriers (*Obstat*)**

Availability is often limited by economic, political, and regulatory factors. These include:

- Cost and resource constraints
- Regulatory hurdles and reimbursement regulations
- Ethical and societal acceptance, including the use of animal models in preclinical research

These systemic conditions can significantly delay or hinder the implementation of new imaging technologies.

An informed society raises a broad spectrum of challenging questions: How many expensive diagnostic innovations are truly necessary? Which needs can be addressed using histological or omics-based biomarkers? Where might more cost-effective radiomics approaches fall short? In which cases are new molecular diagnostics essential, and where would hybrid analyses—combining tracers and radiomics—be most appropriate? Which diagnostic innovations are suitable for clinical implementation?

Molecular imaging in oncology is resource-intensive. The acquisition and operation of the necessary equipment are costly, and device availability remains limited. Moreover, the production and distribution of biomarkers and tracers require significant logistical and labor investment. Adequate time and personnel must be allocated for each patient and imaging study.

The clinical adoption of new methods is further impeded when no corresponding therapeutic option is available. In many cases, the added value of enhanced imaging remains unproven. However, a notable shift is emerging: empirical clinical benefit—developed through real-world practice rather than exclusively demonstrated in prospective randomized trials—is becoming more influential in clinical decision-making.

Regulatory requirements present another substantial barrier to the clinical translation of novel molecular imaging techniques. Regulatory processes are costly and time-consuming, and academic scientists are often unprepared for them. As a result, intellectual property is frequently unprotected, and imaging probes are not designed for scalable production under Good Manufacturing Practice (GMP) standards. Funding to bridge the so-called "valley of death"—to produce GMP-grade probes and complete necessary safety, toxicology, and phase I clinical trials—is limited or entirely unavailable in many countries.

Compounding the issue is the academic system's limited recognition of such translational efforts. Scientific success is often measured by high-impact publications, which rarely result from regulatory or early-phase clinical studies. Meanwhile, industry partners tend to engage only in projects that already show clinical proof of concept (i.e., phase II trials). Demonstrating that a diagnostic probe significantly improves therapeutic outcomes or patient survival—a key requirement for insurance reimbursement—is an additional challenge.

As such, reforms to regulatory pathways and reimbursement strategies are urgently needed to prevent promising molecular imaging innovations from stalling at the preclinical stage.

Advancements in imaging technologies—particularly molecular imaging within the oncologic context—are of significant scientific and clinical relevance. These developments reflect a pragmatic and solution-oriented approach, contributing meaningfully to translational research and precision medicine. Nonetheless, overarching strategic frameworks, such as clinically driven research paradigms and programmatic, goal-oriented research structures, remain insufficiently defined. Redundant or parallel research activities—especially those involving registries—should be minimized to optimize the allocation of time, financial resources, and operational efficiency.

The availability of reimbursement for novel radiotracers is contingent upon their developmental maturity and the robustness of clinical efficacy data. As with any innovative diagnostic modality, demonstration of clinical utility is a prerequisite for integration into standard-of-care pathways. However, the generation of this evidence typically necessitates initial public or institutional funding. Upon validation of clinical benefit, reimbursement decisions—preferably conducted on a case-by-case basis by payers—can be appropriately considered.

In light of demographic changes, rising healthcare costs, increasing life expectancy, and growing public expectations amid limited resources, interdisciplinary collaboration and strategic networking across research and clinical practice are more important than ever.

To enable effective translation from research to clinical application, sustained interdisciplinary collaboration among medical professionals, chemists, pharmacists, computer scientists, and engineers must be fostered. This collaboration should be institutionalized in dedicated translational centers where regulatory and clinical implementation strategies are integrated into research planning from the outset.

4. **Enablers *(Age)***

The transformation towards both improved diagnostic accuracy and efficiency as well as enabling truly personalized treatment strategies will be driven by:

Artificial intelligence and AI-driven radiomics:

- Deep-learning models for robust, automated tumor segmentation and feature extraction across large heterogeneous imaging datasets
- Correlation of radiomic signatures with underlying tumor biology and patient outcomes
- Continuous model refinement via real-world data to ensure consistency across different scanners and populations

Interdisciplinarity and transdisciplinarity:

- Hybrid imaging workflows that fuse metabolic, functional, and anatomical information in one session
- Incorporation of multimodal imaging (including e.g. advanced MRI sequences, photon counting CT, total body PET) and Radiomics for comprehensive tumor characterization
- Development of frameworks to combine imaging features with genomics, proteomics, and liquid-biopsy data to enable holistic tumor phenotyping to account for phenotype plasticity

Federated data-sharing and interoperability:

- Privacy-preserving federated learning networks that facilitate cross-institutional AI development without centralized data-pooling
- Adoption of common data models, standardized ontologies, and interoperable formats for seamless data exchange
- Cloud-based platforms and shared registries that support multicentric trials, external validation of biomarkers, and rapid AI benchmarking

Interdisciplinarity and Transdisciplinarity

Today more than ever, scientific and clinical questions must serve as key drivers for the technical sciences, including medical technology, physics, and engineering. In chemistry and pharmacy, increasing awareness of unresolved clinical challenges and the active search for novel biomarkers represent promising trends that should be further supported and expanded.

Translation and interdisciplinarity are both essential and inherently challenging. Many of these efforts fall under the broader "-omics" umbrella. The suffix "-omics" denotes subfields of modern biology that generate comprehensive, high-dimensional data—such as radiomics, genomics, metabolomics, proteomics, lipidomics, systemomics, transcriptomics, glycomics, fluxomics, interactomics, sensomics, and others.

For translation and interdisciplinarity to succeed, their value must be recognized and embedded across all levels—both in terms of content and human resources. This includes integrating interdisciplinary thinking into education and training, institutional structures, scientific communication (e.g., at conferences, symposia, and seminars), and academic publishing.

Future challenges include the efficient sharing and coordination of information, for example, through centralized registries (such as clinical trial databases), and the prevention of unnecessary duplication of research efforts—all while maintaining rigorous standards for quality and scientific integrity.

Phenotypic Plasticity

Phenotypic plasticity—a hallmark of cancer—can only be partially captured by histological analysis, which typically samples small, potentially unrepresentative tissue sections. Given that many cancers are diagnosed at the metastatic stage, imaging that reflects the gene expression, the dynamic, pathophysiological behavior of tumors and their response to therapy is essential for identifying treatment-resistant lesions and guiding individualized care.

Improving the differentiation between tumor and normal tissue continues to be a key research priority. One longstanding yet underaddressed issue in cancer therapy is spatial tumor heterogeneity, which is equally significant in systemic therapies and radiotherapy (e.g., as the different metastases and the primary tumor may have divergent response profiles). Tumor heterogeneity is frequently a root cause of therapy resistance and local treatment failure and must be better understood and targeted.

Imaging (e.g., diagnostic scans) and tissue characterization (e.g., histological and genetic analyses) can reveal relevant tumor subpopulations that may influence therapy decisions. While radiotherapy planning—such as target volume delineation, local boosting, and dose escalation or de-escalation—remains conceptually unchanged, it increasingly benefits from advanced biological insights.

One example illustrating the complexity of mechanism-driven imaging is tumor hypoxia. Hypoxic regions often require higher radiation doses, a concept dating back to the Warburg effect (1924), which describes the shift to anaerobic glycolysis in tumors. This metabolic adaptation forms the basis of fluorodeoxyglucose (FDG-PET) imaging in oncology. Clinically relevant studies, such as Individualized Radiation Dose Prescription-Fluorine-18 Fluoromisonidazole (INDIRA-MISO)—which explores individualized dosing for head and neck cancers based on hypoxia imaging with F18-fluoromisonidazole FMISO-PET—highlight the potential of such personalized approaches.

The development of immunological markers should also help determine, through indirect mechanisms or tracer-based imaging, whether lesions are immunologically "cold" or "hot." This information is important not only spatially (e.g., in identifying affected tumor regions or specific lymph nodes) but also temporally, across days or weeks. Radiation therapy induces immunological responses that can be harnessed both diagnostically and therapeutically, contributing to immunomodulation strategies.

The identification of highly individualized biomarkers to predict radiation resistance would meet a strong clinical need in radiotherapy, as radioresistant tumor cells are a major cause of recurrences and finally therapy failure. Rational approaches could target mutations such as those involving the p53 protein and its regulatory pathways that lead to evasion of apoptosis.

36.2 Conclusion

Advancements in imaging technologies—particularly molecular imaging within the oncologic context—are of significant scientific and clinical relevance. These developments reflect a pragmatic and solution-oriented approach, contributing meaningfully to translational research and precision medicine.

Molecular imaging offers a distinct and complementary scale of longitudinal, spatial, functional, and quantitative information compared to conventional histopathological and morphological assessments. By enabling the visualization of molecular targets and their microenvironment in vivo, it bridges the diagnostic continuum between macroscopic anatomical imaging, histological analysis, and molecular characterization—thus facilitating more precise tumor phenotyping and therapeutic decision-making.

MIX
Papier aus verantwortungsvollen Quellen
Paper from responsible sources
FSC® C105338

If you have any concerns about our products,
you can contact us on
ProductSafety@springernature.com

In case Publisher is established outside the EU,
the EU authorized representative is:
Springer Nature Customer Service Center GmbH
Europaplatz 3, 69115 Heidelberg, Germany

Printed by Libri Plureos GmbH
in Hamburg, Germany